THE CULTURE-BOUND SYNDROMES

CULTURE, ILLNESS, AND HEALING

Studies in Comparative Cross-Cultural Research

THE CULTURE-BOUND SYNDROMES

Folk Illnesses of Psychiatric and Anthropological Interest

Edited by

RONALD C. SIMONS

*Depts. of Psychiatry and Anthropology, Michigan State University,
East Lansing, Michigan, U.S.A.*

and

CHARLES C. HUGHES

*Dept. of Family and Community Medicine, Medical Center, The University of Utah,
Salt Lake City, Utah, U.S.A.*

D. REIDEL PUBLISHING COMPANY

A MEMBER OF THE KLUWER ACADEMIC PUBLISHERS GROUP

DORDRECHT / BOSTON / LANCASTER / TOKYO

Library of Congress Cataloging-in-Publication Data
Main entry under title:

The Culture-bound syndromes.

(Culture, illness, and healing)
Bibliography: p.
Includes indexes.
1.   Medical anthropology—Addresses, essays, lectures.   2.   Ethno-
psychology—Addresses, essays, lectures.   3.   Mental illness—Social aspects—
Addresses, essays, lectures.   4.   Psychiatry, Transcultural—Addresses, essays,
lectures.   I.   Simons, Ronald C.   II.   Hughes, Charles C. (Charles Campbell)
III.   Series.   [DNLM: 1.   Culture.   2.   Ethnic Groups—psychology.
3.   Mental Disorders—etiology.   4.   Social Environment. WM 31 C9685]
GN296.C835   1985   362.1'042   85-14613
ISBN 90-277-1858-X
ISBN 90-277-1859-8 (pbk.)

Published by D. Reidel Publishing Company.
P.O. Box 17, 3300 AA Dordrecht, Holland.

Sold and distributed in the U.S.A. and Canada
by Kluwer Academic Publishers,
190 Old Derby Street, Hingham, MA 02043, U.S.A.

In all other countries, sold and distributed
by Kluwer Academic Publishers Group,
P.O. Box 322, 3300 AH Dordrecht, Holland.

Printed in the Netherlands

With Appreciation to:

Clyde Kluckhohn
Alexander H. Leighton
Eng-Seong Tan
Nathaniel N. Wagner

TABLE OF CONTENTS

PART II: FOLK ILLNESSES OF PSYCHIATRIC INTEREST IN WHICH A NEUROPHYSIOLOGICAL SHAPING FACTOR IS ONLY SUSPECTED

A. The Genital Retraction Taxon

B. The Sudden Mass Assault Taxon

C. The Running Taxon

PART III: FOLK ILLNESSES USUALLY LISTED AS CULTURE-BOUND PSYCHIATRIC SYNDROMES WHICH SHOULD PROBABLY NO LONGER BE SO CONSIDERED

A. The Fright Illness Taxon

B. The Cannibal Compulsion Taxon

APPENDIX

SOURCES AND ACKNOWLEDGEMENTS

Ronald C. Simons, 'The Resolution of the *Latah* Paradox' originally appeared in the *Journal of Nervous and Mental Disease* **168** (1980), 195–206. It is reprinted here by permission of the Williams & Wilkins Co., Baltimore.

Michael G. Kenny, 'Paradox Lost: The *Latah* Problem Revisited', and Ronald C. Simons' rejoinder, '*Latah* II — Problems with a Purely Symbolic Interpretation', first appeared in the *Journal of Nervous and Mental Disease* **171** (1983), 159–67 and 168–75 and are both reprinted here by permission of The Williams & Wilkins Co., Baltimore.

Emiko Ohnuki-Tierney, 'Shamans and *Imu*: Among Two Ainu Groups — Toward a Cross-Cultural Model of Interpretation', first appeared in *Ethos* **8** (1980), 204–28 and is reproduced here by permission of the Society for Psychological Anthropology.

Joseph D. Bloom and Richard D. Gelardin, '*Uqamairineq* and *Uqumanigianiq*: Eskimo Sleep Paralysis' originally appeared in *Arctic* **29**(1) (1967), and is reprinted here by permission of the Arctic Institute of North America.

Gwee Ah Leng, '*Koro* — A Cultural Disease' first appeared in the *Singapore Medical Journal* **4**(3) (1963) and is reprinted here by permission of the Singapore Medical Association.

O. I. Ifabumuyi and G. G. C. Rwegellera, '*Koro* in a Nigerian Male Patient: A Case Report' first appeared in the *African Journal of Psychiatry* **5** (1979) and is reprinted here by permission of Literamed Publications Nigeria Ltd.

J. Guy Edwards, 'The *Koro* Pattern of Depersonalization in an American Schizophrenic Patient' originally appeared in *The American Journal of Psychiatry* **126** (1970), 1171–73 and is reprinted here by permission of the American Psychiatric Association.

Burton G. Burton-Bradley, 'The *Amok* Syndrome in Papua and New Guinea' originally appeared in *The Medical Journal of Australia* **1** (1968), 252–56 and is reprinted here by permission of The Medical Journal of Australia.

J. Arboleda-Florez, '*Amok*', first appeared in the *Bulletin of the American Academy of Psychiatry and Law* **7** (1979), 286–95 and is reprinted here by permission of the American Academy of Psychiatry & the Law.

Z. Gussow, '*Pibloktoq* (Hysteria) Among the Polar Eskimo' first appeared in *The Psychoanalytic Study of Society* **1** (1960), 218–36 and is reprinted here by permission of the International Universities Press, Inc., New York.

Philip A. Dennis, '*Grisi Siknis* in Miskito Culture' is a shorter version of the article entitled: '*Grisi Siknis* Among the Miskito', which appeared in *Medical Anthropology* **5**, 445–505 and is reprinted here by permission of Redgrave Publishing Co.

Lou Marano, '*Windigo* Psychosis: The Anatomy of an Emic–Etic Confusion' and the 'Commentaries and Replies' following this article originally appeared in *Current Anthropology* **23** (1982), 385–412 and **24** (1983), 120–25 and are both reprinted here by permission of The University of Chicago Press.

We also wish to acknowledge quotations from the following publications:

Alexander H. Leighton, T. Adeoye Lambo, Charles C. Hughes, Dorothea C. Leighton, Jane M. Murphy, and David B. Macklin, *Psychiatric Disorder Among the Yoruba: A Report from the Cornell–Aro Mental Health Research Project in the Western Region, Nigeria.* © 1963 by Cornell University. Reprinted by permission of the publisher, Cornell University Press.

A large quotation from P. M. Yap in M. P. Lau and A. B. Stokes (eds.), *Comparative Psychiatry: A Theoretical Framework*, 1974. Reprinted by permission of the University of Toronto Press.

Parts from the *Diagnostic and Statistical Manual of Mental Disorders*, Third Edition, American Psychiatric Association, Washington, D.C., APA, 1980. Reprinted by permission.

Z. Gussow, 'Some Responses of West Greenland Eskimo to a Naturalistic Situation of Perceptual Deprivation', *INTER-NORD: International Journal of Arctic and Nordic Studies* (December 1970), 227–62. Reprinted with permission.

Joseph P. Reser and Harry D. Eastwell, 'Labelling and Cultural Expectations: The Shaping of a Sorcery Syndrome in Aboriginal Australia', *The Journal of Nervous and Mental Disease* **169** (1981), 303–10. Reprinted by permission of The Williams & Wilkins Co., Baltimore.

PREFACE

In the last few years there has been a great revival of interest in culture-bound psychiatric syndromes. A spate of new papers has been published on well known and less familiar syndromes, and there have been a number of attempts to put some order into the field of inquiry. In a review of the literature on culture-bound syndromes up to 1969 Yap made certain suggestions for organizing thinking about them which for the most part have not received general acceptance (see Carr, this volume, p. 199). Through the seventies new descriptive and conceptual work was scarce, but in the last few years books and papers discussing the field were authored or edited by Tseng and McDermott (1981), Al-Issa (1982), Friedman and Faguet (1982) and Murphy (1982). In 1983 Favazza summarized his understanding of the state of current thinking for the fourth edition of the *Comprehensive Textbook of Psychiatry*, and a symposium on culture-bound syndromes was organized by Kenny for the Eighth International Congress of Anthropology and Ethnology. The strongest impression to emerge from all this recent work is that there is no substantive consensus, and that the very concept, "culture-bound syndrome" could well use some serious reconsideration. As the role of culture-specific beliefs and practices in all affliction has come to be increasingly recognized it has become less and less clear what sets the culture-bound syndromes apart. Does the concept of culture-bound syndromes still retain any utility or is it merely the anachronistic legacy of an ethnocentric and imperial past?

There are many other questions as well, e.g.: how are the individual syndromes best thought of: what concepts derived from which disciplines are the most reasonable and the most useful with which to consider each syndrome? Can they be encompassed in a meaningful collective category? Does biology, especially neurophysiology, have a role in explaining the manifestations of any of the syndromes? Are multi-disciplinary explanations possible, are they necessary, and for which syndromes? How do the syndromes relate to current psychiatric nosology; are they variants of ubiquitous psychiatric syndromes or is each locally unique? What is the role of culture; does it cause something locally unique to happen or is it merely the symbol system for elaborating ubiquitous pathological processes? And in one noteworthy instance, does a syndrome which has been repeatedly described and variously explained even exist, or does it have no actual incidence whatsoever?

This book was originally intended to follow a conference considering these questions which Professor John Carr of the University of Washington and I had planned to arrange. As old friends who views differ almost diametrically on several of the central issues, our plan was to assemble a group of fieldworkers from various

xiii

Ronald C. Simons and Charles C. Hughes (eds.), The Culture-Bound Syndromes, xiii–xv.
© 1985 *by D. Reidel Publishing Company.*

disciplines who had done primary work on the syndromes and to publish both their original descriptive papers and a summary of our deliberations and debates. For a number of practical reasons, the conference could not be held, and though Jack and I for a long time still cherished the plan of publishing a collection of papers representing our two viewpoints, ultimately the press of his duties as acting chairman of the University of Washington's psychiatry department forced him to withdraw from that plan as well. As we had by that time collected the papers that form the nucleus of this volume, I offered a seminar based on this compilation as part of the Medical Anthropology core curriculum at Michigan State University. The more we considered the controversies, the more useful it seemed to publish some compilation such as that which Professor Carr and I had originally envisaged.

Desiring some assistance with the editorial chores and even more importantly some view of the field complementing mine, I thought first of Charles Hughes, from whom I had taken my first course in anthropology a dozen years earlier. I had once discussed a similar project with him, but it had been abandoned when he left Michigan State for a professorship at the University of Utah. Much to my pleasure and relief, Charles was interested; he had also been keeping up his interest in the syndromes and had been puzzling out how they might be related to standard psychiatric nomenclature. We did not fully agree on the most useful way to classify and analyze the syndromes, but we did agree that the time was ripe for a book laying out some of the controversies. Further, we agreed that many of the major conceptual problems had to do with the levels of abstraction in which divergent analyses were couched. All of this history is offered as a way of explaining the somewhat unusual nature of the present collaboration and more importantly, the organization of the pressent volume.

From the vast literature on culture-bound syndromes, this volume contains an illustrative sampling chosen to reflect a wide diversity of viewpoints and analytic conceptualizations. The papers' authors include anthropologists, sociologists, psychologists, psychiatrists, and non-psychiatric physicians. Some of the papers are classic accounts from the literature; many are adapted from more recent journal publications; several were written expressly for this volume; and one is an excerpt from a PhD dissertation. Each of the papers deals with a single syndrome, and the papers have been grouped into subsections based on gross behavioral resemblances within syndrome sets, groupings which I have called "taxa". There are two explicit debates; my debate with Michael Kenny on how *latah* might best be understood and a debate between Lou Marano and his critics on the existence or non-existence of *windigo* as a set of actual behaviors. The book also contains as many implicit debates as we could cram in; contrasting viewpoints with the contrast emphasized by the juxtaposition of papers. This is a volume of controversy, and to that extent at least, a true reflection of the present state of thinking in this field. Charles Hughes' introductory chapter relates the syndromes to current psychiatric nosologic and taxonomic thinking and suggests a new way of considering single instances of any of the syndromes discussed. My introductory chapter suggests a way in which biological, psychological, social, and cultural factors can be considered jointly, and it proposes a taxonomic scheme which I believe could be helpful in bringing some order to the field and in suggesting avenues for future research. The present volume, organized according to this scheme, is intended as a demonstration of its potential utility. Both Dr. Hughes and I stress the need to collect descriptive data bearing on specific unanswered questions, although the data we solicit and the questions we seek to answer differ somewhat.

The last section of the volume is a preliminary, partially sorted listing of culture-bound syndromes, prepared by Dr. Hughes. It is presented in the hope that it will be useful to future researchers and that some may even be tempted by this volume to undertake additional sorting. We also hope that this volume will acquaint readers with the main currents of thought on culture-bound syndromes and will expose them to a wide enough range of sets of data, analytic perspectives and styles of reasoning to make possible preliminary conclusions as to which approaches to future research are likely to prove most useful.

RONALD C. SIMONS
East Lansing, MI
January, 1985

INTRODUCTION

CULTURE-BOUND OR CONSTRUCT-BOUND?

The Syndromes and DSM-III

The several syndromes discussed in this book exist in a kind of "twilight zone" of psychiatric phenomena, having variously occasioned puzzlement, controversy, or dismissal from detailed analysis. The puzzlement about the syndromes has its source in the bizarre characteristics of the behavior displayed. If (as is usually the case) the frame of comparison is the Western-derived system of psychiatric diagnostic categories, these syndromes are, at least phenomenologically, unfamiliar ways of being "crazy". From that point of view, they are instances of *deviant deviance!* The controversy exists over whether such episodes or patterns of behavior are simply culturally-based and different, yet "normal", ways of acting, or examples of "authentic" disease and disorder. And the dismissal may occur when such syndromes are summarily assigned to categories of disorder already established in Western nosology without any fine-tuning to capture possible culture-specific meanings or symbolism of the behavior necessary for a valid categorical assignment.

As a putative class, the syndromes appear to be so much in the "twilight zone" that, for example, they are nowhere to be found in the index nor in the table of contents under any heading suggestive of the term "culture-bound" in any of the three versions of the *Diagnostic and Statistical Manual of Mental Disorders* of the American Psychiatric Association (the latest and greatly revised edition, 'DSM-III', being the most comprehensive and conceptually innovative). Yet there continue to appear case reports of newly-discovered syndromes referred to in this fashion (e.g., Lin 1983a; Lewis 1975) as well as commentaries — including this book — which demonstrate that all has not been put to rest in analysis of the nature of the syndromes or the appropriateness of their assignment to conventional psychiatric diagnostic categories. This suggests at least the following possibilities: (1) the syndromes are simply unusual and striking, but not necessarily pathologic, behaviors (an extreme cultural relativistic position); (2) the standard diagnostic categories in their present form are perfectly able to assimilate these syndromes; (3) the standard diagnostic categories are inadequate because they themselves are so culture-bound they cannot conceptually accommodate the syndromes; (4) there is no conceptual or theoretical justification for establishing this or any other assemblage of syndromes as uniquely and singularly influenced by culture; or, finally (5) that there is such disparity in the semantic referents of terms used, and in the levels of abstraction and analysis employed, that meaningful discussion and comparative analysis is difficult if not impossible. This chapter is a commentary upon these several possibilities.

For convenience the term "culture-bound syndromes" is used in discussion here, but later the suitability of continuing such usuage will be questioned. Indeed, there are numerous ambiguities raised by that term as well as others used to describe the

Ronald C. Simons and Charles C. Hughes (eds.), The Culture-Bound Syndromes, 3–24.
© 1985 *by D. Reidel Publishing Company.*

syndromes, issues which are further reflected in the lack of agreement among commentators regarding the ontologic and diagnostic status of the specifically-named syndromes themselves.

The *folk* nosologic terms by which such syndromes or behaviors are known present almost a Cook's Tour of world cultures, one or another such syndrome being found in every major geographic region (see the Appendix to this volume). In addition, of course, there are locally recognized syndromes of this general nature that do not necessarily have a distinctive indigenous name, such as "malignant anxiety", "thanatomania" or "voodoo death", and possession or trance states.

One reason such syndromes have been of continuing interest is that they highlight important questions relevant to several fields, e.g., psychiatry, psychology, and anthropology, such as the differential contribution of biological and cultural factors in the etiology and shaping of mental disorders, the relativity of meaning across cultural contexts, and the potential generalizability of psychiatric classificatory schemes developed in one culture. That such syndromes might easily capture the psychiatrists' attention, for example, can be seen in the variety of symptoms collectively displayed in three of the more well-recognized syndromes discussed in this book, *latah, amok*, and *koro*: sleep disturbance, prodromal brooding, depression, social withdrawal, anxiety, depersonalization, echolalia, glossolalia, echopraxia, delusions and thought disorder, amnesia, mutism, somatization, and violent or homicidal behavior.

But other types of data are also frequently reported, data especially relevant to unravelling the dynamic interplay between personality functioning and sociocultural context: behavioral and situational precipitants of the episode, demographic characteristics of the victims, "emic" or indigenous cultural explanations for the event, outsiders' analyses of the psychodynamics involved, and procedures for treatment or management of the victim. The purported precipitants are both closely associated in time with the event — such as verbal suggestions, fright, social embarrassment or social disruption — and more distally, as in a recelled traumatic event that had occurred even several years earlier. Emic explanations include the actions of witches and other evil persons, taboo and norm violations by the victim, malevolent actions of ancestors or other spirits, loss of soul by the victim, and occasionally a "naturalistic" explanation. Etic analyses include the episode's serving as a legitimate sick role for the victim, as an institutionalized means of tension-reduction or catharsis, or as "time-out" from a stressful situation. Such analyses also often link the episode to the victim's social marginality. Sometimes the possible role of physiological factors is also explicitly included in the discussion. Forms of therapy include isolation of the victim, use of specialized healers (often in a group context), and the empowering force of social dramatization. Usually included in an account of such a syndrome also are demographic characteristics of the victims, such as relative preponderance of males or females, and differential incidence between adults and children.

As we will see momentarily, such a holistic set of descriptive characteristics directed at assessing the behavior of a person in a particular cultural situation is congruent, in spirit at least, with the enlarged conceptual framework suggested in the DSM-III. The extent to which that contextualizing intent may be translated into congruent specifics remains the question. In this regard, more than a decade ago P. M. Yap, a pioneer in this field (e.g., Yap 1951, 1969), presented a relevant assessment of this subject and a challenge to clarify concepts and dissect the interplay of normal cultural expectation from pathologic response:

Whether or not there are 'new' psychiatric illnesses to be found in folk cultures or non-metropolitan populations is a question that first requires semantic resolution. Undoubtedly there are in certain cultures clinical manifestations quite unlike these described in standard psychiatric textbooks, which historically are based on the experiences of western psychiatrists. In this sense illnesses presenting so strangely may be regarded as 'new'. However, each of the same textbooks also espouses a system of disease classification that by its own logic is meant to be final and exhaustive. From this point of view, no more new illnesses are to be discovered, and any strange clinical condition can only be a variation of something already recognized and described. Two problems then arise: firstly, how much we know about the culture-bound syndromes for us to be able to fit them into a standard classification; and, secondly, whether such a standard and exhaustive classification in fact exists.

It has long been known that there are, in certain cultural groups, peculiar aberrations of behavior which are regarded by themselves as abnormal. Over the years a number of terms taken from indigenous languages have crept into the psychiatric literature to denote these conditions, but many of them do not point to novel and distinct forms of disorder unknown elsewhere. Some are simply generic terms for 'mental disorder' without definite meaning, others refer only to healing rituals, and still others to supernatural notions of disease causation. From a psychiatric point of view the field has, with notable recent exceptions, remained confused and barren. Interest has tended to wither after the syndromes have been disdainfully labelled 'exotic', and the colourful names are then surrendered to the belletrist. To avoid stagnation in this field, it is essential to apply the concepts of clinical psychopathology to the analysis of these disorders, to integrate them into recognized classifications of disease if possible, or to broaden the classification if necessary. (Yap 1974: 86)

The purpose of this chapter is to discuss the utility of a response to Yap's final suggestion based on the categorical system and conceptual approach embodied in the DSM-III. It will also be suggested that progress in understanding the etiology and dynamics of such conditions will be hastened if some of the *mystique* is taken from the term "culture-bound" through a culturally-informed use of this categorizing scheme, and through use of a concept of culture dynamically and not statically defined — i.e., in terms of normative beliefs, values, perceptions, and meanings as they function in *behavior*. We might then be better able to determine whether such syndromes are, indeed, uniquely or relatively more influenced in their etiology and expression by the specific cultural setting in which they occur than are other disorders (hence justifying their designation, by contrast to other syndromes, as "culture-bound"), or are the adventitious victims of the particular constructs used to fix them in thought.

If one accepts the demonstrated depth and pervasiveness of culture in shaping behavior, both in internal ideational models and external motoric manifestations, then it follows that at the phenomenological level there can be culturally distinctive ways of being mentally disordered regardless of the extent of specific organic involvement. In this respect, biology provides the base and culture provides the vehicle, the form for translation of biologic factors into conceptualization at the behavioral level in the same way that anatomic and neurologic factors provide the substrate and mechanism *for* speech, which in its observable form is a distinctive, culturally-programmed *language*. Although it is obviously too simple a formulation, the essence of this position is: learn a language, learn an illness. Edgerton's statement regarding implicit cultural "knowledge" of psychotic symptoms in four East African tribes cogently makes the point: ". . . this catalogue of psychotic behavior was widely known within each society even by people who had never seen a psychotic themselves. In effect there was a known pattern of expectations for psychotic behavior" (1969: 53).

My view is that problems of the analysis and diagnosis of the so-called "culture-bound syndromes" are no different from those encountered in the study of any purported instance of psychopathology when cultural boundaries are crossed — regardless of whether there is a distinctive folk label applied to the behavior. It is a question of familiarizing one's self with the cultural context of norms and conceptualizations of illness relevant to the behavior of the particular person or patient. The considerable body of literature in transcultural psychiatry underscores both the need to do this, as well as the difficulty of the challenge. Lin's commentary on a recently-reported Korean culture-bound syndrome makes the point well, noting that the patients' ". . . culturally determined belief in *Hwa-Byung* profoundly influenced the way they experienced and presented their symptoms, the kind of help they sought, and the treatment results they expected" (Lin 1983b: 1269).

Two earlier examples illustrate the conjunction of both the locally-defined (emic) and outside-analyst defined (etic) ideas of psychopathology. Both persons were patients of native healers among the Yoruba people of Nigeria:

A 50-year-old woman is afraid of being killed. She thinks her brother who brought her to the native healer wants her killed. She is restless, cannot sleep, weeps for no obvious reason, and may refuse food, fearing it is poisoned. She has ideas that she is going to be attacked or arrested. She looks frightened, talks to herself, and seems to hear voices.

A 23-year-old man dances and sings around the town. He expects to be paid for his dancing and gets abusive if he is not. He takes food in the markets and then refuses to pay for it, threatening to stone the sellers if they persist in their demands. He is restless and complains of fear. Sometimes he behaves and talks like an Egungun (violates a taboo by inappropriately imitating a sacred being). (A. Leighton et al. 1963: 107, 108)

With reference to breaking through the cultural masking of the behaviors and discerning whether pathology exists, the authors further note that:

When we reviewed all these symptoms, both those that emerged from general questions about illness types and those from native healers' descriptions of particular cases, none stood out as being unsuited to one or more of the psychiatric symptom categories. Indeed, they have a familiar ring, for they resemble behavior that used to be commonly seen in public mental hospitals before the advent of modern treatment. Although particulars of culture came into the picture in the matter of taboo violations, this was not at a very subtle level or one that was difficult to appraise. The behavior was so obviously wrong by Yoruba standards that members of this society could readily point out and explain it to the stranger. The discrepancies were, furthermore, easily understood by a psychiatrist because they have close parallels in the Euro-American cultural system. (ibid.: 109)

It is of interest that the psychiatric diagnostic categories used in that particular study were those of the *first* version of the DSM, those current twenty years ago. Even then, therefore, when used in conjunction with firm knowledge of the cultural setting of the behaviors, they were of use in providing a point of entry into the issue of psychopathologic versus normal though unusual behavior. The extent to which the DSM-III is an improvement on DSM-I when cultural boundaries are crossed will be examined shortly.

Before doing that, however, let us briefly consider the semantic implications of the several general terms used to denote these maverick behaviors. As will be seen, such an exercise serves an important hermeneutic function, for such terms interpose themselves between the analyst and the specific syndromes, and the emphases suggested in the language used inevitably convey varying predispositional biases that unknowingly may skew analysis of the phenomena.

THE GENERAL CLASSIFICATORY LABEL

Beyond the term "culture-bound", these syndromes have also variously been called the "psychogenic psychoses" (Faergeman 1963); the "ethnic psychoses" and "ethnic neuroses" (Devereux 1956); the "hysterical psychoses" (Langness 1967); and the "exotic psychoses" (Yap 1969), among other terms. Yap attempted a complex designation containing several conceptual elements: the "atypical culture-bound reactive syndromes" (1974), a conceptually variegated label comparable to Arieti and Meth's (1959) "rare, unclassifiable, collective, and exotic syndromes", a title which includes but is not confined to the "culture-bound syndromes".

There are several semantic issues to consider, for in these various proposed major categorical labels ambiguity abounds. For example, can all (or any) of these classes of disorders or behaviors justifiably be considered "psychoses"? For the class, many writers would disagree with such labelling, noting the relatively transient and benign character of most of them. Let us examine the implications of the other descriptive labels.

'Atypical' and 'Exotic'

Both the labels "atypical psychoses" and "exotic syndrome" imply deviance from a "standard" diagnostic base. If something is "atypical" it obviously falls outside the range of what is "typical". Similarly, "exotic" means "foreign", "different", "deviant" from something that is *not* exotic, that is, from something familiar and well-known. So with these two categorial labels, we would be dealing with psychiatric (or imputed psychiatric) syndromes that fall outside the scope of known and described phenomena.

What constitutes that 'scope of known and described phenomena'? On the

basis of historical factors it is those phenomena denoted by the set of concepts
and diagnostic labels which evolved in Euro-American psychiatric thinking for
understanding and treating the varieties of mental disorder. That set of concepts,
that frame of reference, might be those embodied in whatever at any given time
may be the most recent edition of the *International Classification of Diseases*
(currently the 9th), the latest edition of the *Diagnostic and Statistical Manual of
Mental Disorders* of the American Psychiatric Association (currently DSM-III),
or any of the contemporary versions of the numerous formal medical diagnostic
systems Stengel (1959) discussed a generation ago and more recently Spitzer et al.
(1983).

Let us first note that such a categorical system, intended to be universally
applicable, may be ethnocentric in both obvious and subtle ways insofar as, either
in discrete categories or in basic organizing principles, it may be implicitly influenced
by values and beliefs of the particular society in which it evolved. In the long view
that might not necessarily render it invalid, of course, as new knowledge accumu-
lates and new conceptualizations emerge in the scheme itself. But in the shorter
time perspective there may well be problems; for not only is science in general
as we know it a historical product of Western Europe, but so, too, in its explicit
theoretical conceptualizations (though not all of its practice, of course) is Western
medical science and its derivative, psychiatric nosology. Perhaps the clearest example
of an inherited ethnocentric bias in Western medicine and psychiatry is the Cartesian
dichotomy between matter and mind, body and "soul". Seen in cross-cultural
perspective, most cosmological schemes do not make such a separation, but
rather, see human life in terms of unities and completementary systems. But
the "mind/body" dichotomy is, of course, the most fundamental classificatory
distinction made in Western psychodiagnostic schemes.

A comment by Tsung-yi Lin is particularly apt in this regard:

Modern psychiatry was born in the West, and as it grew it was moulded by specifically Western
philosophical and scientific traditions; it developed as a child of Western culture. Considering,
then, the prevalence of ethnocentrism and the untested presumption of clinical universality
in modern psychiatry, it is not difficult to understand why unfamiliar psychiatric phenomena
or folkloric healing practices aimed at mental disorders in non-Western cultures are regarded
as foreign, primitive, uninteresting or even inferior. Quite simply they are considered as phenomena and practices isolated from the totality of the cultural contexts which shape them and
serve to define their real significance. It is the challenge of cultural psychiatry to overcome the
inertia of ethnocentrism while helping modern psychiatry to step beyond its boundaries,
enriched by new materials, new perspectives and new insights. (1982: 235)

It is of interest that on another level analogous to the issue of "ethno"-centrism,
DSM-III has been attacked as being "anthropo-centric" or "male-centric" (Kaplan
1983). It has been asserted that some of the categories of disorder are based upon
the reification into instances of pathology, of socially-selected and culturally-
defined behavioral traits considered differentially appropriate for either female or
males in American society. The trait of dependence is a good example. Traditionally
males have been expected to be adventurous, curious, active, and self-reliant, and

boys are socialized toward that behavioral ideal. Girls, on the contrary, have been expected — and trained — to be compliant, agreeable, self-effacing, and dependent upon others for direction and support. Kaplan claims that these different value sets are accorded different "pathologic" implications in DSM-III, and she presents two admittedly created examples to make her case. But she goes on to assert that "masculine-biased assumptions about what behaviors are healthy and what behaviors are crazy are codified in diagnostic criteria; these criteria then influence diagnosis and treatment rates and patterns" (1983: 786). Whether or not her argument is fully accepted in terms of these particular patterns, the basic point made demands consideration — namely, that the assumptions built into the labels used must be explicitly examined for whether they are rooted primarily in nature or in cultural values.

'Rare'

One sometimes sees these syndromes referred to as "rare". While that may be accurate, determination of whether or not a syndrome is infrequent should be a matter for epidemiological research as to relative rates of the disorder, and not simply be decided by assumption, as is so often done. With a few notable exceptions (e.g., Rubel 1964), epidemiologically-based data on these syndromes are scanty. Further, however, if by "rare" one means that the syndrome is infrequent in a given population (let us say of the order of 1% or so lifetime prevalence), then by the same logic we must say that on the basis of its comparable prevalence, schizophrenia would be in the same category. Perhaps, when the final data on the "culture-bound syndromes" are all in, we will compare the situation in this regard to the search for tropical diseases in the temperature latitudes: they may be rare in frequency in any given population but they are not bizarre or strange to medical knowledge as a whole.

'Culture-Bound' and 'Culture-Reactive'

With the terms "culture-bound syndromes" and "culture-reactive syndromes" there are conceptual issues of a different nature. For something to be "bound" to something else (in this case, the syndrome to the sociocultural setting) can imply several things. For one, it is restricted to that particular setting; i.e., it is "culture-specific" and is not found elsewhere (comparable therefore, to the neurologic disease *kuru*, found only among the Fore people of New Guinea; see Gajdusek 1977); there is an exclusive and unique relationship between the two entities. This is the type of meaning formerly common in the discovery and discussion of these syndromes; for example, the terms "latah" and "amok" are taken from the languages of groups in which the syndromes were first noted and reported, and in each case the usage at least implied that the syndrome was unique to that culture. The latter, of course, has not been found to be true, and the published literature documents the appearance of similar behavior in widely separated locations. The concept of "taxon" (Simons, Chapter 2 in this volume) and the organizational format of this book reflect the non-localized nature of at least some of the syndromes.

To be bound to something may also have an etiological and not simply a distributional component. The syndrome may be *a result* of factors operating in that particular culture. This meaning, of course, is also implied in the other term mentioned above, the "culture-reactive syndrome". The assumption is that there is something in the cultural and social setting — perhaps beliefs and values that shape perception of the world and its mysterious forces; or perhaps particular types of standardized social situations, such as disadvantaged roles — that over time fosters and/or predisposes toward temporary or chronic disorder. Such a condition may (or may not) be noted by locals as a type of "sickness", but may well be regarded by outsiders as psychiatric abnormality.

These two common labels, "culture-bound" and "culture-reactive", suggest a particular emphasis in a theory of psychopathology. In these instances, the psychopathology is rooted, at least in large part, in social environmental forces and/or situations. Biological factors aside for the moment, what one is dealing with is an assumption widespread in dynamic psychiatry, namely that the behavior labelled psychiatric disorder is an attempt by a person to adapt to major problems in his or her life and personality. And when we enlarge the purview to imply that the given disorder is "culture-bound" we may be saying that the person is trying to adapt to problems that, at least in part, stem from definable characteristics of that particular socio-cultural environment.

But does this mean that if *these* syndromes are thus influenced by their cultural setting, then the *non*-"culture-bound" syndromes, the presumably more familiar syndromes, are therefore *not* similarly influenced? *Are* there any such syndromes, or is it merely a matter of degree? One need not be an extreme cultural determinist with regard to the role of culture in the etiology and shaping of mental disorder to question whether it serves any useful purpose so to single out syndromes of this type as having significant or unusual cultural content and structure, thereby implying an exclusivity to that category with respect to the role of cultural factors. To the extent that culture has a role in psychiatric disorder, both in etiology and symptomatology (a position well-supported in the literature), the use of the descriptive phrase "culture-bound" becomes vitiated as a differentiating term referring to a distinctive set of disorders. It is unfortunate that the term itself seems to have taken on a life of its own and, instead of remaining a useful construct that facilitates analysis of empirical events, has become an inhibitor of such analysis, a good example of what Whitehead meant by "the fallacy of misplaced concreteness".

Furthermore, to say that the "culture-bound" syndromes may represent simply another series of examples of those disorders constituted in large part by the sociocultural environment raises other interesting questions. For one, it implies that there might be such syndromes that could be so designated in any of the *industrialized* societies in the same way as one looks, for example, to the particulars of Malay society for precursors and behavioral expressions of *latah*. Combining the notion of (1) an exclusive relationship of a disorder to its sociocultural setting with (2) the idea of prepotency of sociocultural factors in the etiology and behavioral expression of such a disorder, could we say, for instance, that "petism" (see Simons, Chapter 2 in this volume) or "Type A Behavior" might be "culture-bound", "culture-reactive" disorders of American society? These particular examples, of course, may be stretching it a bit, but the logic of the extrapolation stands. Indeed, as Murphy (1977) suggested a few years ago, it is as imperative that the role of cultural factors in the psychodynamics of mental disorder in Western society not simply be taken for granted but should be as fully incorporated into analysis as it is when the therapist is dealing with a patient from a widely divergent culture. Indeed, in words that cheer the anthropologist, he notes that "transcultural psychiatry should begin at home" and stresses that

... the time is overdue when the relationship between cultural backgrounds and psychopathology or forms of therapy in developed countries should be more formally examined, and when we should cease thinking that our behavioral expectations are all 'nature', not requiring re-examination (1977: 390–371).

In the papers included in this volume considerable effort is made to present and analyze the relevant cultural context of each disorder — the particular symbols, meanings, and interpersonal situations that underlie the psychodynamic patterns discussed. In short, the 'behavioral expectations' specifically have *not* been taken for granted, but rather, have been explicitly analyzed in the manner proposed by Murphy. The analysis of culture-bound syndromes, then, driven by perplexity to examine the cultural background of the disorder because the behavior is so strange, may serve as a heuristic model for what should be done with regard to any *non-*"culture-bound" syndrome as well.

It may well be that the dichotomy between "us" and "them" in regard to discussions of culture-bound syndromes has been too quickly drawn; between, that is, the non-western peoples, the "underdeveloped" peoples, the "primitives" (who have the "exotic" and the "culture-bound" syndromes) and the western world, the "developed" world, the "civilized" world. Indeed some would speak in such terms, noting that the allegedly 'less well organized' and 'less complex psyches' of the former groups of people are more easily subject to culturally-derived pathoplasticity than is the person in the industrialized world (e.g., Langness 1967; Kiev 1972; Wittkower and Prince 1974). But regardless of the possibility (and many would disagree), and in agreement with Tsung-yi Lin's earlier comment, it may well not be fanciful to suggest that if the Hopi people, a group which prizes self-effacing, non-competitive interpersonal behavior, were to develop a cross-cultural scheme for the classification of the undesirable = deviant = "sick" behavior, it would include "Type A behavior" as a prime example.

I suggest that the way out of the semantic quagmire created by use of these several terms — "culture-bound", "exotic", and the others — is to abandon altogether the search for an acceptable *general* classificatory term; the phenomena under discussion appear to be neither homogeneous nor distinctive. Different, to be sure, but in the absence of persuasive data to the contrary, one may assume as a working hypothesis that the differences inhere more in the failure of the diagnoses to include a thorough-going cultural analysis (to ascertain how deeply and in what manner the cultural dimension is embodied in the observed behavior), than it does in distinctive pathologic structural differences. One can agree with Wig's telling comment on the issue of the

"culture-bound syndromes" and DSM-III: "It is not very logical to term 'spirit possession' or 'fear about shrinking of the genitals' culture bound when 'fear of being alone or in public places' or 'intense fear of becoming obese' retain the dignified names 'agoraphobia' and 'anorexia nervosa' and find suitable niches in psychiatric classifications" (1983: 87).

Perhaps, if a term is really needed for this collection of unusual disorders, we should simply stay with something like "folk psychiatric disorders", but *only as a term of convenience* and not of analysis. This suggestion is especially strengthened by the assembly of data gathered together in the appendix to this volume, which convincingly vitiates any conceptual distinction between "culture-bound" syndromes and the general category of "folk" taxonomies or systems for recognizing aberrant behavior.

Let us consider how adequately the DSM-III scheme might contribute to further understanding of the syndromes, especially in regard to the ease with which cultural data can be elicited and incorporated into the analysis.

THE "CULTURE-BOUND SYNDROMES" AND DSM-III

As Whitehead once noted, science is

... the thought organization of experience. The most obvious aspect of this field of actual experience is its disorderly character. It is for each person a continuum, fragmentary, and with elements not clearly differentiated. (1949: 109)

A taxonomy, the necessary first step in the scientific search for order among phenonena, is the conceptual instrument by which such 'differentiation among the elements' occurs, grouping as it does those observations into categories each marked off from the others by distinctive characteristics or patterns of observables. Categorizing experience into classes or groups of like-appearing objects is an ancient, universal, and vital human activity that serves both cognitive and social adaptational needs (cf. Raven et al. 1971). The language of a group constitutes its most obvious system of classificatory constructs.

However useful and necessary they are, however, taxonomic schemes can also be the source of error and obfuscation in dealing with nature. The basic categorizing concepts employed, as much as incomplete and fragmentary data on the objects to be categorized, may be the source of mischief and mystery in an attempt to understand, in that such concept-derived perception may so distort the phenomenon being observed that its basic structure or pattern is obscured. With regard to cross-cultural psychiatric issues for example, it has been suggested that lack of sufficient knowledge of the cultural context of the behavior may skew the outsider's interpretation toward pathology when none exists; the classic case of the 'psychotic' Navajo Indian (Jewell 1952) makes the point well. In that instance, an interpretation of behavior that did not take account of the subject's own culturally-defined ways of expressing "normality" led to his extended hospitalization as a diagnosed schizophrenic.

Given the heterogeneous nature of psychiatric and purported psychiatric phenomena, the inability to measure many significant features, the often divergent but undiscussed differences in meaning, and the use of nominal instead of operationalized definitions of terms, it is small wonder that reliability in psychiatric diagnostic schemes has been relatively low, even in the cultural context of a single society (Spitzer et al. 1978; Cantor 1980). Add to the above problems the semantic and conceptual difficulties implied by cultural differences, and the situation becomes even more confused.

There have been — and are — numerous psychiatric diagnostic systems developed in Western society (e.g., Menninger 1963; Stengel 1959; Spitzer et al. 1983); and these concepts have been used, with varying degrees of looseness and reliability, to classify the culture-bound syndromes. What, then, makes the idea of using the DSM-III categories and approach any more promising as a way of bringing order into analysis of these phenomena than was use of earlier systems?

For one thing, its reliability as a classificatory system has been subjected to systematic studies, and the findings are highly encouraging (in part, no doubt, due to the sustained effort made to "operationalize" definitions of the terms used). But in addition, compared to earlier schemes the DSM-III is an attempt to place the diagnosis and assessment of psychiatric phenomena on a more comprehensive, and because of that, innovative basis. Indeed, one might say that DSM-III is a major step toward *meta*-diagnosis; that is, toward going behind the conceptual boundaries of the traditional medical philosophy of diagnosis and looking at the phenomena of interest and the very purpose of such labelling in a new way. DSM-III does, indeed, seem to provide more points of entry for validly and usefully incorporating cultural data — more "receptors", if you will — than did previous versions of the DSM, even though, as seen earlier, DSM-I did not disallow the analyst's making a culturally-informed appraisal of possible psychopathology. And DSM-III, with its greater variety of conceptual "tools", would seem to provide the materials for constructing more adequate models of the observed phenomena in general than has been the case earlier, when the critical step was that of assigning a diagnosis. In traditional thinking, such a label articulated with not only a given set of symptoms but also tended to have etiological and prognostic features in that single conceptual package. The DSM-III format, on the other hand, lays out a constellation of various types of data that bear upon the episode, not simply a diagnosis *per se*.

Moreover, the formulation is explicitly committed to taking a theoretically neutral position with regard to etiology, as well as an explicitly descriptive approach with respect to symptoms, except where the pathophysiologic processes are known (DSM-III: 6). As demonstrated in earlier studies in social psychiatry (A. Leighton et al. 1963; D. Leighton et al. 1963; A. Leighton 1969); such an approach is less likely to confound reliability, at least at beginning stages of inquiry. DSM-III comments "The major justification for the generally atheoretical approach taken ... with regard to etiology is that the inclusion of etiological theories would be an obstacle to use of the manual by clinicians of varying theoretical orientations ..." and

This approach can be said to be 'descriptive' in that the definitions of the disorders generally consist of descriptions of the clinical features of the disorders. These features are described at the lowest order of inference necessary to describe the characteristic features of the disorder. Frequently the order of inference is relatively low, and the characteristic features consist of easily identifiable behavioral signs or symptoms, such as disorientation, mood disturbance, or psychomotor agitation. For some disorders, however, particularly the Personality Disorders, a much higher order of inference is necessary (ibid.).

As will be evident, such an approach bears some resemblance to what is suggested by Simons in the following chapter — that based on a first-order classificatory concept drawn from biology, the *taxon*, which groups objects that show a general resemblance to each other. The DSM-III represents the further evolution of the conventional diagnostic classificatory scheme with mixed levels of conceptualization, and its categories are avowedly atheoretical. Because of the still perplexing nature of these syndromes, it is the belief of the editors of this volume that the convergence of these dual perspectives may help shed light on and stimulate conceptual and theoretical clarification of the behaviors.

But aside from its atheoretical intent, there are other features of the DSM-III, in contrast with its predecessors, that also argue for the attempt to apply this system in an orderly way to the culture-bound syndromes. One is its explicit departure from notions of disease specificity so embedded in traditional reductionistic medical thinking: that there is a distinct diagnosis reflecting a "disease entity" as well as being "the" cause of that disease. This represents a shift from an "ontological" to a "physiological" (Engelhardt 1975) or "processual" concept of disease. Further, the assumption is that disorders may be multicausal, with several factors involved in the etiologic chain as well as outcome. Statements about a "syndrome", then depend not upon finding a single, essential defining characteristic, as has been traditional in medical thinking (Temkin 1963), but rather upon designating a set of correlated or associated features, any given one of which is not a necessary or sufficient "cause" of the disorder. While the concept of syndrome is not new of course, it is an extremely important conceptual tool given the somewhat contentious state of etiology regarding the culture-bound syndromes.

In other language, the approach to categorization embodied in DSM-III is thus a departure from one based upon the search for and use of "ideal types". In psychiatry it is a change from what has been called "typological" thinking to "dimensional" thinking (Straus 1975); or from "classical" types of categorization to "prototype" approaches (Cantor et al. 1980). Earlier this kind of change in the theory of classification was developed in biological taxonomy, with the shift from what Mayr (1963) termed "typological thinking" to "population thinking" — i.e., an approach that inductively derives types, patterns, or syndromes from the data observed and is not based on *a priori* assumptions.

Another feature of DSM-III promising for systematic use with the culture-bound syndromes is that one is not constrained to select a single diagnosis; rather, it is suggested that multiple diagnostic designations be used if the data so indicate. While, to be sure, one lists these in terms of a "principal diagnosis" followed by others, the basic point is that by being able to include other diagnostic features of the behavior and episode, important information about the person and the behavior in a particular situation is not lost. In a comment especially important in inquiry into the somewhat perplexing domain of the culture-bound syndromes, DSM-III (p. 6) pertinently notes:

A common misconception is that a classification of mental disorders classifies individuals, when actually what are being classified are disorders that individuals have. For this reason, the text of DSM-III avoids the use of such phrases as "a schizophrenic" or "an alcoholic", and instead uses the more accurate, but admittedly more wordy "an individual with Schizophrenia" or "an individual with Alcohol Dependence".

Another misconception is that all individuals described as having the same mental disorder are alike in all important ways. Although all the individuals described as having the same mental disorder show at least the defining features of the disorder, they may well differ in other important ways that may affect clinical management and outcome.

The DSM-III dictates that one go beyond simply the "diagnosis" or diagnoses, and develop, instead, an assessment or profile of the person and his or her behavior *vis-à-vis* a life situation, an assessment which includes estimates of severity. In the DSM-III the profile is constructed from several discrete dimensions of the observed person-in-environment behavioral unit. These dimensions are termed "axes". (It is relevant to note here that such an approach was foreshadowed in a multi-dimensional scheme used in some of the initial cross-cultural psychiatric research a generation ago, which not only focused on symptoms rather than diagnoses, but also included an estimate of severity and the psychiatric evaluator's own assessment of relative certainty that the protocol being evaluated did, indeed, give evidence of psychiatric symptoms; cf. D. Leighton et al. 1963; A. Leighton et al. 1963; A. Leighton 1969).

DSM-III contains five such axes. Axis I, labelled "clinical syndromes", represents the more or less traditional mental disorders. It is to be noted that even in this new version of a "traditional" listing of diagnostic categories there are several which, *prima facie*, show potential for being useful in classifying at least some of the culture-bound syndromes — such as "brief reactive psychosis" (298.80), "atypical psychosis" (298.90), "social phobia" (300.23), "atypical anxiety disorder" (300.00), "atypical somatoform disorder" (300.71), "depersonalization disorder" (300.60), "factitious disorder with psychological symptoms" (300.16), or "isolated explosive disorder" (312.35). It should also be noted that every major category in Axes I and II has a residual category of disorders "not elsewhere clas-sified", as well as a final entry in each of those residual categories that provides a slot for the "atypical" example. This, of course, can allow for growth in the number and variety of possible anomalous cases such as the "culture-bound" behaviors.

As with Axis I, multiple diagnoses may be made within Axis II, e.g., diagnoses of multiple specific developmental disorders, or a specific developmental disorder along with a personality disorder. In addition, specific personality *traits* useful in characterizing a person's behavior may be noted even if there is no diagnosis of Personality Disorder.

Axis III is the niche for including physical disorders and conditions in the overall evaluation of a person's behavior. While any given behavior may not be significantly influenced by an underlying physical "cause", when there is an organic condition that may be etiological relevant in assessing the observed pathology, it is obviously critical that such data be recognized in the analysis. An example from an early cross-cultural psychiatric study makes the point. In the Cornell-Aro study of psychiatric disorder among the Yoruba people of Nigeria, a number of symptoms were interpretable as possibly expressing mental disorder, such as bodily weakness or a feeling of worms crawling under the skin. However, at the same time it was known that the burden of physical disease was considerable in that population, e.g., from parasitic infestation, malaria, or malnutrition. Special care was taken, therefore, to parcel out such symptoms to their probable origin, including physical and laboratory examinations of a sub-sample of the overall study population (A. Leighton et al. 1963: 241–262; Collis 1966).

Axis IV and Axis V probably provide the most important innovation for in-corporating the phenomena denoted by the term "culture-bound syndromes" into the body of the literature dealing with mental disorders. Axis IV deals with "psychosocial stressors", clearly an area of prime importance in much discussion of these syndromes. It allows for entry into the total profile of not only particular types of stress, but also a judgement as to their severity. Suggested sources of stress (DSM-III: 28) include conjugal (marital and nonmarital), parenting, other interpersonal, occupational, living circumstances, financial, legal, developmental, physical illness or injury, factors in the family relationships of children and adolescents, and other.

Axis V notes the "highest level of adaptive functioning" during the preceding year, once again *contextualizing* the behavior both longitudinally and situationally. Suggested areas to explore for such an assessment are social relations, occupational behavior, and use of leisure time.

Obviously the *content* areas of both Axes IV and V cited as examples in DSM-III must be used in only a suggestive and not delimiting sense when one is dealing with a person from a different cultural background. And, while use of both of these axes is suggested as optional for clinicians — and apparently is not really catching on; old thought ways die hard (Perspectives 1983: 8) — their importance in research into the culture-bound syndromes cannot be over-stressed. Indeed, it may be asserted (with Murphy 1977) that they are of such significance that their use should be mandated for understanding the non-"culture-bound" syndromes as well.

As noted earlier, use of DSM-III results not in a single "diagnosis", but rather in a *profile* structured by judgements made on these five axes. What does such a "profile" look like? An example of such a "multi-axial examination" shows the range of information summarized for characterizing a person and his problem (DSM-III: 30):

Axis I: 296.23 Major Depression, Single Episode, with Melancholia
          303.93 Alcohol Dependence, In Remission
Axis II: 301.60 Dependent Personality Disorder (Provisional, rule out Borderline Personality Disorder)
Axis III: Alcoholic cirrhosis of liver
Axis IV: Psychosocial stressors: anticipated retirement and change in residence with loss of contact with friends
          Severity: 4 — Moderate
Axis V: Highest level of adaptive functioning past year: 3 — Good

The utility of such a composite profile for getting, at one glance, a better grasp on a person's problems and life situation is quite apparent. And in a comment that has obvious implications for use of a multiaxial format in the study of the culture-bound syndromes, Mezzich notes:

The structural innovation in psychiatric diagnosis represented by the multiaxial model has opened the door to the proposal of new clinical aspects or axes as additions to, or modifications of, those formulated above, keeping in mind issues of manageability of number of axes and need for axial evaluations .... Examples of such other axes are 'family relationships' ... and 'interaction with other individuals and groups' (which together with 'work functioning' and 'functioning in family' attempt to cover the social functioning area) .... (Mezzich 1979: 129)

Let us look at an instance of a 'culture-bound' syndrome and hold it against the DSM-III scheme to test for possible fit. A case report of such a syndrome found among the Greenland Eskimos, *kayak angst*, will be used. (This syndrome, incidentally, well illustrates the dangers of literalness in the interpretation of such terms as "culture-specific". In a strict sense, *kayak angst* could be found only among the Eskimos, for only they, among all the world's peoples, traditionally used kayaks! So the analytic question becomes: at a higher level of abstraction, are the essential features of this pattern of behavior found in other cultural situations also?)

The case report is from a large series of such reports brought together by Gussow (1970: 243):

Malachias L., Sukkertoppen, 47 years old, slight mixed descent. Has a number of relatives who are kayak-dizzy; a mother's brother's son, a father's brother's son and his own son. He used to be a clever catcher and kayak-rower until his condition started about 10 years ago. One October while out hunting he felt his legs getting cold and he thought he heard water forcing its way into the kayak. He checked and found the kayak dry. He nevertheless rowed to shore for fear that water was coming in and he would sink. On shore he was surprised to find the kayak dry. He went out again and felt better this time. A couple of days later he was out one morning in completely quiet weather. He was close to land and was about to turn a peninsula when suddenly he felt blood rushing to his head and he became nervous and started to sweat. He also developed a strong pain in his neck and he wondered what was happening. He had never thought of the possibility that he should become kayak-dizzy. He felt stiff all over and could not raise the oar which seemed extremely heavy. He did not feel that he would tip over, however. The kayak had become too heavy to row. He called for help and when his companion arrived he put his oar over the other kayak which kept the two boats together while the other man rowed both of them forward. After a while he felt better and when he could row again he went and stayed out for the rest of the day. Within the year he got a similar attack when the wind started to blow up and he became frightened to the point of stiffening up completely. About three years ago he found a catcher floating around drowned in his kayak. For several months after that he got an attack every time he went out. Now he has attacks as often as once a week and especially in storms and when there is a following sea. He also gets attacks easily in stormy weather when there are other kayaks around for he is afraid they will collide. When the weather is quiet, however, he prefers to be close to others. Now and then he is able to fight attacks off by refusing to let them affect him. He cannot upright himself if he tips over. He was pushed over by another once but was helped up immediately. He may suddenly and un-expectedly stiffen while in the mountains but he doesn't black out nor do his eyes flutter. He is a very ill-tempered person and now and then brutish. He appears anxious. Examination shows no abnormalities. His use of tobacco or coffee has never been excessive.

In DSM-III format, this might appear as follows:

Axis I: 300.01 Panic Disorder
             (The "... essential features are recurrent panic (anxiety) attacks that occur at times unpredictably, though certain situations, e.g., driving a car [or paddling a kayak?], may become associated with a panic attack .... The panic attacks are manifested by the sudden onset of intense apprehension, fear, or terror, often associated with feelings of impending doom. The most common symptoms experienced during an attack are dyspnea; palpitations; chest pain or discomfort; choking or smothering sensations; dizziness, vertigo, or unsteady feelings; feelings of unreality (depersonalization or derealization); paresthesias; hot and cold flashes; sweating; faintness; trembling or shaking; and fear of dying, going crazy, or doing something uncontrolled during the attack. Attacks usually last minutes; more rarely, hours .... The individual often develops varying degrees of nervous-ness and apprehension between attacks. This nervousness and apprehension is characterized by the usual manifestations of apprehensive expectation, vigilance and scanning, motor disorder may be limited to a single brief period lasting several weeks or months, recur several weeks or months, recur several times, or become chronic. (p. 230) [1]

One might also want to add another diagnostic dimension to this behavior pattern: 300.29 Simple Phobia

             (The "... essential feature is a persistent, irrational fear of, and compelling desire to avoid, an object or a situation other than being alone or in public places away from home ... or of humiliation or embarrassment in certain social situa-tions .... This disturbance is a significant source of distress, and the individual recognizes that his or her fear is excessive or unreasonable. The disturbance is not due to another mental disorder . . . . When suddenly exposed to the phobic stimulus, the individual becomes overwhelmingly fearful and may experience symptoms identical with those of a panic attack . . . . (pp. 228–229)[1]

Axis II: No diagnosis on Axis II

Axis III: Physical examination negative

Axis IV: Psychosocial stressors: No information

             Severity: O – Unspecified

Axis V: Highest level of adaptive functioning past year:

             5 – Poor ("Marked impairment in either social relations or occupational functioning . . ." (p. 29), an evaluation based on data in the case report – "Now he has attacks as often as once a week and especially in storms and when there is a following sea.")

Instances in which a person believes himself the victim of the witchcraft or sorcery (behavior often put in the "culture-bound" category) provide key illustrations of the classificatory problem with regard to these symptoms. Are such people merely playing a socially-appropriate role in a culturally-prescribed scenario, or are they mentally ill? A case reported from the Australian aborigines illustrates the issue (Reser and Eastwell 1981: 306):

Ng was a 19-year-old youth living in a small community deep in the bush. He was escorted to the hospital in an agitated tremulous state. He had the firm conviction that he was soon to die as the result of sorcery from a tribal elder. Noises outside the ward were misinterpreted as evidence of the sorcerer waiting to kill him; he was vigilant and pacing through the night. A classificatory brother who travelled with the patient explained his clansman's concern. He recounted how Ng had suddenly broken off relations with a young woman forbidden to him by tribal law, being convinced that her tribal elders knew about his affair and that punishment would ensue. In precontact times, 30 years ago, the punishment was death by the metal-tipped spear; today, sorcery takes its place. The brother implied that sorcery emanated from the tribal elder whose duty it was to properly bestow the girl, a message already suspected by the patient but now reinforced by his own clansman. Despite the severity of the presenting symptoms, the patient recovered in 2 weeks' treatment with chlorpromazine. Thereafter, he was discharged to relatives who lived some distance from his usual home.

Is the patient being delusional with regard to witchcraft? One possibility, perhaps, the resolution of which is not a simple matter even in a society which supports such beliefs; it depends upon the psychodynamic function of such a belief (cf. Ludwig 1965: 290–291; A. Leighton et al. 1963: 147–148). Once again, perhaps the better diagnostic label for the behavior of this patient is "Panic Disorder" (300.01). The authors themselves, however, citing as the basis for their evaluation the *local cultural meaning* of the entire set of behavioral episodes, would not necessarily rush to such "psychiatric" judgment:

The recurrent nature and characteristic features of the presenting symptoms suggest a culturally institutionalized syndrome. There is a clear consensus within the Aboriginal community as to the nature and identifying characteristics of this "disorder". Such diagnosis appears to be a carefully and culturally scripted role enactment on the part of victim and extended group, in which expected symptoms are enacted and labeled. The behaviors associated with the syndrome reported are neither over-reactions or unwarranted. There is complete consensus on

the gravity of the situation for the victim, and the legitimate nature of his fears, which helps
to validate the contextual definition and labels associated with sorcery. This raises questions
as to the "psychotic" nature of the illness, because premises are in accord with the "assumptive
world" of this society. Diagnosis by the Aboriginal community therefore is in terms of social
conflict with another clan, not individual illness, and the treatment orientation is in terms of
a victim rather than a patient.

The point they make raises one of the most significant issues with respect to
analysis of the culture-bound syndromes, for one might want to take exception
to such a strong statement of "cultural relativism". Was there no hint, no semblance
of *dysfunctional* behavior in the victim's actions? Did the victim himself not feel,
at some level, a sense of "dys-ease" even though he was performing in accordance
with the group's expectations?

Even granting the power of the word to create the "thing", one still may ask
whether labels for mental illness are *merely* labels? To say, as does Szasz, that
mental "illness" is a myth, an artifact of the words used to label it, indicates
either confusion over the adequacy of the model of illness being used (i.e., the
reductionistic biomedical model), or confusion over the basic semantic function of
words. After all, application of a symbolic label to an event does not expunge
that event itself, does not render the sensate qualities null and void; and if there
be pathology or dysfunction at any level — including the psychological — then one
can surely use the term "illness" or a cognate such as "disorder".

But, returning to the victim in the case above, let us assume, with the authors,
that he was not really "sick", but was merely fulfilling social expectations. In
this respect it may be time to raise for further consideration the question whether
some instances of culture-bound syndromes may be comparable to the disease
hypertension, for example, in that it is clear there are no symptoms of the "disease" apparent — the person feels "fine" — although other types of data and
techniques might allow such a diagnosis. However, in the above culture-bound
syndrome the victim apparently does feel a certain level of dysfunction and discomfort (is quite anxious — "tremulous" — at least) even though he may define
his behavior to himself, as it is defined by others, as "quite normal" under the
circumstances.

Perhaps DSM-III can accommodate this behavioral episode by coding it as
some form of situational reaction to extreme stress. But if that is done then the
further question arises whether this could be carried too far? Would there be
any behavior that could escape the net of DSM-III, for most people are at least
occasionally subject to such transient "situational" responses that go beyond the
"normal", the mean, the rational? In this respect some might argue that systematic
use of DSM-III (which has its share of critics even in the sphere for which it was
intended; see Millon 1983; Smith and Kraft 1983) could lead to this being another
instance of an Illichian "medicalization" of all behavioral phenomena. Perhaps
not, however, since with use of the multiaxial system, Axis V (judgment concerning the highest level of adjustment during the preceding year) places the person
and his behavior in a longitudinal perspective and underscores (if that indeed is

the case) the transiency of the particular behavior. The DSM-III format thus seems to provide something of a system of checks and balances against the possible hegemony of any single evaluative dimension.

Furthermore, the DSM-III emphasizes the fluid, continuous, and at times evanescent nature of the boundary between "disorder" and well being: ". . . there is no assumption that each mental disorder is a discrete entity with sharp boundaries (discontinuity) between it and other mental disorders, as well as between it and No Mental Disorder" (p. 6). Such a conceptualization can greatly help resolve the issue of whether the culture-bound syndromes should "really" be classed as "diseases" in the ontologic sense, or as something short of that concept. If, indeed, one sees the disorders as entities not fixed in nature and in the personality, but rather as existing on a continuum (e.g., Menninger 1963) and being influenced in their emergence by both sociocultural, psychological, and biological factors, then perhaps the way is opened for charting their occurrence with greater precision.

Based upon this brief application of the DSM-III concepts to some instances of "culture-bound" phenomena, it would therefore seem promising that use of a multi-dimensional scheme may provide the basis for more informed judgement regarding the ontological status and (eventually) etiology of the culture-bound syndromes. It must quickly be added, of course, that this can occur with use of this scheme, or any other classificatory scheme, only insofar as its categories are appropriately operationalized in terms of the specific sociocultural world in which the person lives, no matter whether that be the world of the Australian Aborigine or the modern Condo-ite.

A culturally-informed use of the DSM-III categories means not only knowing the culture of the person being evaluated in sufficient detail to make a valid behavioral assessment, and not only resisting taking the values and meanings of one's own culture (and social class) for granted when dealing with a patient. It also means recognizing the implicit values and assumptions upon which the diagnostic categorical scheme itself is based and remaining always skeptical, testing for fit against the data observed. In this respect, perhaps, the "culture-bound syndromes" can serve their most significant role by presenting a stern challenge to DSM-III's potential for transcending cultural parochialism. It should be stressed, of course, that this can happen only if one looks at the primary behavioral data, at cases or instances of the purported disorder, and not simply at generalized descriptions of a given syndrome for evaluation in terms of the DSM-III categories. To "diagnose" an already abstract syndrome by use of another abstracted diagnostic construct is to compound the confusion. For this reason, in my commentaries that follow each section, I will attempt to focus on actual behavioral materials included and not on the authors' theoretical and analytic formulations, although the former data are usually not adequate for a complete evaluation in this respect. Perhaps that will change in the future.

REFERENCES

American Psychiatric Association
    1980 Diagnostic and Statistical Manual of Mental Disorders. Third Edition. Washington,
          D.C.: American Psychiatric Association.
Arieti, Silvano and Johannes M. Meth
    1959 Rare, Unclassifiable, Collective, and Exotic Psychotic Syndromes. *In* Silvano Arieti
          (ed.), American Handbook of Psychiatry, Vol. I. New York: Basic Books, Inc.,
          pp. 546–563.
Cantor, Nancy, Edward E. Smith, Rita deSales French, and Juan Mezzich
    1980 Psychiatric Diagnosis as Prototype Categorization. Journal of Abnormal Psychology
          89: 181–193.
Collis, Robert J. M.
    1966 Physical Health and Psychiatric Disorder in Nigeria. Transactions of the American
          Philosophical Society, New Series, 56 (4): 1–45.
Devereux, George
    1956 Normal and Abnormal: The Key Problem of Psychiatric Anthropology. *In* J. B.
          Casagrande and Thomas Gladwin (eds.), Some Uses of Anthropology: Theoretical
          and Applied. Washington: Anthropological Society of Washington, pp. 3–48.
Edgerton, Robert B.
    1969 On the "Recognition" of Mental Illness. *In* S. Plog and R. B. Edgerton (eds.), Chang-
          ing Perspectives in Mental Illness. New York: Holt, Rinehart and Winston, pp. 49–
          72.
Engelhardt, H. Tristram, Jr.
    1975 The Concepts of Health and Disease. *In* H. Tristram Engelhardt, Jr., and Stuart F.
          Spicker (eds.), Evaluation and Explanation in the Biomedical Sciences. Dordrecht:
          D. Reidel Publishing Co., pp. 125–141.
Faergeman, P.
    1963 Psychogenic Psychoses. London: Butterworth.
Gajdusek, D. Carleton
    1977 Unconventional Viruses and the Origin and Disappearance of Kuru. Science 197:
          943–960.
Gussow, Zachary
    1970 Some Responses of West Greenland Eskimo to a Naturalistic Situation of Perceptual
          Deprivation: with an appendix of 60 case histories collected by Dr. Alfred Bertelsen
          in 1902–1903. INTER-NORD: International Journal of Arctic and Nordic Studies,
          December 1970 (11): 227–262.
Jewell, Donald P.
    1952 A Case of a "Psychotic" Navaho Indian Male. Human Organization 11: 32–36.
Kaplan, Marcie
    1983 A Woman's View of DSM-III. American Psychologist, July: 786–803.
Kiev, Ari
    1966 Prescientific Psychiatry. *In* Silvano Arieti (ed.), American Handbook of Psychiatry,
          Vol. III. New York: Basic Books, pp. 165–179.
    1972 Transcultural Psychiatry. New York: The Free Press.
Langness, L. L.
    1967 Hysterical Psychosis: The Cross-Cultural Evidence. American Journal of Psychiatry,
          124: 143–152.
Leighton, Alexander H.
    1969 Cultural Relativity and the Identification of Psychiatric Disorders. *In* William Caudill
          and Tsung-yi Lin (eds.), Mental Health Research in Asia and the Pacific. Honolulu:
          East-West Center Press, pp. 448–462.

Leighton, Alexander H., T. Adeoye Lambo, Charles C. Hughes, Dorothea C. Leighton, Jane M. Murphy, and David B. Macklin
  1963 Psychiatric Disorder Among the Yoruba: A Report from the Cornell-Aro Mental Health Research Project in the Western Region, Nigeria. Ithaca: Cornell University Press.
Leighton, Dorothea C., John S. Harding, David B. Macklin, Allister M. Macmillan, and Alexander H. Leighton
  1963 The Character of Danger: Psychiatric Symptoms in Selected Communities, Vol. III. The Stirling County Study of Psychiatric Disorder and Sociocultural Environment. New York: Basic Books Inc.
Lewis, Thomas H.
  1975 A Syndrome of Depression and Mutism in the Oglala Sioux. American Journal of Psychiatry 132: 753–755.
Lin, Keh-Ming
  1983a Hwa-byung: A Korean Culture-Bound Syndrome? American Journal of Psychiatry 140 (1): 105–107.
  1983b Letter. American Journal of Psychiatry 140 (1): 1268–1269.
Ludwig, Arnold M.
  1965 Witchcraft Today. Diseases of the Nervous System 26: 288–291.
Mayr, Ernst
  1963 Animal Species and Evolution. Cambridge: The Belknap Press of Harvard University Press.
Menninger, Karl
  1963 The Vital Balance: The Life Process in Mental Health and Illness. New York: Viking Press.
Mezzich, Juan E.
  1979 Patterns and Issues in Multiaxial Psychiatric Diagnosis. Psychological Medicine 9: 125–137.
Millon, Theodore
  1983 The DSM-III: An Insider's Perspective. American Psychologist July: 804–814.
Murphy, H. B. M.
  1977 Transcultural Psychiatry Should Begin At Home. Psychological Medicine 7: 369–371.
Perspectives . . .
  1983 Perspectives on the VII World Congress of Psychiatry, Vienna, 1983. Vol. I, National Schools and World Psychiatry. Philadelphia: Wyeth Laboratories.
Raven, Peter H., Brent Berlin, and Dennis E. Breedlove
  1971 The Origins of Taxonomy. Science 174: 1201–1213.
Reser, Joseph P. and Harry D. Eastwell
  1981 Labeling and Cultural Expectations: the Shaping of a Sorcery Syndrome in Aboriginal Australia. The Journal of Nervous and Mental Disease 169: 303–310.
Rubel, Arthur J.
  1964 The Epidemiology of a Folk Illness: Susto in Hispanic America Ethnology 3: 268–283.
Smith, Darrell and William A. Kraft
  1983 DSM-III: Do Psychologists Really Want an Alternative? American Psychologist 38: 777–785.
Spitzer, Robert L., Jean Endicott, and Eli Robins
  1978 Research Diagnostic Criteria: Rationale and Reliability. Archives of General Psychiatry 35: 773–782.
Spitzer, Robert L., Janet B. W. Williams, and Andrew E. Skodol (eds.)
  1983 International Perspectives on DSM-III. Washington, D.C.: American Psychiatric Press, Inc.

Stengel, E.
   1959 Classification of Mental Disorders. Bulletin of the World Health Organization 21:
          601–663.
Strauss, John S.
   1973 Diagnostic Models and the Nature of Psychiatric Disorder. Archives of General
          Psychiatry 29: 445–449.
   1975 A Comprehensive Approach to Psychiatric Diagnosis. American Journal of Psychiatry
          132: 193–197.
Temkin, Owsei
   1963 The Scientific Approach to Disease: Specific Entity and Individual Sickness. In A. C.
          Crombie (ed.), Scientific Change: Historical Studies in the Intellectual, Social, and
          Technical Conditions for Scientific Discovery and Technical Invention, From An-
          tiquity to the Present, New York: Basic Books, Inc., pp. 629–658.
Lin, Tsung-Yi
   1982 Culture and Psychiatry: A Chinese Perspective. Australian and New Zealand Journal
          of Psychiatry 16: 235–245.
Whitehead, Alfred North
   1949 The Aims of Education and Other Essays. New York: Mentor Books.
Wig, Narendra N.
   1983 DSM-III: A Perspective from the Third World. In Robert L. Spitzer, Janet B. W.
          Williams, and Andrew E. Skodol (eds.), International Perspectives on DSM-III:
          Diagnostic and Statistical Manual of Mental Disorders, Third Edition. Washington,
          C.D.: American Psychiatric Press, Inc., pp. 79–89.
Wittkower, Eric D. and Raymond Prince
   1974 A Review of Transcultural Psychiatry. In Silvano Arieti (ed.), American Handbook
          of Psychiatry, 2nd edition. New York: Basic Books, Inc., pp. 535–550.
Yap, Pow Meng
   1951 Mental Diseases Peculiar to Certain Cultures: A Survey of Comparative Psychiatry.
          Journal of Mental Science 97: 313–327.
   1969 The Culture-Bound Reactive Syndromes. In William Caudill and Tsung-Yi Lin (eds.),
          Mental Health Research in Asia and the Pacific. Honolulu: East-West Center Press,
          pp. 33–53.
   1974 Comparative Psychiatry: A Theoretical Framework. M. P. Lau and A. B. Stokes
          (eds.). Toronto: University of Toronto Press.

RONALD C. SIMONS

SORTING THE CULTURE-BOUND SYNDROMES

> Confucius said, "if you look at them from the
> point of view of their differences, then there
> is liver and gall, *Ch'u* and *Yüeh*. But if you look
> at them from the point of view of their same-
> ness, then the ten thousand things are all one."
> − (*Chuang Tzu* 1969: 65)

INTRODUCTION

The present volume contains papers which describe certain of the phenomena
usually classified as "culture-bound psychiatric syndromes", or as "culture-bound
syndromes" with "psychiatric" understood. Both terms have long been used to
refer to sets of remarkable individual experiences and/or behaviors which some
observer has considered to be psychopathological, hence the medical rubic,
"syndrome". Unlike the categories of standard Western psychiatric nosology,
culture-bound syndromes are restricted to specifiable peoples and locales, hence the
term "culture-bound". Thus their full explications require description not only
of the behaviors and experiences which are considered deviant, but also of the
ways those behaviors and experiences are embedded in specific social systems and
cultural contexts.

The category, culture-bound syndrome, is intrinsically ethnocentric, since the
phenomena it lumps together have in common only the fact that they occur some-
place other than Western cosmopolitan society and the fact that they are culturally
elaborated. With increasing recognition that culture-specific factors shape all
afflictions (e.g., Fabrega 1968; Kleinman 1980), the distinction between culture-
bound syndromes and other forms of alleged psychological deviance has blurred.
Rittenbaugh (1982), for example, has recently proposed American obesity as a
culture-bound syndrome. Other Western culture-bound syndromes could readily
be suggested. One example is what might be termed "petism" (Simons 1981).
One regularly reads newspaper accounts of isolated elderly Americans and Britons
who live surrounded by great menageries of dogs and cats. They usually come
to public attention when a neighbor complains about noise, odor, or animal neglect.
The accounts contain a limited number of fairly predictable elements, which I
will not list here. Would not a non-Western nosologist be justified in classifying
obesity (or at least the form of it described by Rittenbaugh) and petism as culture-
bound syndromes? Thus as currently used, the category "culture-bound syndromes"
seems not only ethnocentric, but indefinitely expansible. For these and other
reasons several recent papers have suggested doing away with a term which has
always been at best a residual category (e.g., Hahn in press).

25

Ronald C. Simons and Charles C. Hughes (eds.), The Culture-Bound Syndromes, 25–38.
© *1985 by D. Reidel Publishing Company.*

Manschreck and Petri (1978) included culture-bound syndromes in the category, "Atypical Psychoses", but the culture-bound syndromes are not all psychoses, and "atypical" defines by exclusion; it specifies only what the culture-bound syndromes are not. Favazza (1985) has suggested 'Syndromes Not Seen in Western Culture' , which is clear and straighforward. However, this too is a definition by exclusion, and it rules out of consideration syndromes which are usually considered culture-bound even though they occur in societies which participate in Western culture, e.g. *Jumping*, described in a population of French Canadian descent living in Maine. And neither of these suggestions retains an idea usually considered central to the concept of culture-bound syndromes, the idea that each of these syndromes is to be found only in a specific cultural context.

"Folk illness" is a general and inclusive term used to designate any indigenously perceived illness entity. The culture-bound syndromes are those folk illnesses which include alterations of behavior and of experience prominently among their symptomatology. As the altered experience and behavior of individuals constitutes the claimed field of expertise of psychiatry, a considerable psychiatric literature has grown up about them. Because the constellations of signs and symptoms which constitute the syndromes exist as coherent phenomena by virtue of their indigenous categorization and naming, anthropologists likewise see the culture-bound syndromes as lying within their field of expertise. Clearly it is necessary to understand the nature and operations of culture to understand them. Thus explanatory schemata tend to be polarized into biomedical and anthropological formulations, with the vast bulk of recent literature by both anthropological and medical workers squarely in the latter camp.

Most of the formulations which have been proposed in recent years to explain either single culture-bound syndromes or the category collectively treat the biology of the subject, including his or her neurophysiology, as an undifferentiated ground against which the interplay of psychological, social and cultural factors shape altered experiences and altered behavior. However I believe that in at least some of the syndromes the effects of psychological, social, and cultural factors are mingled with the effects of biological factors in an intricate way. Further, I believe that explications of this mingling are the most revealing and hence the most useful way in which many culture-bound syndromes can be considered. Difficulties in conceptualizing how this may be done when analyzing specific syndromes account in part for the polarization into discipline-centered camps. I believe that this polarization is both unfortunate and unnecessary. It is possible, and I believe in some instances necessary, to consider factors in many disciplines simultaneously.

NATURE AND NURTURE

Most of the papers in the anthropological literature, both classic and recent, consider each culture-bound syndrome to be fully explained by the system of meanings prevalent in the locale where the syndrome is endemic. John Carr has written one of the best argued and most persuasive expositions of this position. Carr argues reasonably that since *amok* is a fully elaborated cultural complex in Malaysia and Indonesia, it can be understood only in the context of the cultures of those societies.

We are now able to return to the concept of the culture-bound syndrome and reconsider its definition in light of our examination of the amok phenomenon. I have demonstrated the important role played by implicit values, belief systems, and social structure in determining the manifest behavior of amok, and to this extent I must concur with Yap's definition (1969). However, I take issue with the position that the behaviors upon which culture exercises so pervasive an influence are only superficial and underneath this facade is the 'real disease', the basic form of which is inviolate and universal in nature. I find no support in the case for amok for this assumption. Further, I would argue that such a definition is nondiscriminating since the case has been made that for every instance of sickness, the illness behavior, as distinct from the disease process, is always culturally determined (Kleinman et al. 1978) (Carr 1978 and this volume).

However, the position alternative to Carr need not be that cultural factors are a "superficial" gloss of a "real disease". Terms like "superficial" and "real" are value laden and obscure rather than clarify the issues. And further, the instrinsic indefiniteness of the concept, "disease", especially as applied to behavioral events (Fabrega 1968) and the current lack of consensus about the way it can most usefully be defined (Hahn and Kleinman 1983) make arguments about whether or not any syndrome is a *bona fide* disease worse than futile. The question, rather, is whether specifiable biological factors must be included to explain an observed behavior, and this is a question which cannot be resolved by deduction; empirical investigation is necessary. I believe that although it is useless to debate whether or not any syndrome is a "real disease", it is extremely useful to ask what in each syndrome the specific contribution of biology, culture and individual psychology may be. In this essay, I wish to discuss this question and to suggest that confusion about the roles of biology and experience has been a major impediment to progress in the study of the culture-bound syndromes.

Though any given culture-bound syndrome is profoundly shaped by the social and cultural realities of the society in which it is found, no amount of description of that shaping disproves the relevance of biology in the shaping of the same syndrome. One can not meaningfully argue that *latah* or *amok* is shaped principally by biological or by experiential factors. Always the problem is to explicate how the observed behavior is shaped by experience and how by biology. What aspects of *latah* and *amok* are shaped in what manner by what aspects of the material and social environment; what aspects are shaped in what manner by what aspects of the subject's biology?

Assertions of cause are always problematic, in part because of the reasons cited above; in part because of metaphysical problems which can never be satisfactorily resolved. Even more than economics, epistemology is a dismal science. Therefore throughout this essay I have used the term "shaped" rather than the term "caused". By "shaping" I mean influencing the specifics of expression. Both the physiology of hunger and culture-specific food preferences shape the specifics of meal taking.

Many influences may shape an observed behavior; the term does not suggest primacy, as does the term "cause".

I disagree explicitly with the approach which holds that culture is, by logical necessity, the sole (or the only interesting) cause or shaper of all culture-bound syndromes (e.g., Kenny 1978 and this volume). In that approach, a hierarchy of disciplines is envisaged, each providing an undifferentiated ground for those above it. Though advocates of that approach usually concede that whatever else they may be, human beings are also corporeal, they allow human corporeality only arbitrary and abstract properties, such as "needs" for food and sexual expression.[2] In contrast, I believe that highly individual and changing aspects of biology greatly influence every person's experience of his or her material and social environments and hence the culture-specific concepts which seek to make sense of that experience. Since humans are not disembodied spirits, both behavioral and conceptual consequences must flow from the specifics of their bodies. And human bodies are not all alike. They differ in ways which profoundly affect how their owners experience existence. Further, each single body exists in many physiological states, which change over minutes, days, months, and decades. My experience of the world varies, reflecting states of my body: whether I have had adequate sleep, whether the tooth that needs the root-canal is quiescent or excruciating, with my age. These changing states markedly influence my social exchanges with others. Is this not true of everyone?

My own thinking about the roles of biology and experience in culture-bound syndromes was greatly clarified by a paper written in another context by the physiological psychologist Daniel Lehrman (1970). In this paper, which has become a classic, Lehrman contrasts his thinking with that of Konrad Lorenz. Lehrman makes two points: the first is interesting, though not unique to Lehrman; the second, a brilliant insight. First, he explains that biology and experience shape behavior simultaneously. Any instance of behavior is 100% determined by the biology of the behaving organism. Change its sensory or motor capacities or the intervening neural linkages between them and you change the resultant behavior. However the same instance of behavior is also 100% determined by the organism's experiential history. Change that history and the resultant behavior is likewise changed. Here is a human example: one never observes a human speaking a generic language. Rather one only hears John speaking English or Jacques speaking French. While it is meaningless to assert that John or Jacques' language behavior is shaped principally by his biology rather than by his linguistic experience, it is equally meaningless to assert that it is shaped principally by his linguistic experience rather than by his biology. Species-typical biology and a specifiable experiential history are both absolutely necessary for any person to speak any language. Neither is sufficient; neither is more important. Lehrman argues that it never makes sense to argue for the primacy of either nature or nurture in shaping *any single instance* of observed behavior.

Here is an example drawn from a culture-bound syndrome. *Old hag* is a syndrome from Newfoundland, described by Ness (1978 and in this volume) and by Hufford

(1982). A victim of *old hag* awakens terrified, unable to move and with a sensation of weight on his chest. This set of sensations has a specific neurophysiologic substrate and has been experienced by persons in many times and places. However it is only in Newfoundland that it is interpreted as the result of "being hagged". This culture-specific interpretation profoundly affects the way that the neurophysiologic event is experienced. One can suffer from *old hag* only if a certain neurophysiologic event occurs and only if one is a member of a society which shares belief in *old hag*. Thus to explain *old hag* one must describe both biological and cultural shaping factors.

Lehrman's second point is that the relative contributions of biology and experience *can* be parceled out *when accounting for a difference between two instances*. Considered with his first point, it immediately suggests avenues for potentially fruitful empirical research. One *can* meaningfully ask whether experience or biology accounts for the *difference* between the language behavior of John and Jaques. One can also meaningfully ask the same question if either begins to stutter or ceases to speak. Lehrman's formulation is that *biology and experience are always equally important in shaping any single instance of behavior but that differences between two instances may be attributable to one or the other*.

Though the forum in which this formulation was developed was the discipline of comparative (animal) psychology, the logic of the argument is equally compelling in the present context. For example, any given episode of *latah* is simultaneously shaped by biology and by experience. However, it is reasonable to ask if a *latah* person differs in experience or in biology from her non-*latah* neighbor. Similarly one may ask if she differs in biology or in experience from a (non-*latah*) American who has an excessively strong startle reaction. And the answers to these two questions are different!

The approach advocated here is problem-centered rather than discipline-centered. Too often discipline-centered approaches have included subtle and sometimes not so subtle attempts to restrict relevancies to Those in which I am Certified Expert (or, more charitably, to Those I Am Competent to Discuss). In reality, relevant data may lie within many disciplines. And these data can seldom be organized hierarchically. Every set of human behaviors exists in a complex matrix of biological, social, psychological, and cultural facts which shape each other. How any portion of this set of facts shapes specific aspects of behavior or experience is a matter which must be discovered empirically, and an accurate analogy is not a layer cake but a marble cake.[3] Since the phenomena called culture-bound syndromes are very disparate, no single causal outline will fit all cases once appropriate data are filled in.

Though the literature explicating the culture-specific meanings of individual syndromes is voluminous, descriptions of the actual behaviors which constitute them are often surprisingly sketchy and tend to focus on features which are highly salient, highly culturally meaningful, or "storyable". What is needed is first a clear separation of accounts of meaning from accounts of behavior. Accounts of behavior should contain detailed description of stimulus side and response side event[4], including what I have referred to as "microdetail" (Simons 1981). Microdetail is the fine detail of the experience or behavior which is to be explained. The voluminous literature on culture-bound syndromes contains astonishingly little detail describing the actual events being explained (Tseng and McDermott 1981: 53). Instead, one finds exhaustive description of cultural context, especially of the culture-specific interpretation of the phenomenon and of culture-specific curative or reparative procedures. Behavioral details are frequently compressed into a few general categories. For example, in explaining the unusual verbal productions of startled *latahs*, Murphy (e.g., 1983) compresses these into the category *coprolalia*, which he then explains as resulting from repressed sexual wishes. However, as I argued in response to Murphy (Simons 1983b: 181), if one records, transcribes, and studies what *latahs* actually say when in *latah* states, it is clear that the simple concept, *coprolalia*, does not adequately encompass it. What they say makes a very interesting list, which includes repetitions of the last word or phrase just uttered by the *latah* or in the *latah*'s hearing, "nonsense" of certain types, deity references, and the names of objects in their immediate visual fields, especially striking or prominent one. If a taboo word is blurted out, it is always the first word after the startling stimulus. It is only when actual *latah* verbalizations are recorded, sorted, and analyzed that one can see that the single general category *coprolalia* fails as an adequate descriptor and that therefore formulations which do not explain the frequent alternatives are necessarily faulty. I believe that *what* happens must be specified in considerable detail before one can come to any valid conclusion as to *why* it happens.

My own work on *latah* has been criticized on many grounds, e.g.: biological reductionism (Kenny 1983 and this volume), insufficient attention to dreams (Murphy 1983), no life histories (Tseng, personal communication), and insufficient description of the cultural setting (Winzeler, in press). However, no one has yet complained about what I see as the work's most significant deficiency: insufficient description of the fine details of *latah* episodes. Though these are shown in the *latah* film (Simons 1983c), I have as yet not provided detailed descriptions of *latah* behavior in print. *Latah* episodes, like episodes of other culture-bound syndromes, vary considerably from one to another. Attention to microdetail counters the tendency to reify syndromes — it is always a variable spectrum of experiences and behaviors which must be explained. I advocate a perspective that includes careful attention to the minutiae of the behavior actually observed and which accepts as adequate explanation only formulations which account for those minute particulars. Microdetail, as in the case of the disturbed speech of *latahs*, often rules out otherwise tenable hypotheses.

Because of the difficulty in seeing, much less capturing with verbal description, an adequately detailed behavioral record, film and video recording is especially desirable. Often repeated study of a filmed record may reveal important regularities which are brief, inconspicuous, or less likely to attract an observer's attention than more dramatic concurrent events. These regularities also need explanation and may be especially revealing about the nature of underlying shaping mechanisms.

Very little work of this sort has so far been done, in part because of practical problems in obtaining the records.[5] There are even fewer data about potentially significant physiologic changes occurring during episodes of culture-bound syndromes.[6] Far from being a dead end, the study of culture-bound syndromes is in its infancy.

The perspective taken in this essay and used in organizing this volume cannot legitimately be dismissed as "reductionistic", "behavioristic", or even "biological". It cannot be equated with searches for underlying diseases, nor is it a form of Sociobiology. It is an approach which I generally refer to as "ethological"[7]. This perspective is avowedly non-Durkheimian; in it "culture" is a useful analytic level, not a system operating with functional independence in the world. The purely intra-cultural study of any type of aberrant behavior is the only means for discovering how that behavior fits into the web of understanding that constitutes the meaning of the ongoing social life of a given society. However, meanings are not the only relevant data. I believe that the purely cultural perspective, though logically impeccable, "solves" some of the most interesting problems of the culture-bound syndromes by ruling them irrelevant.

Occasionally, for example, one reads an allegation that an instance of a culture-bound syndrome has been found in a place far removed from the area in which the syndrome is part of the social-cultural reality. Cases alleged to be *koro* have been reported from England (Barrett 1978), Israel (Hess and Nassi 1977), India (*India Today* 1982), and the United States (Edwards 1970). It is easy enough to define these cases as necessarily not-*koro*, since the victims patently do not share the belief system which is part of the Southeast Asian *koro* syndrome. However, the empirical question remains: have these geographically isolated cases been shaped significantly by any of the same factors responsible for the syndrome in Southeast Asia? How similar are the details of the experience? Do the cases share any hypothesized or demonstrated physiology in common? Someone arguing for a purely cultural perspective can, without difficulty, demonstrate no end of differences between Southeast Asian and geographically remote cases, since the experiences and behaviors of persons from differing cultural settings must differ in significant ways. However differences do not cancel similarities. If there are significant similarities, these too must be explained. Since phenomena are not different *or* similar, but rather different *and* similar, it is necessary to specify and explain both the similarities and the differences. The pattern of these similarities and differences may be especially revealing. In the case of the culture-bound syndromes the similarities will often be biological and the differences cultural. The more similar exemplars are in micro-detail, the more likely it is that they share common shaping influences (e.g., see Simons on *latah*, Ness on *old hag*, and Edwards on *koro* in this volume).

SORTING INTO TAXA

Although the meanings assigned to unusual experiences and behaviors vary markedly from site to site, salient features of those experiences and behaviors are sometimes surprisingly similar in historically unrelated and culturally dissimilar times and places. Thus as I reviewed the culture-bound syndrome literature it became increasingly apparent that many of the folk illnesses which had at one time or another been considered culture-bound syndromes could be sorted readily into phenomenologically similar sets. *Latah* and *imu*, for example, are defined by strikingly similar behaviors: someone is startled, after which he or she says things which are normally socially tabooed, talks in a manner locally considered nonsensical and amusing, matches the movements and words of others, and obeys or defies commands in an exaggerated and stereotyped way. In like manner *old hag* and *uqumairineq* are defined by constellations of strikingly similar experiences: awakening to find oneself terrified and unable to move or cry out. Clearly the behaviors of *latah* are descriptively like those of *imu* and the experiences which define *old hag* are like those which define *uqamairineq*. A logical listing of culture-bound syndromes would group such similar syndromes into sets, separating them from other parallel sets. I prepared such a listing and generated a number of such sets, which I have called "taxa" (singular: "taxon")[8].

The term "taxon", borrowed from biology, denotes a grouping based on similarity without specifying the level of abstraction of that similarity, and it suggests a less than final grouping. In the usage proposed in this essay and in this volume, local terms are retained to designate local culture-specific syndromes and an especially coined taxon name is used to designate the set collectively. Assigning to taxa names which differ from those of any of the constituent syndromes eliminates the ambiguity inherent in a suggestion I made previously to use the lower case to designate the culture-specific local syndromes and an upper case prominent exemplar to designate the taxon (e.g., *latah* and *Latah*, Simons 1980). Among other problems with the previous scheme, meaning is unclear when the term is the first word of a sentence. Thus in the usage proposed here *latah* and *imu* are included in a taxon called *Startle Matching* and *old hag* and *uqamairineq* in a taxon called *Sleep Paralysis*. As illustration of this classificatory plan, the present volume contains seven taxa: *Startle Matching, Sleep Paralysis, Genital Retraction, Sudden Mass Assault, Running, Fright Illness*, and *Cannibal Compulsion*[9]. The taxon name also serves as a rubric for aberrant instances not connected with culturally elaborated beliefs and practices. Thus in the usage proposed, the cases of *latah* in South Africa cited in *Latah II* (Simons 1983a and this volume) and the report of *koro* in an American schizophrenic patient (Edwards 1970 and this volume) would be called instead instances of the *Startle Matching* and *Genital Retraction* taxa respectively. This assignment, I believe, is conceptually useful. The question then changes from the insoluble one of whether or not these are instances of "real" *latah* and "real" *koro* to one of whether their resemblances to SE Asian *latah* and *koro* are significant or merely trivial and coincidental. The question becomes empirical, suggesting a search for correspondence in microdetail, rather than metaphysical and answerable only by definition.

When one uses a few highly salient behavioral or experiential features (often those which indigenously define the syndrome) to sort the culture-bound syndromes into groups, the members of some of the sets which one generates will sometimes be found to share many additional features as well. Often these are features logically unconnected with those on which the sorting was based. Here is an example: if the syndromes in which saying something vulgar and matching the behavior of others after being startled are sorted into a group it will be found that members of this group share an extraordinary number of other features, e.g., that stimuli in any modality will effectively elicit an episode so long as the subject is actually startled, that the nature of the episode will, however, be unaffected by the modality of the stimulus, that catching sight of a snake will be an effective elicitor, that automatic obedience will also be a response feature.

Why do so many small and specific features recur in so many culturally independent sites? Not only the individual culture-bound syndromes which are the constituent members of taxa but also the taxa themselves require explanation. To the extent that members of a taxon share small and specific elements the taxon can be considered a "natural" (i.e., non-arbitrary) grouping. The coincidence of features suggests that in addition to those already discovered, other as yet undiscovered features may also be shared, and it suggests searching for them. For example, because of the sizeable number of known features shared by all members of the *Startle Matching Taxon*, I wonder if in addition subjects with *latah, imu, mali-mali* (etc.) also share a generalized difficulty in habituating to stimuli. This suggests testing *latahs, imus, mali-malis* (etc.) for this phenomenon. Such a finding would support the validity of the taxon as a non-arbitrary assemblage. Cross-cultural sorting suggests the hypothesis; empirical work at several culturally independent sites would be required to support or refute it.

A formulation which explains a taxon will inevitably raise doubt about formulations of any of its constituent syndromes which depend on factors not present in all of the sites where members of the taxon are found. It is this fact that makes me doubtful of formulations that locate the cause of matching and obedience after being startled in aspects of Malay child rearing (Murphy 1976) or in shamanistic practices (Ohnuki-Tierney 1980 and this volume). The fact that the *Startle Matching Taxon* is widespread and has many members suggests that one might better search for shaping causes that operate at a quite different level of abstraction.

In this regard I believe that it is often useful to make a distinction between features which account for a syndrome's descriptive features (its "shape") and those which account for its being endemic to one site and absent from another (its distribution). For example, in the case of *latah*, I believe that matching, obedience, and saying naughty words are determined in large part by physiological processes associated with strong and frequent startles. However I also believe that the presence of *latah* or some member of the *Startle Matching Taxon* throughout virtually all of SE Asia is the result of cultural factors having to do with the treatment of stigmatized others, the absence of a belief that playful startles can injure health (a belief widespread in Latin America and in Africa), etc. It is in explaining distribution that aspects of Malay child rearing or the shamanistic practices of the Ainu may indeed be relevant.

CONSEQUENCES

Rival explanatory formulations can be judged against each other on two grounds: validity and consequence. "Validity" refers to consistency with the most descriptive data and inconsistency with the least. A formulation cannot be valid if it is inconsistent with adequately established data. Dreams with sexual content, for example, cannot be responsible for the onset of *latah* if such dreams are prevalent in only one of the many areas in which *latah* is endemic and even there are denied by two-thirds of the subjects queried about them (Simons 1983b). However, independent of validity, explanatory formulations must also be weighed in terms of their consequences.

Though culture-bound syndromes are not always afflictions, they sometimes are. Some of the persons who perform the behaviors or undergo the experiences of culture-bound syndromes suffer, and sometimes they act in ways which bring suffering to others. Therefore, the syndromes cannot be adequately conceptualized as mere dramatizations, games, or ceremonies. Because the syndromes so often include suffering, explaining a syndrome is an action which has a moral dimension. What is the likely consequence? What will happen to whom if any proposed explanatory formulation becomes widespread or "official"?

It has sometimes been asserted (e.g., Kenny 1983 and this volume) that attending to biological factors in addition to sociocultural ones will inevitably lead to unfortunate consequences for persons suffering from culture-bound syndromes, consequences such as forced treatment or involuntary hospitalization. Like assertions of causality, assertions of consequence may be more or less valid. It is always reasonable to ask what evidence supports the contention that any proposed explanatory formulation will lead to such and such a consequence. Anthropological research has repeatedly demonstrated that it is not possible accurately to predict the effect of any innovation in behavior or thought from general principles. Rather it is always necessary to study local circumstances empirically.

The approach suggested in this essay and in this volume has, at least in some instances the potential for mitigating the suffering of those for whom culture-bound syndromes are afflictions. With due respect to the value of understanding non-Western conceptions of illness, illness groupings, and illness causation, the much maligned Western medical model, when properly applied, can also mitigate much suffering. Indigenous conceptions of illness causality may be ill-informed, and some illnesses indigenously attributed to a frightening experience years past may in fact respond to tetracycline (see Rubel 1984 and this volume). Respect for the perceptions and conceptualizations of others need not blind one to the potential life enhancing utility of Western medicine and empirical science.

Explanatory formulations also have political consequences; this has been true since the syndromes were first described. British colonial writers such as Clifford (1927) and Sweetenham (1895) explicitly and unashamedly cited culture-bound syndromes as evidence morally justifying British rule over less powerful peoples.

As Littlewood and Lipsedge (1982) persuasively argue, current interpretations though subtler, are often no less politically significant, since the behaviors which define the culture-bound behavioral syndromes are almost invariably disvalued ones when seen through Western eyes and not infrequently in the indigenous view as well. Further, since the performing subject steps out of the normal social (and sometimes moral) order, the syndromes are available as culturally legitimized forms of social protest. Thus, it is also necessary to consider the political consequences to real persons which are likely to flow from any formulation. However it is not self-evident *a priori* that reformulations of the culture-bound syndromes which include biomedical considerations will necessarily lead to inequity or oppression. Again, there is no single general answer; the question is always one of situation-specific consequences for real people. Accurate assessment of the likely consequences of any interpretation requires knowledge of specific biology and of local cultural, sociological, and political reality.

CONCLUSION

The argument about how best to formulate the culture-bound syndromes is an argument about the nature of humanity, and therefore not likely ever to be settled to everyone's satisfaction. In this volume I suggest that a distinction be made between the broad general category folk illness and that sub-set of folk illnesses which constitute the culture-bound psychiatric syndromes. I suggest an investigative approach which begins with as exhaustive a description as possible of the actual phenomenon which is being studied, using audiovisual records as a primary data source whenever it is feasible to do so. I suggest that factors which determine why a syndrome occurs in one place and not another are not necessarily the same factors as those which account for its descriptive features. I suggest that the occurrence of similar behavior complexes and experiential states in widely disparate cultural settings necessarily casts doubt on the adequacy of explanatory formulations tied to factors not present in all settings. I suggest that it is feasible and useful to sort the syndromes into sets based on gross descriptive resemblances, ignoring culture-specific meanings. I suggest that when this is done, some of the sets thus generated represent "natural" categories. I suggest that likely consequences of formulations which include biomedical considerations cannot be deduced from general principles, but rather can only be predicted from detailed study of locally specific circumstances. And lastly, I suggest that while it is morally necessary to consider the probable consequences of any proposed formulation, formulations which attend to biomedical or physiologic factors are no more likely to have unfortunate consequences than formulations which ignore them.

This volume contains only a sampling of the scores of entities which have at one time or another been considered culture-bound syndromes. If the concepts and the classification scheme proposed here prove useful, the task of sorting and classifying other culture-bound syndromes into parallel categories remains.

ACKNOWLEDGEMENTS

Much of the argument of this essay was developed in a series of papers presented between 1979 and 1983 at meetings of the Society for the Study of Psychiatry and Culture. I would like to thank Drs. Mary Lynn Buss, Armando Favazza, Robert Hahn, Charles Hughes, and Arthur Kleinman for their helpful comments on earlier drafts.

NOTES

1. I will have more to say about this example in the introduction to the sections devoted to the *Startle Matching Taxon*.
2. Clifford Geertz, for example, in his Distinguished Lecture to the American Anthropological Association at its 82nd annual meeting in 1983 said that he did not deny the relevance of biology, after all, "pigeons can't speak, and men cannot fly". Further than this, however, he was not prepared to go.
3. For non-Western or other readers who may not be familiar with this distinction, let me explain that a layer cake is made up of separate cakes stacked one on top of the other, whereas a marble cake is made of several differently flavored and colored batters swirled together before baking, so that when cut, the resultant cake looks like a slice of marble.
4. Paul Ekman and Wallace Friesen's work demonstrates the usefulness of this approach. They considerably advanced the cross-cultural study of facial expression by separating descriptions of stimulus side events from descriptions of response side events. Although they used terms specific to their research ("elicitors" and "display rules") the principle is a general one (see e.g., Ekman 1973).
5. An attempt by Dennis (1981 and this volume) to obtain videotape recordings of Grisi Siknis was not successful because of overwhelming logistical problems. However, even the still photographs he returned with were extremely useful.
6. The best known prior attempt, Foulks' study of *pibloctoc*, was inconclusive, though it did rule out one otherwise tenable physiologic hypothesis (1972 and this volume).
7. Ethological analyses of behavior investigate how a behavior develops in the life of an individual, what its immediate precipitants are, what effects it has on its performer's environment, and how it has changed from individual to individual over the course of time. When the subject species is *Homo sapiens*, meanings must be considered in answering all these questions.
8. James Edwards (personal communication) has independently used the same term to designate a grouping of semen loss syndromes from E. Asia.
9. I have the most faith in the ultimate utility of the taxon *Startle Matching* and least in the utility of the taxon "running".

REFERENCES

Barrett, K.
    1978 *Koro* in a Londoner. Lancet 2: 1319.
Carr, J. E.
    1978 Ethno-Behaviorism and the Culture-Bound Syndromes: The Case of *Amok*. Culture, Medicine and Psychiatry 2: 269–293. (Reprinted in this volume.)
Chuang Tzu
    1964 Basic Writings, transl. by Burton Watson. New York: Columbia.
Clifford, H.
    1927 The Further Side of Silence. New York: Doubleday.

Dennis, P. A.
1981 *Grisi Siknis* Among the Miskito: Medical Anthropology 5: 4: 5: 504.
Edwards, J. G.
1970 The *Koro* Pattern of Depersonalization in an American Schizophrenic Patient. American J. Psychiatry 126: 1171–1172. (Reprinted in this volume.)
Ekman, Paul
1973 Cross Cultural Studies of Facial Expression. *In* P. Ekman (ed.), Darwin and Facial Expression, New York: Academic Press.
Fabrega, H., J. D. Swartz, and C. A. Wallace
1968 Arch. Gen. Psychiat. 19: 218–255.
Favazza, A.
1985 Anthropology and Psychiatry. *In* H. I. Kaplan and B. Sadock (eds.), Comprehensive Textbook of Psychiatry (4th ed.). Baltimore: Williams and Wilkins.
Foulks, E.
1972 The Arctic Hysterias of the North Alaskan Eskimo. Washington: American Anthropological Association.
Friedman, C. T. H. and K. A. Faguet
1982 Extraordinary Disorders of Human Behavior. New York: Plenum.
Hahn, R. A.
In press Culture Bound Syndromes Unbound. Social Science and Medicine.
Hahn, R. A., and Kleinman, A.
1983 Biomedical Practice and Anthropological Theory. Ann. Rev. Anthropol 12: 305–33.
Hess, J. P. and G. Nassi
1977 *Koro* in a Yemenite and a Georgian Jewish Immigrant. Confinia Psychiatrica 20: 1980–184.
Hufford
1982 The Terror That Comes in the Night. Philadelphia: U. of Pennsylvania.
India Today
1982 *Koro*; Psychological Scare. October 15: 83.
Kenny, M. G.
1978 *Latah*: The Symbolism of a Putative Mental Disorder. Culture, Medicine and Psychiatry 2: 209–231.
Kleinman, Arthur
1980 Patients and Healers in the Context of Culture. Berkeley: U. of California.
Lehrman, D.
1970 Semantic and Conceptual Issues in the Nature-Nurture Problem. *In* L. R. Aaronson et al. (eds.), Development and Evolution of Behavior. San Francisco: Freeman.
Littlewood, R. and M. Lipsedge
1982 Aliens and Alienists; Ethnic Minorities and Psychiatry. Middlesex: Penguin.
Manschreck, Theo C., and Michelle Petri
1978 The Atypical Psychoses. Culture, Medicine and Psychiatry 2: 233–268.
Murphy, H. B. M.
1976 Notes for a Theory on *Latah*. *In* Culture-Bound Syndromes, Ethnopsychiatry, and Alternate Therapies 4. Honolulu: University of Hawaii.
1983 Commentary on 'The Resolution of the *Latah* Paradox'. J. Nervous and Mental Disease 171: 176–177.
Ness
1978 The *Old Hag* Phenomenon as Sleep Paralysis. Culture, Medicine, and Psychiatry 2: 15–39.
Ohnuki-Tierney
1980 Shamans and Imu: Among Two Ainu Groups. Ethos 8: 204–229. (Reprinted in this volume.)

Rittenbaugh, C.
    1982   Obesity as a Culture-Bound Syndrome. Culture, Medicine and Psychiatry 6: 341–
           361.
Rubel, A., C. O'Nell, and R. Collado
    1984   Susto, A Folk Illness. Berkeley: U. of California.
Simons, R. C.
    1980   The Resolution of the *Latah* Paradox. J. Nervous and Mental Disease 168: 195–206.
           (Reprinted in this volume.)
    1981   A Review of Culture-Bound Syndromes. Paper presented at the annual meeting of
           the Society for the Study of Culture and Psychiatry, Mt. Hood, Oregon.
    1981a *Latah II* – Problems with a Purely Symbolic Interpretation; A Reply to Michael
           Kenny. J. Nervous and Mental Disease 171: 168–175. (Reprinted in this volume.)
    1983b *Latah III* – How Compelling is the Evidence for a Psychoanalytic Interpretation;
           A Reply to H. B. M. Murphy. J. Nervous and Mental Disease 171: 178–181.
    1983c *Latah* – A Culture-Specific Elaboration of the *Startle Reflex*. (Film) East Lansing:
           Michigan State University.
Swettenham, F. A.
    1895   Malay Sketches. New York: MacMillan Collier.
Winzeler
           In press. The Study of *Latah* from 1849–1980.

PART I

FOLK ILLNESSES OF PSYCHIATRIC INTEREST IN WHICH SOME EVIDENCE SUPPORTS THE HYPOTHESIS OF A NEUROPHYSIOLOGICAL SHAPING FACTOR

A. THE STARTLE MATCHING TAXON

RONALD C. SIMONS

INTRODUCTION: *THE STARTLE MATCHING TAXON*

The *Startle Matching Taxon* includes those phenomena which I originally lumped under the rubric, *Latah*, using an upper case initial to designate the taxon name, distinguishing it from the (lower case) local instance. This taxon includes syndromes from all over the world which are characterized by an exaggerated startle followed by a variety of odd behaviors locally considered amusing. Matching the words or actions of others is one such frequent and prominent behavior, hence *Startle Matching*. As the first paper in this section is my 1980 report in which *Startle Matching* is more fully described, there is no need for an extensive description here. In that paper I attempt to demonstrate that the factors which account for *latah*'s shape and form (what *latah* looks like, what *latahs* do) include specific aspects of pan-mammalian neurophysiology, and that the *latah* syndrome seen in Malaysia can be considered a local cultural elaboration of that physiology. I suggest that since the same physiology is available for potential elaboration elsewhere, it is not surprising that other societies have elaborated the same elements in ways consistent with their own specific social and cultural realities. I propose that *latah* is best understood as a culture-specific elaboration of the potential of the startle reflex.

This paper elicited several critiques, the most extensive of which, by Michael Kenny, is reprinted as the second paper. Kenny believes that "*latah*-like conditions are best considered in terms of their local meaning within their societies of origin". He demonstrates that the previous literature is open to a variety of readings, and he argues that if one can demonstrate the symbolic meaning of *latah*, the allegation that physiological factors are important in its shaping is logically unnecessary and therefore misguided. The third paper contains my attempts to rebut Kenny's well expressed criticism. Among other issues, both of us consider what the implications each of our interpretations is likely to be for the lives of actual *latahs*.

In the last paper in this section, Emiko Ohnuki-Tierney describes another member of the *Startle Matching Taxon* – *imu*. She points out that persons who were shamans were also *imu* and that persons who were *imu* were also shamans with considerably greater than expected frequency both in her samples and in the samples of others. She discusses the phenomenon of *imu* and the institution of shamanism, and she suggests a way in which they are related. To one reading the papers sequentially, it will be apparent that her formulation is parallel to Kenny's in that it locates the source of the phenomenon exclusively in local meaning. It will also be apparent that I disagree with this interpretation. For example, Ohnuki-Tierney notes that catching sight of metallic washing pans, neon signs, and cats, all introduced by the Japanese, can induce episodes of *imu*. She interprets their common denominator as being that they are "unfamiliar foreign objects which *symbolize* (italics added) the Japanese". To me it is interesting that of the many

Ronald C. Simons and Charles C. Hughes (eds.), The Culture-Bound Syndromes, 41–42.
© 1985 *by D. Reidel Publishing Company.*

objects introduced by the Japanese, only a certain selection induce episodes of *imu*, and I wonder if the physical properties of the pans and the neon lights are not equally relevant; that these objects function in this way, in part, because they are unfamiliar and *shiny*. Cats too are potent startle elicitors since, unlike dogs, they hunt with stealth and a pounce. (I have a sizable cross-cultural collection of cat startle stories; none about dogs.) What of the many introduced objects like scrolls and yukatas which are equally foreign but which do not produce startle or *imu*? Other inducers which she mentions also suggest startle to me. Catching sight of a snake and hearing the shouted word "snake" are both also effective cross culturally. Catching sight of someone eating raw fish or of a writhing just-shot reindeer also can be interpreted as other than symbols as well, since objects or scenes which produce revulsion or horror are also especially effective startle elicitors. Whether these function as stimuli as well as symbols cannot be deduced. The answer, however, could come from detailed descriptions of *imu* subjects' inter-actions with symbol/stimulus objects and empirical analyses of how episodes of *imu* followed thereafter.

Because they both were aware of my disagreement with their formulations, it was especially good of Kenny and Ohnuki-Tierney to allow me to reprint, and here to critique, their studies. Thus, it seems only fair to give Kenny the last word: "Needless to say, I do not consider *latah* part of a taxon, but never mind . . . . Best wishes."

RONALD C. SIMONS[1]

THE RESOLUTION OF THE *LATAH* PARADOX

... *latah* is remarkably congruent with themes which are both unique to and central to [Javanese culture]. If it were not for the presence of *latah* elsewhere in the world, one would be tempted to conclude that the reason for its occurrence in Java is self-evident, that its congruence with Javanese culture sufficiently accounts for its appearance there – Hildred Geertz (1968: 104).

... any one who desires to really account for this affliction must, I am convinced, begin by analysing and examining and explaining the pathology of the common start or 'jump' to which we are all in a lesser or a greater degree subject – Sir Hugh Clifford (1898: 197).

... it may be surprising to hear that the startle reflex of human subjects can be facilitated or inhibited, more or less at will, by applying a very simple paradigm which has been used with rats and rabbits – Frances K. Graham (1975: 238).

Culture-bound syndromes are forms of unusal individual behavior restricted in distribution to discrete areas of the globe. They are considered eccentricities in the cultural systems of societies in which they are endemic, and psychopathologies in the reference system of Western psychological medicine. Most are episodic and highly dramatic. Because of their intrinsic interest as dramatic exotica and their implications for theories of deviance, several have been the subjects of much previous work.

Latah is such a culture-bound syndrome from Malaysia and Indonesia. A person exemplifying the *Latah* syndrome typically responds to a startling stimulus with an exaggerated startle, sometimes throwing or dropping a held object, and often uttering some improper word, usually "*Puki!*" ("Cunt!"), "*Butol!*" ("Prick!"), or "*Buntut!*" ("Ass!"), which may be embedded in a "silly" phrase. Further, he or she may, while flustered, obey the orders or match the words or movements of persons nearby. Since spectators invariably find this funny, a known *Latah* may be intentionally startled many times each day for the amusement of others. In Malay villages in Negri Sembilan and Melaka visited during the course of this research, *Latahs* were common and everyone knew who they were.

Both men and women are affected. Most *Latahs*, however, are women, in middle life when the syndrome begins, and of relatively low status. Whether abrupt or gradual in onset, the syndrome, once begun, continues throughout life. Though *Latah* is frequent in some families, it may also develop in persons with no *Latah* relatives.

Syndromes essentially like *Latah* have been reported from Burma (where it is called *yaun*), Thailand (*bah-tsche*), and the Philippines (*mali-mali*), (*silok*) (Yap 1969). More surprisingly, it also occurs in Siberia (*myriachit, ikota, amurakh*) (Czaplicka 1914), South-West Africa (allegedly unnamed) (Gilmour 1902), Lapland

43

Ronald C. Simons and Charles C. Hughes (eds.), The Culture-Bound Syndromes, 43–62.
© 1980 by The Williams & Wilkins Co., Baltimore.

(*Lapp panic*) (Colinder 1949), and among the Ainu in Japan (*Imu*) (Nakagawa 1973; Uchimura 1956). It was also described in a small group of French Canadians living in Maine in the 1870s (*jumping*) (Beard 1880) and has recently been redis-covered in the same area (Kunkle 1967).

The general explanation for the culture-bound syndromes is that cultures shape hysterical symptomatology in ways congruent with belief systems. This explanation, however, does not sufficiently explain the phenomenon of *latah* [2] since it does not account for the occurrence of such similar behavior complexes in societies having long independent histories and unrelated cultural systems. Further, the peoples involved do not share genetics, diet, or ecologies more generally. In her 1968 paper, Geertz demonstrated how exquisitely the Javanese form of *latah* reflects Javanese values and customs. She therefore labeled the occurrence of *latah* elsewhere a paradox. If *Latah* arises from features specific to Javanese culture, why is it found in unrelated culture areas? The intent of the present paper is to resolve this paradox by showing how the various forms of the *latah* reaction are culture-specific exploitations of a neurophysiologically determined behavioral potential.

THE STARTLE RESPONSE

In 1939 Carney Landis and William Hunt published a comprehensive report of their studies of a:

... complex, almost invariable, involuntary, innate reflex response, clearly demonstrable under the temporal magnification of high or superspeed motion-picture photography. This pattern has two elements, the eye-blink, which is always present in normal adults, and the facial-bodily response, which appears in a more or less complete sequential form (p. 146).

They described this response pattern in detail: a generalized flexion with a characteristic head movement occurring in the first half-second after a sudden intense stimulus. Their usual test stimulus was the sound of a .22-caliber pistol fired close behind each subject, but they also used auditory stimuli of other in-tensities and qualities, bright light, exposure to jets of cold water, and electrical shock. When presented suddenly and with sufficient intensity, all of these stimuli induced startles.

Landis and Hunt observed the startle response replacing the Moro reflex in infants at 4 months and described it in children of various ages, in subjects of both sexes and several ethnic groups, and in patients with a variety of psychiatric and neurological diagnoses. They found an analogous response present with the addition of flexion (laying back) of the ears in the 18 species of mammals they tested and absent in the tested reptiles and amphibian. Birds and fish were not tested.

Testing veteran police marksmen, they found that, although the whole body response was sometimes lost through habituation, the eyeblink never was. Given a stimulus of sufficient intensity, prior knowledge of its imminence did not eliminate the startle response. Landis and Hunt justifiably concluded that: ". . . In place of having recourse to statistical proof of the occurrence of a pattern, we find ourselves in possession of that highly desirable scientific occurrence — a clear-cut stimulus-response relationship of an almost invariable nature" (1939: 146).

As ethology was in its infancy and human ethology had not yet emerged as a discipline when Landis and Hunt did their work, they did not call startle a fixed or modal action pattern (Lorenz 1960; Barlow, 1977), although this is what they described. It is one of the very few so far discovered in *Homo sapiens*.[3]

Landis and Hunt focused their attention almost entirely on the first half-second after the presentation of the startling stimulus. They noted, almost in passing, that some "other responses appear much less logical and seem not to be directed toward the stimulus but to be mere overflow phenomena . . . . Thus some subjects will change their position; others will smile aimlessly or address some remark to the experimenter" (Landis and Hunt 1939: 137). They suggested further investigation of these phenomena.

In 1960 Sternbach reported a study in which subjects depressed a reaction time key as quickly as possible after hearing a pistol shot. Of interest are the comments of his "slow reactors": "I know I was supposed to do something, but I couldn't think of it at first", "it took me a moment to realize what I had to do"; fast reactors made no similar comments, merely saying such things as "I wasn't expecting it so soon", "it was louder than I expected" (p. 147).

Some of the "slow reactors" were confused and flustered. The startling stimulus had not only elicited startle responses but had also deflected their foci of attention, which could be directed back to the assigned task only with difficulty. Tomkins (1962), reviewing this work, concluded ". . . that these secondary responses to startle represent an important area for further investigation in the same detailed way in which Landis and Hunt isolated the startle pattern itself" (p. 520).

THE UBIQUITY HYPOTHESIS

Considering certain of Landis and Hunt's "secondary effects" and the behaviors of Sternbach's "slow reactors", I hypothesized that most or all human populations contain individuals who can be easily and strongly startled and whose ongoing stream of activity can be disrupted by startle. The hypothesis is similar to the observations of both Teoh (1972) and Westermeyer (1973) that though *amok* has long been considered to be a phenomenon restricted to Malay culture, parallel instances of rapidly repetitive, random homicide are frequently reported in the world press from many Eastern and Western societies. Only in Southeast Asia, however, has this behavior pattern been named and institutionalized. I hypothesized startle to be similar to fainting, in that it is frequent in populations whose cultures notice, expect, and shape such behavior, and rare but not absent in populations which do not attend to it.

AMERICAN HYPERSTARTLERS

The first problem in pursuing this hypothesis was to determine whether *latah* equivalents could be found in a society with no named and recognized cultural complex concerning startle. American society being the nearest such society to hand, advertisements were placed in local newspapers asking for easily startled subjects.

Twelve persons who answered the advertisement were interviewed and were videotaped as they responded to startling stimuli. Ten of these persons were born in America, nine Caucasians and one Black. In the formulation which follows they will be referred to as American hyperstartlers. A fuller description of their interviews and behavior will be presented elsewhere; representative excerpts from their interviews follow:

K.B.: The reason I answered that I am a startler is that when I'm alone somewhere and not expecting to be anything but alone and someone comes behind me or into where I am, I have a physical reaction, I jump, maybe I do like this (demonstrates) ... it's just what I do, I'll say something, I might go "Uuuh!!!", like that, I might swear, I might momentarily accuse, I might say to my husband, "Damn you, Ken!" when he has done nothing but come into the house; accuse him of sneaking up on me even when I know he has not, and even though I know he knows that I might do that and so he makes noises that he thinks for sure I'll hear.

K.E.: I was typing in my office, and a person came in behind me, was looking over my shoulder, and I didn't know they were there, and they said, in a kind of normal-to-quiet tone of voice, "You're getting pretty good at that" and I literally went backwards in the chair, it startled me so badly.
  E: Did you say anything?
K.E.: Something like "Oh, my God!" or some exclamation, and he started laughing, and I started laughing. I laugh sometimes when people do that to me, but it's a very uncomfortable feeling, you know. . . . People think it's amusing when they find out they can startle you, they often do try to startle you, and I think it's a pretty uncomfortable sensation.

L.L.: It was my girlfriend's boyfriend, and I had a plate in my hand and I simply dropped it on the kitchen floor as I turned to see a form in the door . . . I continued to scream and they, everyone piled out of their rooms and said, you know, "Just what is the problem?" And they were just accusing me of, you know, all sorts of foolish things. But it was sincere. I don't know why I continued to scream [And I was thinking] that's Wanda's boyfriend; why am I scared, frightened, why am I screaming? . . . Nothing to be frightened about, but that doesn't stop it; the whole thing goes on the same.

E.C.: My little grandmother, she's so prim and proper from Virginia, and we were coming up the hill to her house which scares the daylights out of me because it's straight up. I was with my husband, and I begged him, "Let's leave the car at the bottom of the hill, and we'll walk up". And he says, "Oh, we can make it, it'll be okay. You know we have a good car" and Grandma was in the car. Oh, he started up the hill, and then he pretended like it wouldn't go anymore and pretended it was sliding backward to tease, and it startled me, it really did, because that's my fear! I was really afraid it was going to roll down that hill so, uhm, I said something, I don't remember the word, I doubt it was anything like I just said ["Fuck!"], I think it was like "Shit!" or something. "Why, Elaine!", she couldn't believe that I said that. I was extremely embarrassed.
  E: Were you scared or were you startled?
E.C.: I was startled. When I'm startled I jump, I move, . . . it's different, yes, I jumped up

to the front of the car ... I would say [I'm severely startled] probably at least once every other day.

M.D.: People have told me, you know, like when they come up behind me and say, "Boo!" or "Hi!" all of a sudden I get really red in the face and I sort of well [embarrassed laugh] this is going to sound absurd, but they said I even sort of get into a fighting position, you know, like I'm ready to start fighting or self-defending myself, or something . . . .

Although most of the American Hyperstartlers believed themselves unique, their behaviors, the behaviors of others towards them, and the phenomenology of their experiences are strikingly alike. Further, they are much like those reported by and of *latahs*. Like *latahs* elsewhere, American Hyperstartlers describe being startled extremely easily and hence frequently. They report exaggerated physical and mental responses, including throwing or dropping of held objects, uncontrolled vocalizations, and (rarely) uttering of normally inhibited, situationally inappropriate, and embarrassing language. Like *latahs* elsewhere, they tell of this condition having begun in adolescence or later, and they describe how once this is noticed they are repeatedly intentionally startled for the amusement of others. All this is so, although nothing in American culture describes and names such persons or prescribes the behaviors they report. Thus, the interpretation of this behavior as mere conformity to a culturally prescribed role is suspect. American Hyperstartlers did not report obedience to commands or matching of others' behaviors. Why this is so is discussed below.

Experiments comparing the behavior, physiology, and phenomenology of American Hyperstartlers and normals are in progress. Initial results include the findings that facial responses of the American Hyperstartlers to a standard stimulus are much greater than those of normals and that, unlike those of normals, these facial responses cannot be voluntarily inhibited. American Hyperstartlers also respond to strong stimuli with strong startles even if they know exactly when the stimuli will occur.[4]

COLLECTION OF CROSS-CULTURAL DATA

A major strategy of the present research has been to obtain adequate audiovisual samples of startle phenomena, including *Latah*, *mali-mali*, and *imu*, and to examine minutely the audiovisual record, using the form and differential occurrence of microstructural events to suggest and test hypotheses about macrostructural (social and psychological) ones. Data collected from *mali-malis* in the Philippines and from Malay and Portuguese *Latahs* in Malaysia include 16-mm and super 8-mm sound film footage and taped interviews describing relevant aspects of personal and social histories. Information was collected from non-*latahs* on *latahs* known and *latah* episodes witnessed, local attitudes about *latah*, and stories about *latahs* which reflect cultural perceptions of its cause and significance. Additional documents studied include a print of a film (in the author's possession) made in 1936 by Uchimura of the University of Tokyo of Ainu subjects in Hokkaido demonstrating *imu*, the Ainu form of *latah*, and a second film of *imu* (studied by the author) collected in 1970 by a team from the Medical College of Sapporo headed by Nakagawa and Ishibashi.

FORMULATION: HOW LATAH COMES ABOUT

Unexpectedness and Intensity of Stimulus

Stimuli in any modality can elicit a startle response. Humans, like other mammals, startle at the sudden presentation of auditory, visual, tactile, gustatory, and proprioceptive stimuli. It is the suddenness of the appearance of a novel stimulus in the perceptual field that triggers a startle response (Landis and Hunt 1939). Elegant neurophysiological studies have demonstrated that the strength of a startle response varies greatly with the time from initial appearance to maximum strength of the stimulus (Fleshler 1965). Introspection also confirms that this is the case. Accounts of startles by normals, *Latahs, mali-malis*, and American Hyperstartlers repeatedly refer to the suddenness with which a stimulus appears as a cause of the startle and whatever behaviors are consequent to it. Our film records of *latahs* show clear differences between responses to attempted stimulation by touches which are truly percussive and those in which the pressure gradient of contact appears to be more gradual. Unexpectedness is also a factor, both unexpectedness of occurrence (no potentially significant stimulus expected) and unexpectedness of configuration. Sufficiently intense stimuli can also elicit startles even when expected (Landis and Hunt 1939), although they are responded to with much smaller startles by normals.[4]

Prior State of Subject – Monitoring

Graham and co-workers noted that "in rats, the startle reflex may be predictably inhibited or facilitated when a neutral stimulus, itself ineffective in eliciting the reflex, precedes an effective stimulus by a short interval" (1975a): 161). These studies have been replicated in rabbits, are true for cross-modal stimulation, are not dependent on learning, and are true when the lead stimulating event is the cessation as well as when it is the beginning of a stimulus. In a series of carefully controlled experiments, Graham and co-workers (1975a) demonstrated the same effects in humans. Prestimulation of a subject less than 1/4 second before a startling stimulus decreases the magnitude of the startle response, and *prestimulation more than 1/4 second before a startling stimulus increases its magnitude*. Graham noted that, because the timing of the prestimulation can increase or decrease the magnitude of the subsequent startle, it provides precise control of an involuntary response, the relevant point being that a neural regulatory mechanism exists which, independent of the properties of a stimulus, can significantly increase the strength of a startle.

The reports of normals, *Latahs, mali-mailis*, and American Hyperstartlers and stories about startle from America, the Philippines, and Malaysia consistently assert that the prior state of a subject influences whether or not a given stimulus is adequate to elicit a startle and, if a startle is elicited, its magnitude. Startles are most readily elicited when subjects are in one of two states, seemingly at opposite poles of a continuum of attention. Startles are most readily elicited when subjects are either intensely monitoring their immediate environments or when drowsy or lost in thought. Experimental work is needed to clarify how easily a startle is elicited and how strong it is in each of these two states.

Hypermonitoring may be produced pharmacologically (Callaway 1959). Ingestion of caffeine and certain other CNS stimulants increase arousal, monitoring, ease of startle elicitation, and strength of startle responses. Hypermonitoring of either the environment or of interior states may be transient and situationally specific or may be chronically characteristic of a subject. Persons not previously chronically hypermonitoring or losing themselves in thought may begin to do so in anxious periods, for example, after a significant loss. *Latahs* and *mali-malis* frequently reported that their first episodes of *latah* occurred in a period of anxious worry, often after the loss of a spouse or child.

The neuroanatomical mechanism serving both startles and directed attention is believed to be located in the limbic system, especially the amygdala. Th electrical activity which can be recorded from the amygdaloid complex changes only when a subject animal is startled or when its attention is focused on an environmental stimulus of instinctive or conditioned special significance. Hippocampal ablation, however, leads to changes in the electrical activity recorded from the amygdala in response to *any* novel sensory stimulation (Miller et al. 1960).

Three Types of latah

In Malaysia and the Philippines, three distinguishable types of behavior are called *latah*. The first, *Immediate Response Latah*, consists merely of strong responses to a startling stimulus which others find amusing: violent body movements, assumption of habitual defensive postures, striking out, throwing or dropping held objects, and sometimes "Naughty Talk". In the Philippines and Malaysia, there is a continuum between normal responsiveness to potentially startling stimuli, slight over-responsiveness ("a little *latah*"), and the extreme response which is characteristic of the *latahs* described in Western literature.

In all populations studied, striking out and the assumption of idiosyncratic defensive postures may be modified into a stylized form by prior experience. After judo training, an American Hyperstartler would immediately assume the overlearned judo defensive posture whenever she was startled. Similarly, one subject from the Malay sample, a former teacher of bersilat (the Malay art of self-defense) responded to all startling stimuli, even to an unexpected loss of footing, with a vocalization, an instantaneous strong blow, and the assumption of the bersilat defensive posture. His type of *latah* is locally referred to as *Latah Pendekar* and, needless to say, he is not much teased. Similar behavior is prominent in the Maine Jumpers rediscovered by Kunkle in 1960, the name *Killer Jumper* being applied to those most strongly affected, although no deaths from being hit by a Jumper have ever been reported (p. 356).

A second form, *Attention Capture Latah*, includes matching, the completion of other-initiated actions, and sometimes obedience. In 1959, Easterbrook proposed that increased arousal causes a restriction of the range of cues that an organism uses in the guidance of an action. Considerable and varied evidence supports this hypothesis. Callaway (1959), who manipulated arousal pharmacologically, demonstrated that drugs like amphetamines which increase arousal interfered with the registration of peripheral cues, whereas atropine-like drugs had the opposite effect. Kahneman (1973), reviewing these and related studies, pointed out that it is not that arousal interferes with peripheral vision but rather that it affects the allocation of attention (p. 38). High arousal leads to a focus on the most strongly demarcated cues available in a given stimulus situation. I hypothesize that this arousal-determined narrowing of attention is the neurophysiological basis of matching, completion of other-initiated actions, and obedience.

Latahs become extremely aroused when startled. This is evidenced in our films by a high (increased) frequency of displacement gestures. Matching, obedience, and similar behaviors are then induced by the actions of other persons. To induce compliant behavior in *latahs*, one must not only induce a startle response but must also present the behavior to be matched or the command to be followed in a framed and forceful manner. The presence of an audience, the improper nature of commands, and the presence of higher status persons all increase arousal and hence vulnerability to this capture of attention. *Latahs* and *mali-malis* invariably told me that, when alone and startled, their responses were exaggerated but brief. I observed this to be true whenever the startling stimulus was not followed by forcefully presented commands or models. Not all *Latahs* and *mali-malis* become sufficiently aroused after being startled to allow attention to be thus captured. Their stories and indigenous explanations describe *latah*'s beginning with no more than very strong and flustering startles. They point out that *Attention Capture* develops only when a known hyperstartler comes to be increasingly startled and teased by fellow villagers.

It seems likely that the behaviors of *Immediate Response Latah* can be found in all societies. *Attention Capture*, however, will only sometimes be seen, as this requires the framed and forceful presentation of commands and models, *behaviors of others which are culture-specific*. (However, neurophysiologically equivalent versions, such as a startled person driving an automobile into, rather away from, a suddenly appearing danger, are not unknown in the West.) I suggest that American Hyperstartlers would also obey and match if, after being aroused by a startle, they were to be confronted with adequately presented commands and models. That doing so might have amusing results is not known to their American peers. One would, however, expect occasionally to learn of independent discoveries of the vulnerability to *Attention Capture* of those hyperaroused by startle, especially in populations in which teasing horseplay is permissible. The *latah* of the Maine Jumpers represents just such an independent discovery.

I have called the third form *Role Latah*. In one sense all social behavior is role behavior to the extent that culturally specific cognitive categories provide the performer and witnesses with interpretations and evaluations which specify that behavior's locus in the total set of behaviors and evaluations which constitute the repertoire of the culture. However, by the term *Role Latah* I refer to the practice of selecting behaviors from the categories of *Immediate Response* and *Attention Capture Latah* and elaborating them idiosyncratically into intentionally amusing performances. Although these performances include behaviors approximating the behaviors induced by a startling stimulus, they may be performed after a stimulus inadequate to trigger a startle response, e.g., a gentle nudge. An actual startle may not occur, although an acted version of one is usually performed. The "silly" behaviors of *Role Latah* may include social commentary, teasing of others, and considerable wit and satire. For some, acceptance of the *Latah* role is obviously rewarding. Behaviors which comprise the *Latah* role conflict with those expected of males, and I was unable to find any heterosexual males who performed *Role Latah*. For obvious reasons, reports of witnessed *latah* episodes and descriptions of *latahs* by urban based investigators seeking *latahs* to study are biased in favor of role performances of those willing to perform on cue.

Sometimes persons doing *Role Latah* begin with simulation, but with the arousal their performances engender, and after being repeatedly poked, show actual startles and the phenomena which follow them. Sometimes, *Latah* role acceptors, when startle stimulation by others is insufficient to maintain authentic performances, repeatedly stimulate themselves with an abrupt jerky turn of the head away from the audience and a sharp, abrupt vocalization ("Eh!"). This head turn and "Eh!" is not part of the *latah* behavior of nonrole acceptors and does not occur in the ordinary speech of the role acceptors when not "doing *Latah*".

In societies in which *Attention Capture* is practiced, the behaviors offered to be matched, completed, or obeyed are often those which violate culture-specific rules of propriety. Since the point of the demonstration is, after all, that the just-startled person is in other than conscious volitional control of her own behavior, performing normally tabooed behavior most unequivocally demonstrates this. Such demonstrations also provide an opportunity to perform ordinarily proscribed behaviors which the subject indeed might like to do or that others might like to see done.[5] In Ainu, Philippine, and Malay/Indonesian cultures, the just-startled person is sometimes induced to perform suggestive sexual behaviors, such as disrobing or imitating copulatory movements.

In a continuum of elaborations, the *Role Latah* seen in Malaysia and Indonesia falls somewhere between the situation in the West and that reported from the Ainu. Although play with *Latahs* is a frequent occurrence at Malay weddings and other feasts, this is not by prior arrangement, nor is such play a scheduled feature of the occasion. In contrast, among the Ainu at certain feasts, *latahs* (*imus*) attend with the intention of performing *latah* (*imu*) behavior. Among the Ainu there is a cultural recognition that *Attention Capture* is an interactive process, and not only is the role of the *latah* labeled and culturally demarcated (the *imu bakko*), but also the role of the interactant who is responsible for eliciting the startle and for offering the behaviors or commands which will then be matched or obeyed (the *imu yara*). The *imu yara* is often the *imu bakko*'s best friend (Nakagawa 1973). Nakagawa described *imu* subjects volunteering for and seeking out opportunities to express and demonstrate their *latah* states. He attributed these performances to the importance of a snake god in the Ainu pantheon and hence a positive evaluation of behaviors influenced by this deity.

Naughty Talk

One of the features of the startle response most consistent across cultures is the phenomenon of Naughty Talk. The usual terms "coprolalia" (Greek for "dung babble") and "pornolalia" ("prostitute babble") are somewhat misleading, since when normal persons and *latahs* are startled they do not begin to talk about excrement or sex. Rather, if they vocalize verbally, they usually utter either a deity referent or a single normally prohibited vulgar sexual or excremental referent. In the United States what is usually said is "God!", "Jesus!", "Fuck!", or "Shit!"; in the Philippines, "Jesus-Maria-Joseph!" or "*Uten!*" ("*Prick!*"); in Malaysia "Allah!" or "*Puki!*". An American Hyperstartler who exclaims "Fuck!" when startled is not labeled in any culturally prescribed way. However, the labels "Mali-mali" and "Latah" are applied to Philippinos and Malaysians who perform equivalently.

What deity referents and Naughty Talk have in common is the fact that negative social sanctions follow their appearance in casual speech. The terms themselves and not their meanings are unacceptable; their meanings can readily be expressed in acceptable alternative forms. The common denominator is the sequestration from casual conversational appearance of these terms. That brain-injured subjects, otherwise aphasic, may still be able to utter them forcefully when excited is further evidence that they are neurologically encoded in some special manner.

Since it is this very guarding itself and not the meaning of Naughty Talk terms that defines the category, any instance of lapse which incurs negative sanctions will, by intensifying the guarding, more strongly sequester into the Naughty Talk the term which leaked, thus increasing the likelihood of its appearance in subsequent lapses. This process is important in shaping the stereotyped Naughty Talk responses of *latahs*.

The characteristically prohibited utterance appears as the first word in the series, though it is sometimes preceded by an "Oh!" or "Ah!" Sometimes, within a syllable or so, startled subjects were able to add a context which made their utterances less socially consequential and objectionable. In the Philippines, where the Tagalog word for penis is *uten*, one speaker when startled would characteristically utter "*Utes!*" Although identified to me by others as a *mali-mali*, she denied being one, explaining that *utes* is a nonsense word and has no meaning. In Malaysia, a secretary who was identified to me as a *Latah* because she said "*Puki!*" when startled was once recorded as saying "*Pulut!*" ("glutinous rice!") instead. When the embarrassing word is not modified internally, the violation may be downgraded by various techniques such as by adding an animal referent, as, for example, "*Uten kabayo!*" ("Prick of a horse!"). Both of these techniques are also used by Americans, "Jesus!" being changed, for example to "Cheese and crackers!"

So great is the magical power of certain words that it is likely that even referential use of the magical English equivalents will prove offensive to some readers. However, translating *puki* as "vagina" or "*pudenda muliebre*" is misleading as it suggests that the significance of the use of these terms lies in their specific denotations. Neutral and emotionally less loaded terms with the same denotations are never uttered in contexts in which *puki* is used. Many terms which by dictionary definition have sexual content are used more frequently for emphasis or aggressively.[6] *Puki* is more often used in emphatic/aggressive contexts than in sexual ones, the expression "*Puki emak engkau!*" ("Your mother's cunt!") being perhaps its single most frequent use.

Sometimes what is said after a startle appears to be part of an automatically triggered verbalization sequence, determined by such factors as immediacy of availability for utterance. What is said is often the name of an attribute of something currently in view or a repetition of the last thing previously said by the subject or in his or her hearing. Sometimes *latahs* respond with the name of an object which frequently elicits a startle. One of our subjects who startled regularly on catching sight of a frog frequently said "*Katak, katak, katak!*" ("Frog, frog, frog!") when she was poked.

None of the above is true for *Role Latah* utterances, since these are part of the intentionally amusing performances of acceptors of the *Latah* role. We filmed, for example, a woman *Latah* wittily and appropriately using the occasion of being startled to play at the completion of offered incomplete quatrains (*pantuns*), a feature of traditional Malay culture. On another occasion, we filmed a male homosexual transvestite (*pondan*) role acceptor from the Malacca Portugese community use the occasion of being startled to demonstrate an impressive familiarity with indelicate antique Portugese.

DISCUSSION

Startle as an Emergency Override System

Startle can be thought of as an override system, automatically activated when a sudden unexpected environmental event requires immediate first priority attention (Tomkins 1962). It is the whole-body equivalent of the single-segment spinal reflex that removes a seared fingertip from a hot stovetop. It is not hard to imagine such a system being highly selected for in the course of evolution: a stimulus-triggered arrest of motion with a refocusing of attention on a suddenly presented threat. This would be highly functional in normal persons.

In both the spinal reflex and in startle, potentially injurious stimuli are reacted to without conscious reflection and hence extremely rapidly. In both reflexes, the response behaviors are little affected by configurational properties of the eliciting stimulus; any adequate stimulus triggers a response of more or less set form. In the startle reflex, this includes a series of serially recruited elements, not all of which are included in the response of every individual. What elements are recruited in a given startle depends largely on the prior state of the subject. For the same subject, a stimulus of given intensity may elicit no more than a blink at one time and an extensive response with blink, jump, and vocalization at another. It is a commonplace of Western suspense films to orchestrate loading stimuli judiciously so that when the startle-releasing stimulus occurs it will have maximal effect. As in the build-up to strong orgasmic release, a series of tension-inducing sequences, each resolved without eliciting release, will accomplish this. *Latahs* live in a chronic state of such readiness for startle.

The Social Context

Phenomenologically, startle is a discontinuity in experience. Anyone who has been startled severely will remember a brief period of being flustered and unable to make a situationally appropriate response. It is this similarity between the effect of a startle on a *Latah* and its effect on normal persons which Sir Hugh Clifford remarked on in the quotation introducing this paper (1898). Because the startle response includes characteristic movements of body parts, evidence that a person is undergoing this experiential discontinuity is visible to others and is therefore socially available. In some contexts, as in the joking horseplay of American adolescent males, sudden gestures designed to make a companion flinch are a frequent part of interactive status determining and maintaining byplay.

In America as in many societies, a strong startle response of another person when grossly disproportionate to the degree of perceived danger is considered amusing.[7] Persons who startle especially violently are often intentionally startled by others for the amusement their responses provide. This is sufficiently frequent that it was possible to include as a criterion for the American Hyperstartlers that the subject consider himself or herself not only to be more easily and violently startled than others but also to be especially selected for startle teasing because of this characteristic.

Who in a given society may be so treated depends on class, status, and culturally specific rules such as those having to do with the bodily availability of specific others. In general, these rules follow patterns salient in other aspects of interrelationships. For example, in Malaysia where the most usual intentional stimulus is a sharp poke in the ribs (a *cucuk*), a female informant told me that it would not be right for her to touch an unrelated man close to her own age. However, she added, there was no such prohibition against her children doing so, the children including two daughters in their early twenties, a teenage daughter, and a younger son.

Marginal Social Status

In general, those who may be intentionally startled for the amusement their responses provide onlookers are those who lack power to effectively retaliate. This explains the fact that the few reported instances of *latah* equivalents in the West occur in situations in which hazing forms of teasing are permitted. The American Hyperstartlers reported a high incidence of provocation in situations such as dormitories. Thorn's 1944 paper on "startle neurosis" in the West described *latah*-like behavior in Army recruits. Those persons who can be startled with impunity are also those whose situations engender a high degree of situational monitoring and hence susceptibility to strong startles.[8] A circular incremental pattern may be established: slightly increased responsiveness leading to intentional startles by others, leading to increased monitoring in social situations in which intentional stimulation is probable, leading to increased ease and strength of response.

Culturally specific rules, such as those having to do with the treatment of low status and stigmatized others, determine whether or not persons startling strongly may be stimulated for amusement in a given society. In the Philippines and Malaysia, derogatory nicknames, sometimes acquired in early youth, may follow someone for his entire life, and a person with a limp or otherwise disabled is often given a nickname referring to that infirmity. Thus a native healer in Kampung Padang Kemunting who lost a leg to a shark is universally referred to as Lumun Patah (Lumun the Broken). The exploitation of easy and violent startling for the amusement of others is congruent with the permitted treatment of persons with other stigmata and infirmities. Intentionally startling others for the amusement their strong responses provide is most frequent in peasant societies in which all persons and their life histories are known to all members of the community. It is this fact, rather than other aspects of modernization, that accounts for *latahs* being less frequently observed in big city settings. In a city the fact that one is a hyperstartler is not known to most persons whom one encounters. Furthermore, it is not safe for those who enjoy provoking *latah* episodes to go about intentionally startling strangers.

Asymmetric Sex Distribution

There is a limited range of solutions to the problems engendered by being startled by others for their amusement. One solution is to accept and elaborate on the *latah* role. Another is to provide strong negative sanctions against being so treated. In asking about the differential incidence of *Latah* in men and women in Malaysia, I often received the culturally appropriate answer referring to a difference in the amount of *semangat* or soul substance characteristic of the two sexes, men having more and women less. With equal frequency, however, informants reported that more women were *Latah* because they could be startled with impunity, i.e., it was much safer to startle intentionally a woman than a man who might effectively retaliate. In a case in the Philippines, a woman who was said to have a cardiac condition and who was *mali-mali* was left alone by fellow villagers after her sons threatened severe retaliation against anyone who might molest their mother. In both the Philippines and Malaysia, the general expectation is that one takes such treatment with relatively good will; husbands are not expected to protect their wives from being startled by others. In Malay society, in which children are, by Western standards, relatively indulged (Djamour 1959), the most frequent startlers of *Latah* women are their own children. It is considerably less acceptable for children to provoke episodes of *Latah* in their fathers.

Previous Formulations

The extensive literature on *latah* has been repeatedly summarized, most competently and exhaustively by Yap (1952). With minor exceptions, those who have witnessed *latah* in its various forms describe strikingly similar behaviors, although their interpretations of them vary considerably. A recent paper speaks of *latah* as a "putative mental illness" and excoriates psychiatric investigators for failing to take adequate account of cultural considerations (Kenny 1978). However, the major papers by psychiatric authors, Yap (1952; 1969), Pfeiffer (1971), and Murphy (1973; 1976), nowhere describe *latah* as a mental illness and are careful to discuss culturally relevant information, sometimes with considerable insight and sophistication, and with Yap warning against the interpretative problems resulting from anthropological naiveté.

Yap (1952) classified the seven cases he saw into a mild and a severe group, the three cases in the latter all showing symptoms of organicity, those in the former similar to cases I observed. He also observed *Role Latah* and noted, "It is often difficult to separate the genuine cases from those which are basically histrionic and exhibitionist in nature" (p. 537). He noted the relevance of Hunt's work on startle, relating it to fright and interpreting it in the context of the work of Pavlov and Rivers. He believed that coprolalia was defensive rather than primarily sexual and suggested that it could occur automatically, independent of central volitional processes (p. 548). He recognized that data did not support the then widely held notion of racial defect and believed instead that:

... the environmental [cultural] factor is alone sufficient to cause the disorder without the aid of either individual or racial morbid inheritance (p. 552). ... *Latah* is considered to be essentially an intense fright reaction involving disorganization of the Ego and obliteration of the Ego-boundaries. A theory of automatic obedience and the echo-reactions is given: this states that fright provokes inhibitory processes which bring about "suppression" (Rivers) of perceptual activity; impairment of the perception of local signature leads to a dissolution of the boundaries of the Ego as has been shown by Uexkull, so that the patient's behavior becomes more directly determined by forces in the total behavioral field according to Gestalt principles; this manifests itself in echo-phenomena and automatic obedience (Yap: 561).

Pfeiffer (1971) reported on 22 *Latahs* he saw in Java, nine of whom he observed in *Latah* states. His observations resemble those of Yap and earlier workers, and he concluded that *latah* requires an abnormal startle reaction with a labile state of consciousness, fixing of attention with a tendency towards mimesis (associated with a peaceful, unchanging rural life), the example of others doing *latah*,[9] and conditioning and tension produced by expectation (*Erwartungsspannung*) (p. 98).

Pfeiffer noted that anecdotal clinical observation had generated testable hypotheses and called for systematic research on sociological and cultural factors, neurophysiological factors (including EEGs), and psychological investigations, including analyses of expressions and comparison of *latahs* with normals. He emphasized the fact that strong startles, startle disruption, and behavioral matching are phenomena that occur in normal subjects and deserve investigating in their own right (p. 98).

In contrast, Murphy's work (1973; 1976) for the most part ignores the important advances in the understanding of *Latah* in the works of Yap and Pfeiffer, and, although he cites the works of Landis and Hunt and of Sternbach, Murphy does not use their findings in his formulation. In his most recent paper on *Latah*, Murphy (1976) listed seven factors contributing to the development of a typical case:

1. *Repressed wishes* probably of an infantile sexual character . . . .
2. *Stimulus generalization* leading to non-sexual stimuli being misinterpreted as being sexual.
3. A *masochistic tendency* resulting in a failure to defend against the provocative stimuli . . . .
4. *Dissociative child-rearing practices* conducive to hyper-suggestibility.
5. *The rewarding of hyper-suggestibility in adults*
6. *Suppression of lengthier dissociations* or trance states through which the repressed wishes could obtain fuller expression.
7. *An inflexibility of impulse control* that leads to exaggerated startle reactions . . . and thence to temporary suspension of inhibitions when startle occurs (pp. 16–17).

He went on to say:

. . . one can also interpret the evidence as suggesting that the milder cases of *latah* illustrate a different type of ego-id relationship from that which seems to exist in the milder varieties of Western neurosis. It is this, in my opinion, which makes this quite rare and otherwise unimportant condition of *latah* worthy of attention by psychiatric theorists (p. 17).

Cross-cultural data make Murphy's conclusions untenable. Data from American Hyperstartlers and accounts of *latah* elsewhere show that Murphy's factors are not necessary for *latah* to occur. Further, to the extent that they accurately describe conditions prevalent in Malay-Indonesian culture they apply to all members of Malay and Indonesian societies and do not account for the appearance of *latah* in only certain individuals.

On the other hand, anthropological papers, of which those of Geertz (1968) and Kenny (1978) are representative, are limited to explaining how *latah* behaviors are congruent with other aspects of the cultures in which they are observed, usually locating a complete and sufficient explanation of *latah* in that congruence. Geertz (1968), noting that "we receive a strong impression that *Latah* is a very Javanese way of expressing mental disturbance", listed factors in Javanese culture which *Latah* behavior violates: the importance of highly stylized and formal etiquette, high differential status,[10] reticence about sex, and a dread of psychological shock. She concluded:

Thus it appears that *Latah* is an unusually clear-cut example of how the form of a set of symptoms may be determined primarily, by a cultural tradition, a tradition which persists because of its congruity with basic themes in the wider culture . . . . The way in which culture could be said to "provide" a ready made set of symptoms to a psychological disturbed person may be better understood when a symptom is viewed as a kind of symbol, as a symbolic act by means of which the ill person can express his psychological dilemmas outwardly (p. 101).

However, Geertz noted that the analysis does not account for the appearance of *latah* elsewhere and commented, "A cultural analysis such as this can never explain a psychological disorder . . .". (p. 102).

In his recent paper, Kenny (1978) takes a position similar to that of Geertz but ignores the relevant cross-cultural data. "*If latah is specific to Malayo—Indonesia, as I take it to be* [italics added], the question which then arises is that of the factors specific to this culture area which have led to it" (p. 210). Reviewing historical data on the prevalence of *Latah* and certain other aspects of Malay—Indonesian culture, Kenny concluded that ". . . *Latah* is a symbolic representation of marginality" (p. 209).

CONCLUSIONS

The present investigation was begun in the belief that a proper understanding of the nature/nurture issue could best be derived from the detailed cultural, phenomenological, and biological analysis of specific single behaviors. It is more feasible to untangle the role of cultural and biological components in brief and discrete phenomena than to do the same with larger behavioral categories such as nurturance or bonding. Startle is a particularly suitable phenomenon for such an analysis. Since any instance of startle is localized in time and space, it can serve as a natural analytic unit. It is easily identified by the person to whom it occurs, by other members of a startled person's society, and by investigators. As it is a discontinuity in experience and in the flow of ordinary social interaction, it is culturally marked in many (probably most or all) societies. Cultural elaborations of startle phenomena can be identified, described, and compared more readily than can those of less discrete and longer lasting behaviors.

Startle also lends itself well to biological analysis. Occuring in virtually identical form in lower animals, much of its behavioral biology and neurophysiology has been competently and minutely explicated. Lastly, startled persons and those who witness others being startled can easily provide vivid and detailed accounts of their experiences which can be analyzed phenomenologically. An ethological perspective, starting with an observed behavioral phenomenon and abstracting behaviors encompassing it at multiple levels, can reconcile explanations which, because of disparate levels of abstraction, apparently conflict. For example, Ekman and Friesen (1975) studying facial expression anatomically, neurologically, psychologically, and as used in symbol systems, have enormously added to our knowledge of how the face works. Many other phenomena readily lend themselves to investigations of this sort.

In contrast, approaches confined to single disciplines, no matter how finely analytic, necessarily ignore much relevant data. Which aspects of which phenomena can most profitably be analyzed with the tools of one discipline and which with the tools of another cannot be determined *a priori*. As understanding emerges, one can make intelligent decisions about which elements to investigate more thoroughly with which techniques. Very often a logical chain tracing a single behavioral element, e.g., responses to snake stimuli, will cross several disciplines. Natural experiments may exist which can be studied and experimental contingencies can be devised. For example, both observational and phenomenological data collected cross-culturally suggest that the sudden presentation of a sinuous line, especially if it is moving, is a potent elicitor of the startle response and that this may require little or no previous experience with snakes. Controlled experimentation is necessary to distinguish among various logically tenable explanations of this fact. Parallel experiments are planned with human volunteers and with subjects of other species.

The defect in purely cultural explanations of *Latah* such as Geertz' and Kenny's lies in what they do not explain (a) the correspondence of so many small and specific features of the *latah* syndrome in persons living in societies unrelated historically and culturally; and (b) its occasional appearance in persons in societies without a cultural tradition to account for *latah* behavior. The *latah* paradox disappears when *latah* is understood to be the culture-specific exploitation of a neurophysiological potential shared by humans and other mammals. Which facets of the behavioral biology of startle are exploited and which ignored, what cultural themes startle phenomena illustrate and exemplify, who may tease whom within what limits, are all culture specific. Cultural congruences such as those noted by Geertz and Kenny permit and shape local elaborations.

The present formulation is consistent with all of the known facts about *latah* — a claim which could not be legitimately asserted earlier.

NOTES

1. Departments of Psychiatry and Anthropology, Michigan State University, East Lansing, Michigan 48824.

The author is grateful for the generous support of the Harry Frank Guggenheim Foundation, which supplied the major portion of the costs of the investigation. This work was supported in part by the University of California International Center for Medical Research Grant AI 10051 from the National Institutes of Health, United States Public Health Service.

This work has benefited immensely from talks with James Anderson, George Barlow, Wallace Friesen, Brigitte Jordan, Lawrence Van Egeren, Sherwood Washburn, and most especially Paul Ekman, without whose insightful suggestions and repeated material and moral assistance the study could not have been carried out.

Helping the author immeasurably at one or another stage of the investigation were Mr. and Mrs. Jesus Cortez, Polly Crisp, Sidang Husain bin Dalip, Brian Kost-Grant, Leslie Lintern, Enche Yusoff bin Mohamad, Nakagawa Hidezo, Josefina Nazarea, Enche Amat bin Ngah, Ogata Motoi, Enche Jaafar bin Omar, Gunter Pfaff, Richard Schmidt, Betsey Shipley, Sandra Teel, the Latahs and other residents of Kampung Padang Kemunting and surrounding area, members of the Malacca Portuguese community, and many persons in and around the towns of Bay and Guagua in the Philippines.

The author thanks the Director, Institute for Medical Research, Kuala Lumpur, Malaysia, for permission to publish this article.

An abbreviated version of this paper was presented at the Annual Meeting of the American Psychiatric Association, Chicago, 1979.

2. To permit unambiguous reference, *Latah* (capitalized) will be used to refer only to the cultural elaboration of startle phenomena found in the Malay peninsula, the Indonesian Archipelago, and contiguous areas where *Latah* is the local term. Similarly, local terms for *latah* occurring elsewhere will be capitalized, and the general form will be denoted *latah*, with a lower case "l". [This usage has been superseded. See p. 32, this volume.]

3. Barlow (1977), because of the variability in the expression of these patterns, suggested the term "modal action pattern" to replace Lorenz's (1950) "fixed action pattern". He cited the following as characteristic of MAPS: "(1) The behavior patterns are stereotyped in appearance. (2) The pattern is produced by a functionally organized system in the central nervous system (CNS). (3) Once triggered, the behavior is able to run to completion without further environmental control, i.e., without exteroceptive feedback. (4) The behavior is spontaneous; its occurrence lowers the probability that it will soon recur. and its nonoccurrence increases its probability so much that the behavior may happen without apparent stimulation. (5) The directional (taxic) component accounts for much of the variation and is not a part of the core CNS coordination. (6) Though genetic differences may produce differences in spatiotemporal patterning, this patterning is little affected by experience" (p. 99, slightly modified by Barlow in a personal communication).

4. Ekman, P., Friesen, W. V., and Simons, R. C. *In press*. The Boundary Between Emotion and Reflex: An Examination of Startle. Journal of Personality and Social Psychology.

5. Among the Dusun Rungus, where female interest in and knowledge about sexuality is not acknowledged, the Naughty Talk after a startle is one of the few ways in which a woman publicly identifies herself as a sexual being (George Appell, personal communication).

6. E.g., the classic Army story: "So I meets this fucking girl, and we go to her fucking place, and we has intercourse".

7. In a collection of cartoons from the Lansing, Michigan. *State Journal* Sunday comics, some person being startled was present in one cartoon or another most weeks. The points to note here are that, in the United States as in Malaysia, Japan, and the Philippines, strong startle responses are regularly found to be amusing, and that there are American cultural elaborations of this fact (Simons 1979).

8. Even where not culturally exploited, this consequence of marginality (equivocal status) has been regularly noted, e.g., the following senryu from Japan published in about 1800:

> The second wife
>
> Jumps
>
> Even if a rat appears. (Blythe 1959: 351)

9. I have so far collected reports from three Westerners, two women and a man, who, living long among people with *latah* in their cultural repertoires, began showing mild forms of *Immediate Response Latah*, although they all tried to suppress it. None were subjected to techniques for *Attention Capture*. When a larger series is collected, these data will be analyzed and reported on.

10. In the course of discussing this, Geertz noted that, in Java as in several other societies in which *latah* has been found, "seizures" appear to be more easily provoked in the presence of higher status persons.

REFERENCES

Barlow, G. W.
  1977 Modal Action Patterns. *In* T. A. Sebeok (ed.), How Animals Communicate. Bloomington: Indiana University Press.

Beard, G. M.
  1880 Experiments with the *Jumpers* or *Jumping Frenchmen* of Maine. Journal of Nervous
         and Mental Disease 7: 487–490.
Blythe, R. H.
  1959 Oriental Humor. Tokyo: Hokusaido.
Callaway, E.
  1959 The Influence of Amobarbital (Amylobarbitone) and Metamphetamine on the Focus
         of Attention. Journal of Mental Science 105: 382–392.
Clifford, H. C.
  1898 Some Notes and Theories Concerning *Latah*. *In* H. C. Clifford (ed.), Studies in
         Brown Humanity. London: Grant Richards.
Collinder, B.
  1949 The Lapps. New York: Greenwood Press.
Czaplicka, M. A.
  1914 Aboriginal Siberia: A Study in Social Anthropology. Oxford: Clarendon Press.
Djamour, J.
  1959 Malay Kinship and Marriage in Singapore. *In* J. Djamour (ed.), London School of
         Economics Monographs on Social Anthropology. London: University of London.
Easterbrook, J. A.
  1959 The Effect of Emotion on Cue Utilization and the Organization of Behavior. Psy-
         chological Review 66: 183–201.
Ekman, P. and W. V. Friesen
  1975 Unmasking the Face. Englewood Cliffs, N.Y.: Prentice Hall.
Fleshler, M.
  1965 Adequate Acoustic Stimulus for Startle Reaction in the Rat. Journal of Comparative
         and Physiological Psychology 60: 200–207.
Geertz, H.
  1968 *Latah* in Java: A Theoretical Paradox. Indonesia 3: 93–104.
Gilmour, A.
  1902 *Latah* Among South African Natives. Scottish Medical Journal 10: 18–20.
Graham, F. K.
  1975 The More or Less Startling Effects of Weak Prestimulation. Psychophysiology 12:
         238–248.
Graham, F. K., L. E. Putnam, and L. A. Leavitt
  1975 Lead-stimulation Effects on Human Cardiac Orienting and Blink Reflexes. Journal of
         Experimental Psychology (Human Perception) 1: 161–169.
Kahneman, D.
  1973 Attention and Effort. Englewood Cliffs, N.Y.: Prentice-Hall.
Kenny, M. G.
  1978 *Latah*: The symbolism of a Putative Mental Disorder. Culture, Medicine and Psy-
         chiatry 2: 209–231.
Kunkle, E. C.
  1967 The *Jumpers* of Maine: A Reappraisal. Archives of Internal Medicine 119: 355–
         358.
Landis, C. and W. A. Hunt
  1939 The Startle Pattern. New York: Farrar & Rhinehart Inc.
Lorentz, K. Z.
  1950 The Comparative Method in Studing Innate Behavior Patterns. Symposia of the
         Society for Experimental Biology 4: 221–268.
Miller, G. A., E. Galanter, and K. Pribram
  1960 Plans and the Structure of Behavior. New York: Holt, Rinehart and Winston.
Murphy, H. B. M.
  1973 History and Evolution of Syndromes: The Striking Case of *Latah* and *Amok*. *In*

        M. Hammer, K. Salzinger, and S. Sutton (eds.), Psychopathology. New York: John
        Wiley & Sons.

1976   Notes for a Theory on *Latah*. *In* W. Lebra (ed.), Culture-Bound Syndromes, Ethno-
        psychiatry, and Alternate Therapies, Vol. 4. Honolulu: University Press of Hawaii.

Nakagawa, H.

1973   *Imu* of the Ainu. (Lecture privately published honoring the retirement of H.
        Nakagawa [in Japanese]). Sapporo, Japan: Sapporo Medical College.

Pfeiffer, W. M.

1971   Die *Latah*-artigen Reaktionen. *In* W. M. Pfeiffer (ed.), Transkulturelle Psychiatrie.
        Stuttgart: Thieme.

Simons, R. C.

1979   Elaboration of Biologically Significant Aspects of the Startle Reaction in Two
        Cultures. Presented at the annual meetings of the Animal Behavior Society/Interna-
        tional Society for Human Ethology. New Orleans: Tulane University.

Sternbach, R.

1960   Correlates of Differences in Time to Recover from Startle. Psychosomatic Medicine
        22: 143–148.

Teoh, J.

1972   The Changing Psychopathology of *Amok*. Psychiatry 35: 345–351.

Thorne, F. C.

1944–1945 Startle Neurosis. American Journal of Psychiatry 101: 105–109.

Tomkins, S. S.

1962   Affect-Imagery-Consciousness, Vol. 1. New York: Spring Publishing Co.

Uchimura, V. Y.

1956   *Imu*, eine psychoreaktive Erscheinung der Ainu-Frauen. Der Nervenarzt 12: 535–540.

Westermeyer, J.

1973   On the Epidemicity of *Amok* Violence. Archives of General Psychiatry 28: 873–
        876.

Yap, P. M.

1969   The Culture-Bound Reactive Syndromes. *In* W. Caudill and T. Lin (eds.), Mental
        Health Research in Asia and the Pacific. Honolulu: East-West Center Press.

1952   The *Latah* Reaction: Its Pathodynamics and Nosological Position. Journal of Mental
        Science 98: 515–564.

MICHAEL G. KENNY[1]

PARADOX LOST: THE *LATAH* PROBLEM REVISITED

R. C. Simons recently examined in this Journal (1980) the Malay–Indonesian condition known as *latah* in the hope of resolving a question posed by the anthropologist, Hildred Geertz (1968). The *latah* pattern is typified by susceptibility to sudden fright and is commonly described as a "startle reaction"; startle in turn leads to temporary dissociation accompanied by compulsive obscenity and/or mimesis. Throughout the area sudden fright or loss of poise are believed to render one open to the intrusion of erratic forces and hence, although there are degrees in this, *latah* is held to be involuntary. The pattern is a highly stereotypic, culturally labeled state which locally is differentiated clearly from insanity. Geertz, basing her observations on an extended period of fieldwork on Java, found that *latah* appears to have an intimate internal relationship to the most valued norms of Malayo–Indonesian culture — that it draws its energy and possibly its psychic motivation from its very contrast to these norms. Indonesian culture emphasizes order, self-control, and courtesy, and the *latah* — generally an older woman — contravenes all three.

Yet a paradox arose when it was noted that *latah*-like performances are reported from other cultures as well. Why, Geertz asked, if *latah* is so closely tied to the values of Indonesia, should it also occur in far distant and historically unrelated areas such as Mongolia, Siberia, or even Maine? It is this question to which Simons addressed himself and to which, in opposition to Simons, I address myself in turn.

Briefly put, Simons' position is that *latah* represents a universal human psychophysiological startle response which some cultures have seen fit to elaborate and label, sometimes to the point where it may assume role-like stereotypic qualities; but, in origin, startle is an instinctive pattern resulting in a "narrowing of attention" which can lead to mimesis and the eruption of socially unacceptable words or phases. Simons also holds that, whether or not it is culturally elaborated, all societies have some members — "hyperstartlers" — who are prone to exaggerated startle, and who therefore may provide a model for more general application (1980: 197). In support of this claim, he provides a sample of American subjects who reported responses analogous to those of the Malay *latahs*, including involuntary utterance of usually proscribed words. Although the Americans did not show compulsive mimesis, Simon believes that they could be made to do so if "after being aroused by a startle, they were to be confronted with adequately presented commands and models" (1980: 200). Given the presumed generality of this startle response, Simons proposes to use the term *latah* (lower case "l") when speaking of it cross-culturally, and *Latah* (capital "L") when in the context of Malaya alone (1980: 196, footnote 2); he then goes on to examine certain general social and cultural factors which affect its appearance in practice.[2] His final conclusion is that "the

63

Ronald C. Simons and Charles C. Hughes (eds.), *The Culture-Bound Syndromes*, 63–76.
© 1983 *by The Williams & Wilkins Co., Baltimore.*

latah paradox disappears when *latah* is understood to be the culture-specific exploitation of a neurophysiological potential shared by humans and other mammals"
(1980: 205).

Simons' case rests on a certain hypothetical interpretation of Geertz's paradox.
If this paradox either does not exist or can be explained with equal plausibility
in other ways, then his argument loses its force or at least its interest. The issue
is of some importance because it brings to focus certain of the basic difficulties
implicit in cross-cultural psychiatry, especially with regard to the interpretation
of the so-called "culture-bound syndromes" (Yap 1969). Here a basic question is
whether these are truly culture-bound or can in fact be explained in more general
ways. Simons' belief is that *latah* can be understood in terms of a biomedical
reduction to universal principles which resolve Geertz's paradox; my view, on the
other hand, is that the *latah* pattern can be fully explained in terms of its meaning
within specific social and cultural contexts. These alternatives are of significance
because of their implications for the nature of clinical practice; this dichotomy
between the biomedical and the cultural-meaningful, unnecessary as it should be,
nonetheless pervades Western psychiatry, and takes a particularly acute form when
Western theories are to be applied in non-Western situations.

My own contribution to the *latah* debate (1978) is based on Geertz's position
that the condition has a profound internal relation to Malayo—Indonesian culture,
and on the observation that psychiatric and anthropological interpretations of
latah and kindred states have, with little exception, been impossibly superficial. I
explored in detail the contextual significance of *latah* in Malaya and Indonesia,
and found that it is related to local witchcraft beliefs, to midwifery, to shamanism,
to folk art, and to fundamental ideas pertaining to the gaining of religious insight
and power through loss of self. In sum, I see the meaning of *latah* through its
position in an implicit system of relationships between elements of Malayo—
Indonesian culture. This meaning is complex and depends on the situations in
which *latah* is manifested or elicited; but the fundamental underlying pattern
is one which signifies marginality, disorder, and even transcendence. *Latah* is a
peculiarly appropriate means of communicating such marginality to others, which
it does in a number of ways. As in the case of midwives and shamans, it may be
an attribute of roles involving contact and mediation with supernaturals; some
people may use it to communicate their own marginality and distress, and in doing
so to publicly force acknowledgment and redress of their situation; still others
manifest *latah* for the gain involved in the ribald amusement which it arouses,
and may be employed as jesters at weddings. Hilarity, disorder, marginality, supernaturalism, transition, and loss of self are all intimately connected within the
cultural matrix of the *latah* pattern.

There is general agreement that "loss of self" — or, as it may be termed in
the West, "dissolution of ego boundaries" (Yap 1952: 544—545) — is a central
attribute of *latah*. I accepted this, but then, because an absence within a system
of communication is just as significant as a presence, I proceeded to examine the
metaphysical and sociological correlates of loss of self as such. The general finding

was that such "loss", as expressed symbolically through disordered behavior, can be put to culturally santioned use in demonstrating the presence of liminal marginality: an ambiguous boundary condition within the framework of ritual or within the related framework of an individual life. Such "disorder" can express pain and distress and hence be part of a pathological process but, equally, it can be put to uses in which pathology has no part at all, and so find a place in situations in which marginality or change of state is a culturally ascribed attribute: weddings, funerals, initiations, communion with the spirits, and so on. These conclusions in turn point to the meaning of the involuntary mimesis and obscenity of the *latah* who, virtually by definition, stands in a mirror relationship to specific norms of order, decency, courtesy, and poise. And this is the essence of Geertz's paradox, for, if *latah* is a parody or mirror-image of Malayo—Indonesian values — and is "funny" precisely for this reason — then why is it that this performance is also found in Siberia and elsewhere?

To rephrase the original question in this way — replacing *latah* by "performance" — suggests an interpretation which contrasts markedly to Simons'. Simons, we have seen, wishes to derive *latah* from a culture-specific exploitation of a neurophysiological potential. In contrast, I see *latah* as a culture-specific exploitation of a meaning potential implicit in a limited human repertoire of concepts pertaining to order, disorder, and self-identity.

The term "performance" is chosen because, in its neutrality — and unlike words like "reaction", "syndrome", or *latah* — it presupposes little about the meaning, cause, or psychopathological significance of its referent, while at the same time calling attention to the social nature of the display. This is not the case for Simons' proposal to use *latah* (lower case "l") as a label for what he evidently considers to be based on a homogeneous generic reality. The dangers of such an approach are shown by similar taxonomic mismanagement in the history of anthropology. Exotic words have been adopted and applied to apparently analogous phenomena outside of their culture of origin (the "totem" of certain native American groups becomes "totemism"; the "tabu" of the Polynesians becomes "anything which must be avoided", etc.). The general result of this process has been the delusion that such reifications actually refer to something, and once this is accomplished no further detailed attention to the facts is needed. In other words, the danger of adopting a term such as *latah* is that its application will blind us to possible differences between the things to which it is applied, this, of course, is the danger hidden in all taxonomies and nosologies, as the problem of "schizophrenia" amply shows.

However, Simons is working within a biomedical paradigm which stresses human biological and ethological universals and which requires concepts which are cross-culturally applicable. This necessity is manifest in Simons' desire to treat the Malay concept of *amok* in the same way that he has treated *latah*. He says, for example, that "though *amok* has long been considered to be a phenomenon restricted to Malay culture, parallel instances of rapidly repetitive, random homicide are frequently reported in the world press from many Eastern and Western socieites.

Only in Southeast Asia, however, has this behavior pattern been named and insitutionalized" (1980: 197). I find the assertion that *amok* is somehow the same as these other outbursts of homicidal violence to be quite astonishing. The stereotypic *amok* pattern is clearly labeled in Malaya, pertains to concepts of masculine honor specific to the area, and as such preexists any specific manifestation of it. Simons, however, is saying that *amok* behavior preceded its cultural selection and labeling, but — given the evident origins of *amok* in the warrior ethic of the old Malay kingdoms — this is unbelievable and, in any event, unprovable.

Simons is more clearly wrong with regard to *amok* than *latah*, and now I examine the latter in more detail. Performances strikingly similar to the *latah* pattern are indeed reported from a number of widely separated areas, but most consistently from northern Asia. Malay and non-Malay conditions began to be conceptually assimilated at quite an early date, and it is primarily material from Siberia and Mongolia which led to Geertz's initial puzzlement. Nonetheless, in my own paper on *latah* I emphasized its cultural specificity, while being aware of the grounds for Geertz's sense of paradox; Simons, on the other hand, states that I "ignore" relevant cross-cultural data, which is inaccurate, since I *dismissed* it on grounds of insufficiency and still do. Yet Simons is willing to generalize the *latah* concept on the basis of surface similarities and so I had best outline what these are. In neutral language, but consistently with local data, the performance pattern may be superficially characterized as follows:

1. Reduction in powers of self-control caused by sudden fright or startle leads to:
2. Involuntary and normally inappropriate acts which may include one or more of the following:
   a. Mimicry
   b. Compulsive obedience to commands
   c. The utterance of affect-laden words generally pertaining to sexuality.

This schema contains a number of elements and relations between them, each of which would ideally have to be understood in its cultural and social context before any claim could be made to truly comprehend the whole. The first factor is perhaps the most significant: (a) What local concepts define the nature of the "self", its powers, and those factors which diminish them? What are the phenomenological correlates of these beliefs? These questions are logically followed by: (b) How is fright conceived, and by what signs is it subjectively and objectively manifest? What things are considered "frightful" and why? (c) What role do mimicry, obedience, sexuality, and obscenity have in relation to the culture as a whole? (d) What other actions and experiences are held to be involuntary, how do these pertain to concepts of self-structure, and what causes them?

Answers to these questions would provide the ideological background to all the personal and social factors which have already been observed to contribute to the appearance of Malay *latah* itself. Of course, all specific cultural detail could be taken as a local version of what is actually the outcome of processes rooted in a universal biological substratum. Measles or smallpox, for example, are clearly identifiable disease entities, but receive very different cultural interpretations. Is this also true for *latah, amok*, and other ostensibly culture-bound syndromes? In short, are *latah*-like startle responses best considered as the "exploitation of a neurophysiological potential" or are they *themselves* more plausibly considered as the outcome of social rather than biological factors? If the latter proposition is the more acceptable, then the solution of the so-called *latah* paradox is effectively contained in the answers to the four sets of questions in the paragraph above, as considered in the dramatic framework of the *latah* performance. Hildred Geertz herself provided a step to this solution in pointing out "that Javanese are no more easily startled than anyone else, but what I am describing is a particular view of human nature which they hold" (1968: 100; see Kenny 1978: 215).

The Siberian material, though not truly adequate — and all of it quite old — allows certain tentative conclusions to be drawn about the local meaning of *latah*-like performances. As I have said, it is this northern and central Asiatic material which inspired the statement of Geertz's paradox in the first instance and so led to Simons' attempted resolution of it. In fact, both Geertz and Simons utilized secondary sources; Geertz drew on a widely cited paper by David Aberle (1952), and Simons employed Czaplicka's *Aboriginal Siberia* (1914) which, itself a synthetic account, derived from primary ethnographic sources, explicitly draws parallels between Malay *latah* and certain Siberian conditions. So, neither Geertz nor Simons looked closely at the Siberian data, though Geertz was certainly aware that better data might invalidate her senses of paradox: "This is the sort of paradox, obviously, which arise either where there is insufficient data or inadequate conceptualization" (1968: 104). I submit that Simons has not consulted the Siberian material because he is already caught in the conceptual box of universal lower case "l" *latah*.

There are earlier passing accounts of compulsive mimesis in Siberia, but most information about these interesting conditions comes from Russian enthnographers whose fieldwork was carried out in this century, before the Russian Revolution. Aberle cited three sources which provide detail on *latah*-like behavior: Jochelson's *The Koryak* (1908) and *The Yukaghir* (1926), and Shirokogoroff's *The Psycho-mental Complex of the Tungus* (1935).

I will use these same sources when commenting upon the cultural matrix in which Siberian *latah*-like performances take place, and judge the acceptability of Simons' hypothesis in terms of the results. There are interesting similarities between the Malay and the Siberian conditions. For example, Jochelson describes a certain form of "arctic hysteria" among the Yukaghir of northern Siberia: "Extreme susceptibility to fright is one of the symptoms of arctic hysteria. . . . At the least knock, shout, and generally at any unexpected noise, the patient shudders or falls backward. It is remarkable, however, that the fright usually evokes from the patient the most obscene words or phrases connected with the names of the sexual male or female organs" (1926: 33). The same pattern recurs among the Koryak of the eastern Arctic, where it is labeled by a word translated "to startle" (1908: 417); this is true again for the Tungus who label such behavior with a word derived from a verb translated "to be suddenly frightened" (Shirokogoroff 1935: 244). Simons therefore has a *prima facie* case, but let us consider the question more deeply by reference to the four sets of cultural factors which pertain to my neutral description of the common pattern.

As seen, the first and perhaps most significant cultural factor is that of the nature of the "soul" as it is locally conceived. What may be generally said, and this is true of Malayo—Indonesia as well, is that "startle" or "fright" is held to precipitate soul-loss which may then lead to the intrusion of evil spirits (Jochelson 1908: 101; Shirokogoroff 1935: 134–136). This process is objectively detected in disordered behavior, illness, and ultimately in death; phenomenologically it is represented as debility and loss of control. Children, in particular, are seen to be in jeopardy; this is a reflection of their general vulnerability expressed through the belief that children are more easily startled than adults. The Yukaghir provide a useful example of the context in which such soul concepts actually function: "The head-soul does not usually leave of its own accord, but on account of its fear of evil spirits which enter the body of a man and cause diseases. In such cases then the absence of the head-soul is not the cause but one of the consequences of the disease" (Jochelson 1926: 157). The Koryak theory of disease causation focuses in a similar way on a set of cannibal monsters who frighten the soul away and prey on its material residue. Curative practice accordingly concentrates on the shamanic expulsion of evil spirits and the enticing of the soul back into the body. "Fright" is a generalized folk etiology which, without clearly distinguishing between the "physical" and the "mental", explains how it happens that one becomes ill; as such, this theory figures in *post hoc* causal reconstruction of a process in which no actual emotion may have been experienced at all, and is only surmised from its putative result — illness. Given this theory, it may be seen that special conditions involving mimesis and obscenity are parts of a much more inclusive whole in which "startle" only ambiguously figures as a causal agent. Illness is considered due to the departure of something — the soul; but the cause of its departure must be construed as "fear" not "startle". Fear has an object, something which one would like to avoid or leave behind, and therefore is a mediated and culturally conditioned response, whereas "startle", as Simons presents it, is an involuntary and objectless mobilization reflex. Where, it might be asked, does one stop and the other begin?

Difficulties increase when mimesis and obscenity are themselves considered. Even in Malaya the degree to which "startle" precipitates individual cases of *latah* remains unclear. It is reported that some who manifest the condition first experienced dreams with unusual but stereotypic content, and then subsequently developed the typical *latah* performance pattern. A more potent example is that of the midwives who are held to have developed *latah* after taking up this occupation "since midwifery involves communication with supernatural entities" (Kenny 1978: 220). Therefore, susceptibility to hyperstartle is in some cases the *consequent* of other events. To the extent that this is true, it follows that *latah*-like performances often result from the self-fulfilling belief that certain people or kinds of people are unusually sensitive to influences which bring about alterations in powers of self-control. As Simons and others have shown, Malays believe that entire social categories — men, women, or children for example — have differing quantities of the soul-substance which renders them more or less liable to startle, soul loss, and spirit intrusion. However, these facts in themselves are not fatal to Simons' hypothesis as he also shows that some persons, for purely social reasons, may become educated into what he calls "*Role Latah*". Nonetheless, Simons maintains that this is simply the institutionalization of the universal hyperstartle response, and I now consider the truth of this in terms of the Siberian material.

The same difficulties found in the Malay literature also pertain to the Siberian, and again the basic problem is that of whether the components of hyperstartle should best be considered as prior to specific cultural institutions or as their result. Testimony in favor of the latter answer comes from the most systematic examination of *latah*-like performances in the Siberian literature, that of Shirokogoroff on the Tungus. These displays are called *olon* and may include mimesis, obscenity, or both. The ethnographer, however, concluded that "after a continuous observation and hundreds of experiments . . . I have come to the conclusion that in exceptionally rare cases there is a really 'pathological' condition of . . . 'imitative mania', while the rest of the cases are all due to the possibility of a manifestation of sexual [factors] or of a social 'rebellion' under the cover of olonism" (Shirokogoroff 1935: 247). Thus, in a culture with the institutionalized *olon* response, it is difficult if not impossible to separate the startle response from the social and cultural factors which affect its appearance. Shirokogoroff has shown how imitation and obscenity are socially conditioned — that they are indeed "performances" which, like Malay *latah*, may be used for a variety of ends (1935: 255) — and that, as such, they do not derive by any obvious route from observation of a preexisting startle response. This conclusion is reinforced by the fact that women who have been forced into mimetic behavior implore their tormentors to stop, even while they carry out outrageous acts at their instruction: "It is evident that there again is an element of consciousness in the continuing state of imitation, and it is only supposed by the *subject* to be an uncontrollable state" (1935: 250, my emphasis); the same odd mixture of consciousness and compulsion is reported from Malaya. Simons supposes that such compulsiveness — which he calls *Attention Capture Latah* (1980: 200) — results from a "narrowing of attention" brought about by hyperarousal. Yet Shirokogoroff shows that this supposed compulsiveness is merely the product of a culturally based attitude which the *olon* victim has *herself* tacitly accepted. Of course, given the procrustean quality of Simons' thesis, it can also be supposed that cases of this nature are really *Role Latah* derived from true *Attention Capture Latah*, but this is for Simons to demonstrate.

Tungus *olonism* is only indirectly related to supernaturalism, but is in a way similar to Malay *latah*. Shirokogoroff states that: "I have been frequently told by the Tungus how the person may become *olon* without any interference on the part of spirits" (1935: 244). However, he also shows how a "fearful" person is in danger of having his psychic equilibrium shaken by sudden contact with spirit beings (1935: 139), and how submission to a spirit may buy remission from the attack (1935: 206). The ethnographer also relates how he was able to compel verbal mimesis and compulsive utterance of spirit-names by merely mentioning spirits associated with solitary places or derived from the souls of suicides (1935: 139—140). Jochelson induced "nervous fits" in Yukaghir women by simply showing them a carved wooden figure in which a spirit was held to reside (1926: 167). *Latah* could be induced in Malay shamans by saying in their presence the names of animals, such as the tiger, with mystical connotations (Kenny 1978: 219); but such shamans are also credited with the ability to transform themselves into were-tigers, and the instability of *latah* is only an aspect of their general liability of form.

The effect of power-laden words suggests a view of the nature of Siberian "obscenity" which is at variance with Simons', though his own views on this question are less than clear. He points out that the involuntary obscenity of the *latah* involves words which "have in common . . . the fact that negative social sanctions follow their appearance in casual speech" (1980: 201). He believes that such emotive terms are "neurologically encoded in some special manner" and that they reappear verbally when the "guarding" which normally keeps them in the dark is temporarily removed under the impact of a strong stimulus.

The Siberian material again leads to a more complex view. Shirokogoroff does not say which words and phrases were typical of Tungus *olonism*, but he does discuss the relativity of the concept of "obscenity" itself. First calling attention to the normality of "obscene" sailor-talk, he then shows that *olonism* utterances are only "obscene" for younger child-bearing women and not for their older sisters; in fact, the latter tease and fluster the former into using them. Once more the social matrix of the performance is the key to the appearance of the phenomenon. In the same way, the "obscenity" of *latah* is not out of place in the context of the *latah* performance itself. My view was that this so-called obscenity is an aspect of marginality, of loss of control, of humor, and — given the mystically flavored sexual content of *latah* onset dreams — even of contact with supernaturals. The same logic can easily be applied to Siberia.

The actual content of involuntary obscenity is known for the Yukaghir and Koryak. It features exclamations translated as "vulva!" or "penis!" and phrases such as "the penis hangs; the vulva hangs!" or "the vulva splitted!" (Jochelson 1926: 33; Jochelson 1908: 417). In order to attain a provisional understanding of the meaning of this, it is necessary to consider the words themselves and the way in which power words are used. A good deal is known about the latter because of the place of words in exorcisms and spells. The Tungus, for example, believe that certain spirits flee "in fright" from the human voice (Shirokorogoff 1935: 140), and the Koryak belief is that words as such have an autonomous power, "that the course of events may be influenced by spoken words, and that the spirits frequently heed them . . . . In this way, diseases are treated, amulets and charms are consecrated, animals that serve as food-supply are attracted, and spirits are banished" (Jochelson 1908: 59; cf. p. 117). Koryak incantations dealing with the banishment of disease-causing cannibals are in the hands of older women who thus are the keepers of an oral literature which often is Rebelaisian in the extreme; this in itself calls into question the degree to which Koryak startle expressions can actually be regarded as "obscene" at all. Women and shamans are the mystical protectors of Koryak well-being, and a variety of techniques are available to expel or repel spirits, including the ritual use of excrement and the giving of unpleasant names to children so that spirits will not be attracted to them (Jochelson 1908: 60–61).

Jochelson does not delve into the possible meaning of startle-induced sexual exclamations, and states only that "Koryak women, when frightened, generally shout in this manner, and it must be considered as a symptom of hysteria" (Jochelson 1908: 247). He does, however, record a great number of stories in which the sexual organs figure in surprising ways, and which have in common the notion that the genitalia have a quasi-autonomous power in their own right but yet are also part-for-whole representations of their possessors.[3] Various mythic beings transform their sexual organs into persons or animals (Jochelson 1908: 139, 165, 168, 183). Elsewhere genitalia are said to have ritual uses, as when it is found that a shaman's drum has a vulva attached to it, and that its drumstick is a penis which, when played together, grant powers of weather control. In the hands of the shaman these "instruments" are used to alter the world. The sexual organs thus "speak" — that is, they act and work changes (Jochelson 1908: 20–26): "Even such things as the voice of an animal, sounds of the drum, and human speech, have an existence independent of that of the objects which produce them" (Jochelson 1908: 117).

I conclude that the sexual content of Siberian startle-utterance is mainly defensive or invocative in nature. These utterances assert the self-identity of their authors and offer defense against spirits which are frightened at being confronted by words which invoke the power of the things they represent. An example which Simons uses to demonstrate the ubiquity of the hyperstartle response — *Lapp panic* — reinforces this point. It was believed that a Lapp woman, if she were to suddenly encounter a bear, should expose herself to it, because "this gesture makes the bear ashamed" (Collinder 1949: 219).[4] "Indecency" was also believed to have been used by Malay witches to frighten spirits into submission (Kenny 1978: 219). In lieu of exposure we see sexual expletives in which the word is as good as the thing itself.

Facts such as these do not lead to great confidence in Simons' views concerning the releaser function of startle, nor is it obvious that the utterances so released need be considered as "naughty talk" at all. If the parts of a hypothesis are so questionable, what then is to be made of the whole? I maintain, as before, that the cultural meaning of situationally dependent displays such as mimesis and obscenity must be themselves understood before anything can be credibly said about their place in a sequence of putatively involuntary automatisms.

And the central issue in this whole problem is the sense in which *latah*-like performances are involuntary or originate in reflex-like processes which can be understood psychophysiologically. The cultures with which I have been dealing relate the genesis of such states to "fear" or "sudden fright" which, I emphasize again, is not necessarily the same thing as "startle", nor is "startle" itself necessarily a clear-cut reflex. Anyone who has been "slapped in the face" by an insult will know how "startling" such a culturally rooted assault can be, and that an immediate symbolic response is required to it. The Malay shaman who even verbally is exposed to contact with the tiger may respond abruptly, and so less stereotypically, with *latah*; Tungus exposed to lost souls automatically invoke a series of spirit names in response. Such events are permeated with meaning, and they are no less context-dependent and meaningful on account of their supposed involuntary quality.

"Fear" itself is socially conditioned, and (in English) is a complex notion which ranges from "fear" of loss of face, to "fear" of ghosts, to "fear" of heights, and so on. I would imagine non-English equivalents to be equally multivalent, and hence equally difficult to relate to any one set of perceptual or neurophysiological antecedents. If, then, a particular cultural tradition relates a given psychic aberration to "fear", one had better be quite sure just what is meant by it, and so far as I know none of the literature on *latah*-like states has made this attempt. *Latah*, *olon*, and their kin, are also complex notions which only partially involve behavior observably produced under the impact of sudden fright. Mimesis and command automatism, for example, may occur without any "startle" at all, and it is not clear whether, in many instances, it was ever even putatively a causative factor in initiating the pattern.

The body is a symbol. Its appearance and actions point beyond itself to an inner world, but also beyond itself to a total life situation. The body expresses a state of being, and the degree to which it is "controlled" represents this state. It is notoriously difficult to uncouple the psychic and the somatic, and the folk medical theories considered here do not really try as they make no precise recognition of the distinction. Soul loss due to fright explains a multitude of afflictions, and is a belief which does not unequivocally point back to "startle" as the model on which it was founded. Nor, if one looks further, is soul loss necessarily due to fear alone; the Siberian shaman cultivates the ability to "leave" his own body, which remains behind in a dramatically incapacitated state while his soul goes off to the spirit world. The shaman must show unstable and uncontrolled qualities in order to be publicly recognized. The entranced shaman, the *latah*, and the *olonist* demonstrate a modified state of being, indicating in doing so that they are in some way out of the ordinary and liable to contact with forces sharing this attribute. The performance then is publicly reinforced through the interest taken in it by others (Shirokogoroff 1935: 255). I would therefore say that proclivity to startle is a *sign* that the performer is in an unusual condition; as in the case of Malay *latah* this may then force re-evaluation of the actor. As with the fool in Elizabethan tragedy, the *latah*-performer steps outside the normal and makes transcendant comments on it in the process; startle provides but one cue to take this step.

This overt lack of control in bodily or verbal behavior is reflected in the inner state of the actor, for here we are dealing with "method" acting in which the performer becomes the part. Internal experience registers external expectation, and if there is social expectation that an act is performed involuntarily, then that is the way in which it comes to be felt. This is the key to the involuntary quality of the *latah* performance, as well as to the nature of the basic difference which separates my views from those of Simons. A more familiar example should make this distinction clearer.

Hypnosis, in western folk culture, is analogous to *latah* in that the subject's actions and self-experience are held to be under the control of the hypnotist. However, the only truly valid conclusion about this state is that the hypnotic performance is shaped by the expectations of the participants in it and by the sociological constraints of the hypnotic situation itself.[5] The hypnotist steers the experiences of his subjects, and they respond according to their conviction that something genuine is happening; the roots of this conviction reach into the 18th century. In hypnosis there is the experience of "ego-dissolution" without startle; rather, we have the opposite, ego-dissolution brought about by the induction of a state popularly regarded as resembling sleep. In neither the cases of *latah* and hypnosis do I see any necessity for supposing that these culturally rooted phenomena are built on the model of some universal neurophysiological response.

The boundaries between the "voluntary" and "involuntary" are, in large measure, culturally established. The difficulty in accepting this proposition stems from a naive view of the nature of the "ego". We say, in our everyday manner, that the self simply *is*, and fail to take account of the social contexts in which it functions and receives feedback about its own nature. "Consciousness", including "self-consciousness" is positional and cannot be considered as a reified abstraction. It is supposed, both in Malaya and Siberia, that persons in given situations are involuntarily open to certain experiences and, as with hypnosis, these duly make their appearance in accord with local expectation. If I look at my experiences in a certain way, I could easily say that they are *all* involuntary: my body moves itself down the street, my thoughts just come to me, I just say things without knowing why, etc. However, others insist that I take responsibility for most of my actions, and I come to view them as responsible self-created acts. But if others say that I am not responsible for certain things, then this is equally acceptable, and so I become educated into the experience of the involuntary: certain things may be said and done while drunk, while spirit-possessed, or while *latah*. When the occurrence of the involuntary is culturally sanctioned or even labeled, then it must be understood through its relationship to the norms of order from which its meaning is symbolically derived.

I conclude that the *latah* paradox does not exist.[6] Indeed, there are similarities between Malaya and Siberia with regard to certain of the features of the *latah* performance. It still has to be demonstrated how frequently these features occur elsewhere. Both Malaya and Siberia have hit on similar ways of indicating marginality; both have institutions, such as shamanism, in which loss of self is actively cultivated, and to which the *latah* pattern is related; but it is not clear to me just how far-reaching these similarities are. Siberia lacks the politeness pattern which makes true *latah* so evocative and hilarious in Malayo–Indonesia; Siberian obscenity seems instead to have locally specific invocative functions. On the other hand, both *latah* and *olon* seem to have the capacity to function as vehicles for symbolic protest on the part of marginal or otherwise disadvantaged persons; how such protests develop is a matter for future investigation.

Simons' hypothesis has a historical dimension; various cultural traditions are taken to have exploited the startle reaction in the development of certain institutions. But it must be said, even if my reasoning is otherwise quite misguided, that his hypothesis is destined to remain such, as the facts which might serve to establish it are not forthcoming and never will be. Of course, perhaps there is no problem here at all, and *latah* in its cross-cultural distribution is no more of a paradox than is the fact that all people have hands, but only some cultures have exploited the fact in requiring them to be shaken in formal greeting. If this is the case, then the *latah* performance is taken out of the province of biomedical reductionism and is seen in what I take to be its true light — as theater.

Yet the involuntary quality of *latah* has led to its being viewed as pathological; *latah*-like conditions have been persistently regarded as medical problems in spite of the fact that they are not particularly dysfunctional in their cultural milieu. Simons states that I "excoriate" psychiatric investigators for failing to take proper account of cultural considerations (1980: 203) and to this I plead guilty. Simons, in this context, is defending various investigators, such as Yap (1952), who he believes to have adequately dealt with *latah*-like conditions in cultural as well as medical terms. He seems to imply that these authors do not see *latah* as pathological; but this is not the case. For example, Simons states that Yap did not deal with *latah* as an "illness"; this is true — he called it a "disease" and did so in the first line on the first page of his seminal paper on the *latah* reaction. I reject the "disease" model of *latah* just as I reject Simons' more neutral and noncommittal neurophysiological and ethological approach.

This, in the end, is why: neither approach takes cultural factors adequately into account, Simons' claim notwithstanding, and therefore neither is in a position to understand *latah* performances in human terms, that is, in terms of their meaning within the systems of communication whereby people negotiate the quality and significance of their lives. In the entire history of the problem, no case of *latah*, with the partial exception of Kessler's Malay widow (1977), has been documented with sufficient care to penetrate its full meaning; in other words, no case study has successfully combined an analysis of *latah* as symbol and performance with a thoughtful examination of the social and psychological position of the person manifesting it. This easily documented lack of psychological depth and sensitivity is of particular note, as much of the *latah* literature is derived from the observations of psychiatrists; I take this situation to be a product of inadequate psychiatric models. Even Geetz, who herself noted the absence of detailed case studies, applied Aberle's psychoanalytic model of mimetic *latah* without in fact testing the truth of it against her own cases in the field. Aberle's and Geertz's interpretations, as well as those of psychiatry, are essentially deduced from propositions supposed to hold good for anomalous mental states in the West; but, if understanding of *latah* in its cultural context is as superficial as I take it to be, then clearly any attempt to interpret it in terms of Western psychological theory is premature at best. Psychiatric labeling theory indicates the further dangers which may accrue if *latah* is accepted as a nosological entity; it will then become something to be treated in the mental hospitals of Malaya, Indonesia, and elsewhere: but in what terms?

I do not deny the universality of the startle reflex, but it seems to be basically irrelevant to the understanding of *latah*. The consequences of adopting this or any other biomedical formulation are potentially great in that they may blur perception of the human content of the phenomena. I can only repeat what was said in 1898 by one of the earliest, and still one of the best, commentators on *latah*: "It is doubtless difficult for a medical man to always bear in mind that a patient is a human being in the first instance, and a 'case' purely incidentally" (Clifford 1898: 187).

NOTES

1. Department of Sociology and Anthropology, Simon Fraser University, Burnaby, British Columbia V5A 1S6, Canada.

    The author thanks Philip Moore, H. S. Sharp, and Yasmeen Jiwani for comments and criticism.
2. I use *latah* with a lower case "l" throughout this paper, but this should not be taken as adoption of Simons' terminology.
3. This idea has also occurred to the Malays, as *latah* induction dreams often feature detached but quite lively male organs; other beliefs also emphasize the detachability of body parts (Kenny 1978: 223).
4. The *latah*-pattern in Siberia presents a special problem. Such conditions appear to be widely reported right across northern Asia, from the Ainu of the northern islands of Japan in the east to the Lapps of Scandinavia in the west. This sort of consistent cultural similarity is worthy of ethnological investigation; the bear cult is also widely distributed.
5. I have elsewhere examined this process with regard to the perception and shaping of multiple personality phenomena (Kenny 1981).
6. Geertz accepted Aberle's essentially psychoanalytic approach to *latah*. On the basis of purely deductive reasoning they saw it as a defense in which the victim identifies with the aggressor. This hypothesis seems to me no more necessary than the neurophysiological.

REFERENCES

Aberle, D.
    1952 *Arctic Hysteria* and *Latah* in Mongolia. Transactions of the New York Academy of Science 14: 291–297.
Clifford, H.
    1898 Studies in Brown Humanity. London: Grant Richards.
Collinder, B.
    1949 The Lapps. New York: Greenwood Press.
Czaplicka, M. A.
    1914 Aboriginal Siberia. Oxford: Clarendon Press.
Geertz, H.
    1968 *Latah* in Java: A Theoretical Paradox. Indonesia 3: 93–104.

Jochelson, W.
    1908   The Koryak. Leiden: Brill.
    1926   The Yukaghir and the Yukaghirized Tungus. Leiden: Brill.
Kenny, M. G.
    1978   *Latah*: The Symbolism of a Putative Mental Disorder. Culture, Medicine, and Psy-
           chiatry 2: 209–231.
    1981   Multiple Personality and Spirit Possession. Psychiatry 44: 337–358.
Kessler, C.
    1977   Conflict and Sovereignty in Kelantanese Malay Spirit Seances. *In* V. Crapanzo and
           V. Garrison (eds.): Case Studies in Spirit Possession. New York: John Wiley and
           Sons.
Shirokogoroff, S. M.
    1935   The Psychomental Complex of the Tungus. London: Kegan Paul, French & Trubner.
Simons, R. C.
    1980   The Resolution of the *Latah* Paradox. Journal of Nervous and Mental Disease 168:
           195–206. (Reprinted in this volume.)
Yap, P. M.
    1952   The *Latah* Reaction: Its Pathodynamics and Nosological Position. Journal of Mental
           Science 98: 515–664.
    1969   The Culture-Bound Reactive Syndromes. *In* W. Caudill and T. Lin (eds.): Mental
           Health Research in Asia and the Pacific. Honolulu: East-West Center Press.

RONALD C. SIMONS

LATAH II – PROBLEMS WITH A PURELY SYMBOLIC
INTERPRETATION

A Reply to Michael Kenny

It began when my mother died. I was very sad. I was sitting quietly like this, thinking 'my mother is gone'. Someone came from behind. He grabbed me and said, 'What's up!' I was startled! My body trembled like this. My mind went blank. When my body stopped trembling he again suddenly poked me in the ribs. I picked up a stick and hit him. I couldn't think – what could I know? Later, wherever I went, people liked to watch me. They thought I was just pretending. They startled me with pokes in the ribs over and over again until I became ill. – Hajjah Misah Bani, a *Latah*

If we don't startle them with pokes in the ribs they don't become *Latahs*. If we keep poking a normal person like that he'll become a *Latah*. It doesn't take long; five days of poking over and over, little by little by little a person gets quite flustered. – Pawang Lumun, an indigenous healer

Any explanation of behavior which excludes what the actors themselves know, how they define their actions, remains a partial explanation that distorts the human situation. – James Spradley (1979: 13)

In 1980, I published in this *Journal* a paper entitled, 'The Resolution of the *Latah* Paradox' (Simons 1980). This was the first report of a series of investigations into *Latah* which was begun in 1975 and which continues to the present time. In the paper, I suggested an interpretation of *Latah* which seemed to me not only to account for the peculiar and specific constellation of behaviors which constitute the *Latah* syndrome but also to explain a hitherto puzzling fact, the occurrence of virtually identical behavior complexes in places as widely separated as Malaysia, Japan, Siberia, South Africa, and the state of Maine. In his present critique, Kenny challenges my interpretation and denies the very existence of the puzzling distribution my paper purports to explain. Instead, he argues for an alternative interpretation, first argued by him in a paper entitled, 'Latah, the Symbolism of a Putative Mental Disorder' (1978).

The present paper, a response to Kenny's critique, will contrast our two interpretations of *Latah*, the data from which they were derived, and the investigative techniques that have led us to such widely disparate interpretations of the same phenomenon. In it I will attempt to demonstrate that the investigative techniques and the interpretive framework which I use and which I term "ethological"[1] more adequately explain the data and are more useful than the techniques and the interpretive framework suggested by Kenny. I believe that the debate between us has significance beyond its immediate object, clarification of the nature of an uncommon culture-bound syndrome. Special features of *Latah* make it an especially useful exemplary case from which more general conclusions regarding

77

Ronald C. Simons and Charles C. Hughes (eds.), The Culture-Bound Syndromes, 77–89.
© 1983 *by The Williams & Wilkins Co., Baltimore.*

the usefulness of our two investigative techniques and ways of reasoning about data can reasonably be inferred.

DOES SYMBOLIC SIGNIFICANCE PRECLUDE BIOLOGICAL SIGNIFICANCE?

Kenny's critique, like his previous paper on *Latah* (1978) seems to me to rest on two fundamental misconceptions. First is his notion that by demonstrating that a behavior has symbolic meaning one has also demonstrated that biology is irrelevant in its causation. Since *all* human behavior is imbedded in cultural contexts and is therefore multiply symbolic, a logical extension of this position is that therefore *no* human behavior has a biological cause. With a caveat which I will discuss below, I am impressed with the literature review in which Kenny lays out the symbolic gloss for Siberian *olonism*. However, it says nothing about the presence or absence of biological factors in the etiology of *olon*. Biologically significant behaviors are always culturally elaborated and interpreted in ways perfectly congruent with all of Kenny's gloss. The argument that biology is irrelevant in the causation of any behavior with demonstrated symbolic significance is a non sequitur. Whatever a sneeze may symbolize, e.g., that the soul has temporarily left the body, or that the next statement uttered will be true, etc., sneezing is nevertheless more frequent in ragweed season.

The second misconception is that deductions from the literature somehow cancel out or refute the findings of present empirical investigations. It is more useful to consider such deductions as hypotheses which must stand or fall depending on what one discovers by empirical testing. In the present case my conclusion that *Latah* is a culture-specific elaboration of the startle reflex was not deduced but rather is based in large part on discoveries made by ethnographic investigation focused on this point and by the inductive analysis of films of hyperstartling Americans and of Malay, Ainu, and Philippine *latahs* doing *latah* behavior.

Kenny's summary of my formulation seems to me to be on the whole a fair one. It might be restated thus: I believe that *Latahs, mali-malis, imu-jaras, jumpers*, American hyperstartlers, etc. (persons exhibiting *latah* with a lower case "l") share a physiological peculiarity which differentiates them from their non*latah* peers. These persons are all hyperstartlers, persons who startle readily and violently. I believe that the physiology of the startle reflex explains why the behaviors that constitute the *latah* syndrome constellate as a set in Malaysia and also why essentially identical behavior sets are found wherever social and cultural conditions encourage the startle-teasing of vulnerable hyperstartling persons. The complex of behaviors associated with hyperstartling is always elaborated in culture-specific ways and is always imbued with specifically local meanings. However, as the physiology of hyperstartling is everywhere the same, the same set of behaviors is observed wherever social and cultural conditions encourage the frequent startling and subsequent teasing of hyperstartling persons.

Any anthropological argument must stand and fall on its own merits irrespective of whether the proposer was ever on site. However, there are some real consequences of the fact of my having gleaned my strongest impressions of *Latah* from having lived in Malaysia, having traveled in the Philippines for several months interviewing about *latah* and observing instances of it, and having studied films of the Ainu form of it collected by investigators in northern Japan. My field data include extensive interviews with *latahs*, relatives of *latahs* and other villagers, collections of stories about *latah*, genealogies, and, most importantly, repeated observations and film recordings of *latahs* in and out of *latah* states. In contrast, Kenny draws his conclusions by deduction from his study of previous ethnographic sources, not ever having, himself, seen or described any *latah* person or any *latah* episode. This circumstance does not affect the validity of either of our arguments, but it may explain why I find *latah* rather more complex and multifaceted than he. His formulation, "the *latah* pattern can be fully explained in terms of its meaning [marginality] within specific social and cultural contexts" (Kenny 1983: 160), is simple and elegant. However, no less a scientist than Einstein has observed that a theory should be as simple as possible, but no simpler. I believe that Kenny's formulation is far too simple and that it does violence to observed data. Kenny has not conducted an independent investigation and discovered that *latah* is not associated with hyperstartling persons. Rather his argument is that since *Latah* in Malaysia is embedded in and shaped by local meanings, no data whatsoever could be adduced to establish either the importance of physiology in its causation or the cross-cultural consistency of the behavior set which constitutes it. I submit that Kenny's reasoning does not make the interesting empirical data go away.

Although I believe that others looking at the film I have published [2] will also see what I saw, it is logically possible to imagine another analysis resulting in different findings. I can also conceive of another investigator collecting films which do not show what mine show (although I strongly doubt that this would be the case). Either would be a strong counterargument to the formulation which I have proposed. However, I do not see how any reading of previous ethnography can refute a present empirical finding.

IS STARTLE IRRELEVANT TO THE UNDERSTANDING OF *LATAH*?

Kenny flatly denies that the startle reaction is in any way connected with *latah* and categorically asserts, "I do not deny the universality of the startle reflex, but it seems to be basically irrelevant to the understanding of *latah*" (1983: 166). He supports this position by a highly idiosyncratic reading of a restricted selection from the relevant literature. In contrast, my conclusion, that an understanding of startle is central to the understanding of *latah*, is based on empirical research. Although I base this conclusion on empirical research, it will be useful to examine what the literature actually says. The literature describing the *latah* syndrome is voluminous, and although interpretations of *latah* vary considerably, descriptions of the observable behaviors which constitute it are remarkably similar. All accounts describe *latahs* as hyperstartlers, and all relate episodes of *latah* to a prior startle. Rather than pitting my authorities against Kenny's authorities I will confine my literature citation to three of the investigators Kenny cites as supporting his position: Aberle (1952), Clifford (1898), and Shirokogoroff (1935).

In the paper by Aberle which Kenny cites as supporting his contention that *Latahs* do not differ physiologically from most of the population, this is what Aberle actually wrote:

The severe *latah* seems *always to show a strong reaction to being startled or frightened* [italics added]. He may jump violently or freeze, or flee, or turn on the source of his surprise and attempt to destroy it . . . . This startle reaction, especially when there is coprolalia, is considered a mild form of *latah*. Severe *latahs* may first respond to a stimulus with the startle reaction and then proceed to imitation, but some seem to show the startle reaction alone on occasion, and some pass into imitation without first being startled on occasion . . . (1952: 292).

Thus Aberle reported that all severe *latahs* are hyperstartlers, that their responses may include a violent startle ("jump") and hitting out, that a strong startle reaction itself, especially with coprolalia, is locally considered a form of *latah* (which I have called *Immediate Response Latah* [1980: 199]), that when imitation occurs it usually follows a startle (*Attention Capture Latah* [1980: 200]), and the interesting and puzzling fact that though they are always hyperstartlers, "some pass into imitation without being startled on occasion" (*Role Latah* [1980: 200]). In short, although his interpretation differs, Aberle's description of the behaviors which constitute *Latah* is wholly congruent with mine.

Kenny also misrepresents the conclusion of Sir Hugh Clifford. Clifford observed that *Latah* and startle were intimately related:

Latah is an affliction, a disease, one hardly knows what name to give it, which causes certain men and women to lose their self-control for longer or shorter periods as the case may be, whenever they are startled, or receive any sudden shock . . . . A complete stranger, by startling a *latah* man or woman can induce the condition, of which I speak, accidentally and without exercising any effort of will (1898: 189).

The book by Shirokogoroff which Kenny cites, *The Psychomental Complex of the Tungus* (1935), discusses a variety of conditions and is largely theoretical. In the section on *olonism* (his term for the Tungus' form of *latah*), reports of actual incidents are extremely abbreviated and say little about stimuli but rather focus on response. Nevertheless, and although Shirokogoroff's interpretation is, as Kenny observes, that *latah* is "an ethnographic complex", the fact that startle is important in its causation is embedded in his description, too:

From the observation of a great number of facts and evidences published by other observers it may be supposed that the first moment, immediately after the loss of psychomental equilibrium due to unexpectedness of some change in the situation, e.g., when a person of the milieu in which the subject finds himself, makes a sudden movement or produces an unexpected sound or complex act, – there is a moment of shaken consciousness when the act of 'imitation' is committed (Shirokogoroff 1935: 250).

In this excerpt Shirokogoroff cites "other observers"; his paper, however, also contains observations of his own in which *latah* behavior was produced by a knife failing down suddenly in front of a man (who seized it and stabbed with it), and by intentional actions toward another person "which would suddenly attract his attention", etc. I have quoted here only authors cited approvingly by Kenny. I leave it to any interested reader to examine the rest of the *latah* literature.

The Malay informants I interviewed also related *Latah* to startle, as, for example, in the interview excerpts which begin this paper. In fact all Malaysians interviewed (villagers, city-dwellers, *Latahs*, non-*Latahs*) made this same association and supported it with a wealth of corroborative detail about stimulus side and response side events. For lack of space I will quote only two more:

At first one is merely startled. One sees a centipede or snake or a coconut leaf falls, and one is startled. Then someone sees that happen. Later when he sees me again perhaps he'll poke me in the ribs. After a while something can happen. Take an ordinary person like Betsy here – if she's startled – Whenever you see her you startle her with a poke in the ribs. After a while she'll get very flustered! She'll say whatever comes out. If you tell her to dance, she'll dance. If you startle her with a poke in the ribs whenever you see her, she'll do this too [demonstrates] That's what it's like.   Cik Layut binti Ali, a *Latah*

Ethnographer (R. C. S.): "If someone startled you with a poke in the ribs every day, would you become *Latah* or not?" Informant: "If it were done face to face like this, I think not. But if it were done from behind, and over and over I think I'd become a *Latah* too." – Sidang Hussain bin Dalip, village headman

Most importantly, there is the empirical evidence gathered in the research which led to the findings I reported. When I traveled in the Philippines and in Malaysia searching for persons with *latah* and observing *latah* episodes I found these to be invariably precipitated by startle, and local informants invariably used startling stimuli of various types to induce *latah* behaviors. The stimuli used were sudden unexpected loud noises, sudden pokes in the ribs, objects suddenly thrown, on one occasion a photographer's flash bulb, and so forth, their only common denominator being that they all were startle elicitors. I filmed every episode of *latah* that I could and studied these films. Without exception the films show episodes to be preceded by strong startles. In addition I studied the film records of *latah* (*imu*) made in Hokkaido in 1936 and in 1972. These *imu* episodes are also invariably induced by startling stimuli and begin with the *imu* subjects exhibiting exaggerated startles.

MARGINALITY

I believe that Kenny is most likely correct in his assertion that *Latah* is overrepresented in marginal persons, though neither he nor anyone else has presented corroborating survey data. Much anecdotal evidence in the literature supports this contention, and it is congruent with impressions I received in both the Philippines and Malaysia.

It is, however, a great leap to conclude from that probable association that marginality is the cause of *Latah*. Why any correlation has been observed is always a question to be anwered; it can never be assumed that an observed correlation results from direct causal association. In the case of *Latah* and marginality there are several reasons why the association cannot be a simple causal one. First, there is the fact that by any definition of marginality only a miniscule fraction of marginal persons are *Latahs*. Why these and not the others? Second, some *Latahs* are persons who by no stretch of the imagination can be considered marginal. If marginality is the cause of *Latah*, how is it that these persons are *Latahs*? Marginality is neither necessary nor sufficient to produce *Latah*.

As I argued in the 1980 paper, I believe that the association between marginality and *Latah* results from two sets of factors. The first set is psychological and physiological: marginal persons tend to monitor their environments more continuously and more intently than nonmarginal ones (Chance and Larson 1976). Because wariness leads to strong and easily elicited startles, other things being equal, marginal persons tend to startle more readily and more violently than their nonmarginal peers. The second set of factors is social and cultural. In cultural contexts in which startle-teasing is encouraged, those who lack the power to retaliate receive a disproportionate share of such teasing. As marginal persons on the whole are less likely than others to be able to exert effective negative social sanctions, marginal persons are more likely to receive startle teasing than others. Thus in Malaysia the persons who are most likely to startle readily and strongly for physiological reasons are the very ones who are intentionally startled most frequently for social and cultural reasons.[3]

THE PARADOX

I have accused Kenny of ignoring relevant data from other parts of the world which fail to support his thesis. In his present rebuttal Kenny says that he has not ignored these data but rather has "*dismissed*" them (italics in original). Lack of space precludes extensively quoting the voluminous literature so dismissed; let me give but two examples. The first is from the state of Maine:

One jumper when standing by a window, was suddenly commanded by a person on the other side of the window, to jump, and he jumped straight up half a foot from the floor, repeating the order. When the commands are uttered in a quick loud voice the jumper repeats the order. When told to strike, he strikes, when told to throw it, he throws it, whatever he has in his hands. Dr. Beard tried this power of repetition with the first part of the first line of Virgil's Aeneid and the first part of the first line of Homer's Iliad, and out-of-the-way words in the English language, with which the jumper could not be familiar, and he repeated or echoed the sound of the word as it came to him, in a quick sharp voice, at the same time he jumped, or struck, or threw, or raised his shoulders, or made some other violent muscular motion . . . . It was not necessary that the sound should come from a human being: any sudden or unexpected noise, as the explosion of a gun or pistol, the falling of a window, or the slamming of a door, provided it be unexpected and loud enough, would cause these jumpers to exhibit some, one or all of these phenomena . . . . All of the jumpers agree that it tires them to be jumped and they dread it, but they were constantly annoyed by their companions (Beard 1880: 487).

The second is from South Africa:

"In all three (subjects) sudden auditory, tactile or visual stimuli produced the diseased condition. Sudden and unexpected noises caused them to imitate these sounds, while words, musical
notes, etc., were accurately repeated by the men. A sudden touch appeared to make them
lose control of themselves, while all movements made by the experimenter were copied without
fear of consequences. In this way a practical joker by shooting out his arm would cause the
latah man to involuntarily follow his example, even though he knew he would strike a more
powerful man standing beside him . . . .

"Consciousness and intellect remained clear, but the mimicry was unwilling, even though
every effort was exerted by the subject to escape from his tormentor. These men were conscious of and ashamed of their infirmity, but in no instance was any effort made by the victims
to retaliate at any time on those amusing themselves at their expense and they were frequently
the butt of practical jokers of all ages . . ." (Gilmour 1902: 19).

"Native traditions and superstitions are usually supposed to determine the type the psy-
chical disease will assume in various races. It is therefore peculiar to find the cases seen in South
Africa so closely resembling the cases of *Latah* described in the Malay peninsula, where obviously folklore and custom so widely differs. In the three cases mentioned above no influence
of religion or superstition could be traced, and no native name could be found applied to the
disease . . ." (Gilmour 1902: 20).

I do not see how correspondences such as these, repeatedly described by many
observers, can be dismissed. Kenny refers to my thesis as "procrustean", referring
to the giant who stretched unfortunate travelers who were too short to fit his bed.
It will be remembered that Procrustes also had a way of dealing with travelers who
were too tall for it; he cut their legs off. I leave it to readers to decide whether in
dealing with data I or Kenny more closely resembles Procrustes.

Kenny refers to these correspondences as "superficial", and he considers cross-
cultural examples of *latah* to have only "surface similarities". What he means by
"superficial" and "surface similarities" is that only the behaviors correspond;
the meanings attributed to them differ in the different cultural settings. But this
is precisely the key to understanding *latah*. Hidden behind the pejorative terms
"superficial" and "surface" is the observation that in different cultural settings,
the behavior sets correspond even though the meanings attributed to them do not!
It is this very observation that forces one to conclude that each behavior set cannot
be fully accounted for by its specifically local meanings.

Kenny says that he finds the correspondence of these behavior sets unremarkable
("no more remarkable than that all people have hands").[4] Because what anyone
finds remarkable is a personal matter, Kenny has a legitimate right to his apathy.
However, I for one would not have expected to find as improbable a set of behaviors
as hyperstartling, automatic obedience, matching the behavior of others, and (often)
uttering normally tabooed words associated in such a diverse set of places.[5] To me
and to most previous investigators this has been a great puzzle. To one who believes
latah to be adequately explained in terms of purely local meanings *latah*'s distribution *ought* to be a paradox.

Geertz, who first used the term "paradox" in this context (1968: 104), is quoted
in the preface to my 1980 paper, *q.v.* Here let me quote Aberle:

"Comparison of accounts of Malay *latah*, the imitative form of *arctic hysteria*, the North Africa condition, and the French Canadian (or mixed French Canadian and American) Jumpers of Maine, with the Mongol *belenci*, etc. and *acting belenci* indicates that all of these syndromes are identical, symptom by symptom, except that coprolalia is not mentioned for the Jumpers or for North Africa. The condition is found in Arabs, Negroes, and 'mixed' (Arab-Negro?) individuals in North Africa as well as in one Maltese" (1952: 294).

[Aberle lists other areas and peoples and concludes]: "Theories relating to culture areas, social structural features, or to childrearing practices, which will cover this range of cultures, are hard to conceive of at this point" (1952: 295).

In his 1978 paper, Kenny suggested a symbolic explanation for the occurrence of the set of behaviors which constitute *Latah* in Malaysia, and in his present rebuttal he has suggested a second explanation for Siberia. Thus, even dismissing the cross-cultural data from elsewhere, he is forced to account for the correspondence of the behavior sets in these two culture areas; the paradox cannot be escaped. He resolves his "mini-paradox" thus: "Both Malaysia and Siberia have hit on similar ways of indicating marginality" (1983: 166). I submit that "have hit on" is not an adequate explanatory concept and hence not a viable alternative to the explanation I have proposed.

AMOK AND OTHER CULTURE-BOUND SYNDROMES

Space precludes a complete answer to the question of whether *amok* is also a culture-specific exploitation of a universal neurophysiological human potential. Here it will be possible to merely sketch out the reasoning involved; a more complete discussion of the problem of *amok* will be published elsewhere. In brief I argue that Kenny's explanation of *amok*, perhaps most fully and cogently argued by Carr (1978), is a tautology. Kenny, like Carr, argues that the meaning of *amok* can be "fully" understood only in the context of Malay culture, an assertion that is indisputable. All behavioral phenomena are embedded in local systems of meaning which powerfully influence their expression and shape. Yet as with *latah* a phenomenon exists which local meaning does not fully explain. That phenomenon is the fact that in many times and in many places persons, always or almost always men, after some loss or insult which is taken to heart, do not seek revenge on the person(s) responsible for their loss but instead embark on a rampage of indiscriminate killing. Purely local explanations are inadequate for phenomena of widespread occurrence. There is a body of knowledge concerned with rage and aggression in humans and other animals. I do not find compelling the logic of an explanation which considers only local systems of meaning and rules out *a priori* the possible relevance of that body of knowledge.

IS KENNY'S ARGUMENT SOUND ANTHROPOLOGY?

Kenny frames his argument as a conflict between medical and anthropological models of reality, the former preoccupied with the body, cases, and pathology, the latter with the symbolic meaning of events. As I have pointed out above, this is a dichotomy I cannot accept, as there is no necessary logical tension between interpreting any event as both embodied and symbolically significant. The body and its vagaries are the kind of raw stuff of which symbols are made. I also believe that a fair-minded reader of other investigators of *latah* with psychiatric backgrounds (e.g., Yap [1952; 1969], Pfeiffer [1971], and Murphy [1973; 1976]) would show them to be far more cognizant of the anthropological significance of *latah* behavior than Kenny alleges and also to consider anthropological and psychiatric perspectives as complementary rather than alternative. But even if one were to accept the proposition that *latah* must be understood only "anthropologically", the question remains, how sound is Kenny's anthropology. I think not very.

The first problem is the illogic of holding that if a behavior can be shown to be symbolic one has thereby shown that it is *only* symbolic. Next there is the highly selective reading of the relevant literature which allows Kenny to dismiss or misrepresent both the extraordinarily well documented association of *latah* with startle and the incidence of *latah*-like behavior sets in culture areas other than Siberia and Malaysia. Sound anthropology does not ignore relevant data to make points.

Furthermore, there are all the problems inherent in the culture-at-a-distance approach. The Malaysia that Kenny speaks of is an amalgam of many sites and several centuries of culture change. I cannot recognize in his characterization (e.g., "gaining of religious insight and power through the loss of self" [1983: 160], indecency used by Malay witches to frighten spirits, *latah* as symbolic protest, etc.) anything that corresponds to the reality of the villages in Melaka and Negri Sembilan I studied. I am not competent to discuss the ethnography of Siberia, but I find Kenny's description of Siberia suspect for the same reason.

Kenny has not *discovered* the symbolic meaning of *latah* in Malaysia to be "marginality"; rather he has *deduced* that this is what it must mean from 8000 miles away. In contrast, when I collected Malay stories about *Latahs*, and when I tape-recorded, transcribed, and studied descriptive histories and anecdotes, other themes emerged. The recurrent themes in actual *Latah* stories deal with social vulnerability, the laughableness of not being in control of oneself, and to a surprising extent (and one not at all justified by actual events but especially interesting in this cultural context) the danger of being in other than full and proper control of oneself and the danger of being in the presence of someone who is not in control.

The *latah* paradox could be reformulated in symbolic terms as "How is it that this particular set of symbols has been used repeatedly with a variety of meanings in a variety of cultural contexts?" Kenny's best gloss is that the Malays and Siberians "have hit on" them. No less an anthropologist than Raymond Firth has stated that "One of the main tasks of anthropology is the reduction of arbitrariness as it appears in symbolic allocation . . ." (1973: 62—63). My work could be understood as an attempt to reduce that arbitrariness by specifying why *latah* behaviors regularly constellate as a set.

"CASES", THE MEDICAL MODEL, CONSEQUENCES, AND
A HUMANE VIEWPOINT

Kenny says, "The body is a symbol", an irrefutable proposition. But the body is also a body. Even the common cold may be legitimately considered as theater so long as it is not claimed that it is theater only. Although I do not fluster easily, I have been flustered often enough to have no difficulty in empathizing with the state *latahs* described to me. Sir Hugh Clifford put it thus:

The man who is the victim of a sudden fright or nervous shock loses for a moment all control over his body, as completely as the Malay on whom *latah* has won its firmest grip. The difference which exists between him and the *latah* man is only one of degree, and that difference may be more trifling than that which separates one *latah* subject from another. Imagine a start or 'jump' infinitely prolonged, and you have the *latah* state about which so much has been said and written (1898: 196).

In America too, startled persons, even without a belief in startle-caused soul absence, sometimes do and say things that they had not planned, occasionally with socially embarrassing results. Kenny's argument about voluntary and involuntary behavior does not cancel the common observation that sometimes there is a difference between what one blurts out when startled and what one meant to say. It should be noted, moreover, that his argument is not merely against the proposition that *latahs* sometimes behave involuntarily, but rather against any behavior by anyone ever being so considered.

Kenny makes much of the issue of whether *Latah* has ever been considered a disease or an illness and points out that at least it has sometimes been so considered by authors such as Yap. However, the question is not how *Latah* can be classified in one or another scheme. Difficulty in classifying hard cases perplex all classificatory schemes. A phenomenon like *Latah*, so complex and multifaceted, will find itself classified ambiguously with great regularity. Clifford used the term "affliction". It is often that.

I routinely asked *Latahs* whether, if a medicine were available, they would wish to take it to stop their excessively strong startles and hence their *Latah*. Although few expressed any convincing desire for such treatment, some of those few were very convincing. I myself saw how cruel the teasing to which they were subjected could be, and I had no difficulty in understanding their desire for anything that would reduce their susceptibility. Most of these were men who found the *Latah* role extremely uncongenial and who had established a more reclusive way of life than they desired in order to avoid social situations in which they were vulnerable. To offer such persons the option of a treatment, deconditioning or a medication, seems not at all unreasonable, and in some instances a great charity. Is Kenny arguing that because *Latah* is culturally meaningful, treatment should be withheld from those requesting it?

In his abstract Kenny raises the question of the practical consequences of our two viewpoints, and in the body of his critique he says, "Psychiatric labeling theory indicates the further dangers which may accrue if *latah* is accepted as a nosological entity; it will then become something to be treated in the mental hospitals of Malaya, Indonesia, and elsewhere . . ." (1983: 166). His argument is that accepting the view that *latah* has a physiological substrate will inevitably result in unfortunate consequences for those so labeled: they will be rounded up and herded into asylums for involuntary treatment. But clearly this is polemical and a *non sequitur*. Persons with conditions described by biomedical nosology – colds, toothaches, phobias – may or may not choose any sort of treatment, and when chosen, treatment is not tantamount to involuntary incarceration in mental hospitals. Kenny's argument is also based on deduction rather than on the ethnography of disturbed behavior in Malaysia. Aberle's comment is instructive on this point: "Ellis [Medical Superintendent of the Government Asylum at Singapore and someone who believed *Latah* to be caused by neurophysiological pathology] said that he had only one *latah* in his psychiatric ward, and she was his head nurse, a thoroughly competent and sane individual" (1952: 292).

Kenny concludes by accusing me of failing to recognize that a *Latah* is a human being and not "a case". When I reflect on my life in the village I do not think that accusation justified. In the village, I did my best to observe local etiquette, entered into a pattern of reciprocal favors and obligations according to local custom, and tried hard to understand the nature of the life experience of those defined locally as *Latahs*. But, perhaps Kenny means something less personal. Seeing all human activity in terms of its symbolic value only, he construes any alternative explanation in terms of clinical and "cases". I do not accept this dichotomy. While recognizing that all human activity has important symbolic dimensions, I nevertheless believe that emotions and other bodily states (e.g., hunger, thirst, lust, love) can be experienced as real and not merely as the raw material for dispassionate symbolic elaboration. All humans startle. For those who startle excessively and whose behavior and experience are therefore radically disrupted when they are startled, managing startles is socially problematic. How problematic depends on where, how, and how often they are startled. This is determined by society and culture. Thus in cultural contexts in which there are no sanction against startling them repeatedly, they are faced with a very human predicament. I could go on, but the argument is given in fuller detail in my earlier paper. This seems a perfectly human, humanistic, and humane way of looking at *latah*; in contrast seeing *Latahs* as disembodied bearers, markers, or tokens of some symbolic system seems to me to leave out their humanness altogether.

An empirical inductive approach such as that which I have taken has many advantages. First, it seems intuitively obvious that if the question is what is the nature of that behavioral entity locally termed *Latah*, the logical investigative strategy is to go to the place where it is endemic, inquire about its local definitions and meaning, and to look at it. This clearly seems preferable to selectively analyzing previous ethnographies from a predetermined theoretical perspective.

Second, an empirical inductive approach allows one to discover new facts not predicted by the theory that determines the investigation. In the present case, for example, I learned how Malay villagers believed *Latah* to be induced by their repetitive poking of hyperstartling persons, that when role-performing *Latahs* perform a kind of sham startle to justify otherwise inappropriate behavior, that villager friends of *Latahs* quiet them by inducing them to limit incoming stimuli (by ordering them to pretend to sleep or to cover their faces) when they are considered to be excessively stimulated, that villagers hesitate to poke and startle men, etc., etc., etc. Although I could predict none of these observations before I went to the field, all had to be accounted for by the unifying formulation I ultimately derived.

Last, an empirical inductive approach produces data which can be examined and evaluated by others. I recorded every instance of *Latah* I could film. Excerpts from these films have been released and hence are available for independent viewing.[2] They show all instances of *Latah* to be preceded by real or enacted startles and they show those persons who are defined locally as *Latahs* to have exaggerated startle reactions. Those who on theoretical grounds knew that there could be no more than seven planets refused to look through Galileo's telescope. Will Kenny refuse to look at my film? Kenny concludes by quoting Sir Hugh Clifford, whom he identifies as "one of the earliest and still one of the best commentators on *latah*" (1983: 166). Let me conclude by quoting him also:

... anyone who desires to really account for this affliction must begin by examining and explaining the pathology of the common start or 'jump' to which we are all in a lesser or a greater degree subject. This must be the starting point . . . . (Clifford 1898: 197).

NOTES

1. This interpretive framework has been powerfully used by Engel, who refers to it as "the biopsychosocial perspective" (1977). Barkow, taking a hermaneutic perspective, has written of "vertically integrated explanations" (1980). For reasons which I will elaborate on elsewhere I prefer the term, "ethological".
2. '*Latah*, A Culture-Specific Elaboration of the Startle Reflex', 16 mm, color, optical sound, 38 minutes, available for rental or purchase from the author.
3. Vulnerable persons may receive startle teasing virtually any time they appear in public. See the quotes from Malay informants cited in this paper.
4. I believe Kenny is here being disingenuous. As he has devoted one paper to explaining why the behaviors that constitute *Latah* occur in Malaysia and a good portion of another (his present critique) to explaining why they occur in Siberia it can reasonably be inferred that he finds these behaviors at least a trifle remarkable.
5. Microcorrespondences are even more convincing. One finds, for example, observers from quite diverse times and places noting that commands must be presented immediately after the startling stimulus and in a framed and forceful manner or they will not be followed.
6. Department of Psychiatry, Michigan State University, East Fee Hall, East Lansing, Michigan 48824.
   The author is grateful for the generous support of the Harry Frank Guggenheim Foundation which provided the major portion of the costs of this investigation, and thanks Mary Lynn Buss, Frederick Erickson, Anne Millard, and Lawrence Van Egeren for their comments on an earlier draft.

REFERENCES

Aberle, D.
  1952 *Arctic Hysteria* and *Latah* in Mongolia. Transactions of the New York Academy of
       Science 14: 291–297.
Barkow, J.
  1980 Sociobiology: Is This the New Theory of Human Nature? *In* A. Montague (ed.),
       Sociobiology Examined. New York: Oxford University Press.
Beard, G. M.
  1880 Experiments with the *Jumpers* or *Jumping Frenchmen* of Maine. Journal of Nervous
       and Mental Disease 7: 487–490.
Carr, J.
  1978 Ethno-Behaviorism and Culture-Bound Syndromes: The Case of *Amok*. Culture,
       Medicine and Psychiatry 22: 269–293. (Reprinted in this volume.)
Chance, M. R. A. and R. R. Larson
  1976 The Social Structure of Attention. New York: John Wiley & Sons.
Clifford, H.
  1898 Studies in Brown Humanity. London: Grant Richards.
Engel, G.
  1977 The Need for a New Medical Model: A Challenge for Biomedicine. Science 196:
       129–137.
Firth, R.
  1973 Symbols Public and Private. Ithaca, N.Y.: Cornell University Press.
Geertz, H.
  1968 *Latah* in Java: A Theoretical Paradox. Indonesia 3: 93–104.
Gilmour, A.
  1902 *Latah* Among South African Natives. Scottish Medical Journal 10: 18–20.
Kenny, M. G.
  1978 *Latah*: The Symbolism of a Putative Mental Disorder. Culture, Medicine and Psy-
       chiatry 2: 209–231.
  1983 Paradox Lost: The *Latah* Problem Revisited. Journal of Nervous and Mental Disease
       171: 159–167. (Reprinted in this volume.)
Murphy, H. B. M.
  1973 History and Evolution of Syndromes: The Striking Case of *Latah* and *Amok*. *In*
       M. Hammer, K. Salzinger, and S. Sutton (eds.), Psychopathology. New York: John
       Wiley and Sons.
  1976 Notes for a Theory on *Latah*. *In* W. P. Lebra (ed.), Culture-Bound Syndromes,
       Ethnopsychiatry, and Alternate Therapies, Vol. 4. Honolulu: University Press of
       Hawaii.
Pfeiffer, W. M.
  1971 Die *Latah*-artigen Reaktionen. *In* W. M. Pfeiffer (ed.), Transkulturelle Psychiatrie.
       Stuttgart: Thieme.
Shirokogoroff, S. M.
  1935 The Psychomental Complex of the Tungus. London: Paul, Trench, and Trubner.
Simons, R. C.
  1980 The Resolution of the *Latah* Paradox. Journal of Nervous and Mental Disease 168:
       195–206. (Reprinted in this volume.)
Spradley, J. P.
  1979 The Ethnographic Interview. New York: Holt, Reinehart & Winston.
Yap, P. M.
  1952 The *Latah* Reaction: Its Pathodynamic and Nosological Position. Journal of Mental
       Science 98: 515–564.
  1969 The Culture-Bound Reactive Syndromes. *In* W. Caudill and T. Linn (eds.), Mental
       Health Research in Asia and the Pacific. Honolulu: East-West Center Press.

EMIKO OHNUKI-TIERNEY

SHAMANS AND *IMU*: AMONG TWO AINU GROUPS
Toward a Cross-Cultural Model of Interpretation

The Tungic term *saman* has long been with us in anthropology and other disciplines in Western academia. During the first half of the 20th century, however, shamans, as the term became anthropologized or Anglicized, were regarded primarily as "primitive" magico-religious specialists who carried out so-call individual rituals. They were regarded as less important or impressive than monks, priests, and other religious specialists who represented a body of people or a religious institution and who officiated in elaborate rituals. With respect to individual personalities, shamans were often regarded as mentally ill, although anthropologists were quick to recognize that many of the technologically less advanced peoples were more tolerant than their highly industralized neighbors in not ostracizing their deviants, but rather providing them with a culturally sanctioned role.

In the recent past, there have been significant findings and insights both in the study of shamanism and mental disorders in general and culture-bound reactive syndromes in particular. Scholars continue to be concerned with the individual personality of shamans as well as with culture-bound reactive syndromes despite a rapid decrease in the frequency of their occurrence. If there is a possibility that shamans are psychologically disturbed on one hand, and that the culture-bound syndromes are expressions of psychological problems on the other, then there is a need to look closely at the relationship between the two. Yet we have seldom seen such studies.

The aim of this paper is to suggest possible ways of understanding the interrelationships between shamans and culture-bound syndromes as well as to examine the sociocultural correlates of these phenomena. While I hope that the present interpretation may serve as a model with cross-cultural applicability, my immediate goal is to understand these phenomena among the Ainu. For this purpose, I compare two Ainu societies – the Ainu of the northwest coast of southern Sakhalin and the Ainu of the Saru River region in Hokkaido. Remarkable contrasts are seen between these two Ainu groups both in the nature of shamanism and in *imu:*, which scholars have referred to as the culture-bound syndrome of the Ainu.

While the topic of this work lies at the interface between anthropology and psychology or psychiatry, the nature of evidence presented in this paper is more anthropological than psychological, with the purpose of interpreting significant correlations in cultural institutions.

The data on the Ainu of the northwest coast of southern Sakhalin were obtained during three separate periods of fieldwork in Wakasakunai and Tokoro in Hokkaido (one year in 1965–1966, three months in 1969, and another three months in 1973). The shamanistic practices and associated cultural phenomena discussed in this paper are those of the Ainu who, during the first half of the 20th century,

Ronald C. Simons and Charles C. Hughes (eds.), The Culture-Bound Syndromes, 91–110.
© 1980 *by the Society for Psychological Anthropology.*

inhabited the northwest coast of southern Sakhalin, extending from north of Rayčiska (Japanese designation: Raichishika) to the former Russo-Japanese border. Together with the rest of the Sakhalin Ainu, they are now relocated in Hokkaido. Information on the Hokkaido Ainu of the Saru River region is derived from various published sources. Although publications on the Hokkaido Ainu are almost innumerable, the bulk of work pertains to the Ainu of the Saru River region in the Hidaka-Tokachi region of Hokkaido during the first half of the 20th century. The largest concentration of the Hokkaido Ainu has been found in this region and their Ainu way of life has remained intact much longer than elsewhere in Hokkaido.

My discussion starts with a brief description of the two Ainu societies, followed by a presentation of major characteristics of shamanism and *imu*: in these two societies. In the last section of this paper, I present hypotheses regarding the interrelationship between the phenomenon of shamanism and that of *imu*: in these two societies so as to offer a cross-cultural model. Throughout the paper, I use the ethnographic present.

THE SOCIETIES

Despite a common assumption that Ainu culture is monolithic, not only are there significant differences between the three major Ainu groups — the Hokkaido, Sakhalin, and Kurile Ainu — but there also are significant intracultural variations within each group. All of the Ainu, however, share some basic cultural features, such as the high development of oral tradition and the basic subsistence economy which consists of hunting, fishing, and gathering plants. My presentation here is confined to major differences between the northwest coast Sakhalin Ainu and the Hokkaido Ainu of the Saru River region in Hokkaido as they relate to shamanism and *imu*:. In what follows, the two groups will often be referred to simply as the Sakhalin Ainu and the Hokkaido Ainu, unless further specification is necessary.

The Ainu on the northwest coast of sourthern Sakhalin are semisedentary, engaging at least in seasonal migration between their coastal summer settlement and the interior winter settlement. Their population is extremely small with most settlements consisting of less than five nuclear families. The Hokkaido Ainu of the Saru River region, on the other hand, enjoy the largest population of all Ainuland. A few settlements there consist of close to 30 families, and the population of more than half of the settlements in the valley exceeds 5 families (Izumi 1952: 34; Watanabe 1972: 264).

The nuclear family is the basic social unit among both the Sakhalin Ainu and the Hokkaido Ainu. A settlement in both regions consists of male agnates as the core members with patrilineal descent and patrilocal postmarital residence as the rule.

As a corollary to the small size of the population, formal political structures and social stratification of any kind are little developed among the Sakhalin Ainu. Even in the case of larger settlements, two communities may share a common political organization. In contrast, the formal political structure is more developed among the Hokkaido Ainu, each settlement having its autonomous political organization.

There has been no systematic study of the status of men vis-à-vis that of women in any Ainu society. Scholars note that men as a group enjoy a much higher status than women in Hokkaido (Kindaichi 1961: 44) and that the difference of status between men and women is greater among the Hokkaido Ainu than among the Sakhalin Ainu (Chiri 1973: 153). We might guess that the presence of a more formalized political structure among the Hokkaido Ainu necessarily creates a greater power differential between women and men, who alone have access to the political authority. In other words, the distance between the public and the domestic sphere becomes greater in such a situation (for the definitions of "domestic" and "public", see Rosaldo 1974: 23). Among the Sakhalin Ainu, meager development of the formal political structure structurally reduces the distance between the two spheres. Furthermore, greater flexibility in role assignments and in other structural features which govern the lives of men and women in society is required by the ecological conditions. These conditions include the small population size, necessitated by the environment in which the Ainu live and by their methods of hunting and gathering, and the semisedentary settlement pattern which results from the climate and the fluctuation in available resources.

It must be stressed, however, that unlike the assumption of some scholars that all hunting-gathering populations enjoy sexual egalitarianism, the Sakhalin Ainu are highly sexist in their ideological norm. There is an explicit ranking based upon sex and age, with male elders on top of the apex and young females at the bottom. The ideological norm is meticulously supported by daily behavioral rules such as the seating arrangement at the hearth in the house and various other manners. In other words, political power vested in males is of no great significance due to the meager development of political organization, and, therefore, the formalized power differential between men and women is not great; yet their ideological structure which governs the day-to-day behavior of the Ainu is quite nonegalitarian, placing males as a group above women. (For details of the differences between the two Ainu groups, see Ohnuki-Tierney 1976; for details of the social ranking, see Ohnuki-Tierney 1974: 84–85.)

SHAMANISM

Shamanism Among the Sakhalin Ainu

Among the Sakhalin Ainu, shamanism receives high cultural valuation. The shaman's rites are performed only after sunset inside the house beside the hearth with glowing embers as the only source of light. The Ainu regard the hearth as a miniature universe as well as the residence of Grandmother Hearth, without whose mediation no human prayers would ever reach the deities. A shaman, male or female, starts a rite by beating a drum, whose sound invites good spirits to aid the shaman and chases away evil spirits which attempt to interfere with the rite. Amidst smoke and aroma produced by three plants (a branch of spruce or larch, a mildly narcotic plant called *nuhča*, and a minced dried leek)[1] placed on embers and aided by a salty drink (sea water or river water with tangle coated with salt)[2] which the shaman takes, he or she reaches the climax. At this point he or she becomes possessed by a spirit and reaches a state of trance or at least semitrance. The spirit, then, speaks through the shaman delivering messages from the deities about the illness or whatever matter for which the rite is performed. Characteristically, a spirit decides upon which particular shaman to possess and a shaman has no say in the matter. Although these spirits are difficult to identify, they are mostly small animals; major deities of the Ainu pantheon such as bears do not become spirits in shamans.

Descriptions of shamanistic performance reveal that the Ainu shamans carry out at least four roles, all of which may be in operation simultaneously. Shamans are theatrical performers, religious specialists, health care specialists, and also covert politicians. Of the four roles, only the one of religious specialist and that of health care specialist are formalized; they are given "formal status and recognition" by the Ainu (see Chiñas' definitions of formalized and nonformalized roles in Chiñas 1973: 93–94; the nonformalized roles may be referred to as "functions" or "dimensions").

Shamans as theatrical performers have received much attention in recent anthropological literature (e.g., Beattie 1977; several articles, especially Leiris, in Beattie and Middleton 1969; Firth 1966–1967). Indeed, Ainu shamanistic rituals are the only type of regular communal entertainment for which almost everyone in the settlement gathers at the beat of the shaman's drum which announces the commencement of a rite. The performance of miracles in particular has a large element of theatrical performance. These performances include such feats as fetching the soul of a sick person that has already migrated to the world of the dead, fetching the mouthpiece to a pipe lost in a sea storm, and the like (for details of these performances, see Ohnuki-Tierney 1973). In the past they played an even more important part in the repertoire of male shamans, and their legends seem to provide a significant proof of the power of shamans in general.

As religious specialists, shamans are unimpressive. They are passively possessed by spirits, which are minor members of the Ainu pantheon. They perform the rites only as individuals for individual clients in a house. Their "humble" status becomes obvious when contrasted with a male elder, a politico-religious leader of the community, who holds an elaborate ceremony for the supreme deity, the bear. Not only the entire community, but also members of adjacent settlements and even distant east coast communities are invited to participate in the ceremony, which lasts for several days. The elder, acting as host, receives much admiration from all the participants for his generosity in holding the ceremony.

Shamans are also the only kind of health care specialist available in northwest coast Ainu society. Although the role of medical doctor is critical in any society, there is an additional dimension in the Ainu shaman's role as a medical doctor. Thus, Ainu shamans are doctors for the illness of an individual but they are also in charge of the healing of social ills. This dimension becomes apparent when we take a close look at Ainu definitions of illnesses for which shamans are consulted and the process by which diagnoses are reached. Ainu shamans are asked to diagnose and cure illnesses, all of which are characterized by the involvement of most of the important members of the Ainu universe — demons, deities, souls, and spirits — in the etiology, as pathogens or sources of cures. For example, *kamuy iramohkari* (punishment by the wrath of a deity) strikes when an Ainu engages in some form of disrespectful behavior towards a deity. Or, *aymawko ahun* (entrance of the spirit of an arrow) takes place when a member of the community utters angry words about someone else in the community. The words then become an arrow which is shot into the victim's body, thereby causing this illness. These illnesses are usually not characterized by a standard set of symptoms and only shamans can identify and provide the cures. Or, even when a set of symptoms immediately identifies the illness, the particular etiological circumstance which led to this instance of the illness must still be identified by a shaman who then can provide instructions for the cure. In all of these cases, however, the victim who falls ill may not necessarily be the one who violates the Ainu moral and social codes. (For details of these illnesses, which I label "metaphysical illness", see Ohnuki-Tierney 1980a, 1980b.)

The definitions of these illnesses clearly indicate that they are seen as expressions of disjunction in the network of social relations among the beings of the universe, caused by human misconduct. Thus, in the Ainu medical scheme, an illness of an individual is an expression of a social ill (cf. Turner 1975: 159). The role of shamans is to examine the behavior of their fellow Ainu to locate the seat of these disarticulations. As judge of the moral and social behavior of fellow Ainu, however, a shaman cannot be autocratic. Before reaching a diagnosis, shamans ask their patients about their dreams, feelings, and thoughts about themselves and others. They may also receive pertinent information for diagnosis from others in the community. When a shaman reaches a diagnosis, it must be convincing not only to the patient but also to the rest of the community. The process of diagnosis thus indicates that the diagnostic ability of shamans rests heavily on their knowledge of the behavioral patterns and personalities of the members of the settlement and of interpersonal relations among them. For example, anybody who is ill tempered, apt to provoke others verbally, or generally antisocial must be a likely suspect in the case of *aymawko ahun*, the illness caused by harsh words. For shamans to blame some other type of person is not convincing, and may cause the loss of their credibility and even their profession. Ainu shamans, therefore, must be skillful social analysts, although this ability may not have to be as extensive as that of the Ndembu doctor (Turner 1967: 359—393) and the Chinese soul raiser (Elliott 1955: 134—140), who operate in much larger societies.

This discussion leads us to another important role which Ainu shamans play — their role in social control. They can even act as covert politicians, subtly direct-ing the course of events in the community by evaluating the conduct of others, thereby affecting the behavior of offenders of Ainu moral codes and nonoffenders who are nevertheless reminded of the outcome of misconduct. Their nonformalized power in this area takes on even greater significance when we consider the absence of elaborate legal codes and the meager development of a formal political structure. It should be reiterated, however, that the role of the shaman as politician is a covert and nonformalized role, which some shamans can play if they so choose.

Although an individual must receive a call before becoming a shaman, both men and women can become shamans. The Ainu do not regard shamans either as cunning, mysterious, or abnormal in any negative sense; they are simply ordinary Ainu who have a special gift for interacting with the spirits and deities.

Until recently, male and female shamans were equal in number, but since World War II, female shamans far outnumber male practitioners, possibly as a result of the more rapid acculturation of Ainu men than women. Although my sample is too limited to suggest it as a rule, Ainu men barred from access to the regular routes for political success are attracted to a shaman's career. For example, a noted shaman of the Rayčiska settlement was blind and therefore could not engage in hunting, fishing, and other male activities which provide the means for males in Ainu society to achieve power. The Ainu situation corresponds with the involvement of politicially peripheral males in shamanistic/medical professions in other societies (Lewis 1971: 100–105; Mair 1969: 216; Needham 1973, 1976; Turner 1967: 371; Worsley 1968: ix–xxi). Shamanistic practices provide the practitioners neither with economic gains nor with political power. Only when a male shaman happens to be already politically powerful does his shamanistic ability add to his reputation and power. This was the case with a political leader at the Hurooči settlement. (For details of northwest coast shamanism, see Ohnuki-Tierney 1973, 1980b.)

Shamanism Among the Hokkaido Ainu

Very little information is available on Hokkaido Ainu shamanism, due in part to the lack of significance assigned to shamanism both by the Ainu themselves and by outsiders. Scholars point out that Hokkaido Ainu shamanism is not as developed as Sakhalin Ainu shamanism (e.g., Kindaichi 1944: 299; Hanihara et al. 1972: 178). Among the Hokkaido Ainu, shamans are reportedly all women (Kindaichi 1961: 45; Segawa 1972: 192), although in the past there were some male shamans (Chiri 1973: 23; K. Wada 1971: 19). Batchelor (1927: 275–285), on the other hand, notes that he met both male and female shamans. Hokkaido shamans also enter into a possession trance. In sharp contrast with the possession trance of Sakhalin Ainu shamans, a Hokkaido Ainu shaman becomes possessed only if a male elder induces it in her by offering prayers to the deities (Kindaichi 1961: 45; K. Wada 1971: 18–19). Their role is also to diagnose illnesses. It is to be noted, however, that their function is confined to diagnosis, after which male elders take over and engage in the healing process (Munro 1963: 10; Uchimura et al. 1938: 36).

Available information on Hokkaido Ainu shamanism, then, suggests two major features which distinguish it from Sakhalin Ainu shamanism. First, it is the exclusive territory of women at least during the recent past (roughly during the 19th century and early 20th century). Second, Hokkaido Ainu shamans play a much more minor role — they are no more than assistants to male elders and are not autonomous or full-fledged specialists in medicine or religion.

Shamanism in Ancient Ainu Society

In order to further interpret the shamanism in these two Ainu groups, I now refer to information available about shamanism in the past. Using oral tradition, Chiri advances an interpretation that the culture hero, who is a central figure in the Ainu oral tradition in most regions, represents Ainu political leaders who necessarily were shamans in the ancient society of the Ainu (Chiri 1953: 90; 1960: 111). As Chiri (1973: 19) points out, a shaman-chief is often accompanied by his "sister", who is also a shaman. These female shamans are the ones who, during their possession trance, deliver instructions from the deities with regard to political, economic, and other decisions that males were about to make. At that time, the shamanistic ability of a wife, sister, mother, or of any close female relative was essential for the success of a male who was or who strived to be politically successful (cf. Kindaichi 1961: 45—46). In the recent past, however, major decisions have been made by the males without the consultation of shamans, thus demonstrating the diminishing importance of shamans in the workings of Ainu society. Chiri (1973: 8) places a special emphasis on the fact that at the time of shaman-chiefs, an element of theatrical performance was much greater. Chiri (1973: 23) suggests that shamanism lost its importance in Ainu culture between the 17th and 18th centuries.

Even in northwest coast Sakhalin Ainu Society, in which shamanism continued to enjoy a favorable cultural valuation up to the ethnographic present, there are some indications that shamanism received even higher cultural valuation in the past. In a tale from the oral tradition of the northwest coast, two brothers, who lived at the Rayčiska settlement at the beginning of the world and are regarded by the Ainu as their great ancestors, are said to have been powerful shamans. One of them was married to the Goddess of the Sun and Moon and could travel to the sky while performing a shamanistic rite. In a sacred tale from the east coast, the culture hero during his battle with female demons is saved by a woman whom he subsequently marries. She is depicted as being a "deity-like" young woman with shamanistic ability (Kindaichi 1914: 103—104). In another story, also from the east coast, the culture hero himself is described as being a powerful shaman (Pilsudski 1912: 149—155). The story implies that he is expected to excel in miracle performances rather than in the ordinary curing of illnesses.

In shart, both in Hokkaido and Sakhalin, it seems that shamanism received a high cultural valuation in the past and that shamans enjoyed high social standing. Also, there were both male and female shamans. Although male shamans alone were at the same time political leaders, female shamans played an integral and vital role in the decision-making processes of male shaman-chiefs.

Although a reconstruction of the ancient society of the Ainu must remain speculative, there is enough evidence to suggest that Ainu societies in the past were very small; on the basis of historical resources, Watanabe (1973: 93–100) presents an excellent summary of demographic figures of Ainu settlements in the past, which ranged between a few to a dozen houses in a settlement.

Figure 1 summarizes the information presented so far on shamanism in three Ainu societies: (1) ancient society; (2) the society of the northwest coast of southern Sakhalin; and (3) the society of the Saru River region in Hokkaido. When the society is small, as in the case of the ancient society and the northwest coast society, both men and women are shamans. Significantly, in both societies, shamanism receives high cultural valuation. An important distinction between the two societies is that male shamans were also political leaders in the ancient society, while the two roles are independent in the northwest coast society. In fact, some male shamans are politically marginal, since shamanistic ability is not automatically translated into political power. Disparity between political authority and shamanistic power, however, is not as significant as it may seem, since, as a corollary to small population size, formal political structure is not well developed and hence not as much authority is vested in political leaders. Although the ideological norm of the northwest coast Ainu subscribes to sexual stratification, as I discussed earlier, political power vested in males is not great, and therefore inequality between the sexes is reduced in practice. Furthermore, basic flexibility rules required by ecological factors necessarily mitigate the degree of stratification of any kind in the society. Since it shared similar ecological conditions, my guess is that, in regard to political structure and sexual stratification, a similar picture holds true for the ancient society.

Society	Ancient Ainu	Northwest coast of southern Sakhalin	Saru River valley in Hokkaido
Size	small	small (5–25 people)	larger (25–150 people)
Political organization	meagerly developed	meagerly developed	well-developed
Sexual stratification	meager development?	meager development	well-developed
The sex of shamans	men and women	women and (politically marginal) men	women only
Shamans and political arena	politically central	politically marginal	outside of political structures
Cultural valuation of shamanism	very high	high	low

Fig. 1. Shamanism in three Ainu societies.

Shamanism as a cultural institution in the society of the Saru River Ainu in Hokkaido, on the other hand, is significantly different. In this larger society, with a more developed political organization, all shamans are women and shamanism receives low cultural valuation.

This three-way comparison of shamanism suggests a possible cross-cultural generalization in terms of the relationship between shamanism and political power. In a very small society shamanistic ability is an important component of political power. When a society becomes larger and a group religion or an institutionalized religion develops, as in the case of Hokkaido Ainu society in the recent past, the group religion (e.g., the bear ceremony) takes over political functions and shamanism loses its high cultural valuation. In a larger and more complex society, the distance between the public and the domestic domain is greater, with the public domain receiving much higher cultural valuation. The allocation of activities often starts to follow the sex line more strictly, relegating the activities in the public domain exclusively to men. As a corollary, the role of shaman is assumed by women who have no access to the political arena, whereas males claim the leadership in group religions that lie in the public domain. The northwest coast Ainu society occupies a position midway between ancient Ainu society and Hokkaido Ainu society. In the northwest coast society, this separating out of the political from the shamanistic power is already starting to take place, but shamanism continues to receive high cultural valuation and is open to both sexes.

IMU: – A CULTURE-BOUND REACTIVE SYNDROME OF THE AINU

In order to discuss its possible relationship to the personality of shamans, I describe in this section a temporary psychobehavioral departure from the norm, referred to as *imu*: in Ainu. At least a brief description is justified because details of *imu*: have been published only in Japanese (for more detail than space permits in this paper, see Ohnuki-Tierney 1980b: Appendix III). Of particular interest to the topic of this paper is that, as in the case of shamanism, the nature of *imu*: demonstrates several significant differences between the Sakhalin Ainu and the Hokkaido Ainu – a fact that has never been systematically pursued in any language. In what follows, I rely primarily on my own data on the northwest coast Sakhalin Ainu and the data gathered by Uchimura et al. (1938) for the Hokkaido Ainu, although all other available sources have been consulted and are presented when pertinent.

The meaning of the Ainu word *imu*: is not clear (Chiri and Wada 1943: 67; see also Uchimura et al. 1938: 9–10). Neither the northwest coast Sakhalin Ainu, nor the Hokkaido Ainu regard *imu*: as any type of illness. They simply regard the behavior during an *imu*: seizure as amusing, and they often make fun of it. If a respected shaman or a political leader happens to be a victim of *imu*:, it in no way affects the respect which the person commands; the others laugh at the victim of *imu*: only during the seizure. In this regard, the Ainu attitude is similar to the one held by the Eskimos toward *pibloktoq* (Wallace 1972: 374, 379) or the Malay and Indonesian attitude toward *latah* (Kenny 1978: 209).

Not being an illness, *imu:* requires neither diagnosis nor cure among the north-west coast Sakhalin Ainu. Among other Sakhalin Ainu groups, however, *imu:* is said to be caused by possession by a spirit, called *imu: kamuy (kamuy* = deity) (K. Wada 1964: 112). The Niputani Ainu in the Saru River region of Hokkaido, under Munro's investigation, also link *imu:* with possession by a snake. Thus an *imu:* victim would usually consult a shaman and "a frequent diagnosis is that the illness is due to possession by an evil snake spirit" (Munro 1963: 161). It is some-what unclear whether *imu:* is identified as an illness by the Niputani Ainu or its reference as an illness is done by Munro himself.

The Sakhalin Ainu see two distinct categories of *imu:*. The first category in-volves a mild state in which an individual becomes surprised, but not necessarily frightened, and mumbles meaningless sounds. Each individual *imu:* Ainu, when surprised, almost always utters the same nonsensical phrases, such as "Ačikapahse", which has no meaning in Ainu. While in the field, I once stood up, bumped my head on a bare light bulb hanging from the ceiling, and uttered an English exclama-tion, "Oops". Those Ainu present thought that I was experiencing an *imu:* state, since they had never heard the English expression which was of course meaningless in either Ainu or Japanese. (In fact, this incident precipitated a series of discussions on *imu:* which provided rich ethnographic information.) The manner in which an *imu:* victim reacts to a mild shock is seen as analogous to the way in which a seed pod of a certain plant snaps open and expels the seeds; this plant has been identified by Chiri (1953: 81) as *Impatiens noli-tangere* L. The plant is thus named *imu: kina (kina* = grass in Ainu). Individuals with an *imu:* tendency seem to become *imu:* whenever they are surprised. One informant stated that she became more susceptible to an *imu:* stimulus when she was tired.

The second category of *imu:* constitutes a more severe state during which the individual loses touch with reality and has no control over him or herself. The Sakhalin Ainu refer to these individuals "who do *imu:* in a grand way" as *sikutu,* and terminologically distinguish them from the milder *imu:* Ainu. Each individual exhibits a definite pattern during the *imu:*. According to B. Wada (1956: 45), the Sakhalin Ainu *imu:* is characterized by manifested automatic obedience — doing what one is told to do. In the samples listed by Uchimura et al. (1938), the compulsive imitation of what one observes (echopraxia) and compulsive imita-tion of what one hears (echolalia) are also noted.

The symptoms of the Hokkaido Ainu *imu:* are more varied. According to B. Wada (1956: 45), the Hokkaido Ainu *imu:* is characterized by negative automatic obedience, thus being in sharp contrast to the Sakhalin Ainu *imu:*. Although Uchimura et al. (1938: 13) report one case of manifested automatic obedience among their Hokkadio Ainu samples, their description of symptoms of individuals is so incomplete that it is hard to conclusively affirm or deny Wada's statement. Other symptoms include echolalia and echopraxia, as well as copropraxia and coprolalia — involuntary utterances or behavior that is obscene or sexual in nature. Chiri's examples of coprolalia include "A filthy looking person had diarrhea", or "Let your penis have a drink" (Chiri 1952: 56, 1953: 84—85). Uchimura et al.

(1938: 26) report that coprolalia and copropraxia take place usually at a drinking session. (For further discussions of symptoms, see Tsuboi 1889: 457–458; Uchimura et al. 1938: 19–28; K. Wada 1965: 264–265; Winiarz and Wielwaski 1936: 184.)

In regard to the precipitating factor or stimulus, there is a marked difference between the Sakhalin Ainu and the Hokkaido Ainu. In the case of the milder form of *imu*: for the Sakhalin Ainu, the stimulus for induction seems to be a mild but unexpected shock incurred by various phenomena and objects. In the case of the more severe *imu*:, a verbal suggestion alone seems to suffice to incite the individual into the *imu*: state. For example, in the case of a male *imu*: whose initial occurrence of *imu*: took place at the sight of a writhing reindeer which he had shot, he immediately entered the state of *imu*: when someone asked, "What happened to the reindeer you shot?" In contrast, the precipitating factor for the Hokkaido Ainu *imu*: seems to be almost always the sight of a snake or the Ainu word for snake, *tokoni*. Thus, for all of the 77 Hokkaido Ainu *imu*: individuals listed in Figure 1 by Uchimura et al. (1938: 10–13), the stimulus was the hearing of the word *tokoni* or seeing a snake, a toy snake, or a picture of a snake. Uchimura et al. (1938: 28, 46) report a case of a male Hokkaido Ainu who talked about a snake by referring to it as "a long worm" or "an abominable worm", without being incited into an *imu*: state, until one of the investigators asked if he meant *tokoni*, using the Ainu term for snake, upon which he became seized with *imu*:. Other items which serve as a stimulus to some Hokkaido Ainu include a frog, an octopus, and a crab.

An important category of stimuli is foreign objects that are newly introduced or otherwise unfamiliar to the individual. For example, metal washing pans newly introduced from the Japanese at the time of investigation or neon signs which an Ainu saw for the first time while visiting Tokyo served as stimuli (Uchimura et al. 1938: 29). Unfamiliar foreign objects serve as stimuli also for the Sakhalin Ainu, as in the case of a Sakhalin Ainu woman whose initial occurrence of *imu*: took place at the sight of a Japanese domesticated cat which she had never seen before.

The Sakhalin Ainu do not regard *imu*: as sex-linked, although out of nine cases described to me, seven were women. On the other hand, the two males also had severe cases of *imu*:. This situation again contrasts with the Hokkaido Ainu, among whom Uchimura et al. (1938: 29) found no male *imu*: Ainu, although they do refer to other scholars' observations which testify very infrequent cases of males in the past. Jimbo (1901: 1) also states that *imu*: afflicts only women. It should be pointed out that one of the two males in my sample had originally come from Hokkaido when he was young, perhaps before his first seizure of *imu*:. Thus it seems that although *imu*: affects some men, especially in Sakhalin, it affects women with a much higher frequency among any Ainu group.

The age of those who suffer from *imu*: is decisively old. In fact, the mental image which the Sakhalin Ainu have of these individuals is that of people in their late 50s or 60s. When the age of individual *imu*: Ainu was examined, however, it was found that some had begun to have seizures as early as in their 40s. Among the Hokkaido Ainu at Hidaka, out of 45 cases, 17 were in their 50s, 14 were in their 40s, and 10 were in their 60s, although the onset of *imu*: takes place predominantly in people who are in their 20s and 30s (Uchimura et al. 1938: 33). According to Jimbo (1901: 7–8), of 12 individuals under his investigation, 3 experienced the first seizure in their teens. Evaluation of Jimbo's information is somewhat difficult since his investigation is fairly limited in scale and depth.

My data are too inconclusive to provide meaningful speculation about the percentage of *imu*: in the total population of the northwest coast of southern Sakhalin. The investigation of Uchimura et al. (1938: 15) shows the highest frequency, 3.91%, at the Piratori settlement in the Hidaka district, 2% elsewhere in the Hidaka area, and less than 1% outside of the Hidaka area of Hokkaido. The Hidaka district exhibits the highest density of Ainu population in Hokkaido, and its Piratori settlement is referred to as the Ainu capital because of its large Ainu population and high retention of the Ainu way of life in the community.

As the highest frequency of *imu*: at the Piratori settlement suggests, there seems to be a definite correlation between its frequency of occurrence and the degree of integrity of Ainu way of life; the retention of the Ainu way is often facilitated by the great distance of the settlement from a Japanese city, as in the case of the Piratori settlement (Kumasaka 1964; Uchimura et al. 1938: 13–14). As a corollary, with the rapid process of Ainu acculturation into the Japanese way of life, *imu*: is quickly disappearing, at least in its classical form, just as in the case of *latah, amok*, and other culture-bound syndromes elsewhere, When Suwa and his colleagues carried out an investigation in 1958, they located only four *imu*: Ainu in the Niputani settlement in the Piratori district of Hidaka (Suwa 1963). Figure 2 summarizes the above information.

There are some marked differences in the nature of *imu*: between the Sakhalin Ainu and the Hokkaido Ainu. I will try to interpret the occurrence of *imu*: among the Hokkaido Ainu first. Recent studies indicate that certain psychobehavioral disorders, many of which are culturally sanctioned, are prevalent among the members of a social group for whom culturally important rights and positions are not accessible. Such studies as Foulks (1972), Kenny (1978), Lewis (1971), Obeyesekere (1970), Rubel (1964), and Spiro (1977), demonstrate the prevalence of psychobehavioral disorders among women in societies in which women, regardless of their ability and personality, not only are deprived of rights and privileges of high cultural esteem, but are expected to meet strict and rigorous role expectations. Thus, one can speculate that low status in a society can result in psychological stress beyond the individual's capacity to resolve it, but that the culture provides a way for these individuals to resolve it in a culturally sanctioned manner such as *imu:, latah*, demonic possession, and so forth. Culture thus provides simultaneously both pathogenic/etiological agents as well as healing agents (cf. Wallace 1970).

Sociocultural factors such as the marginal position of the individual or strict role expectations provide at least a partial expalnation for *imu*: occurrence among women in Hokkaido Ainu society. The fact that negative automatic obedience, coprolalia, and copropraxia are characteristic behavioral patterns of Hokkaido

	Sakhalin Ainu	Hokkaido Ainu

Symptoms	(A) Non-sensical utterances
	(B) Echolalia; echopraxia
	(C) Manifested automatic
	    obedience
	(D) Sudden violent actions
		(A) Echolalia; echopraxia
		(B) Coprolalia; copropraxia
		(C) Negative automatic
		    obedience; (manifested
		    automatic obedience)
		(D) Sudden violent actions

Stimulus	(A) Startle in general
	(B) Hearing verbal suggestions
	(C) (Seeing unfamiliar
	    foreign objects)
		(A) Catching sight of a snake,
		    frog, octopus, or crab
		(B) Hearing the word *tokoni*
		    (snake)
		(C) Seeing unfamiliar foreign
		    objects

Sex of the victims	Women; some men	Women exclusively (a few men in the past)
Age of the victims	Middle age to old age	Middle age (forties and fifties)
Frequency per population	?	c̄ 4—1%

Fig. 2. *Imu:*.

Ainu *imu:* but are not symptoms of Sakhalin Ainu seems to support this line of interpretation. As noted earlier, there is a greater distance between men and women in Hokkaido Ainu society than there is in Sakhalin Ainu society, and women's modesty, especially with regard to their body, is extremely emphasized. Also of importance here the some of the stimuli. The snake, the primary precipitating factor for Hokkaido Ainu *imu:* is not a consciously perceived phallic symbol among the Hokkaido Ainu according to Chiri (1962: 223—228); instead, a turtle is called *ečinke* (one whose head looks like a penis) in one of the Hokkaido Ainu dialects (Chiri 1962: 223). While the snake may or may not symbolize a threat posed by men, Japanese washing pans and neon signs are clearly symbols of the threat of the Japanese to Ainu society just as *latah* is, at least in part, a response to new European overlords (Murphy 1976). Note that Japanese washing pans became the major stimulus for *imu:* in the Tokachi district of Hokkaido when they were first introduced to the Tokachi Ainu (cf. Uchimura et al. 1938: 29). Thus, there is at least partial evidence that the *imu:* among Hokkaido Ainu women is linked to their marginal status vis-à-vis Ainu males who form the dominant group in Ainu society. It is also linked to their status vis-à-vis the Japanese who constitute the dominant group in a larger universe, the Ainu having become a minority group in Japanese society. Even in the case of Sakhalin Ainu *imu:*, such stimuli as a domesticated cat of the Japanese or raw fish-eating introduced by the Japanese (see Cases 2 and 3 described at the end of Appendix III in Ohnuki-Tierney 1980b), suggest that their *imu:*, too, may also be related to the minority status of the Ainu in Japanese society.

In short, the data indicate that the etiology of *imu:* may relate to threats from the social environment. Among the Hokkaido Ainu, there is greater patterning in that the dominant group, either men or the Japanese, poses or at least is seen to pose, the threat to the victims who are almost exclusively women. In the case of the Sakhalin Ainu, the etiology of *imu:* may be more individualistic, although in some cases it may also relate to the threat of the Japanese.

RELATIONSHIP BETWEEN *IMU:* AND SHAMANS

On the basis of etymological analyses and information from the oral tradition of the east coast Sakhalin Ainu and the Hokkaido Ainu, Chiri (1952) and K. Wada (1965) propose that in the past the Ainu saw a close association between *imu:* and shamanism. However, present-day Ainu, either in Sakhalin or Hokkaido, do not consciously relate *imu:* to the personality of shamans. However, when I checked a list of individuals who were victims of *imu:*, more than half of them were also shamans. Of the 13 Hokkaido Ainu shamans and 1 Sakhalin Ainu shaman investigated by Uchimura et al (1938: 39), 9, including the Sakhalin Ainu, were also *imu:* victims. Uchimura et al. also report that for 20% of their sample the initial occurrence of *imu:* related to shamanism, for during a major illness these individuals consulted a shaman who diagnosed the cause of the illness to be a possession by a snake. In each case the individual was cured by an elder on the condition that she would eventually become an *imu:* sufferer after the recovery from the illness. They indeed started to periodically experience *imu:* shortly after the recovery (Uchimura et al. 1938: 35–36). Among the Niputani Ainu of Hokkaido, Munro (1963: 161–163) records two prayers which attempt a "transmutation of an incapacitating or distressing neurosis to Imu [sic]" and two other prayers which aim at "transmutation to *tusu* shamans in case of a severe neurosis where *imu* [sic] could not be obtained".

It is fairly certain to conclude that there is an overlap between shamans and *imu:* victims and but that the overlap is only partial – not all shamans suffer from *imu:* and not all *imu:* victims are shamans. In order to probe into this question of partial overlap, it is now necessary to examine the nature of spirit possession which characterizes the Ainu shamanistic ritual. As noted earlier, Ainu shamans become possessed by spirits when the spirits wish; the possession is not subject to the shaman's will. The spirits act and speak through the shaman's body. During a possession trance, therefore, shamans are not held responsible for their behavior. It is for this reason that Ainu sorcerers are not held responsible for their acts (see Ohnuki-Tierney 1973).

Possession, therefore, can serve as a culturally sanctioned mechanism with a definite therapeutic function for the individuals who, either because of their personality or role constraints, cannot otherwise express themselves in the manner that is possible during a possession trance. As Spiro (1965) eloquently expressed a number of years ago, religion serves as a "culturally constituted defense", and provides a "non-pathological resolution of the conflicts" (Spiro 1965: 107). In discussing Burmese shamans, Spiro (1977) successfully demonstrates that the availability of a variety of *nats* makes it possible for these Burmese female shamans, who have a variety of personality types, to dissolve their various types of frustrations through the *nat* possession. Similarly, using as an example a case of demonic possession in Sri Lanka, Obeyesekere (1970) illustrates how the role resolution is accomplished through a culturally sanctioned means of temporarily deviating from the norm. Obeyesekere (1970: 102) states:

The adoption of a new status, and its attendant role, which utilizes and acts out the psychological problem of the individual in a positive matter, would be considered a normal way of "coping".

Similar reasoning is behind Wallace's (1970) explanation of the process of becoming a shaman as one example of the process of mazeway resynthesis, during which a confusing and anxiety-provoking world starts to make sense.

While the psychological conficts which some individuals resolve through the culturally sanctioned possession trance may arise from "deprivation in personal satisfaction", they may also relate to "deprivation resulting from low social status or lack of power" (Bourguignon 1973: 328). An often cited work by Lewis (1971) emphasizes this link between status deprivation and possession trance. Lewis (1971: 31) explains:

For all their concern with disease and its treatment, such women's possession cults are also, I argue, thinly disguised protest movements directed against the dominant sex. They thus play a significant part in the sex-war in traditional societies and cultures where women lack more obvious and direct means for forwarding their aims.

In contradition to the sex-war interpretation of Lewis, Wilson (1967) asserts that illness and possession are caused by tension and frustrations between the members of the same sex arising from competition for the same goals and rewards, such as competition for the husband's attention among co-wives. According to Wilson, they are not due to tension between the sexes. It seems to me that Wilson's interpretation in fact reinforces the interpretation by various scholars, including Lewis, cited above, which links sociocultural deprivation to possession, illness, and various culturally normative departures. If culturally defined rewards and goals are narrowly defined for women, then competition becomes sharper and thus causes greater anxiety on the part of the individual.

These two types of sources of psychological conflict which the possession trance serves to alleviate explain the differences between the Sakhalin Ainu and the Hokkaido Ainu in regard to the shamanism and *imu*: phenomenon in each respective society. I interpret that some, but not all, Ainu shamans may indeed by psychologically disturbed and we see a partial overlap between shamans and *imu*: victims. The case of the Hokkaido Ainu, on the other hand, is more closely correlated with status deprivation and role constraints imposed by Ainu culture upon women (cf. Bourguignon 1973; Greenbaum 1973). For this reason, women alone are shamans and *imu*: victims among the Hokkaido Ainu, and their *imu*: symptoms include negative automatic obedience, coprolalia, and copropraxia. In short, there is a partial overlap in the etiology and function between *imu*: and the spirit possession of shamans. In order to explain a partial, and not complete, overlap between shamanism and *imu*: and to probe into the relationship between shamanism and other types of behavioral disturbances, we must have a much more extensive picture of psychobehavioral disorders of the Ainu.

The interpretation that some shamans may indeed be individuals with psychological difficulties should in no way preclude the possibility that some shamans may be stable or "healthy" individuals without major psychological problems, as Kennedy (1975) suggests. Here I must emphasize the multiple roles of shamans discussed in an earlier section of this paper. Shaman-chiefs in the ancient society of the Ainu may indeed have been "healthy" and perhaps strong-minded individuals who learned the art of possession. For that matter, it seems not at all contradictory to see a strong-minded person with a desire to exercise formalized or nonformalized power occasionally manifest temporary departures from the norm. Given the complexity of the multiple roles which shamans carry out, and given the fact that at least half of the population – that is, women – are politically peripheral and have only a marginal status in society, we must allow room for "perfectly healthy" individuals to enter the career for other reasons, such as the exercise of nonformalized power. A female sorcerer in pre-Communist China who became an eloquent village representative (Yang 1969: 132) is an example of a "healthy" and "strong-minded" magico-religious practitioner who, if given the opportunity, would have used a legitimate route.

SUMMARY

On the basis of data from a small society of the Sakhalin Ainu and a larger society of the Hokkaido Ainu, I have attempted to understand the interrelationships between shamans and *imu*: victims. Although data are limited and thus interpretations remain highly speculative, my study suggests that we must assume that shamanism is an extraordinary complex cultural institution which is highly variable in nature from culture to culture, but which is closely related to the structure of the society in which it operates. The cultural valuation it receives and the social position of shamans are thus explainable in terms of the structure of the society.

I speculate, as a gross generalization, that when a society is small, shamanism often receives high cultural valuation and shamans are not confined to certain personality types, certain statuses in the society, or one biological sex. In a larger society, shamanism is culturally insignificant and consequently is an arena for the socially marginal, including women. As a corollary, a greater number of shamans are individuals with psychological difficulties which they in turn resolve through the experience as shamans, and in particular, through the possession trance. Relevant sociocultural factors that are responsible for such a configuration of shamanism in these larger and more complex societies include the presence of such cultural features as an institutionalized religion, social stratification, a great distance between the public and the domestic domains, ascribed statuses, strict role allocation, rigidity of role expectations, and several other related factors. In the case of the Ainu, the shamanism of the northwest coast Sakhalin Ainu used to be that of a small society in which it was an important cultural institution, while the shamanism of the Hokkaido Ainu typifies that of a large and complex society. Northwest coast Ainu shamanism during the ethnographic present represents shamanism which falls somewhere between the two types.

Another factor which further increases the complexity of shamanism is the fact that shamans in any society are at least potentially capable of carrying out multiple roles — healers, religious specialists, covert politicians, and theatrical performers. They may be perfectly "healthy" shamans who enjoy exercising nonformalized power or who enjoy entertaining an audience. It is perhaps for this reason that the scholars' interpretation of shaman's mental state ranges from those who view them as having psychological disorders (e.g., Lebra 1964, 1969; Lévi-Strauss 1967: 161–180; Spiro 1977) to those who consider them to be well balanced (Kennedy 1973: 1151). This is another reason why there is a definite but partial overlap between shamans and the victims of psychological disorders, such as the culture-bound syndrome of *imu:* [3]

NOTES

1. The three aromatic plants are (listed here in order of their closeness to the embers) a branch or two of Yesso spruce or, if the shaman is a woman, of larch; a plant called *nuhča*; and minced dried leek. Yessor spruce is *Picea jezoensis* Carr (Chiri 1953: 236) and is *sunku* in Ainu. Larch is *Larix dahurica* Turcz (Chiri 1953: 237) and is *kuy* in Ainu. *Nuhča* is *Ledum palustre* var. *dilatatum* Wahlb (Chiri 1953: 53), and is reported to be narcotic (Miyabe and Miyake 1915: 308). The Ainu use this plant for tea and also as medicine and it does not seem to be strongly narcotic, although to my knowledge there is no chemical analysis of this plant available in publication. Leek is *Allium victorialis* var. *platyphyllum* Makino (Chiri 1953: 195) and is called *kito* in Ainu.
2. They use sea water during the warm season. During the cold season when they are in the settlement further inland, they use river water in which dried tangle coated with salt is soaked. Tangle is *Laminaria ochotensis* Miyabe (Chiri 1953: 253) and is *ruru kina* in Ainu.
3. Although the concept of multiple etiology, as suggested by Foulks (1972) as an explanation of the Polar Eskimo *pibloktoq* is a useful tool of interpretation, sociocultural factors seem to be more basic than that of a biochemical basis for the etiology of *imu:*. Since most female *imu:*, both among the Sakhalin and Hokkaido, are found to be in their 40s and 50s, one might postulate that hormonal and other biological changes are responsible. However, since women of other ages are also *imu:* victims and, especially in the past, some men also suffered from *imu:*, a biological explanation of this sort may be considered at best only one of multiple factors in the etiology of *imu:*.

REFERENCES

Batchelor, John
    1927 Ainu Life and Lore. Tokyo: Kyobunkwan [sic].
Beattie, John
    1977 Spirit Mediumship as Theatre. Royal Anthropological Institute News No. 20 (June
          1977): 1–6.
Beattie, John and J. Middleton (eds.)
    1969 Spirit Mediumship and Society in Africa. London: Routledge & Kegan Paul.
Bourguignon, Erika.
    1973 An Assessment of Some Comparisons and Implications. In E. Bourguignon (ed.),
          Religion, Altered States of Consciousness, and Social Change. Columbus: Ohio State
          University Press, pp. 321–339.
Chiñas, Beverly L.
    1973 The Isthmus Zapotecs – Women's Roles in Cultural Context. New York: Holt,
          Rinehart & Winston.
Chiri, Mashio
    1952 Jushi to Kawauso (The Magician and the Otter). Hoppo Bunka Kenkyu Hokoku
          7: 47–80.
    1953 Bunrui Ainugo Jiten (Classified Dictionaries of the Ainu Language). Vol. I:
          Shokubutsuhen (Plants). Tokyo: Nihon Jomin Bunka Kenkyujo.
    1960 Kamui Yukaru – Ainu Jojishi Nyumon (Kamuy Yukaru – Introduction to Ainu Epic
          Poems). Sapporo: Aporo Shoten.
    1962 Bunrui Ainugo Jiten (Classified Dictionaries of the Ainu Language). Vol. II:
          Dobutsuhen (Animals). Tokyo: Nihon Jomin Bunka Kenkyujo.
    1973 Chiri Mashio Chosakushu (Collected Works of Mashio Chiri). Vol. 3. Tokyo:
          Heibonsha.
Chiri, Mashio and Bunjiro Wada
    1943 Karafuto Ainu-go ni okeru Jintai Kankei Meii (Body Terms in the Sakhalin Ainu
          Dialect). Karafutocho Hakubutsukan Hokoku 5(1): 39–80.
Elliott, Alan J. A.
    1955 Chinese Spirit Medium Cults in Singapore. London: London School of Economics.
Firth, Raymond
    1966–1967 Ritual Drama in Malay Spirit Mediumship. Comparative Studies in Society
          and History IX: 190–207.
Foulks, Edward
    1972 The Arctic Hysterias. Washington, D.C.: American Anthropological Association.
Greenbaum, Lenora
    1973 Possession Trance in Sub-Saharan Africa: A Descriptive Analysis of Fourteen
          Societies. In E. Bourguignon (ed.), Religion, Altered States of Consciousness, and
          Social Change. Columbus: Ohio State University Press.
Hanihara, Kazuro, Hideo Fujimoto, Toru Asai, Masakazu Yoshizaki, Motomichi Kono, and
Yoichi Nyui
    1972 Shimpojumu Ainu (Symposium on the Ainu). Sapporo: University of Hokkaido
          Press.
Izumi, Seiichi
    1952 Saru Ainu no Chien Shudan ni Okeru Iwor [The Iwor and the Territorial Group of
          the Saru Ainu]. Minzokugaku Kenkyu, Vol. 16, Nos. 3–4: 29–45.
Jimbo, Saburo
    1901 Imbakko ni tsuite [About the Imbakko]. Tokyo Igakukai Zasshi XV (4): 1–15.
Kennedy, John
    1973 Cultural Psychiatry. In J. Honigmann (ed.), Handbook of Social and Cultural Anthro-
          pology. Chicago: Rand McNally & Company, pp. 1119–1198.

Kenny, Michael G.
    1978 *Latah*: The Symbolism of a Putative Mental Disorder. Culture, Medicine and Psychiatry, Vol. 2, 209–231. (Reprinted in this volume.)
Kindaichi, Kyosuke
    1914 Kita Ezo Koyo Ihen (An Epic Poem of Northern Ezo). Tokyo: Kyodo Kenkyusha.
    1944 Ainu no Kenkyu [The Study of the Ainu]. Tokyo: Yashima Shobo.
    1961 Ainu Bunkashi (A History of Ainu Culture). Tokyo: Sanseido.
Kumasaka, Y.
    1964 A Culturally Determined Mental Reaction among the Ainu. Psychiatric Quarterly 38: 733–739.
Lebra, William P.
    1964 The Okinawan Shaman, *In* A. H. Smith (ed.), Ryukyuan Culture and Society. Honolulu: University of Hawaii Press, pp. 93–98.
    1969 Shaman and Client in Okinawa. *In* W. Caudill and Tsung-Yi Lin (eds.), Mental Health Research in Asia and the Pacific. Honolulu: East-West Center Press, pp. 216–222.
Lévi-Strauss, Claude
    1967 Structural Anthropology. New York: Doubleday.
Lewis, Ioan M.
    1971 Ecstatic Religion. Harmondsworth, England: Penguin Books.
Mair, Lucy
    1969 An Introduction to Social Anthropology. New York: Oxford University Press.
Miyabe, Kingo and Tsutome Miyake
    1915 Karafuto Shokubutsushi (Plants in Sakhalin). Toyohara: Karafutocho.
Munro, Neil Gordon
    1963 Ainu Creed and Cult. New York: Columbia University Press.
Murphy, H. B. M.
    1976 Notes for a Theory on *Latah*, Culture-Bound Syndromes, Ethnopsychiatry, and Alternate Therapies. *In* W. P. Lebra (ed.). Honolulu: East-West Center Press, pp. 3–21.
Needham, Rodney
    1973 Right and Left in Nyoro Symbolic Classification, Right and Left. *In* R. Needham (ed.). Chicago: University of Chicago Press, pp. 109–127.
    1976 Nyoro Symbolism: The Ethnographic Record. Africa 46 (3): 236–245.
Obeyesekere, Gananath
    1970 The Idiom of Demonic Possession. A Case Study. Social Science and Medicine 4: 97–111.
Ohnuki-Tierney, Emiko
    1973 The Shamanism of the Ainu of the Northwest Coast of Southern Sakhalin. Ethnology XII (1): 15–29. Abstracted in Human Behavior (June 1973): 54–55.
    1974 The Ainu of the Northwest Coast of Sourthern Sakhalin. New York: Holt, Rinehart & Winston.
    1976 Regional Variation in Ainu Culture. American Ethnologist 3 (2): 297–329.
    1980a Ainu Illness and Healing – A Symbolic Interpretation. American Ethnologist 7 (1): 132–151.
    1980b Illness and Healing among the Sakhalin Ainu – A Symbolic Interpretation. Cambridge: Cambridge University Press, forthcoming.
Pilsudski, Bronislaw
    1912 Materials for the Study of the Ainu Language and Folklore. Cracow: Spólka Wydawnicza Polska.
Rosaldo, Michelle Zimbalist
    1974 Woman, Culture and Society: A Theoretical Overview. *In* M. Z. Rosaldo and L. Lainphere (eds.), Woman, Culture and Society. Stanford: Stanford University Press, pp. 17–42.

Rubel, Arthur J.
    1964 The Epidemiology of a Folk Illness: *Susto* in Hispanic America. Ethnology III (3):
          268–283.
Segawa, Kiyoko
    1972 Ainu no Konin [Marriage among the Ainu]. Tokyo: Miraisha.
Spiro, Melford E.
    1965 Religious Systems as Culturally Constituted Defense Mechanisms. *In* M. Spiro (ed.),
          Context and Meaning in Cultural Anthropology. New York: Free Press, pp. 100–
          113.
    1977 Burmese Supernaturalism. Philadelphia: Institute for the Study of Human Issues.
          Expanded edition.
Suwa, Nozomu, Shonosuke Morita, Wataru Yamashita, Tomoatsu Kuroda, and Masaharu
Ishigane
    1963 *Imu* ni tsuite – Saikin no Chosa ni yoru Chiken [*Imu* – Its Recent Findings]. Seishin
          Igaku 5 (5): 397–403.
Tsuboi, Shogoro
    1889 Ainu no Fujin [Ainu Women]. Tokyo Jinruigaku Zasshi, 42: 453–459.
Turner, Victor
    1967 The Forest of Symbols. Ithaca, N.Y.: Cornell University Press.
    1975 Symbolic Studies. *In* B. J. Siegel, A. R. Beals, and S. A. Tyler (eds.), Annual Review
          of Anthropology, Vol. 4. Palo Alto, C.A.: Annual Reviews Inc., pp. 145–161.
Uchimura, Y., H. Akimoto, and T. Ishibashi
    1938 Ainu no *Imu* ni tsuite [*Imu*: of the Ainu]. Seishin Shinkeigaku Zasshi, 42 (1): 1–69.
Wada, Bunjiro
    1956 Ainugo Byomei to sono Igi [Ainu Terms of Illness and Their Meaning]. Nihon Iji
          Shimpo, No. 1969: 43–45.
Wada, Kan
    1964 Ainugo Byomei ni tsuite – Wada Bunjiro Iko (1) Names of Illnesses in Ainu –
          Manuscripts Left by the Late Bunjiro Wada (1). Minzokugaku Kenkyu, 29 (2):
          99–112.
    1965 Imu ni kansuru Jakkan no Mondai [Some Problems of *Imu*:]. Minzokugaku Kenkyu
          29 (3): 263–271.
    1971 Ainu no shamanizumu [Ainu Shamanism]. Shunju, No. 127: 17–21.
Wallace, Anthony F. C.
    1970 Culture and Personality, 2nd ed. New York: Random House.
    1972 Mental Illness, Biology and Culture. *In* F. L. K. Hsu (ed.), Psychological Anthro-
          pology, New ed. Cambridge, M.A.: Schenkman, pp. 363–402.
Watanabe, Hitoshi
    1972 Ainu Bunka no Seiritsu – Minzoku Rekishi Koko Shogaku no Goryuten [The
          Developmental Stages in Ainu Culture – Ethnological, Historical, and Archaeological
          Approaches]. Kokogaku Zasshi 58 (3): 251–268.
    1973 The Ainu Ecosystem. Seattle: University of Washington Press.
Wilson, P. J.
    1967 Status Ambiguity and Spirit Possession. Man 2 (3): 366–378.
Winiarz, W. and J. Wielawski
    1936 *Imu* – A Psychoneurosis Occurring among Ainus. Psychoanalytic Review, 23: 181–
          186.
Worsley, Peter
    1968 Groote Eylandt Totémism and Le totémisme aujourd'hui. *In* E. Leach (ed.), The
          Structural Study of Myth and Totemism. London: Tavistock, pp. 141–159.
Yang, C. K.
    1969 Chinese Communist Society: The Family and the Village. Cambridge, M.A.: MIT
          Press.

THE STARTLE MATCHING TAXON

Commentary

As illustrated in the preceding discussions of *latah* and *imu*, the *Startle Matching Taxon* consists basically of the presentation of a stimulus which for the given person is so traumatic that it precipitates an episode of unusual and involuntary behavior. Moreover, the power of a startling stimulus to elicit such behavior is a chronic feature of the personality, a factor which has important social and interpersonal implications.

The first issue to be decided with respect to whether *latah* and *imu* can be accommodated within the DSM-III framework is whether the attempt should be made at all. Though unusual, is this behavior *pathological*? Enough analysts have suggested the possibility that it seems an appropriate working hypothesis. I should note, however, that the attempt here and in subsequent sections is obviously exploratory, and it goes without saying the following evaluations may well be different from those arrived at by others using the DSM-III format to order and systematize the primary data for theoretical analysis. But if nothing else, my attempt may sufficiently provoke those who disagree that they will undertake the same challenge.

Assuming that there may be something of psychiatric relevance involved, the second issue is what is the unit of analysis? If both the startle reaction itself and the ensuing behavior are taken together as the unit, then DSM-III diagnostic categories do not appear helpful; they do not, in any straightforward sense, provide for such a syndrome per se. For example, even one diagnostic category that might suggest itself does not seem appropriate (Brief Reactive Psychosis) defined as

... the sudden oneset of a psychotic disorder of at least a few hours' but no more than two weeks' duration, with eventual return to pre-morbid level of functioning. The psychotic symptoms appear immediately following a recognizable psychosocial stressor that would evoke significant symptoms of distress in almost anyone. The precipitating event may be any major stress ... (p. 200).

But in most cases the symptoms are not of sufficient severity to justify this diagnosis; and data from cases indicate that the usual stressful stimulus is not one that would adversely affect "almost anyone".

If, however, the startle response itself is accepted as a normal (and, indeed, universal) neurophysiological pattern, one perhaps varying in threshold of excitation, as Simons suggests, then one might consider the subsequent behavior as potentially having psychiatric relevance. And in some cases that behavior may fall within the broad domain of the abnormal, while in other instances it may not. In this light, the provactive stimulus, the startle reaction, can be seen as the *precipitating* factor for certain abnormal behavior in some people in the same way that

111

Ronald C. Simons and Charles C. Hughes (eds.), The Culture-Bound Syndromes, 111–113.
© 1985 *by D. Reidel Publishing Company.*

psychological trauma is the precipitant of a grief reaction in some persons but not others.

If such an argument is accepted, then the multiaxial evaluative system of DSM-III may provide concepts for incorporating this syndrome; for, taken apart from the initiating stimulus, the observed behavior itself (the flustered, involuntary uttering of normally forbidden phrases, the repetitive echoing of what other people say or mimicking of what they do) is noted by most writers as evidencing a type of hysterical reaction. In DSM-III terms, therefore, this taxon would seem to fall in the general class of Dissociative Disorders: "The essential feature is a sudden, temporary alteration in the normally integrative functions of consciousness, identity, or motor behavior" (p. 253). However, a more specific diagnostic category is less clear. The general features do not fit Psychogenic Amnesia, Psychogenic Fugue, or Multiple Personality, for example (the specific sub-types discussed; pp. 253–259); and they only imperfectly correspond to the Depersonalization Disorder, in which the "... essential feature is the occurrence of one or more episodes of depersonalization that cause social or occupational impairment" and "various types of sensory anesthesias and a feeling of not being in complete control of one's actions, including speech, are often present. All of these feelings are ego-dystonic, and the individual maintains grossly intact reality testing" (p. 259). Perhaps the most appropriate of these sub-categories is the Atypical Dissociative Disorder, "... to be used for individuals who appear to have a Dissociative Disorder but do not satisfy the criteria for a specific Dissociative Disorder. Examples include trance-like states ... ". (p. 260).

But there are also other symptoms commonly included in this behavior pattern, such as echopraxia, echolalia, coprolalia, and coprophagia. Where might they be assigned in this scheme? Given DSM-III's allowance for mulitple diagnostic notation of symptom patterns, in a given instance one might record that these are catatonic in character: "... marked psychomotor disturbance, ... stupor, negativism, rigidity, excitement, or posturing .... Associated features include stereotypies, mannerisms, and waxy flexibility" (p. 190); but the rest of the clinical picture may not conform with definitional elements for the pattern of the Catatonic Type (295.2x) of the Schizophrenic Disorders. On the other hand, some of these symptoms may be referrable to the Residual Type (295.6x) of the schizophrenias or to the clinical features of the Brief Reactive Psychosis pattern (298.80), the latter including "behavior that is grossly disorganized or catatonic among its symptoms" (p. 201).

It is clear that we need a concrete case to look at with regard to possible DSM-III categories. Unfortunately in the preceding papers space did not allow presentation of case instances with sufficient detail for making such an evaluation. In order to do so, then, I will take a case from Yap's classic monograph (1952: 534):

A *nonya* (woman of Chinese racial extraction who for two or three generations have taken largely Malay speech, customs and manners), aged about 40, in Malacca, she had long been regarded as eccentric, and was called *goreng pisang* (fried banana) by way of a nick-name. She was employed as an odd-job cook during festivals, etc., and had a daughter and son, who was also regarded as "silly". Her husband was a stall-holder, selling sweetmeats.

She was markedly histrionic and sensitive to attention. When persuaded she would, after a show of reluctance, start to walk about with exaggerated swaying of the hips and dance the *ronggeng* (a recognized folk-dance). At the same time, she sang snatches of a love song, facing me all the time. After a little while she stopped, saying in a mischievous way that her testicles were dropping. When asked to bow she did so repeatedly, advancing all the while, and incidentally raising hails of laughter from those around. When tickled, she would start to strut about as though making determined and demonstrative attempts to stride away. She was not echolalic, but when she wanted to leave and was, with some physical pressure, made to remain, she showed some confusion in speech which is typical of persons in the *latah* state: she had been playing cards and had hoped to win some money, and kept on reiterating this idea: "Good-night, *eh*, good-night, *untong-lah, kanah lottery, eh, kanah lottery, eh, good-night . . .*" (which may be rendered: "Good-night, eh, good-night, shall have to owe money then, win a lottery, eh, win a lottery, eh, good-night . . . ").

She had developed these peculiar mannerisms and exhibitionistic personality traits from childhood, and her *latah* symptoms hardly ever went beyond this. She appeared to be a gay, mischievous and fairly intelligent person, not unusually nervous or anxious. The most genuine symptom she showed was decomposition of speech when embarrassed or discomfited.

In terms of DSM-III one might characterize this person as follows:

Axis I   300.15 Atypical Dissociative Disorder
            295.6x Residual Type (of the Schizophrenic Disorders) (?)
Axis II: 301.50 Histrionic Personality Disorder (". . . overly dramatic, reactive,
            and intensely expressed behavior and characteristic disturbances in inter-
            personal relationships"; p. 313) (Primary Diagnosis)
Axis III: Son also regarded as "silly" (congenital linkage?)
Axis IV: *Psychosocial stressors*: "long been regarded as eccentric"; called by a
            nick-name; employed as odd-job cook.
            Severity: 2 − Minimal
Axis V: *Highest level of adaptive functioning past year*: 3 − Good (Operationally
            defined as "no more than slight impairment in either social or occupa-
            tional functioning" − she appeared to be a gay, mischievous . . . person;
            embarrassed or discomfited at decomposition of her speech.)

REFERENCE

Yap, P. M.
   1952 The *Latah* Reaction: Its Pathodynamics and Nosological Position. *The Journal of Mental Science* XCVIII (new series 377): 515–564.

B. THE SLEEP PARALYSIS TAXON

RONALD C. SIMONS

INTRODUCTION: *THE SLEEP PARALYSIS TAXON*

In several of the sections of this volume I attempt to make a case for investigating the possible relevance of neurophysiologic factors in shaping a syndrome. When this is done, the research problem is re-formulated in the following way: First there is the question of how physiologic factors are expressed in behavior, and second, how they are subjectively experienced. These questions can, of course, also be asked in the reverse direction: how do experience and behavior alter neurophysiology? And there are the additional questions: how do the experiences and behaviors of individuals shape social interactions and their cultural interpretations, and how do social and cultural factors shape the neurophysiological responses of individuals?

I have suggested that it may be useful to consider not only members of the *Startle Matching Taxon,* but also some other culture-bound syndromes as culture-specific elaborations of specific aspects of human neurophysiology. I was particularly delighted, therefore, to encounter the papers of Bloom and Gelardin and of Ness which describe *uqamairineg* and *old hag* as culture specific elaborations of sleep paralysis. Bloom and Gelardin's paper describes a culture-bound psychiatric syndrome experienced by Eskimos in Alaska, and Ness's a similar syndrome in a population of English descent in Newfoundland; areas separated by 3,300 miles. Both papers mention parallel phenomena in other culturally unrelated areas, and Ness's describes a cultural elaboration in the Carribean. In his discussion, Ness asserts: "I will systematically establish a congruence between the experience known as the *old hag* and a specific medical syndrome. *Following this, I will show how this congruence furthers our understanding of the old hag as well as of the medical syndrome*" (ital. added). After describing how the physiology shapes the experience, Ness goes on to ask "how does the experience influence the nature of folk beliefs about etiology, prevention, and cure?" Bloom and Gelardin raise the question of a relationship between the high frequency with which they have found sleep paralysis in their Eskimo population and aspects of Eskimo culture and individual Eskimo psychology which are discussed more extensively by Foulks and others in the papers on *pibloctoc.*

Incidentally, it may be noted that unlike many reports of *incubi* and *succubi*, Bloom and Gelardin's does not mention their subjects' feeling pressure on the chest. The literature on culture-bound syndromes, however, is such that it is not safe to conclude that when a significant symptom is not mentioned it is not present. To assert that a symptom found ubiquitously is not present in a specified geographic area requires a specific investigation for its presence or absence. Absence can not be deduced from lack of mention.

After this section was planned and the papers which were to be included had been selected, I came across a remarkable volume by David Hufford. Hufford's

115

Ronald C. Simons and Charles C. Hughes (eds.), The Culture-Bound Syndromes, 115–116.
© 1985 *by D. Reidel Publishing Company.*

book (which contains discussions of the Bloom & Gelardin and of the Ness papers) presents massive evidence that the physiology of sleep paralysis shapes *old hag* extensively. Though Hufford considers his work a study in "applied folklore" (he first presented his discovery at a folklore meeting in 1973), he notes that it has medical and psychiatric relevance. He quotes from Cotton Mather's *On Witchcraft: Being the Wonders of the Invisible World* (1692), the testimony of a Richard Coman, who had been "annoy'd with the Abberation of the bishop and two more that were strangers to him who came and oppressed him so that he could neither stir himself nore wake anyone else and that he was the night after, molested again in the like manner". And he quotes Ernest Jones' *On the nightmare* which in turn contains a paragraph from the *Daemonologie* (1597) of King James I of England: "Epistemon: No, that is but a natural sickness which the Mediciners have given that name of Incubus unto, *Ab Incubando*, because it . . . makes us think that there is some unnatural burden or spirit, lying upon us, and holding us down". On the basis of his study of *old hag*, Hufford concludes (in part) that:

(1) The phenomena associated with what I have been calling the *old hag* constitute an experience with a complex and stable pattern, which is recognizable and is distinct from other experiences. (2) This experience is found in a variety of cultural settings. (3) The pattern of the experience and its distribution appear independent of the presence of explicit cultural models. (4) The experience itself has played a significant, though not exclusive, role in the development of numerous traditions of supernatural assault. (5) Cultural factors heavily determine the ways in which the experience is described (or withheld) and interpreted. (6) The distribution of traditions about the experience, such as those involving the *old hag* or the Eskimo *augumangia*, has frequently been confounded with the distribution of the experience itself. (7) The frequency with which the experience occurs is surprisingly high, with those who have had at least one recognizable attack representing 15 percent or more of the general population. (8) The state in which this experience occurs is probably best described as sleep paralysis with a particular kind of hypnagogic hallucination.

The jacket of Hufford's book features a reproduction of *The Nightmare*, painted in 1781 by Henry Fuseli, a print of which hangs in Freud's study in Vienna, a gift of Ernest Jones.

NOTE

In his paper on *lanti*, Hart briefly describes *ngarat*, a member of the *Sleep Paralysis Taxon* from the Philippines. See especially his description at the top of p. 388 (this volume).

REFERENCES

Hufford, David J.
    1982 The Terror That Comes in the Night. Philadelphia: University of Pennsylvania Press.
Hufford, David J.
    1976 A New Approach to the Old Hag. *In* W. D. Hand (ed.), American Folk Medicine: A Symposium. Berkeley: University of California Press.

JOSEPH D. BLOOM AND RICHARD D. GELARDIN

UQAMAIRINEQ AND *UQUMANIGIANIQ*:
ESKIMO SLEEP PARALYSIS

INTRODUCTION

Over the years, studies of clinical syndromes in the North in relation to native peoples' cultures have been of three main kinds. First came descriptions of the so-called culture-specific disorders; the major example of these among the Eskimos was the *pibloktoq* syndrome and its variants (Brill 1913; Murphy and Leighton 1965), but there was also the phobic-like syndrome *kayak-angst* as it appeared in western Greenland (Gussow 1963). Secondly, and more recently, there has been a study of mental disorders as they are conceptualized within particular Eskimo tribes; and both Murphy (1965), working in western Alaska, and Vallee (1960), working in central Canada, have made contributions to it. A third, and still more recent and promising line of research has been developed by Briggs (1970), who describes the shaping of the aggressive drives in an Eskimo family. As these drives are modified by cultural demands one can see the development of what might be called psychoneurotic phenomena within the Eskimo child as it comes to appreciate the aversion exhibited by its elders to the open expression of anger.

The objective in the present paper is to describe and analyse the syndrome of sleep paralysis as it appears among the Eskimo people of Alaska; to relate it to the literature of Eskimo personality dynamics and to traditional Eskimo explanations of phenomena of the same type involving the non-empirical world and, indirectly, shamanism; and to indicate the importance of culturally relevant data in the clinical treatment of mentally-disturbed people of ethnically diverse origin.

DESCRIPTION OF THE SYNDROME

A very detailed description of this sleep paralysis is available from the original case notes concerning a 30-year-old married Eskimo woman who presented herself for help at the Counselling Office of the Anchorage Community College. Originally from a village in northwestern Alaska, she had come to live in Anchorage with her Eskimo husband and their children. She said she had first experienced her trouble before the age of eleven, but had not gone to the doctors in the Alaska Native Health Service (a branch of the Indian Health Service of the U.S. Public Health Service) until she was eighteen.

She provided the following description of an attack:

Just before going to sleep and waking up, I get paralysed. Sometimes it starts with a buzzing. Sometimes I can almost see something and it scares me. My grandparents told me it was a soul trying to take possession of me, and to fight it.

117

Ronald C. Simons and Charles C. Hughes (eds.), The Culture-Bound Syndromes, 117–122.
© *1976 by the Arctic Institute of North America.*

After the buzzing sound I can't move. Sometimes I really start feeling like I am not in my body anymore, like I am outside of my body and fighting to get back. If I don't get back now I never will. I really get panicky. It takes me a long time to move sometimes, like forever. I feel like if I don't get back into my body that I am going to die. That is the first thing that I think of. I finally wake up and move and my heart is just pounding, and I am all shaken up and frightened."

She continued with a description of her visit to the Alaska Native Health Service:

I told the doctors the native name for this and that lots of natives have this . . . no impression except funny looks by doctors . . . I was put on valium and chloral hydrate and tranquilizers. Saw Dr. B. who did an EEG (electro-encephalogram) and he had Dr. R. read it and he said sleep paralysis. Dr. B. continued the valium and chloral hydrate and I relaxed at first and got right to sleep but now and then still had paralysis and had headaches the next day. Dr. B. left and Dr. S. said he didn't believe in drugs and referred me to a neurologist, Dr. J., and a psychologist, Miss A.; Dr. J. said I was getting addicted to the valium and wants me to see Dr. J. again for an exam and spinal tap.

I feel my muscles are so tense, my muscles twitch, my eyes don't feel clear. I don't know what to do if I am addicted. I don't trust the doctors if I am an addict, but then who can I trust? I feel depressed and scared, like I don't know what to do and the doctor said you know that you're getting addicted. When I get up I am so tense that I can hardly move. My husband rubs me and gives me a hot bath. I feel like I am going to explode. I had sleep attacks last week over and over. I feel funny like shaking outside, uncoordinated. I am waiting for someone to show . . . . In class I look to see when someone comes in the door. I don't like to be alone because I might kill myself. My kids would be better off if I were dead.

Following the initial examination, it was decided to conduct what may be referred to as a cross-cultural interview with the object of analysing the patient's statements, to confirm that she was suffering from a condition well-known to Eskimos from her area, and to learn as much as possible about that condition, how common it was, how conceptualized, how other counsellors handled cases of it and, finally, how people recovered from it, and whether the shaman was involved in treatment. In the process, speakers of the two basic Eskimo dialects of Alaska — the northern Inupiaq and the southern Yupik — were interviewed.

The results of the cross-cultural interview served to confirm the statements made by the patient. The syndrome occurs when an individual is going to sleep or waking up. It is characterized by an inability to move, an awareness of surroundings, a clear consciousness, and a feeling of great anxiety bordering upon panic. The person has no control over his body, may attempt to call out, but finds that he cannot utter a sound. The attacks may be accompanied by some prodromal warning; in the case cited the patient almost always experienced a buzzing sound prior to the attack and usually lasting through it. Other persons interviewed had experienced a smell or a clanging sound prior to an attack. Attacks usually ended spontaneously after a variable interval of time, but could also come when the person afflicted was touched by another person aware of his struggles.

The syndrome appears to be well-known and may be fairly prevalent among the Eskimos of Alaska. Aside from the initial informant, sixteen people were asked about it — eight Inupiaq-speaking and eight Yupik-speaking — with ages ranging from thirteen to eighty. All of them had heard of the syndrome and some had experienced it.

Although it is difficult to be certain about the meanings of words in the two dialects, or how they should be spelt, it appears that *uqumanigianiq* is the word most closely descriptive of the syndrome in Inupik, and *uqamairineq* in Yupik.

Traditional explanations for the events of the syndrome were discussed openly. The symptoms were explained by the relationship between man and the spirit world. There is a belief that when people are entering sleep, sleeping, or emerging from sleep, they are more susceptible to influences from the spirit world. The existence of a relationship between man and the spirit world is for many an accepted part of life. One of the informants felt that if an individual did not believe in the spirit world he would be challenged; "a spirit would come to you and make you realize that there are spirits". Another wrote, after hearing a tape-recording of the initial interview:

This sleeping thing can happen to anybody, if he or she knows that the certain place is haunted or if there's a spirit of someone in the certain place. . . . I didn't know about this room till I told one of the workers about my sleeping paralysis, previous to that year there was someone died that used to stay in that room and even used to stay on that bed.

In the sleep cycle, the soul is believed to be more vulnerable to influences from spirits and more likely to leave the body. As indicated in the description cited above, the patient first interviewed felt during an attack that she was not in her body, and that she was fighting to get back in. Apparently, the paralysis relates to the body which has been left by its soul, and so is without the quality essential for life. There was clear implication that if the state of paralysis continued it would result in death.

Other people explained the sleep paralysis syndrome as a possession state in which a spirit enters the body of the susceptible person. The paralysis is related to the fact that the sufferer is "controlled" by the spirit and thus cannot initiate movements of his own.

The symptoms of sleep paralysis were not always easy to distinguish from other phenomena associated with sleep. There are different Eskimo words for bad dreams, nightmares, and sleep walking. Although these matters were not investigated in detail in connection with the present study, it may be surmised that similar phraseology may be in use in explanations of all sleep-related phenomena.

Any discussion of the relationship between sleep paralysis and shamanism was met with resistance. This is not surprising in view of the fact that shamanism was driven underground earlier in the present century, especially by church organizations. The present authors feel that with more exploration the link between the sufferer and the shaman would become more clear.

Several things were said in relation to treatment. The first patient stated that her grandparents always told her that "if you see any spirits, tell the people about it". There was the implication that discussion of the events with other people would be helpful. Another person wrote:

Last of all, I would like to say how you should control yourself while having sleeping paralysis. From my parents I have learned that, when I have such things, I should be patient and try to take it easy. If I can't move and am stiff, I should try to move one of my joints, especially try to move my finger joints and toes. As soon as something moves you'll be relaxed. I have known about this ever since I was a kid, so does my fellow natives.

It was also suggested that the syndrome was related to the manner in which a person conducted his life. The "good" person would suffer from this condition less than the "bad" person. The psychological exploration of what might constitute good and bad was not undertaken in this study.

DISCUSSION

Rushton (1944) describes the essential elements of the sleep paralysis syndrome as follows:

Sleep paralysis is a transient, benign paralysis at the beginning or end of sleep and usually associated with a clear consciousness. The paralysis always occurs during the transition between wakefulness and sleep or vice versa . . . Even though he may have experienced previous attacks and may realize that he will recover soon from this one, he usually cannot suppress a feeling of great fear . . . Recovery may be spontaneous or induced. If the latter, it is always by bodily contact. At times vigorous shaking is needed, but often a light touch is sufficient to dispel the attack within a few seconds. The frequency of attacks may vary from several times a week to once in six months or more.

The aetiology of the sleep paralysis syndrome is apparently unknown; however, it is often associated with the narcolepsy-cataplexy syndrome. West (1966) classifies sleep paralysis as a "disassociative experience related to sleep". He feels that the condition may be related to spontaneous wakening during REM (Rapid-Eye Movement) sleep during which time the muscular relaxation related to this type of sleep is still in force. He also feels that there has not been "sufficient systematic studies to gain any good idea of its incidence or of its degree of correlation with other dissociative symptoms in the same person".

Rushton's description of sleep paralysis fits very closely with that reported by the Eskimo persons interviewed in connection with the present study. What is surprising is that sleep paralysis, which is described as a rare condition, seems from first report to be quite prevalent among Eskimos.

The fact that the syndrome may be classified as a dissociative type of a hysterical reaction may provide some clues to its seeming prevalence among the Eskimo population. Hysterical mechanisms have been postulated in the literature as a basic Eskimo reaction pattern. Brill (1913) sees them as the basis of the *pibloktoq* syndrome, and Parker (1962) sees an evident tendency toward hysterical type behaviour as a basic reaction pattern in Eskimo psychopathology. It has been the present authors' experience that hysterical behaviour, especially dissociative reactions associated with alcohol use and the breakthrough of anger, are very common phenomena. Certainly more systematic study of the sleep syndrome, in which account is taken of psychological, and possible organic, factors will have to be accomplished in order to shed further light on its aetiology.

Regardless of aetiology, the traditional explanation of this phenomena deserves further comment. The spirit world has existed and continues to exist as a reality for many Eskimo people. Burch (1971) has detailed the extent of the "non-empirical environment" of the north Alaskan Eskimos. He describes a total range of phenomena including "a wide variety of entities that range from human-like creatures at one pole to totally invisible beings at the other". The description of the sleep paralysis syndrome is thus consistent with the total range of Eskimo relationships with non-empirical events.

Some other elements of the syndrome are also of interest. There is little in the literature regarding the meaning of sleep to Eskimos. Spencer (1959), in his study of the North Alaskan Eskimos, reports that dreaming is experienced as the wandering of the soul. This also seems to be the major mechanism in the sleep paralysis syndrome. The other explanation – of a possession state – does not seem to be as significant here. Soul wandering, or soul loss, has been extremely important in both the causation and cure of disease. Murphy (1964) points out that it was at night, when the soul was considered to wander, that it was susceptible to influences which could cause disease. The possibility for the separation of body and soul was, on the other hand, an extremely important matter for the Eskimo shaman. It was his supposed ability to have his soul leave his body and travel about with his "familiar" spirits which provided the basic mechanism for him to seek out the causes of disease.

Separation of body and soul also relates to the concept of death. Lantis (1960), in interviews conducted with Nunivak Island Eskimos, records the following statement:

That time, when I looked at the sick man, I saw two men: the body of the man and his shadow right next to him . . . A shaman told me that the shadow was the man's soul. When a person is going to die, his soul starts to leave.

The traditional explanations detailed above shed light on Eskimo world views, the relation of man and the spirit world, and the relation of the spirit world to symptom formation. The importance of understanding in this area is clear in the case presented in this paper in that the original patient lived in Anchorage, far from her home village, and was an "acculturated" person in all outward respects. However, she obviously retained an inner set of beliefs and explanations which were a reality to her. The possession of this information is of crucial importance to any mental health worker attempting to treat such a woman. Furthermore, the act of eliciting the information is an effective way of reducing the distance which may exist between such a patient and those charged with helping her.

CONCLUSION

More will have to be done in the future in an attempt to further delineate the syndrome of sleep paralysis. It is not, however, natural to clinicians to ask the questions which would elicit the type of material described in this paper, and so persons will have to be trained to ask different types of questions. As the questions change so will the data and, hopefully, the patient may be able to experience a form of therapy which strengthens his internal sense of reality and continuity rather than contributes to its destruction.

REFERENCES

Briggs, J.L.
  1970 Never in Anger: A Portrait of an Eskimo Family. Cambridge, Mass.: Harvard University Press.
Brill, A.A.
  1913 *Piblokto* or Hysteria Among Peary's Eskimos. Journal of Nervous and Mental Disease 40: 514–520.
Burch, E. S., Jr.
  1971 The Non-Empirical Environment of the Arctic Alaskan Eskimos. Southwestern Journal of Anthropology 27: 148–165.
Gussow, Z.
  1963 A Preliminary Report of *Kayak Angst* Among the Eskimos of West Greenland: A study of Sensory Deprivation. International Journal of Social Psychiatry 9: 18–26.
Lantis, M.
  1960 Eskimo Childhood and International Relationships. Seattle: University of Washington Press, p. 120.
Murphy, J.
  1964 Psychotherapeutic Aspects of Shamanism on St. Lawrence Island in Alaska. *In* A. Kiev (ed.), Magic, Faith and Healing. London: Free Press of Glencoe, pp. 53–84.
Murphy, J. and A. Leighton
  1965 Native Conceptions of Psychiatric Disorder. *In* J. Murphy and A. Leighton (eds.), Approaches to Cross Cultural Psychiatry. Ithaca, N.Y.: Cornell University Press, pp. 64–107.
Parker, S.
  1962 Eskimo Psychopathology in the Context of Eskimo Personality and Culture. American Anthropologist 64: 76–96.
Rushton, J. G.
  1944 Sleep Paralysis. Medical Clinics of North America 28: 945–949.
Spencer, R.
  1959 The North Alaskan Eskimo. Washington D.C.: Smithsonian Institute Press.
Vallee, F.
  1966 Eskimo Theories of Mental Illness in the Hudson Bay Region. Anthropologica 8: 53–83.
West, L.
  1966 Dissociative Reaction. *In* A. Freedman and H. Kaplan (eds.), Comprehensive Textbook of Psychiatry. Baltimore: Maryland: Williams and Wilkins, p. 896

ROBERT C. NESS

THE *OLD HAG* PHENOMENON AS SLEEP PARALYSIS:
A BIOCULTURAL INTERPRETATION

If you only heard of it and never had it, you could hardly take it all in, could you? – Northeast Harbour postmistress

INTRODUCTION

There is a set of psychological and physical experiences involving paralysis of arms and legs, as well as hallucinations, which have traditionally been interpreted in Newfoundland as a syndrome called the *old hag* or *ag rog*. The broad purpose of this paper is to present a description and analysis of this phenomenon. Within this context, the objectives of this report are four-fold. First, an ethnographic description of the *old hag* phenomenon based on extensive interviewing within a Newfoundland coastal community is presented. Second, the ethnographic description is followed by an analysis of the *old hag* in terms of the clinical syndrome called sleep paralysis. Third, the relationship between attacks of the *old hag* and other sets of physical and emotional complaints is explored by analyzing illness complaint scores derived from the *Cornell Medical Index* (Brodman et al. 1949). Finally, the implications of viewing the *old hag* as sleep paralysis are discussed within the context of current theoretical issues in transcultural psychiatry. The paper concludes with a review of issues raised by the *old hag* phenomenon which require further research.

THE RESEARCH SETTING

The information presented in this report was collected during 13 months (May1973 –June 1974) of field research in Northeast Harbour, a community of approximately 400 people on the northeast coast of Newfoundland. The first permanent European settlers in Northeast Harbour, primarily second-generation immigrants from 'west-country' England, moved into this community from other areas of Newfoundland in the late 19th century to exploit the coastal fishing banks. Until recently most men in Northeast Harbour supported their families by selling codfish, herring, mackerel, and salmon. During the winter months (December through April) many individuals turned to sealing or 'woods work' with a lumber company to supplement their incomes. Inheritance of property and patterns of residence continue to reflect strong patrilineal and patrilocal themes characteristic of Newfoundland fising settlements.

In the early 1960's several decisions by the provincial government and business interests to promote the economic development of northern Newfoundland initiated a series of construction projects that have had a profound impact on the occupa-

123

Ronald C. Simons and Charles C. Hughes (eds.), The Culture-Bound Syndromes, 123–145.
© *1978 by D. Reidel Publishing Company.*

tional structure of coastal communities like Northeast Harbour. In 1964 a road was completed which provided easy access to large towns from these previously isolated communities. By 1973 about 70 percent of the men from Northeast Harbour were commuting to work at a copper mine 14 miles away. The road also improved access to a regional health center, located 30 miles from Northeast Harbour, which opened in 1964. Medical services provided by this facility, in addition to the non-prescription drugs obtained at local stores and Pentecostal faith-healing practiced in the community, represent the major forms of health care utilized by people in Northeast Harbour as they cope with the effects of illness and injury (Ness 1976).

INDIGENOUS PERSPECTIVES ON THE *OLD HAG*

This section describes the *old hag* or *ag rog* experience and indigenous theories about its etiology and treatment within Northeast Harbour, based on reports supplied by (a) 43 adults who had experienced an attack of the *old hag*, (b) seven individuals who had witnessed attacks of the *old hag* and (c) 26 adults who knew about the *old hag* but had not experienced it.[1]

Victims of an attack of the *old hag* typically report that they suddenly awake feeling unable to move or speak. This experience is reported to occur most frequently shortly after falling asleep. Concurrent with the paralysis, victims often feel as though a heavy weight is pressing on their chest. Some victims report seeing the figure of an animal or human astride their chest. People who have experienced the *old hag* insist they are fully conscious during the attack and can see or hear other people in the household. In spite of strenuous efforts to overcome their feeling of paralysis, they remain unable to move until someone touches or shakes them or calls their name.

Informants who have had attacks of the *old hag* report profuse sweating and feelings of exhaustion when the experience ends. Victims say that an attack may be preceded by a dream, but they report that it is equally possible to experience an attack without dreaming first. The attack itself, however, is described as very different from dreaming in that the person feels that he is fully awake during an attack. Most people claim that falling asleep while lying on their backs greatly increase their risk of 'being hagged'.

People who have witnessed attacks of the *old hag* report that some victims emit high-pitched groans or low moans. The eyes may be open or closed. The person's body is motionless and breathing appears normal. After the attack the victim usually perspires heavily and appears exhausted.

There are a wide variety of viewpoints concerning the etiology of the *old hag* experience. For ease of presentation these viewpoints can be grouped into three classes. The most common explanation suggests that a person's blood 'stagnates', especially if a person sleeps on his back. The attack is believed to be potentially fatal if the victim is not shaken out of the paralysis. A 45 year-old miner who had experienced the *old hag* explained:

It can happen anytime; your blood has a lot to do with it . . . it gets right like steel in your body and you can't move. Don't put anything on their chest or they'll surely die. All you gotta do is move 'em or call their name, just even bend their finger and that will do it. It's common, it can happen to anyone and it has nuthin to do with your health.

A 65 year-old woman who has witnessed many of her husband's attacks of the *old hag* said: "Ya gets it when you're on the broad of your back. Old timers say it's your blood standin' still. You're awful sweaty and tired when you come out of it, I'll tell you!"

A second local interpretation suggests that the *old hag* will most likely occur when a person has worked too hard. Many men, for example, recall experiencing and witnessing attacks while they were working at lumber camps. A 40 year-old man recalls: "We used to put splits of wood on fellas' chests and have a good laugh when they got it (the *old hag*). You works hard and your blood gets thin, see; you're in the woods all hours trying to beat the fella next to ya and you push yourself too far." Another man, 61 years old, expressed a similar view: "The way I figures it, back in those days everyone punished their bodies, didn't sleep right or get the proper food. That's what I think does it, but they say it's your blood. Ya don't see it in the younger crowd much." Finally, a 30 year-old housewife noted: "I finds it when I'm over tired. I had it a lot when we were first married . . . you sure feel bad afterwards."

A third view of the *old hag* emphasized that the attack can be precipitated by another person who may harbor hostile feelings toward the victim. This view is expressed by older men and women in the community, although almost all adults in the community will admit that they are aware of this interpretation. A 62 year-old retired fisherman explained: "It's just like you're tied up. Ya know there is some people can put it on you, like a charm, if they think somethin' about ya, or you can get it on your own. It's not your blood. While ya have it you think you're bawling' out, but you're not."

While people discuss their *old hag* experiences, someone is likely to ask: "Do ya know who it was 'agged ya?" An 83 year-old retired fisherman who claimed he had been "agged' several times explained: "Sometimes ya see 'em, they put this over ya." This indigenous theory of victimization is highlighted in the following case illustration of a man who has had frequent attacks of the *old hag*.

CASE ILLUSTRATION

George P., a 50 year-old bachelor, has been a fisherman since he was ten years old. He lives with his elderly parents and two younger brothers who have also remained bachelors. George pursues the inshore fishery with one younger brother and the eldest, who is the only married brother.

All the members of George's household except his youngest brother have experienced attacks of the *old hag*. George cannot recall when he had his first attack, but he claims to have the experience about once a month. A typical attack of the *old hag* was described by George in the following terms:

I can feel it comin' on, ya know it's a real uncomfortable feelin' like a fear spreadin' over ya. I can bawl out when I have it and I can get it when I'm lyin' on my chest, or with my hand along side. I'll say, "Call me! Call me!" Sometime I get all tangled up with cats, horses, or fallin' of cliffs. I was 'agged just a few weeks ago . . . ya know those TV chipmunks or TV puppets or whatever you call' em. I was watchin' those and went to bed and they 'agged me.

One of George's most vivid attacks occurred in 1964 before the road reached the community:

I came up late from the stage [storeroom for fishing gear]. We had beach stones up the path then and I went in and lay down like this [reclining in a chair] and before long I heard steps comin' up the path on those rocks. The outside door opened, then the inner door and I wondered who was comin' in, bein' so late. Then I saw a woman all in white come across the kitchen. She came around the stove and came over to me. Then she put her arms out and pushed my shoulders down. And that's all I know about it. She 'agged me.

George could not recognize the woman, but said that he "was chasin' a few girls around the harbour then." He also noted that "I've dreamed about 'em before and young girls have 'agged me, but I suppose they didn't know it just the same."

Listening to our conversation, George's brother added: "Sometimes ya'll see someone comin' in the room and they'll 'ag ya. I've had it when the person gets hold of your privates and you'll wake up all sore and tender. Boy, that's some punishment!"

The interview materials and case illustration presented above indicate that three distinct theories concerning the etiology of the *old hag* are present in Northeast Harbour. Most adults are familiar with the competing views on the subject and have developed their own opinions. A 40 year-old miner, for example, summarized his position in these terms: "What power do I have to put a thing like that on you? I think it's your blood. I don't think it's when ya get tired . . . according to that I know lots of fellas would have it all the time."

It is important to note, however, that the belief that one's blood stagnates is not thought to be incongruous with the proposition that other people may 'ag you. More specifically, informants may view blood stagnation as the *proximate* cause and a hostile individual as the *ultimate* cause. That is, biological and social-psychological explanations may be offered by informants as complementary, rather than contradictory, viewpoints concerning the etiology of the Old Hag experience. This point is clearly illustrated in the following explanation offered by an 81 year-old fisherman:

It's stagnation of the blood. You think you're bawlin' out but more often you're not. You can see what's goin' on around ya, ya know. Nancy [ethnographer's wife] can 'ag rog ya' and my wife too, she's 'ag rogged me plenty o' times. You'll see she comin' in the room and come right down on top of ya and she'll 'ag rog ya. To prevent it put a Bible under your head; I never been 'ag rogged so long as I does that. It's like a stroke I suppose, but the doc can't do nuthin' for it."

Ideas about prevention of the *old hag* are as varied as theories about its cause. The most common advice given to me was to avoid sleeping on my back. Other preventive practices included sleeping with a Bible under the pillow or repeating a favorite hymn backwards to avoid having a dream which might precede being 'agged. Measures recommended for disrupting the *old hag* experience include touching or shaking the victim, calling the victim's name backwards, or spelling the victim's name backwards on his forehead. Most informants claimed that simply bending the victim's toe or finger would quickly end the *old hag* experience. All informants emphasized that it was possible for a person to die from the attack if they were not 'brought out of it', although no one could cite an example of someone dying from the *old hag*. No individuals within the community specialized in treating or preventing attacks of the *old hag*.

In Northeast Harbour the *old hag* is not considered an illness or a symptom of an illness. People laughed at my suggestion that they consult a physician about their attacks of the *old hag*. Moreover, discussions with the staff physicians providing in-patient services at the regional health center failed to uncover a single case in which symptoms of the *old hag* syndrome were presented as the primary complaints. (One physician could recall a few patients mentioning symptoms resembling the *old hag*, but the patients never specifically related their symptoms to the *old hag* nor did they request treatment for those symptoms.) The chief physician, who has worked at the center since it opened ten years ago, had never heard the term *old hag*.

Nurses may also be unaware of the *old hag* syndrome. One informant who had spent several months in a provincial sanitarium recalled finding his roommate in the middle of an attack of the *old hag*, surrounded by several nurses who were convinced the patient was having a heart attack: "I knew it was the 'ag and gave him a shake, the nurses screechin' at me. When he came out of it he said he could see me (during the attack) but couldn't say nothin'."

These observations are confirmed by the results from a weekly household survey spanning seven months (November 1973—May 1974). This systematic survey was undertaken in Northeast Harbour to ascertain (1) the range of illness complaints appearing within the community, as well as (2) the strategies people used to cope with illness. During the survey 443 illness complaints were reported by 220 people, but there were virtually no reports of symptoms resembling the *old hag* (Ness 1976: 84—92). This finding is remarkable because during the last month of the survey (May) I began asking specifically about *old hag* symptoms and found that people were experiencing these symptoms. Asked why they did not report the *old hag* symptoms during the household survey, respondents assured me that the *old hag* had "nothing to do with being sick".

EPIDEMIOLOGY OF THE *OLD HAG*

I questioned 69 adults in Northeast Harbour about their experience with the *old hag*.[2] In conjunction with questions dealing with the nature of the *old hag* attack, I asked the informants: (1) if they had experienced an attack of the *old hag* during the past month (May) and (2) if they had ever experienced at least one attack of

TABLE I
TABLE I
Reported cases of the *old hag* in Northeast Harbour

sex	No. reporting attack in May, 1974[a]	No. reporting one or more attacks in past	No. reporting no attacks	total
male	4	26	6	36
female	1	12	20	33
total	5	38	26	69
Mean age				
male	56	51	38	
female	52	47	39	

[a] All of these individuals reported attacks 'in the past', but they are not included in the figures reported in column two in order to separate current and past cases.

the *old hag*. The number of affirmative answers to each question along with denials are classified by sex and average age and presented in Table I above.

The figures in Table I indicate that 62 percent (43 adults among 69 questioned) acknowledge having one or more attacks of the *old hag*. The precise number and timing of these attacks was difficult for respondents to recall, but seven percent (five adults among 59 questioned) recalled an attack during the previous month of May. Approximately 70 percent of the people who reported attacks of the *old hag* in the past are males ($n = 30$) and 30 percent are females ($n = 13$).

The mean ages of males and females reported in Table I indicate that those men and women acknowledging attacks of the *old hag* are older than those men and women who report no attacks. Specifically, the mean age of all respondents reporting attacks of the *old hag* is 50.5 years, while the mean age of those respondents denying attacks of the *old hag* is 38.5 years. The difference between these two means is statistically significant ($p = 0.003$, two-tail test). This finding supports the observations of several informants who felt that the younger people in the community were not experiencing attacks of the *old hag*.

In an attempt to explain part of the distribution of *old hag* experiences in Northeast Harbour, I hypothesized that social-psychological stress associated with marrying into Northeast Harbour would place female 'outsiders' at greater risk for experiencing attacks of the *old hag*. A comparison of in-marrying women and locally-born women revealed, however, no differences in the number of reported attacks of the *old hag* between the two groups.

INTERPRETATION OF THE *OLD HAG* AS SLEEP PARALYSIS

The materials presented above bear directly on a number of issues within transcultural psychiatry, especially discussions of the so-called 'culture-bound' syndromes. One issue concerns the relationship between these syndromes and Western medical nosology. Anthropological reports of syndromes such as *amok, latah, koro, piblo-ktoq* have rarely applied Western medical or psychiatric nosology because the behavioral manifestations of these syndromes have appeared so bizarre to field-workers that no clear congruence with Western psychiatric nosology could be seen (Kiev 1959; 107–109; Kiev 1972; Yap 1969).

Some transcultural psychiatrists, however, have sought to establish a congruence between the culture-bound syndromes and the diagnostic categories employed by Western psychiatrists (see, for example, Kiev 1965; Yap 1969). In a recent review, for example, Wittkower and Prince (1974: 543) argue that the culture-bound syndromes are basically the standard syndromes described in the American Psychiatric Association Manual. Establishing such congruity should not, however, be taken as an end in itself. Unless fundamental similarities between a behavioral-affective experience heretofore viewed as a culture-bound syndrome and a psychiatric diagnostic category are employed to broaden our understanding of the ethnographic syndrome as well as the medical diagnosis, the effort to establish such similarities is essentially unproductive (von Mering 1970: 280).

In this section I will systematically establish a congruence between the experience known as the *old hag* and a specific medical syndrome. Following this effort I will show how this congruence furthers our understanding of the *old hag* as well as the medical syndrome. During the final part of the paper additional issues in trans-cultural psychiatry will be examined.

The problems of disease classification notwithstanding (Fabrega 1974), there appears in this case to be a fundamental similarity between the experience described above as the *old hag* and a well-described category in modern medical nosology. A review of the literature on sleep disorders suggests that the experience known as the *old hag* in Newfoundland bears a striking resemblance to the clinical syndrome called 'sleep paralysis', as indicated by the following descriptive summary of the essential features of sleep paralysis:

The term sleep paralysis denotes a condition that occurs in the transition between sleep and wakefulness whereby the individual feels subjectively awake and aware of his surroundings, yet is incapable of voluntary movement. The condition ordinarily lasts from several seconds to several minutes and usually is terrifying. If hypnagogic hallucinations are present the anxiety may be heightened even more by the experience of hearing voices, bells, etc., or seeing animals, objects or people (Liddon 1970: 1028).

Similar clinical features of sleep paralysis have been described recently by Hishikawa (1976) as well as a number of previous authors (Chodoff 1944; Everett 1963; Freedman, Kaplan and Sadock 1972; Goode 1962; Payn 1965; Schneck 1952; 1960, 1969; and Yoss and Daly 1957). Abstracting from these accounts, the core features of sleep paralysis may be summarized as: (1) An inability to perform voluntary movements upon awakening (usually shortly after falling asleep), often accompanied by (2) vivid hypnagogic hallucination which last several minutes (usually less than ten minutes). These episodes (3) end spontaneously or may be terminated by someone touching or speaking to the victim. Finally, (4) the sequelae of sleep paralysis are transitory: exhaustion, anxiety, and sweating.

Most of these features of sleep paralysis are evident in the following report by a woman diagnosed as suffering from sleep paralysis in the United States. Her report clearly resembles informants' accounts, described above, of the *old hag* syndrome experienced in Northeast Harbour.

When I awake I notice that I am unable to move. I try to speak but cannot, I can hear very clearly everything that goes on about me and sometimes my eyes are open enough to see immediately in front of me. I am unable to open my eyes farther or to look about. Sometimes I am frightened and try to struggle to come to ... Sometimes a slight touch is sufficient to bring me out of the spell, but at other times I must be shaken vigorously. If no one is about I try not to be frightened and the spell passes away (Lichtenstein and Rosenblum 1942: 153–154).

More recently, a psychiatrist in New York has published a summary of a 27 year-old patient's experience with repeated attacks of sleep paralysis. His description of her experiences also closely resembles informants' reports about the *old hag*:

On falling asleep or awakening, she would find herself completely paralyzed. She would feel partially awake and partially asleep and would manage to open her eyes partially. She would feel someone climbing onto her bed and on top of her ... The pressure of this weight on her would be great, yet no one could be seen ... As her eyes remained open she would hallucinate other figures in the room ... She would attempt ineffectively to shout, but at most she would be capable of moaning. She would be aware of her surroundings, knowing for example that her daughter was home, hearing her: ... She would make unsuccessful efforts to move her head and arms. Suddenly her attacks would terminate spontaneously ... On occasions her daughter or husband might hear her moan, touch her, and abort the episodes (Schneck 1960: 1129–1130).

The author concludes his description by noting that the patient clearly differentiated these attacks from 'other nightmares'.

In diagnosing a set of symptoms as sleep paralysis it is crucial, in fact, to distinguish sleep paralysis from other sleep-related experiences such as nightmares. This distinction has been described most succinctly by Schneck (1969: 726):

The inability to scream, the sleeper's awareness of his actual location in bed, full recollection of the events of the episodes, and the invariable paralysis that does not necessarily occur in ordinary nightmares, all point up some of the differences between sleep paralysis and descriptions of sleep terror in children and the nightmares of adults.

Virtually all informants in Northeast Harbour insisted that there was a qualitative difference between a nightmare and suffering an attack of the *old hag*. One fisherman, for example, compared these experiences in the following terms: "When I've been 'agged I know where I am. I can smell the coffee in the kitchen and hear my wife but I can't move or speak. When I dream it's not all clear and my wife says I yell sometimes." Statements such as this clearly support the proposition that the *old hag* experience can be interpreted as an attack of sleep paralysis.

Further evidence that the *old hag* resembles sleep paralysis rather than a nightmare can be derived by comparing the accounts provided by victims of the *old hag* with information provided by observers of these victims. Two conclusions are noteworthy: (1) Observers' reports often confirm the victims' perceptions during the *old hag* attack (e.g., the sounds of people, the smell of food); and (2) Observers' reports corroborate that the *old hag* attack actually occurs in the setting claimed by the victim (e.g., a particular room in the victim's home).

Before concluding this discussion of the phenomenological correspondence between the *old hag* and sleep paralysis, a brief review of recent research on hypnagogic hallucinations and sleep paralysis is instructive. Ribstein (1976) has reviewed the literature on hypnagogic hallucinations and notes that these hallucinations typically occur at the first sleep onset in the evening. When accompanied by sleep paralysis, the paralysis is *not* hallucinated but co-exists with the hallucinations; these are almost always visual but occasionally auditory hallucinations are reported. Hallucinations involving smell or taste are rarely reported. Patients reporting these hallucinations typically claim they were not dreaming; they often report not losing their 'temporal or spatial bearings' even while involved in the hallucination (Ribstein 1976: 149). These findings clearly support the experiences reported by informants living in Northeast Harbour.

Finally, a comprehensive survey of types of sleep disorders recently published by Kales and Kales (1974) discusses sleep paralysis as an auxiliary symptom of narcolepsy, a neurological disorder in which people pass suddenly and unexpectedly into a sleep state for a short period of time. The authors note, however, that attacks of sleep paralysis alone may also occur (Kales and Kales 1974: 491; see also Hishikawa 1976: 98). Goode (1962), for example, surveyed 359 individuals comprising medical students, nurses, and hospital in-patients and reported 17 cases (4.7 percent) of primary or idiopathic sleep paralysis. Everett (1963) found that eight of 42 medical students (15.4 percent) questioned about sleep paralysis gave a positive history of that complaint not associated with narcolepsy. My research in Northeast Harbour indicates that without exception the people who reported attacks of the *old hag* did not report symptoms which would suggest that they were also suffering from narcolepsy.

Based on the close correspondence between informants' descriptions of the *old hag* and the clinical features of sleep paralysis reviewed above, as well as the absence of narcoleptic symptoms among my informants, the remainder of this paper proceeds with the cautious assumption that the experiences described above as the *old hag* can be classified reliably as cases of primary or idiopathic sleep paralysis. In other words, unlike some other culture-bound syndromes, such as the arctic hysterias (Foulks 1972) or *malgri* (Cawte 1976), which cover a range of phenomena classified separately by Western nosology, the *old hag* appears to be congruent with a particular Western diagnosis. Extending this theme, the next section examines data from Northeast Harbour which bears directly on discussions about the epidemiology and etiology of sleep paralysis.

THE RELEVANCE OF THE *OLD HAG* FOR THE STUDY OF SLEEP PARALYSIS

In a comprehensive review of the literature Hishikawa (1976: 98) has recently concluded that "only scanty data on ... incidence, distribution, and natural history are available" on idiopathic sleep paralysis. What is currently known about idiopathic sleep paralysis has been derived primarily from groups of patients and students; no epidemiological studies of natural communities have been reported (Hishikawa 1976). Thus the data from Northeast Harbour are of considerable relevance to current discussions of sleep paralysis.

With regard to etiology, there have been a series of reports over the years, based on selected clinical cases, which implicate chronic emotional disturbances as predisposing factors in the expression of sleep paralysis. Rushton (1944), for example, views sleep paralysis as a manifestation of a psychoneurosis. Van der Heide and Weinberg (1945) explore twelve life histories of men which implicate intra-psychic conflicts generated by "passive-submissive sexual needs". More recently, Payn (1965) and Schneck (1960, 1961, 1969) argue that sleep paralysis represents an expression of intense personality conflicts involving feelings of hostility and aggression on the one hand and a need for inactivity, passivity, and dependency on the other. These authors believe that sleep paralysis simultaneously provides a psychic defense against aggressive feelings and fosters the individual's dependency feelings. Finally, Liddon (1970) has presented two case histories of psychotics with sleep paralysis. The author concludes that intense anxiety related to a fear of death in his patients may have generated their episodes of sleep paralysis. In spite of this provocative clinical material, the relationships between forms of emotional disturbance and sleep paralysis, as well as the true prevalence of these associations, have not been investigated within a community setting.

Paralleling these reports, there are a number of publications indicating that idiopathic sleep paralysis may also occur in individuals who are emotionally and physically healthy (see, for example, Mitchell 1876; Goode 1962; and Everett 1963). Although this conclusion appears sound (Hishikawa 1976), the survey research supporting this generalization typically questions presumably 'healthy' populations without systematically measuring physical and psychological parameters of all individuals participating in the study (Goode 1962; Everett 1963).

My opportunity to live and work for 13 months with people who had experienced attacks of the *old hag* convinced me that they were not suffering from any distinctive form of chronic or episodic emotional disturbance. In order to assess the the accuracy of this impression, I analyzed responses to the *Cornell Medical Index* (CMI) provided by the 69 adults who had been interviewed about the *old hag*.[3] Nine CMI sections were selected as possibly relevant for distinguishing differences between those people who had experienced attacks of the *old hag* and those who had not. Specifically, CMI sections measuring complaints in the (1) cardiovascular, (2) digestive, and (3) nervous systems, as well as sections measuring feelings of (4) inadequacy, (5) depression, (6) anxiety, (7) sensitivity, (8) anger, and (9) tension were selected for analysis.[4] The mean number of 'yes' answers for each CMI section was computed for several different classifications of respondents and *t*-tests were conducted to determine if the means were significantly different. The following groups of respondents were compared: (1) people who reported one or more *old hag* attacks vs. people who did not report any *old hag* attacks; (2) male respondents vs. female respondents; (3) males with no *old hag* attacks vs. males with *old hag* attacks; and (4) females with no *old hag* attacks vs. females with *old hag* attacks. The results of the *t*-tests are presented in Table II.

The results reported in Table II show that on seven of the nine CMI sections, those respondents with no history of *old hag* attacks do not have mean scores significantly different from the mean scores of those respondents who do have a history of *old hag* attacks. However, on the CMI sections eliciting complaints about digestion and tension, those respondents with no history of the *old hag* do have statistically significant higher means than respondents with a history of attacks. These findings are explained by the fact that the majority (76 percent) of the respondents with no history of the *old hag* are women. Women in Northeast Harbour have statistically significant higher mean scores than males on the digestion and tension sections of the CMI, as well as CMI sections measuring complaints about nervousness, anxiety, sensitivity, and anger (see column two, Table II). In other words, the sex variable is a confounding influence when respondents are grouped and compared simply in terms of the presence or absence of a history of *old hag* attacks.

The relationship between mean responses to the CMI sections and a history of presence or absence of attacks of the *old hag* is clarified in columns three and four of Table II. When sex is controlled, there are no significant differences between the mean scores of respondents with a history of *old hag* attacks and the mean scores of respondents without a history of the attacks.[5] I conclude, therefore, that respondents with a history of *old hag* attacks in Northeast Harbour do not report significantly more emotional or physical complaints (as measured by specific CMI sections) than respondents with no history of attacks.

This conclusion is further substantiated by an analysis of responses to specific CMI questions selected because of their possible relevance for pinpointing specific conditions which might be associated with the experience of sleep paralysis. The number of 'yes' responses to six specific CMI questions was tabulated for each of four groups of respondents: (1) males with no history of the *old hag*; (2) males with a history of the *old hag*; (3) females with no history of the *old hag*; and (4) females with a history of the *old hag*. The results are reported below in Table III.

The figures in Table III indicate that none of the six CMI questions clearly distinguishes one group of respondents from the other groups. The only possible exception to this conclusion is the fact that two males with no history of the *old hag* reported a history of fits and/or epilepsy. This finding is actually the opposite of what some early researchers have argued, namely, that sleep paralysis is form of epilepsy (Rushton 1944; Ethelberg 1956). It is important to note that the percentage of respondents acknowledging 'bad dreams' is approximately equal in all four groups of respondents. As I described earlier, informants always drew a clear distinction between dreaming and the *old hag* experience and felt there was no causal relationship between the two experiences.

These results provide the first epidemiological support for previous clinical and

TABLE II

The results of *t*-tests comparing groups of respondents on nine sections
of the Cornell Medical Index

CMI sections	attacks vs. no attacks [a]	males vs. females [b]	males, attacks vs. no attacks	females, attacks vs. no attacks
cardiovascular	NS	NS	NS	NS
digestive	$p = 0.016$; no attacks	$p = 0.041$; females	NS	NS
nervous	NS	$p = 0.062$; females	NS	NS
inadequacy	NS	NS	NS	NS
depression	NS	NS	NS	NS
anxiety	NS	$p = 0.006$; females	NS	NS
sensitivity	NS	$p = 0.003$; females	NS	NS
anger	NS	$p = 0.038$; females	NS	NS
tension	$p = 0.039$; no attacks	$p = 0.053$; females	NS	NS

[a] Two-tail probabilities are reported in columns one, three, and four because the direction of the difference between the means was not predicted in advance.
[b] One-tail probabilities are reported in column two because the direction of the difference was predicted in advance.

survey reports indicating that idiopathic sleep paralysis may occur in healthy individuals.[6] A comprehensive understanding of sleep paralysis will have to integrate this conclusion with the clinical data demonstrating that sleep paralysis may also accompany a variety of intense emotional disturbances. There may, in other words, be several etiological pathways leading to sleep paralysis. This integrative effort has not proceeded far, although considerable understanding of the physiological mechanisms involved in sleep paralysis has been achieved (Hishikawa 1976).

A second finding corroborated by this study is the uneven sex ratio described by Goode (1962: 231). In his survey of medical and nursing students, as well as some hospitalized patients in the United States, Goode (1962) found that 80 percent of the respondents who had experienced sleep paralysis were males and 20 percent were females. These figures are comparable to the sex ratio displayed in Table I above which shows that 70 percent of the sample from Northeast Harbour experiencing the *old hag* (sleep paralysis) were males while only 30 percent of the females in the sample reported the same experience. The stability and meaning of these sex ratios across cultural groups obviously warrants further replication and study.

Two further findings from Northeast Harbour should be noted here. First, the figures in Table I indicate that the mean age of respondents reporting an *old hag*

TABLE III

The number of 'yes' responses to six CMI questions in four groups of respondents[a]

CMI question number[b]	males				females			
	no attacks		attacks		no attacks		attacks	
	n	%	n	%	n	%	n	%
087	0	0	1	3%	1	5%	0	0
090	2	33%	1	3%	0	0	0	0
094	0	0	0	0	0	0	0	0
139	1	17%	4	14%	5	25%	4	33%
168	0	0	1	3%	1	5%	1	8%
192	2	33%	7	24%	4	20%	2	17%

[a] The size of each group is: Males, no attacks: $n = 66$
                               Males, attacks: $n = 29$
                               Females, no attacks: $n = 20$
                               Females, attacks: $n = 12$
One male and one female did not complete the CMI.

[b] The CMI questions are as follows:
   087: Was any part of your body ever paralyzed
   090: Did you ever have a fit or convulsion (epilepsy)?
   094: Are you a sleepwalker?
   139: Do you usually have great difficulty in falling asleep or staying asleep?
   168: Did you ever have a nervous breakdown?
   192: Are you often awakened out of your sleep by frightening dreams?

attack is twelve years greater than the mean age of those not reporting an attack. This situation does not conform with Hishikawa's (1976: 98) statement that sleep paralysis is most frequent in adolescence. Unfortunately, those respondents who experienced the *old hag* were not able to recall their age when they had their first attack. The finding does suggest, however, that the age of onset may be highly variable across different cultural settings. Finally, there are some reports (Goode 1962; Hishikawa 1976: 123) that idopathic sleep paralysis may have a familial occurrence. No systematic information on this aspect was collected in Northeast Harbour, but my impression was that two families had more frequent attacks distributed among more family members than did the other 73 families in the community. Further research is clearly needed on this aspect of the phenomenon.

Concluding this section on the relationship between the *old hag* and sleep paralysis, it is important to compare victims' responses in Northeast Harbour with the published material describing people who report idiopathic sleep paralysis. In Northeast Harbour, recall that victims do not evaluate the *old hag* experience as a sign of illness. Following this viewpoint, people in this Newfoundland community do not seek help from either indigenous healers or professionals at the regional health center. This evaluative response and behavior is strikingly similar to descriptions based on 'normal' populations in the United States who are not experiencing additional emotional or physical problems (Goode 1962; Everett 1963;

Hishikawa 1976: 99). This uniformity in response to sleep paralysis will be analyzed below along with other features of the *old hag* syndrome.

THE *OLD HAG* REVISITED

Having established that the *old hag* syndrome may be equivalent to the experience labelled sleep paralysis, what can be accomplished? That is, from an anthropological perspective, what is the significance of viewing the *old hag* syndrome as sleep paralysis?

The question usually addressed in studies of culture-bound syndromes is: How does the culture influence the symptomatology and course of the syndrome? This question is particularly appropriate when the behavioral-affective experience is a public performance which can (1) be learned by others in the community and (2) employed as instrumental behavior (see, for example, Newman 1964). In the case of sleep paralysis, however, I suggest that an equally appropriate question is: How does the experience influence the nature of folk beliefs about etiology, prevention, and cure? I accept, in other words, von Mering's (1970: 277) challenge that "the anthropological study of disease and treatment tries to account for elements of belief contained in the outcome". But I would add that elements of belief regarding etiology and treatment should also be explained, not simply described.

First, it seems to me that any outside observer attempting to understand this intense, subjective and essentially non-public experience is aided considerably by interpreting the phenomenon as sleep paralysis. Especially difficult to understand otherwise are the victims' assertions that they are totally paralyzed, fully awake, and 'seeing' figures that no one else sees at the time of the attack. While other labels, such as 'schizophrenic', may come to mind, they founder on the fact that the victims in Northeast Harbour appear to enjoy good physical and emotional health, or are at least free of intense symptomatology. More benign terms, such as 'nightmares' also fail because they do not capture the essence of the attack, the feelings of wakefulness and paralysis.

Beyond this general point, an analysis of the *old hag* as sleep paralysis assists an anthropological interpretation because five ethnographic features of the *old hag* syndrome are more clearly understood: (1) the intra-community variability in folk theories about causation, coupled with a unitary understanding of a particular 'risk factor'; (2) the uniformity in the symptoms reported, in spite of the fact that the attack is typically a non-public event; (3) the individualistic approach to prevention coupled with a single approach to cure; (4) the evaluation of the *old hag* as an episode unrelated to illness; and (5) certain folk observations about the epidemiological distribution of *old hag* attacks within Northeast Harbour.

Unlike many ethnographic accounts of culture-bound syndromes, the descriptive material derived from interviews in Northeast Harbour reveals a rich diversity in opinions about the cause of *old hag* attacks; there is no single theory commonly given by informants. In fact, there is considerable on-going debate, even arguing, about 'what brings it on'. In the midst of this heterogeneity there is, however, one stable belief: that lying on one's back greatly increases the chances of having an attack.

I believe the diversity of opinions in Northeast Harbour about causation is related to the fact that episodes of the *old hag* are usually private events rarely witnessed by (or reported to) more than a few people. Patterns of 'causal' association, then, between *old hag* attacks and other more public events are not easily detected or assessed by community members. Development of a consensual folk theory is consequently very difficult.

In addition to the non-public nature of *old hag* attacks, there is probably considerable 'indeterminacy' in the onset of these attacks, viewed as sleep paralysis. Hishikawa (1976), for example, has developed strong evidence that sleep paralysis may be generated by sleep-onset REM sleep. On the other hand, it has been demonstrated that sleep paralysis is *not* inevitably associated with a period of REM sleep at sleep-onset (Hishikawa 1976; 105, 108, 111). This 'indeterminacy' makes it difficult for even victims to develop or confirm ideas accounting for their own attacks.

Thus, there is considerable 'noise' between events or conditions that community members or victims might recognize as 'causal' and the onset of an *old hag* attack. This situation is quite different from other culture-bound syndromes, such as *pibloktoq* (Foulks 1972) or "wildman behavior" (Newman 1964), which are usually accessible to observation by the communities in which they occur.

It is striking, for example, that there is no coherent body of folk theory implicating 'social stress'.[7] Based on a survey of ethnographic materials, Kiev (1969: 108) has asserted that "native definitions of specific entities (culture-bound syndromes) have invariably been defined in terms of stressful social events preceding the onset of symptoms, rather than in terms of specific symptoms or combinations of symptoms present". That statement may apply where the onset of symptoms is a public event, allowing cause and effect associations to be developed, but Kiev's formulation cannot be supported by material from Northeast Harbour. In fact, *contra* Kiev, informants are much more likely to agree about the specific symptoms of an *old hag* attack than the cause of the attack. This situation is precisely what we might expect when the onset and expression of symptoms is as invariably private and strongly conditioned by physiological processes as is the case with sleep paralysis (Hishikawa 1976; 105–115).

In the midst of diverse opinions regarding etiology, the recurring belief that lying on one's back places a person 'at risk' for having an attack is curious. Even informants believing that other malicious persons can cause an *old hag* attack will emphasize this 'risk factor'. This stable element in the belief system corresponds with statements made by victims described in the literature on sleep paralysis (Lichtenstein 1942; Ethelberg 1956). More recently, Hishikawa (1976; 102–103) has shown in laboratory work that the sleep position of narcoleptics influences the frequency with which they experience sleep-onset REM sleep, a condition thought to be closely related to the onset of sleep paralysis (Hishikawa 1976: 112). This finding regarding sleep position may, in turn, be generalizable to 'normals' and would explain why my informants view sleep position as a 'risk factor'.

Another area of considerable cognitive variability is found in approaches to prevention of the *old hag*. This situation I interpret as functionally related to the fact that there is no unified body of theory about causation. In spite of these disagreements about ultimate cause and prevention, there is widespread agreement about how to cure a person who is suffering an attack of the *old hag*. Victims, as well as those who have observed attacks, report unanimously that touching or shaking the victim would 'bring them out of it'. Many informants emphasized that only a slight touch was necessary for the desired effect. Again, this element in the belief system corresponds dramatically with published accounts of sleep paralysis (Goode 1962; Schneck 1960; Payn 1965) and has been observed in laboratory work (Hishikawa 1976: 101). Although the precise physiological dynamics are not understood, the stable belief about cure in Northeast Harbour can be viewed as more than simply 'folk culture'.

I turn now to the fact, described earlier in this paper, that people do not evaluate attacks of the *old hag* as episodes of either physical or mental illness. I also noted earlier that this evaluation is similar to observations made by a number of authors describing sleep paralysis within the United States. This similarity is, I believe, related to three fundamental features of sleep paralysis: (1) the attacks are unrelated to the onset of other symptoms of illness; (2) the attacks are usually only a few minutes in lenth; and (3) victims are not impaired physically or mentally after an attack.

The lack of serious or long-lasting sequelae associated with the *old hag* is probably the most significant feature in understanding the lack of concern among victims that they have 'an illness' requiring treatment. D'Andrade (1976), for example, has found that people commonly think about illnesses in terms of connotative attributes such as 'seriousness', and 'curability' rather than in terms of distinctive definitions. Although his work is based on a sample of American students, the results may be generalizable to at least English-speaking peoples. Certainly within the context of Northeast Harbour the *old hag* is thought of as a transient experience with no untoward consequences. It is logical, therefore, that victims neither describe symptoms of the *old hag* to health professionals nor seek treatment for such symptoms.[8]

Finally, certain folk observations about the epidemiology of *old hag* attacks are clarified by viewing the experience as sleep paralysis. Although there is considerable variability in notions about etiology, many informants argued that 'hard work' might predispose individuals to have *old hag* attacks. Within this context, fishermen and men doing 'woods work' are often singled out as groups particularly vulnerable to these attacks.

The validity of such folk observations is supported if the *old hag* syndrome is viewed as sleep paralysis. To begin, a current hypothesis congruent with experimental data suggests that sleep paralysis is experienced when there is REM sleep at sleep-onset (Hishikawa 1976). The mechanisms underlying sleep-onset REM sleep are not completely understood, but Hishikawa (1976: 115) cites research indicating that the deprivation of REM sleep generates REM sleep at sleep-onset in normal subjects (see also Rechtschaffen and Dement 1969: 123). Within Northeast Harbour fishermen and woodsmen may be 'at risk' groups for *old hag* attacks because they may be chronically REM-deprived. Such deprivation, I would hypothesize, has two sources. First, men in these groups arise very early, typically at three or four in the morning. This practice may deprive those men of some REM episodes which are known to be longer toward the end of nocturnal sleep in normal individuals. Second, men in these groups are engaged daily in hard physical labor. Strenuous exercise over prolonged periods is known to increase the amount of slow-wave (NREM) sleep in man (Baekeland and Lasky 1966). Thus, men in these two groups may have chronically increased proportion of NREM sleep to REM sleep, a condition placing them 'at risk' for attacks of the *old hag* (sleep paralysis). The folk observations are therefore congruent with the argument that *old hag* attacks and sleep paralysis are similar phenomena. Further research is obviously needed to fully assess the causal chain developed above.

TRANSCULTURAL CONSIDERATIONS

The previous two sections have examined how our understanding of idiopathic sleep paralysis and the *old hag* syndrome is improved by viewing them as congruent phenomena. This section concludes the paper by briefly examining the consequences of viewing sleep paralysis as a potentially panhuman experience and suggesting future avenues of research.

There are a number of reports indicating that sleep paralysis has a wide occurrence in time and space. Mitchell (1876) described the experience in the United States a century ago as 'night palsy'. Payn (1965) notes that sleep paralysis has been identified in Germany as delayed psychomotor awakening (*"verzögertes psychomotorisches Erwachen"*) and in France as awakening cataplexy (*"cataplexie du réveil"*). Hishikawa (1976: 9) lists additional labels that have been employed in France and Germany and briefly cites the research done in these countries. If sleep paralysis is a common occurrence within normal populations in the United States (Hishikawa 1976) then similar reports can be expected from within other cultural settings as well.

Published reports on sleep paralysis have not, however, examined the indigenous evaluations of and responses to sleep paralysis. Field research is clearly needed to fully document the cross-cultural distribution of sleep paralysis and the interpretation of this experience in different cultural settings.[9] Wallace (1961: 270) has argued, for example, the " . . . incipient neurological disfunction is susceptible to different interpretations by the victim and has associates and can therefore precipitate different overt responses, depending on particular customs of the individual and group." One broad hypothesis that should be investigated is that cultural interpretations of sleep paralysis, as well as the ideational content of the hypnogogic hallucinations, are functionally related to indigenous theories of witchcraft.

There are features of the *old hag* syndrome, for example, that appear related to witchcraft symbolism. The term *hagged* itself is defined by Webster's Third New

International Dictionary (1971) as "bewitched, enchanted; resembling a witch or a hag". The etymology of the term *hag* places its origin in the Old English term *haegtess* meaning harpy or witch. In addition, there are a number of surveys of English folklore connecting the term *hag* with witches (Simpson 1973: 72, 87), a destructive female giant (Hunt 1968: 464), and a class of spirits (Hardy 1895: 77). The people of Northeast Harbour share close cultural ties with the British Isles (Ness 1976) and their use of the term *old hag* reflects these historical affinities. Derived from this same cultural heritage there is also a healthy belief in witchcraft among the elderly in Northeast Harbour, who typically suspect that the *old hag* can be 'put on ya' by another person.

The ideational content of the hypnagogic hallucinations occasionally accompanying sleep paralysis in Northeast Harbour requires further analysis before relationships with witchcraft beliefs can be fully established. Several older informants did, however, report 'seeing' ugly old women during their attacks, a fact congruent with the image of witches within this community.

In addition to examining relationships between witchcraft beliefs and the phenomenon of sleep paralysis, research in other cultural settings should investigate the extent to which core features of sleep paralysis influence the nature of folk beliefs about the onset, course, and cure of the experience. Within specific communities, for example, are folk beliefs about cause and prevention highly variable? Is there a relatively uniform understanding of a 'risk factor' and a 'cure'? Finally, is the hypothesis that chronic REM-deprivation places individuals or groups 'at risk' supported by cross-cultural studies?

Ethnographic material recently obtained in the Caribbean area, for example, indicates that an experience similar to sleep paralysis is recognized by people living near St. Lucia, in the West Indies. One intriguing aspect of this material is the fact that the attacks, called *kokma*, are caused by unpredictable supernatural beings;

The attack comes at the time that an individual is just falling asleep or just waking up, and the individual's sensations include a pressure on the chest, inability to move, and anxiety ... (the experience) is referred to as *kokma*. A *kokma* is the spirit of a dead baby that haunts an area, and will attack people in bed. They jump on your chest and clutch at your throat. To get rid of them the attacked person struggles to cry out, or in some way gets another person's attention, who will scare off the *kokma* ... The informants who have given me a description of *kokma* have always talked about the babies actually clutching at their throats ... the attacks are always by dead, unbaptized babies. The *kokma* cannot be controlled, they 'grab' people just for the hell of it (Dressler 1977).

The unpredictable nature of the dead baby's spirit and the attack itself reflects, it seems to me, a fundamental fact about sleep paralysis described earlier; namely, that this experience has an 'indeterminacy' that prevents victims or observers from developing a causal explanation with predictive clarity at the individual (victim) level of analysis, It is understandable, therefore, that a capricious supernatural agent is held accountable for these attacks within the St. Lucia setting. Further research in St. Lucia and other cultural settings is needed, of course, to establish cross-cultural regularities between core features of sleep paralysis and indigenous con-ceptualizations of this experience.

Many years ago Tylor (1871) suggested that man's capability to dream might provide the experiential base for the development of folk theories about super-natural worlds. It may be that sleep-related experiences such as sleep paralysis, involving intense feelings of paralysis and vivid hallucinations, are far more potent experiences than dreams in initiating and/or sustaining strong beliefs about the activities of a wide range of natural and supernatural beings.[10]

ACKNOWLEDGEMENTS

Northeast Harbour is a pseudonym. The research was supported by a training grant from the National Institutes of Health, Washington, D.C., administered by the Social Sciences and Health Services Training Program in the Department of Community Medicine and Health Care, University of Connecticut Health Center. I wish to thank my wife Nancy for her exten-sive field research relevant to this paper, and to acknowledge and constructive comments offered by Ronald M. Wintrob, M.D. and Harry Fiss, Ph.D. on several earlier versions.

NOTES

1. Older men and women use the term 'ag rog'. People characteristically drop an initial *h* so that *old hag* is typically spoken of as the '*old 'ag*' or simply 'the '*ag*'. The precise distribu-tion of the *old hag* concept in Newfoundland is not known, but I suspect the idea is wide-spread throughout the province. A survey by Hufford (1976) found that approximately 50 percent of the students questioned at the Memorial University in St. John's, Newfoundland had heard about the *old hag*. This figure is impressive because students at Memorial Univer-sity are drawn from throughout the province.

2. My sample represents the group of adults scheduled to complete the *Cornell Medical Index* (CMI) during my last month in the community. The order in which respondents were selected for interviewing was based solely on their house numbers assigned during my first week in the community.

3. The CMI is a 195-item questionnaire designed to elicit information about the respondent's past and present physical health, as well as the respondent's feelings about his state of mind and general health (Brodman et al. 1949). The instrument has been used in the United States in studies of various normal, psychiatric outpatient, hospital, military, and student groups (Arnoff 1956; Brodman et al. 1952a, 1952b, 1953, 1954; Croog 1961; Lawton 1959; Matarazzo et al. 1961; White et al. 1958). The questionnaire has also been used to measure changes in physical and mental health in situations of social change in Alaska (Chance 1965), the eastern United States (Cassel and Tyroler 1961), and South Africa (Scotch and Geiger 1963). The CMI consists of 18 different sections composed of questions answered 'yes' or 'no' about perceived complaints in different parts of the body (e.g., eyes, ears, digestive tract) and patterns of mood and feeling (e.g., depression, anxiety).

4. Thus, all of the psychological questions on the CMI were used plus three sections registering psychophysiological complaints.

5. Similar results were obtained when the remaining nine CMI sections not reported in this paper were analyzed.

6. One may argue that the CMI is inadequate for assessing the existence of emotional distur-bances which may predispose people to experience sleep paralysis. The CMI has, however,

been shown to yield more information on patients' symptoms than are uncovered by the typical clinical history taken by a physician (Brodman et al. 1951, 1952a, 1952b, 1953; Erdmann et al. 1952).

7. The idea that some individuals can cause an *old hag* attack may be seen as an exception to this statement, but this folk theory is not widely accepted; the emphasis, moreover, is on persons with special abilities rather than 'stress' which precipitates the attack.

8. It is also relevant to point out that 'seeing' other individuals, whether dead or alive, is an acceptable and expected experience in Northeast Harbour. This experience may occur within the context of Pentecostal church activity or during daily activities when 'a token' or image of someone may appear. Thus, within this cultural context, hallucinatory experiences such as those occurring during an *old hag* attack are defined as normal happenings, not signs of emotional instability.

9. So far, however, novelists have provided more descriptive data than ethnographers. One of the clearest descriptions of sleep paralysis can be found in Thomas Hardy's *Wessex Tales* (1896: 73–77) where a woman experiences hypnagogic hallucinations and paralysis. Other descriptive statements within well-known pieces of English literature have been analyzed by Schneck (1962: 1971).

10. Disorders such as cataplexy and narcolepsy may also be important experiences in some cultural settings. Weidman (1973), for example, has described an experience called 'falling out' among Southern Blacks and 'blacking-out' among Bahamians living in Miami. Except for the fact that such episodes may occur at any time of the day without warning, these experiences appear to share many similarities with sleep paralysis as well as cataplexy (Guilleminault 1976). Careful comparative analysis of these experiences and their respective folk interpretations may reveal basic similarities.

REFERENCES

Arnoff, Franklin N., LaVerne Strough, and Richard R. Seymour
    1956 The Cornell Medical Index in a Psychiatric Outpatient Clinic. Journal of Clinical Psychology 12: 263–268.
Baekeland, F. and Lasky, R.
    1966 Exercise and Sleep Patterns in College Athletes. Perceptual Motor Skills 23: 1203–1207.
Brodman, Keeve, A. J. Erdmann, and H. G. Wolff
    1949 Cornell Medical Index Health Questionnaire Manual. New York: Cornell University Medical College.
    1951 CMI Health Questionnaire II: As a Diagnostic Instrument. Journal of the American Medical Association 145: 152–157.
    1952a CMI Health Questionnaire III: The Evaluation of Emotional Disturbances. Journal of Clinical Psychology 8: 119–124.
    1952b CMI Health Questionnaire IV: The Recognition of Emotional Disturbances in a general Hospital. Journal of Clinical Psychology 8: 289–293.
    1953 CMI Health Questionnaire VI: The Relation of Patients' Complaints to Age, Sex, Race, and Education. Journal of Gerontology 8: 339–342
Brodman, Deeve, et al.
    1954 CMI Health Questionnaire VII: The Prediction of Psychosomatic and Psychiatric Disabilities in Army Training. American Journal of Psychiatry 11: 37–40.
Cassel, J., and H. H. Tyroler
    1961 Epidemiological Studies of Culture Change. Archives of Environmental Health 3: 25–33.
Cawte, John E.
    1976 *Malgri*: A Culture-Bound Syndrome. *In* William P. Lebra (ed.), Culture-Bound

Syndromes, Ethnopsychiatry and Alternate Therapies. Honolulu: University of Hawaii Press.

Chance, Norman
1965 Acculturation, Self-identification, and Personality Adjustment. American Anthropologist 67: 372–393.

Chodoff, Paul
1944 Sleep paralysis with Report of Two Cases. Journal of Nervous and Mental Disease 100: 278–281.

Croog, Sidney H.
1961 Ethnic Origins, Educational Level and Responses to a Health Questionnaire. Human Organization 20: 65–69.

D'Andrade, Roy G.
1976 A Propositional Analysis of U.S. American Beliefs About Illness. *In* Keith H. Basso, and Henry A. Selby (eds.), Meaning in Anthropology. Albuquerque: University of New Mexico Press.

Dressler, William
1977 Personal communications from St. Lucia, West Indies.

Erdmann, Albert J., et al.
1952 CMI Health Questionnaire V: The Outpatient Admitting Department of a General Hospital. Journal of the American Medical Association 149: 550–551.

Ethelberg, S.
1956 Sleep Paralysis in Medical Students. Journal of Nervous and Mental Disease 136: 283–287.

Fabrega, Horacio Jr.
1974 Problems Implicit in the Cultural and Social Study of Depression. Psychosomatic Medicine 36: 377–398.

Foulks, Edward F.
1972 The Arctic Hysterias. Washington, D.C.: American Anthropological Association.

Freedman, Alfred M., H. I. Kaplan. and B. J. Sadock
1972 Modern Synopsis of Comprehensive Textbook of Psychiatry. Baltimore: Williams and Wilkins Co.

Goode, G. Browns
1962 Sleep Paralysis. Archives of Neurology 6: 228–234.

Guilleminault, Christian
1976 Cataplexy. *In* C. Guilleminault, W. C. Dement, and Pierre Passouant (eds.), Narcolepsy. Advances in Sleep Research, Volume 3. New York: Spectrum Publications, Inc.

Hardy, James (ed.)
1895 The Denham Tracts Vol. II. London: David Nutt.

Hardy, Thomas
1896 Wessex Tales. New York: Harper and Brothers.

Hishikawa, Yasuo
1976 Sleep paralysis. *In* C. Guilleminault, W. C. Dement, and Pierre Passouant (eds.), Narcolepsy. Advances in Sleep Research, Volume 3. New York: Spectrum Publications, Inc.

Hufford, David J.
1976 A New Approach to the *Old Hag*: The Nightmare Tradition Re-examined. *In* Wayland D. Hand (ed.), American Folk Medicine; A Symposium. Berkeley: University of California Press, pp. 73–85.

Hunt, Robert (ed.)
1968 Popular Romances of the West of England. Third Edition. London: Benjamin Blom.

Kales, Anthony, and Joyce D. Kales
1974 Sleep Disorders. New England Journal of Medicine 290: 487–499.

Kiev, Ari
    1965 The Study of Folk Psychiatry. International Journal of Psychiatry 1: 524–552.
    1969 The Concept of Culture-Bound Syndromes. *In* S. C. Plog and R. B. Edgerton (eds.),
          Changing Perspectives in Mental Illness. New York: Holt, Rinehart and Winston.
    1972 Transcultural Psychiatry. New York: The Free Press.
Lawton, M. Powell
    1959 The Screening Value of the Cornell Medical Index. Journal of Consulting Psychology
          23: 352–356.
Lichtenstein, Ben W., and A. H. Rosenblum.
    1942 Sleep Paralysis. Journal of Nervous and Mental Disease 95: 153–155.
Liddon, S. C.
    1970 Sleep Paralysis, Psychosis and Death. American Journal of Psychiatry 126: 1028–
          1013.
Matarazzo, R. G., J. D. Matarasso, and G. Saslow
    1961 The Relationship Between Medical and Psychiatric Symptoms. Journal of Abnormal
          and Social Psychology 62: 55–61.
Mitchell, S. W.
    1876 On Some of the Disorders of Sleep. Virginia Medical Monthly 2: 769–781.
Ness, Robert C.
    1976 Illness and Adaptation in a Newfoundland Outport. Ph.D. dissertation. Anthropology
          Department, University of Connecticut.
Newman, P. L.
    1964 "Wildman" Behavior in a New Guinea Highlands Community. American Anthropolo-
          gist 66: 1–19.
Payn, Stephen B.
    1965 A Psychoanalytic Approach to Sleep Paralysis. Journal of Nervous and Mental
          Disease 140: 427–433.
Rechtschaffen, Allen, and W. C. Dement
    1969 Narcolepsy and Hypersomnia. *In* Anthony Kales (ed.), Sleep: Physiology and Path-
          ology. Philadelphia and Toronto: J. B. Lippincott Co., pp. 119–130.
Ribstein, Michel
    1976 Hypnagogic Hallucinations. *In* C. Guilleminault, W. C. Dement, and Pierre Passouant
          (eds.), Narcolepsy. Advances in Sleep Research, Volume 3. New York: Spectrum
          Publications, Inc., pp. 145–160.
Rushton, J. G.
    1944 Sleep Paralysis. Medical Clinics of North America 28: 945–949.
Schneck, Jerome M.
    1952 Sleep Paralysis. American Journal of Psychiatry 108: 921–923.
    1960 Sleep Paralysis Without Narcolepsy or Cataplexy: Report of a Case. Journal of the
          American Medical Association 173: 1129–1130.
    1961 Sleep Paralysis. Psychosomatics 2: 360–361.
    1962 Disguised Representation of Sleep Paralysis in Ernest Hemingway's *The Snows of
          Kilimanjaro*. Journal of the American Medical Association 182: 318–320.
    1969 Personality Components in Patients with Sleep Paralysis. Psychiatric Quarterly 43:
          343–348.
    1971 Sleep Paralysis in F. Scott Fitzgerald's *The Beautiful and the Damned*. New York
          State Journal of Medicine 71: 378–379.
Scotch, Norman A., and H. J. Geiger
    1963 An Index of Symptom and Disease in Zulu Culture. Human Organization 22: 304–
          311.
Simpson, Jacqueline
    1973 The Folklore of Sussex. London: B. T. Batsford Ltd.

Tyler, Edward B.
   1871 Primitive Culture. London: J. Murray.
Van Der Heide, Carl, and J. Weinberg
   1945 Sleep Paralysis with Combat Fatigue. Psychosomatic Medicine 7: 330–334.
Von Mering, Otto
   1970 Medicine and Psychiatry. *In* Otto von Mering and Leonard Kasdan (eds.), Anthropology and the Health Sciences. Pittsburg: University of Pittsburgh Press.
Wallace, Anthony C.
   1961 Mental Illness, Biology, and Culture. *In* F. Hsu (ed.), Psychological Anthropology. Homewood, Illinois: The Dorsey Press.
Weidman, Hazel H.
   1973 Implications of the Culture-Broker Concept for the Delivery of Health Care. Paper presented at the annual meeting of the Southern Anthropological Society. Wrightsville Beach, North Corolina.
White, C., M. Reznikoff, and J. W. Ewell
   1958 Usefulness of the Cornell Medical Index Health Questionnaire in a College Health Department. Mental Hygiene 42: 94–105.
Wittkower, Eric D. and Raymond Prince
   1974 A Review of Transcultural Psychiatry. *In* Gerald Caplan (ed.), American Handbook of Psychiatry 2nd Ed., Vol. 2. New York: Basic Books, Inc.
Yap, P. M.
   1969 The Culture-Bound Reactive Syndromes. *In* W. Caudill, and T. Lin (eds.), Mental Health Research in Asia and the Pacific. Honolulu: East-West Center Press, pp. 33–53.
Yoss, Robert E., and David D. Daly
   1957 Criteria for the Diagnosis of the Narcoleptic Syndrome. Proceedings of the Staff Meetings of the Mayo Clinic 32: 320–328.

CHARLES C. HUGHES

THE SLEEP PARALYSIS TAXON
Commentary

The most salient symptom in this syndrome is that of the person's suddenly feeling unable to move or speak when in a borderline sleep state, although remaining fully conscious of surrounding events and people and being able to recall events after the experience. Other symptoms also mentioned in cases in the two papers included here are great agitation and anxiety, sometimes a feeling of weight on the chest (as of someone sitting astride the person – the *old hag* spoken of by Ness), or of the sense that the self is dissociated from the body and is struggling to re-unite into a whole, all this followed by exhaustion. The similarities in symptomatology are striking, although the two papers deal with the syndrome in widely different groups. It is in the cultural explanations regarding etiology and the specific content of the perceptual experiences that the differences lie.

Both papers discuss the syndrome in terms of a phenomenon labelled *Sleep Paralysis* in the psychiatric literature, which as described appears remarkably similar to symptoms manifested in the cases reported here. They also make passing reference to the "hysterical" phenomena and terminology so often found in connection with the "culture-bound" syndromes. With the authors of the two papers both agreeing that sleep paralysis conforms to a recognized pattern, there would seem to be no problem integrating the syndrome into DSM-III. Except that such a diagnosis per se cannot be found in DSM-III – again illustrating one of the problems that initiated this attempt to standardize diagnostic categories.

In terms of a broad type of disorder, the charactersitics of the syndrome seem to conform generally to the "Somatoform Disorders", the

... essential features [of which] are physical symptoms suggesting physical disorder ... for which there are no demonstrable organic findings or known physiological mechanisms and for which there is positive evidence, or a strong presumption, that the symptoms are linked to psychological factors or conflicts (p. 241).

The data given in cases presented here, however, are not full enough to be confident about the implication of psychological conflicts.

To be more specific within this broad class of disorders, one might think of Conversion Disorder (300.11), formerly called "Hysterical Neurosis", which has as its essential feature

... a clinical picture in which the predominant disturbance is a loss of or alteration in physical functioning that suggests physical disorder but which instead is apparently an expression of a psychological conflict or need. The disturbance is not under voluntary control, and after appropriate investigation cannot be explained by any physical disorder or known pathophysiological mechanisms .... The most obvious and "classic" conversion symptoms are those that suggest neurological disease, such as paralysis .... (p. 244)

147

Ronald C. Simons and Charles C. Hughes (eds.), The Culture-Bound Syndromes, 147–148.
© 1985 *by D. Reidel Publishing Company.*

But there are also other symptoms included here not accounted for by this diagnostic label, such as the anxiety and hallucinations, and the feeling of depersonalization expressed by some victims. This suggests the need for concomitant diagnosis in the manner allowed for in DSM-III.

With the first case discussed by Bloom and Gelardin, for example (see p. 117), the data reported would suggest the following DSM-III formulation:

Axis I: 300.11 Conversion Disorder ("Just before going to sleep and waking up, I get paralysed . . . . I can't move").
300.01 Panic Disorder (in which ". . . in which the essential features are recurrent panic (anxiety) attacks that occur at times unpredictably . . . . The panic attacks are manifested by the sudden onset of intense apprehension, fear, or terror, often associated with feelings of impending doom"; p. 230 — Patient reports ". . . it scares me . . . . I really get panicky . . . . I feel like if I don't get back into my body that I am going to die . . . . I finally wake up and move and my heart is just pounding, and I am all shaken up and frightened . . . . I feel like I am going to explode . . . .")
300.60 Depersonalization Disorder (". . . an alteration in the perception or experience of the self so that the usual sense of one's own reality is temporarily lost or changed. This is manifested by a sensation of self-estrangement or unreality . . ."; p. 259 — Patient reports "Sometimes I really start feeling like I am not in my body anymore, like I am outside of my body and fighting to get back . . . . If I don't get back now I never will . . . .")

Axis II: Insufficient data, although some of the discussion in the paper would suggest Dependent Personality attributes (301.70) as being involved.

Axis III: No Data

Axis IV: *Psychosocial stressors*: patient undergoing conflicts of acculturation
Severity: 4? — Moderate (Operationalized definitional example is "new career")

Axis V: *Highest level of adaptive functioning during past year*: 5 — Poor (Marked impairment in either social relations or occupational functioning, *or* moderate impairment in both". Patient indicates that she ". . . had sleep attacks last week over and over . . . . In class I look to see when someone comes in the door. I don't like to be alone because I might kill myself. My kids would be better off if I were dead.")

PART II

FOLK ILLNESSES OF PSYCHIATRIC INTEREST IN WHICH A NEUROPHYSIOLOGICAL SHAPING FACTOR IS ONLY SUSPECTED

A. THE GENITAL RETRACTION TAXON

RONALD C. SIMONS

INTRODUCTION: *THE GENITAL RETRACTION TAXON*

The entities in this taxon have as a common feature severe anxiety associated with the perception that the genitals are retracting into the body. As culturally elaborated syndromes, members of this taxon are found most frequently in Southeast Asia and in China. But, as is true in the case of *Startle Matching* and *Sleep Paralysis*, one regularly encounters isolated instances which seem to parallel the culturally elaborated cases but which occur in areas geographically and culturally remote.

The first paper included in this section, by Gwee Ah Leng, was published in the *Singapore Medical Journal* in 1963. It is a straightforward account of three cases of the Chinese form of *Genital Retraction Syndrome*, here called *koro*, and it describes the responses of others, including physicians, to it. The interpretation Gwee offers is probably that most prevalent in both psychiatry and anthropology: *koro* is an "acute hysterical panic reaction, brought on by auto- or hetero suggestion and conditioning by the cultural background". The second paper, by Ifabumuyi and Rwegellera, describes a similar panic in a Nigerian, and the third, by J. Guy Edwards, " acute anxiety associated with a sensation of penile shrinkage" experienced by an American schizophrenic patient. Neither the Nigerian nor the American had ever heard of *koro*.

These two non-Asian cases are not unique. As James Edwards notes, similar isolated instances have also been reported from Israel, Sudan, India, Thailand, France, Britain, and French and English Canada. It seems futile to debate whether or not the remote incidents represent "true *koro*" or not. Clearly, if by *koro* one means both the experience and a specific cultural gloss, these can not be true exemplars (see Carr's argument *re amok*). But this line of reasoning solves an empirical problem by defining it away; it circumvents rather than resolves the question of whether a specific physiologic substrate shapes or does not shape the experience of a suffering person. James Edward's masterful paper discusses not only the cultural context of Southeast Asian and Chinese genital retraction, but offers some novel suggestions about the relationship between an hypothesized underlying physiological substrate and its subsequent cultural elaboration. The argument he makes parallels the arguments made in this volume about *latah* and sleep paralysis. The fact that genital retraction symptomatology has been reported in association with amphetamines (Dow and Silver, 1973), in the presence of a brain tumor (Lapierre, 1972) and in confusional states from epilepsy, heroin withdrawal and cerebral syphilis (Yap, 1965), also suggests that further investigation of a physiologic substrate is warranted.

Parallel instances of panic associated with the perception of genital retraction

151

Ronald C. Simons and Charles C. Hughes (eds.), The Culture-Bound Syndromes, 151–153.
© *1985 by D. Reidel Publishing Company.*

occur and are reported regularly in persons without any major psychiatric disease. Thus in *The Lancet* Barrett (1978) described the case of a thirty-three year old Englishman who awakened one morning

with an intense feeling of impending doom. This was associated with the physical awareness that his penis had become very small and was shrinking into his body. Palpitations, sweating, nausea and other symptoms of the classic panic attack rapidly developed. But the feeling he was about to die was inextricably linked with the recession of his penis. As a result of this he sought to alleviate his anxiety by pulling the organ in an attempt to restore it to normality.

Aside from occasional mild nonspecific anxiety attacks, the man was otherwise psychologically healthy and without psychiatric symptomatology. Barrett concluded, "whilst a patient's ability to cope psychologically with his *koro* . . . may be culture linked, the psychophysiological syndrome itself is perhaps global".

In societies in which the belief in *koro* is endemic, some men will be especially anxious about their penile states and hence will monitor them especially carefully. Many men, from time to time experience the sensation of their penises shrinking as if retracting more than usual. (In the West, there are a number of jokes relating this experience to exposure to cold, usually cold water.) In cultural contexts which include a belief in *koro*, that experience will generate anxiety. Since the physiology associated with anxiety includes as one of its manifestations reduction of blood flow to the penis and consequent further penile retraction, perception of this retraction will further increase anxiety, frequency of monitoring, and frequency of receiving The Bad News. Frequently receiving The Bad News will even further increase anxiety and its effects. This is an example of a self-incrementing causal loop.

The specific meaning structure in which this loop is embedded will vary in differing cultural contexts. For this reason instances of the *Genital Retraction Taxon* will be most frequent in societies in which the endemic meaning structure most magnifies the anxiety. At times, for example when a rumor of a *koro* epidemic is circulating, this sequence of events will be experienced by enough men to generate a *koro* epidemic. However, since the originating experience is ubiquitous in all societies, similar instances will occur sporadically elsewhere, whenever the cognitive state of subjects for any reason generates anxiety sufficient to drive the loop.

James Edwards suggests using the term *Genital Retraction Syndromes* for the general case and proposes to restrict culture-specific names such as *koro* to the culture area where such names are in fact used. He argues for a multidisciplinary approach which includes the kind of sophisticated historical and cultural analysis such as that which he himself presents but which does not exclude neurophysiologic data *a priori*. Like James Edwards, Ifabumuyi and Rwegellera and J. Guy Edwards distinguish between the experience and its culture-specific interpretation. The 1965 paper by Yap, cited by all authors, is superb and is highly recommended to anyone interested in pursuing this topic further.

REFERENCES

Dow, Thomas W., and Daniel A. Silver
1973 Drug-induced *koro* Syndrome. J. Florida Med. Assoc. 60: 32.
Lapierre, Y.E.
1972 *Koro* in a French Canadian. Canadian Psychial Assoc. J. 17: 333.
Yap, Pow Meng
1965 *koro* — A Culture-bound Depersonalization Syndrome. British J. of Psychiatry, III: 43—50.
Barrett, Ken
1978 *Koro* in a Londoner, Lancet II: 1320.

KORO – A CULTURAL DISEASE

It has been know for quite a long time that a strange disease occurred amongst the Chinese, especially in those who originated from Southern China. Those afflicted presented with a picture of having experienced a sudden feeling of retraction of the penis, and were beset with a great fear that should the retraction be permitted to proceed, the penis would eventually be drawn into the abdomen with a fatal outcome. In their anxiety to prevent such a mishap, they held on to the penis either manually or with instrumental aid. In some instances, relatives took turn to hold on to the penis to curb its supposed "wanderings", in others, a clamp, a cloth peg, a loop of string, or even a safety pin was employed to restrain the recalcitrant member. Occasionally, the pans (lie-teng-hok 鳌裎鑓) of a small weighing instrument used by jewellers were employed to grasp the penis (Strong 1915). In spite of the fears, however, a fatal outcome was unknown, although many instances of trauma to the penis, in some cases quite severe, had been seen.

It is also generally accepted that this is a form of neurosis although the psychodynamics are not clearly known and the natural history of the complaint has not been worked out.

Stitt[1] stated that it was a form of anxiety neurosis seen amongst Buginese and Macassarians in the Celebes and North Borneo, and also occurred among the Chinese, who called it *shook yong*.

Manson-Bahr[2] ascribed the original description to Blonk in 1895 and stated that the sufferers were generally neurotic and the anxiety arose out of sexual conflicts.

The following is a report of 3 cases followed up for 7 years:

Case 1. C.C.H. Male Chinese, schoolboy aged 8. On 27.7.56, he had an insect bite on the penis. A couple living in the house inspected the penis and detected some retraction of the penis going on. Immediately, the penis was held on to and vigorous local applications of balms began. The boy was fed several spoonsful of brandy which was regarded as a "heaty" medicine by the Chinese. The condition abated after 1 hour. Next day, in the evening, the boy thought the penis was again retracting. Straightaway, the penis was anchored with a loop of string and he was brought to the outpatient department of the hospital. The doctor in charge gave him 3 injections one after another and he improved. Two days later, at night, he woke up with the complaint. The penis was clamped with a pair of chopsticks and local applications of balms given with good effect. Next day, however, he had the attack again with pain in the hypogastrium and was brought to the hospital, and referred for consultation by the doctor in the outpatient department. When seen, the boy had a

155

Ronald C. Simons and Charles C. Hughes (eds.), *The Culture-Bound Syndromes*, 155–159.
© 1963 *by the Singapore Medical Association.*

loop of string round the mid-shaft of his penis, and his right hand held on to the string. The penis was bruised, but no serious injury was seen. He was obviously very frightened and his parents accompanying him looked every inch as alarmed as he was. No sexual hair was evident, and both the testes were descended. The boy and the parents were reassured, and after several hours of lengthy persuasion, the symptoms abated and he never had an attack again up till the time this report was written.

Case 2. H.K.F., a male Chinese, aged 34, was seen on 24.3.56. He was at a cinema show when he felt the need to micturate. He went out to the latrine in the foyer, and as he was easing himself, he felt suddenly a loss of feeling in the genital region, and straightaway, the thought occurred to him that he was going to get penile retraction. Sure enough, he soon noticed that the penis was getting shorter. Intensely alarmed, he held on to his penis with his right hand and shouted for help which however was not forthcoming as the latrine was deserted during the show. He felt cold in the limbs, and was weak all over, and his legs gave way under him. So he sat down on the floor, all this time holding on to his penis. About half an hour later, the attacks abated. He went to see a medical specialist and was prescribed some pills. Since then he became nervous and jittery especially when coming face to face with a member of the opposite sex. He was single and a subject of spermatorrhoea during defaecation for several years, and in his school days was generally nervous. At the age of 15, he had his first "wet" dream, and felt very weak after it. Nevertheless, he had regular "wet" dreams. At 24 years of age, he exposed himself to a prostitute, and was infected with gonorrhoea, and since then he abstained himself. He heard of *shook yong* from his friends and also heard about some fatalities during intercourse previous to the present attack.

Treatment: He was vigorously reassured and given some talk on sexual anatomy. No further attack occurred.

Case 3. N.C., male Chinese, aged 38, and married for 16 years with 7 children.

His first attack began at the age of 18 when he took a purgative which acted so vigorously that his penis retracted. The attack however was transitory and did not occasion much alarm. In the last 2 years, he has been feeling very weak, and each time he defaecated, he thought there was a tendency to penile retraction which did not materialise but caused great fear and distress. He had no extramarital affair, and had regular intercourse with his wife, but felt that each time he was considerably weakened physically. He heard about *shook yong* during school days and had also understood it to be very dangerous and likely to be fatal.

Present attack occurred during intercourse a few months ago. He recovered spontaneously after holding on for 20 minutes. Since then, he dared not have intercourse again for fear of a new attack.

On examination: A mentally sedate and well-oriented man. Physical examination showed normal sexual development with no organic disease. The penis was of average size.

Treatment: He was given several talks on sexual anatomy and reassured, and he began to have a normal sexual life again and was free from attacks for the last 8 years. However, he had cut down the frequency of his intercourse and thought he felt better as a result.

DISCUSSION

Koro may have deen derived from the Malay word "kuru", meaning to shake, but the real origin was not ascertainable locally from Malay scholars. On the other hand, the Chinese terms *shook yang, shook jong* have been in use for some time, and in a book known as New Collection of remedies of value (驗方新篇)[3] allusion is made to the term " 縮陽 " (*shook yang*), also referred to as Yin type of cold affliction (陰症傷寒).

This book was published in the Chin Period, and its description was as follows:

During intercourse, the man may be seized suddenly with acute abdominal pain. The limbs become cold and the complexion dusky, the penis retracts into the abdomen. If treatment is not instituted at once and effective, the case will die. The disease is due to the invasion of cold vapours (寒氣) and the treatment is to employ the "heaty" drugs (熱藥).

In later periods, sporadic accounts, mostly folklore and old wives' tales, reported instances of *shook yang* with fatal or near fatal results. The general description is one of sudden onset in a male, usually but not necessarily associated with the sexual act. The attack may come on spontaneously with micturition or defaecation, but characteristically during or soon after the act, *but never before*, and always accompanied by intense alarm with pallor, sweats, coldness in limbs, and occasional abdominal pain. Because of its frequent association with the sexual activity, it is also referred colloquially by the Cantonese as "Seon-Ma Fuun" (a seizure of vapour during the act of mounting a horse, 上馬風 being an allusion to the sexual activity).

In Singapore and Malaya, cases of this nature are frequently seen practically all in the Chinese, and a patient may have one attack only, or several recurring ones. No fatality has been observed, although instances of sudden death during intercourse were frequently cited as being due to the complaint. Fortunately, sudden deaths in Singapore and Malaya were liable to postmortem examinations, and so far of 4 cases stated to be of this nature traced by me in Singapore, death had been due to coronary thrombosis in 3 and cerebral haemorrhage in one, and also there was no real account in these cases to show that they did exhibit the characteristic picture of *koro* prior to death.

From the three cases reported above, and the information gleaned locally, it seems reasonable to assume that *koro* or *shook yang* is an acute hysterical panic reaction arising as a result of a deluded belief which has been current in folklore. The patient learns through hearsay that the retraction of the penis can result in death; and under circumstances favorable to the development of the condition, the slightest subjective feeling in the genitalia sets in motion the fear that this particular complaint is afoot! Thereupon, he grasps his penis and summons aid, and the mounting anxiety together with a sympathetic crowd of relatives sharing a common belief does the rest.

PSYCHODYNAMICS

It will be easy to attribute the aetiology of such a complaint to half a dozen psychological reasons. In fact psychological reasons are as a rule so facile that it would be strange if reasons could not be found to explain away any condition. However, it is interesting to note that castration is practised in China to create eunuchs for the Court, and also that in ordinary conversation, children are frequently threatened with castration for misdemeanour in micturition habits. Further, promiscuity is frowned upon by Chinese culture in spite of the public sanction of multiple wives, and literature abounds in exhortations to avoid illicit sexual relationships, with all sorts of supposed ills that may arise as a result of such practices. Also, Chinese medicine, which has a wide appeal, attaches great importance to the spermatic fluid, stating that 10 grains of rice form a drop of blood, and 10 drops of blood form a drop of spermatic fluid, and that a Man's health can be seriously jeopardised if there is an excessive loss of spermatic fluid. In fact, a Han emperor (漢成帝)[4] was said to have died after taking some aphrodisiacs because his spermatic fluid flowed continuously! The formation of spermatic fluid is supposed to the attributable to the kidneys, and round about the kidneys is situated a mysterious point referred to as the Gate of Life (命門). Hence it can be seen that as far as Chinese culture goes, the ground is adequate to give rise to the concept that sexual excesses, apart from being a social and religious taboo, can literally through the loss of the spermatic fluid result in the loss of life.

It remains to be discussed why should the belief of penile retraction occur.

In very old Chinese medical books,[5] the retraction of penis with distension of abdomen (probably peritonitis with abdominal wall oedema) was described as a certain sign of death. In books on calisthenics, a boxer is said to achieve near invulnerability when he, by dint of hard work and complicated training, manages to toughen up his hide so that it can withstand blows from clubs and knives, and also that he could withdraw his testis into his abdomen so that they could not be attacked. A blow on the testis is regarded as fatal, and a particular kick – Liau Yin Tui – (撩陰腿) aiming at the genitals of the opponent is listed as a lethal weapon. Fatality and retraction of penis seem therefore well correlated in the Chinese mind for many years, and a bit of imagination on the part of a physician can easily conjure up such a condition. Thus it would appear that the disease is probably a result of the free play of imagination of a physician on top of a culture which links fatality with genital retraction and sexual activity with risk to life. The popular appeal of Chinese medicine soon propagates such a belief until it becomes a common knowledge found in popular books of household remedies like the New Collection of remedies of value.

A study of the 3 cases reported above together with other cases seen from time to time would seem to suggest that this condition is one of acute hysterical panic reaction brought on by auto- or hetero-suggestion and conditioning by the cultural background. In the first case of the boy, he was taught the concept of *koro* by a couple, and soon he learned to develop the complaint *at home in the evenings.* and his condition was on each occasion reinforced by the sympathy, alarm and anxiety of his parents. In the other two cases, prior information about *koro* was obtained through hearsay, and the first subjective feeling in the genitalia led to a realistic attack.

Thus the cycle of the disease would appear to be as follows:

Information about *koro* on hearsay plus some sexual fears and subjective sensation in genitalia either of a normal nature such as associated with sexual act, defaecation or micturition or of an abnormal nature such as an insect bite plus fear → *koro* → fear → *koro*.

The rapid improvement and case of radical cure following education would indicate that the condition is not psychotic, but more like a conversion hysteria which is usually radically cured. The only difference between it and conversion hysteria is that in the latter, the motivation is not apparent and the patient's emotional content towards the disability is one of indifference, whereas in *koro*, the active cause is frankly sexual in most cases with the belief that sexual activity is bad or weakening and the emotional state is one of extreme alarm amounting to panic.

SUMMARY

3 cases of *koro* were reported after a followup of some years. A brief discussion of the possible mechanism of the disease in Chinese was made.

The opinion is expressed that this is an acute hysterical panic reaction brought on by auto- or hetero-suggestion.

ACKNOWLEDGEMENT

I am grateful for having had access to some of the cases of Prof. G.A. Ransome in the course of this study, and for valuable advice from Prof. E.S. Monteiro.

REFERENCES

1. Strong, R.P. (1945). Stitt's Diagnosis, Prevention and Treatment of Tropical Diseases, 7th Ed. Maple Press Co., U.S.A., p. 1145.
2. Manson-Bahr, Sir Philip Henry (1881). Manson's Tropical Diseases a Manual of the disease of warm climate, 14th Ed. London, Cassel.
3. 驗方新編：卷七 ── 陰症傷寒
4. 飛燕外傳
5. 中藏經

O. I. IFABUMUYI AND G. G. C. RWEGELLERA

KORO IN A NIGERIAN MALE PATIENT: A CASE REPORT

INTRODUCTION

Koro is an acute anxiety characterised by the patient's fear that his penis is shrinking and will disappear into the abdomen. When it occurs in the female it is associated with fear that the vulval labia and breasts are shrinking and will disappear (Linton 1956). To prevent this from happening the patient grips his penis very firmly; and at times he is helped in doing this by anxious and bewildered relatives. Fellatio practised immediately by the wife has been said to be of help. The Chinese employ various devices for this purpose including the application of special wooden clasps and the use of a male factor "yan". The Chinese believe that the illness is a result of imbalance between "yan", the male, and "Yin" the female, factors.

Koro occurs almost exclusively among the peoples of the Malay archipelago and South China (Leng 1963). The Chinese name for this syndrome is *suk-yeong*. Few cases have been reported from other parts of the world. Dow and Silver (1973) reported a case of *koro* in a 20-year-old Canadian who was also intoxicated with amphetamine, and Lapierre (1972), reported one case in a 55-year-old man with a brain tumour.

Koro is a rare syndrome. Thus, Yap (1951) could find only 19 cases after a comprehensive survey of the literature over a period of 15 years. The aetiology of this illness is unknown. Various precipitating factors have been suggested by previous authors. Yap (1951, 1965) mentioned coitus, sudden exposure of the penis to cold air or water, while excessive indulgence in, or inappropriate coitus has been blamed by others. Yap (1965) saw the illness as a depersonalisation and distortion of the body image. However, the inter-action between social and cultural factors and the premorbid personality of the individual would appear to be important factors in the causation of this syndrome.

CASE HISTORY

M. A. is a 36-year-old married father of four children, two boys and two girls. He was referred for psychiatric treatment as a result of recurrent acute anxiety with multiple hypochondriacal symptoms.

His illness started suddenly about a year prior to his referral with a feeling of pain in both shoulders and the waist and heat at the centre of the head. This was followed usually by extreme fear and panic reaction during which the patient feared desperately that his penis was shrinking into his abdomen. At the height of his anxiety he would run into the bush only to be pursued and brought back by relatives and friends.

Prior to his referral, he had consulted several indigenous healers, who prescribed

161

Ronald C. Simons and Charles C. Hughes (eds.), The Culture-Bound Syndromes, 161–163.
© 1979 *by Literamed Publications Nigeria Ltd.*

various herbs which he had to apply to his penis. It was at the height of the second attack that the patient was referred for psychiatric treatment.

Investigation into his personal and marital history revealed that he had been married for about ten years. He described the marriage as satisfactory with "full" sexual gratification. (He refused to mention the frequency of sexual intercourse.) Since his first attack, for which there was no obvious precipitating factor, sexual intercourse with his wife had diminished, and at the time of examination, the patient was worried that he might lose his wife if he became sexually non-functioning as a result of his retracting penis.

There was no history of drug or alcohol abuse. Physical and neurological examinations revealed no evidence of organic illness. Interview with the wife revealed no evidence of marital problems. The patient also denied any extra-marital affair. The patient was, prior to the onset of his illness, happy at his job as a gardener.

DISCUSSION

To the best of the authors' knowledge, *koro* has not been reported among Nigerians. Anumonye and Adaranijo (1978) reported four cases of feeling that the penis was getting smaller in two university undergraduates and two clerks who had previous histories of veneral diseases. As the authors stated these cases were quite dissimilar to the classical *koro* syndrome as described above. The syndrome is rare, only about 21 cases have been reported to date. Prior to the two cases reported from Canada, the illness was believed to be limited exclusively to the Malay archipelago and South China, although Kraepelin had in his textbook mentioned shrinkage of the penis among the hypochondriacal delusions of the depressive states of manic-depressive psychosis.

The aetiology of this condition is largely unknown. Kraepelin's cases showed that features of this syndrome can occur in other psychiatric disorders and other cultures. Lapierre's (1972) case of a 55-year-old man with a frontotemporal tumor and Dow and Silver's (1973) case of amphetamine intoxication suggest that *koro*, like other anxiety state, can be associated with organic mental states in other cultures. The interesting thing about our patient is that he is the only one so far described outside the Malay Archipelago and South China, in whom the main features of the syndrome are not associated with any organic or psychiatric disorder other than anxiety.

This does raise a number of important questions which will need to be answered if we are to advance our knowledge in this field. One question is whether it is correct, to call *koro* a "Culture-Bound" syndrome. Since it occurs in such diverse cultures, this would appear not to be correct, unless we define more precisely the aspects of each culture which are associated with it. The other question is what part, if any, does "culture" play in the causation of this syndrome? All the evidence we have strongly suggests that culture, or at least those relevant aspects of culture, like premorbid personality, has a pathoplastic (moulding) effect on this condition. It lends colour to, but does not cause the illness.

That *koro* has not been described before among Africans should not surprise anyone who is acquainted with the psychiatric scene in Africa. Psychiatrists are few and far between, and most of them work in mental hospitals or asylums, which are also few and inadequately staffed and can only admit the very disturbed psychotic patients. Secondly, the stigma associated with mental illness is still rampant among people in Africa. Going to a mental hospital or an asylum is one sure way of stigmatising oneself and the family. So that even those patients who eventually come to see a psychiatrist try traditional healers first as this particular patient did. This means that the patients seen by psychiatrists in Sub-Sharan Africa are a selected group and a small fraction of those who are mentally ill. Many such "rare" syndromes are probably lost in this way.

ACKNOWLEDGEMENT

The authors would like to thank the Director of the Institute of Health, Ahmadu Bello University, for permission to publish this paper.

G.G.C.R. would like to thank the Regional Director for W.H.O,, Brazzaville, for allowing him to publish this paper. It must, however, be pointed out that the views expressed in this paper are those of the authors and not those of W.H.O. or the Institute of Health.

REFERENCES

Anumonye, A. and H. Adaranijo
    1978 Chronic Non-specific Urethritis As Psychological Reaction Among Nigerian Neurotic Patients. Nigerian Medical Journal 8: 3.
Dow, T. W. and D. A. Silver
    1973 Drug-induced *Koro* Syndrome. Journal of Floridal Medical Association 60: 32.
Lapierre, Y. D.
    1972 *Koro* in a French Canadian. Canadian Psychiatry Association Journal 17: 333.
Leng, G. A.
    1963 *Koro* − A Cultural Disease. Singapore Medical Journal 4: 119.
Linton, R.
    1950 *In* G. Devereux (ed.), Culture and Mental Disorders.Thomas: Springfield, Illinois.
Yap, P. M.
    1951 Mental Disease Peculiar to Certain Cultures: A Survey of Comparative Psychiatry. Journal of Mental Science 97: 313.
    1965 *Koro*: A Culture-Bound Depersonalization Syndrome. British Journal of Psychiatry 3: 43.

J. GUY EDWARDS[1]

THE *KORO* PATTERN OF DEPERSONALIZATION IN AN AMERICAN SCHIZOPHRENIC PATIENT

Koro is a psychogenic syndrome in which a subjective experience of penile shrinkage occurs in association with acute anxiety. The literature on the phenomenon does not make it clear that there are two components. There is the experience of shrinkage of the penis, and the cultural interpretation of this experience – namely, that the penis will disappear into the abdomen with a fatal outcome. The syndrome has been defined by some authors in such a way that both components are mentioned (Arieti and Meth 1959; Mun 1968), while Kline (1968) questions the propriety of diagnosing *koro* in the absence of the folk interpretation, which he thinks is an essential requisite of *koro*.

On the other hand, *koro* has been described without any mention of fear of disappearance of the penis into the abdomen (Yap 1965b). Further, if one considers *koro* along a descriptive axis, various degrees of severity of the experience of penile shrinkage can be found. Only when the experience is severe does the subject panic and fear that the penis will disappear into the abdomen.

Yap (1968) attempts to resolve this difficulty by distinguishing the "*koro* pattern of depersonalization" from the folk illness known by the Indonesian–Malay name *koro* and by the southern Chinese (Cantonese) name *suk-yeong*. He regards the "*koro* pattern of depersonalization" as a "neurotic state with depersonalization involving the penis", but thinks the fear of retraction of the penis into the abdomen is necessary for the diagnosis of *koro*, the folk illness. Thus, one can say that the depersonalization experience (perhaps body image disturbance would be a more descriptive term) is the basic phenomenon and may be universal in its distribution; but it is the exotic interpretation of its outcome in certain cultures that has attracted the attention of psychiatrists and has led to its description as a "culture-bound syndrome". Yap has summarized his views on the nosology of *koro* in an academic lecture delivered in Australia (Yap 1967).

While the folk illness *koro* is endemic in certain Eastern countries and has even occurred in epidemic form (Mun 1968), cases of the "*koro* syndrome" have been sporadically described in Occidentals by Kraepelin (1921), Schilder (1935), Bychowski (1952), and Yap (1965b) in association with depression and a variety of other somatic symptoms. Yap (1965a) has also described *koro* occurring against a background of schizophrenia, but no such case has been described in a Westerner. Because of its implication for cross-cultural comparative psychiatry, the following case report is presented:

CASE REPORT

The patient, aged 40, was born in Greece but has lived in the United States since he was a few

165

Ronald C. Simons and Charles C. Hughes (eds.), The Culture-Bound Syndromes, 165–168.
© 1970 by the American Psychiatric Association.

months old. At the present time he is a patient in the early clinical drug evaluation unit. Research Center, Rockland State Hospital, New York.

There was no family history of mental illness. Prior to becoming ill the patient had been inhibited and immature, and these traits were also evident in his psychosexual life, which was frustrated by impotence. When he was 18 years of age, he became preoccupied with the small size of his penis, and on two occasions he dreamed that "there was a vagina where the penis should be". He had also shown such obsessional traits as perfectionism and compulsive checking.

His schizophrenic illness began when he was 22 years old, and at various times during its course he had had formal thought disorder, thought blocking, flattening and incongruity of affect, delusions, and auditory hallucinations. At the time of writing he said he wanted to forget his past life and asked everyone to call him "Nameless". On an isolated occasion, when one of the attendants accidently called him by his real name, he suddenly experienced acute anxiety associated with a sensation of penile shrinkage. This lasted for approximately an hour, but for several weeks after wards he could only get "two-thirds of an erection".

He had never previously heard of *koro* and had not encountered other patients with genital symptoms. It has not since been possible to induce *koro* by calling him by his proper name.

DISCUSSION

Although 20th century Westerners do not suffer from *koro*, the folk illness, even as part of the heterogeneous symptomatology of schizophrenia, the examples cited above and the case described show that they do experience the "*koro* pattern of depersonalization".

Subjective ideas of genital change are more common than generally realized. Gittleson and Levine (1966) found that 14 out of 70 schizophrenic men had experienced ideas of change in the size or shape of their genital organs. In addition, of the control group of 45 patients, three, over the age of 60 and suffering from endogenous depression, thought that their genitals were shrinking with increasing age and general illness. None of these experiences had the qualities of *koro* (Gittleson 1968) and they seemed to be in the nature of delusional or "delusion-like" ideas. But this does not mean that more frequent and detailed questioning would not reveal more examples of the "*koro* pattern of depersonalization".

The prevalence of the belief in the existence of a fatal illness due to disappearance of the penis into the abdomen predisposes certain anxious individuals to self-scrutiny and overconcern with their genitalia. This could account for the higher incidence of the "*koro* pattern of depersonalization" in the East, and for the etiological role played by suggestion in certain patients, such as those who experienced the sensation of penile shrinkage after hearing *koro* discussed (Yap 1965) and those in the recent Singapore epidemic (Mun 1968).

The interpretation of subjective experiences differs from country to country and age to age. In 20th century Western culture a common interpretation is in terms of physical illness. In days gone by, however, a similar experience may have been regarded as resulting from demoniacal possession or witchcraft.

As early as 1608, Brother Francesco Maria Guazzo (1929) described in his *Compendium Maleficarum*, in the Second Book "... dealing with the various kinds of witchcraft and certain other matters which should be known", how witches exerted their evil influences upon men's and women's sexual potency. The "seventh" way, "rarer" than the others, included "a retraction, hiding or actual removal of the male genitals. This kind of witchcraft is of two sorts, one temporary and the other permanent. It is temporary when it is only to last for a certain time." Interpreted in the light of 17th century ideology and religious belief as being due to the evil influences of witchcraft, it is possible that some of these "temporary" influences are examples of the "*koro* pattern of depersonalization".

In conclusion, it can be said that folk belief pathoplastically molds "sexual anxiety" into the *koro* form of expression, while in the West the etiological factors are derived from idiosyncratic psychopathology (Yap 1967). However, here cultural belief does not allow for more than the experience of penile shrinkage.

NOTE

1. At the time this paper was written J. Guy Edwards was affiliated with the Rockland State Hospital Research Center, Orangeburg, N.Y. Currently he is a consultant psychiatrist, Knowle Hospital, Fareham, Hampshire, England.

The author expresses his appreciation to J. W. S. Angus for drawing his attention to the case described, to P. M. Yap for his help in the preparation of the paper, and to Mrs. June Rogers for her secretarial assistance.

REFERENCES

Arieti, S. and J. M. Meth
    1959 Rare, Unclassifiable, Collective, and Exotic Psychotic Syndromes. *In* S. Arieti (ed.), American Handbook of Psychiatry. New York: Basic Books.
Bychowski, G.
    1952 Psychotherapy of the Psychoses. New York: Grune & Stratton.
Gittleson, N. L.
    1968 Personal Communication.
Gittleson, N. L. and Levine, S.
    1966 Subjective Ideas of Sexual Change in Male Schizophrenics. British Journal of Psychiatry 112: 779–782.
Guazzo, F. M.
    1929 *In* E. A. Ashwin (transl.), Compendium Maleficarum. London: John Rodker.
Kline, N. S.
    1968 Personal Communication.
Kraepelin, E.
    1921 *In* R. M. Barcley (transl.), Manic-Depressive Insanity and Paranoia. Edinburgh: E. & S. Livingston.
Mun, C. T.
    1968 Epidemic *Koro* in Singapore. British Medical Journal 1: 640–641.
Schilder, P.
    1935 The Image and Appearance of the Human Body. London: K. Paul, Trench & Trubner.
Yap, P. M.
    1965a *Koro* – A Culture-Bound Depersonalization Syndrome. British Journal of Psychiatry 111: 43–50.

1965b *Koro* in a Briton. British Journal of Psychiatry 111: 774–775.
1967   Classification of the Culture-Bound Reactive Syndromes. Australian and New Zealand
         Journal of Psychiatry 1: 172–179.
1968   Personal Communication.

JAMES W. EDWARDS

INDIGENOUS *KORO*, A GENITAL RETRACTION SYNDROME
OF INSULAR SOUTHEAST ASIA: A CRITICAL REVIEW

INTRODUCTION

Koro, one of the least known culture-bound syndromes of Southeast Asia, is characterized by complaints of genital hyperinvolution and fear of impending death. Current medical and psychiatric literature describe the syndrome as endemic only among Chinese populations, especially in Southeast Asia. But the term and the syndrome were first introduced to Western science as a malady indigenous to southern Sulawesi, formerly known as Celebes, an island of Indonesia (Blonk 1895). Blonk's short report rapidly engendered a psychodynamic analysis (Brero 1896a, 1896b) and a second case report (Vorstman 1897), but *koro* received no further attention until the 1930's, when another brief spate of articles appeared (Slot 1935; Mulder 1935; Wulfften Palthe 1934, 1935a, 1935b, 1936, 1937). Since then, *koro* rarely has been noted among the non-Chinese peoples of Southeast Asia.

The temporal distribution of reports of indigenous *koro* poses some interesting questions. Is the distribution a product of the idiosyncratic interests and experience of the foreign observers, or did *koro* only appear in highly localized (temporal and spatial) epidemics? If *koro* was not endemic within the wider Malay–Indonesian cultural sphere, what biomedical or sociocultural data account for its limited manifestation? Is indigenous *koro* no longer manifested, and if not, why? That cases of genital retraction among Chinese are concentrated in Southeast Asia poses another question: is indigenous *koro* a product of cultural diffusion, as Wulfften Palthe (1936) proposed?[1] To begin to seek answers to these questions it becomes necessary to address ethno-historical issues which have been inadequately and unsystematically presented: the emic constructs and ethnographic distribution of indigenous *koro*. Anthropological and biomedical insights need to be integrated with the only interpretation thus far offered, the psychiatric. Though the quantity and quality of the data base leaves much to be desired, a systematic, critical review of the *koro* literature is of heuristic value; as will be argued, disciplinary biases may be responsible for the failure of field and clinical researchers to recognize *koro*-related phenomenon as worthy of analysis and reporting. Indigenous *koro* may be more widespread and common (though still an atypical malady) than previously assumed.

ORIGIN OF THE WORD *KORO*

Since Gwee (1963) in Singapore and Yap (1965a) in Hong Kong applied the term *koro* to manifestations of the syndrome among Chinese, the term has become

169

Ronald C. Simons and Charles C. Hughes (eds.), The Culture-Bound Syndromes, 169–191.
© *1984 by D. Reidel Publishing Company.*

the internationally accepted label for patients' fear of penile shrinkage. The term also encompasses the comparable, but rarer, female complaints of labia, breast and mammilla hyperinvolution. *Koro* is not a Chinese word, nor is it recognized by Chinese speakers; the equivalent Chinese term is, in present orthography, *suoyang* (*suo* = retract, shrink; *yang* = penis, genitals). *Koro* is a Malay term of uncertain origin. B. F. Matthes' Buginese dictionary of 1874 contains the first known reference to the term: *koro* means "to shrink", and *lasa koro* is defined as "a shrinking of the penis, a sort of disease that is not unusual amongst the natives and must be very dangerous" (Wulfften Palthe 1936: 536). Blonk's (1895) informant stated that *koro* was the term used by the Buginese and Macassarese peoples of southern Sulawesi; Wulfften Palthe (1936) gave the full Macassaran term as *garring koro*.

The term is said to be of uncertain origin, for *koro* in Macassaran and Buginese dialects has no clear cognate in standard Malay and Bahasa Indonesian speech. Gwee (1968) noted several Malay terms, e.g., *kuru, kerukul, keroh*, and *keruk* as possible origins; of these, he chose the last, meaning "shrink" as the most probable origin. Linguistic investigation of terms related to "shrink" may, however, be misplaced. An alternate explanation, originally provided by an elderly Chinese, a long term resident of the archipelago, was subsequently affirmed by various Malay speaking peoples; Wulfften Palthe (1936: 536) wrote:

According to him the word is not *koro* at all but *kuro* or *kura* meaning a tortoise. Now both the Malays and the Chinese use 'head of a tortoise' as a usual expression for the penis and especially for the glans penis .... The fact that the tortoise can withdraw its head with its wrinkled neck under its shell literally into its body suggested, then, the mechanism so greatly dreaded in *koro* (*kura*) and gave it its name.

In modern Malay and Indonesian, *kura* or *kura-kura* means tortoise (Wilkinson 1932; Wojowasito and Poerwadarminta 1974); in Macassarese *koero* means tortoise (Slot 1935). Most significantly, as we shall see, avoidance of the tortoise figures in native belief regarding penile shrinkage.

The folk explanation may be the most meaningful, but not the only alternative that can be advanced. *Koro* is a term native to the northwest sector of central Sulawesi; it is the name of a river, the surrounding valley, and the local subgroup of Western Toradja peoples (Adriani and Kruijt 1912; Le Bar 1972). Perhaps the syndrome was somehow associated with this area. But whatever the 'true origin' of the term may be, it is clearly inappropriate to expect that *koro* will be recognized by all the various Malay speaking peoples. Wulfften Palthe spent eight unproductive years enquiring about *koro*, but once "sufficiently conversant with the subject" was able to obtain information (Wulfften Palthe 1936: 538). Was a search for *koro* as opposed to the actual syndrome a hindrance to his research, as it was to other investigators? The opposite side of the coin is the field researcher's unfamiliarity with *koro* as a culture-bound syndrome and research topic. For example, Kenneth Payne (personal communication) collected data on, but did not rigorously investigate, cases of shrinking penis among the Tagabawa Bagobos, a Malayo—Polynesian peoples of Mindanao; only after his return to the United States did he learn of *koro* and the importance of his field data. I don't intend this as a personal criticism, but rather to indicate that the syndrome's exoticness, especially in sexual content, masks its true distribution and prevalence; knowledge of the syndrome has filtered little beyond transcultural psychiatry. The riddle of the origin of *koro* (the term) and *koro* (the syndrome) may only be solved after the ethnographic record has been adequately detailed. For reasons that will become clear, I will use native terminology for genital retraction complaints (e.g., *koro* among Indonesian peoples, *suoyang* among Chinese).

EMIC CONSTRUCTS AND CASE DESCRIPTIONS

The major deficiency of the indigenous *koro* literature is the disproportionate focus on psychoanalytic interpretation at the expense of ethnographic description and localization. This is especially true in the writings of Wulfften Palthe who, judging from the frequency of citation, is the main source of other researchers' knowledge of indigenous *koro*. Moreover, very little of the ethnographic details have been culled from the Dutch language articles when these are cited. Thus extensive review of the native concepts and case descriptions is not unwarranted. The best account of native beliefs was provided by Slot (1935), who published the verbatim report of two native researchers' interview of a traditional healer in the Macassaran area of Sulawesi. The following synopsis generally adheres to the original report (Slot 1935: 814–816), but some data have been re-arranged for consistency in presentation.

Definition

Koro is a Macassaran word meaning "to shrink". *Koro* is a nervous disease, so named because the patient feels that his nerves are contracting.

Etiology

Koro attacks are unpredictable, but usually appear after a shock which made the patient anxious or frightened, after performing strenuous manual labor or no labor at all, or as a result of immoderate nocturnal partying. People say that these irregular lifestyles and work habits effect the nerves. Some believe that accidents, such as falling off a horse, can result in *koro*; if this happens, the first thing to do is to check the penis. The fear is that the penis will disappear into the body and death will follow.

Symptoms

In the initial stages of an attack the patient becomes tense, the hands and feet are cold, the heart rate increases, the face pales, there is clammy sweating, vague anxiety, and a loss of feeling in the extremities and limbs. Then the nerves contract and faintness sets in; the crisis of the attack is characterized by a stiffening of the

the body, the eyes bulge out and the pupils are barely visible, and the patient makes gurgling sounds. In extreme cases, the patient may lose consciousness. The attack, which is never accompanied by fever, can last about an hour.

Therapy

At signs of an impending attack, the patient grabs and pulls on the penis, shouting for help. The patient is anxious not to be left alone, for without help death will occur. Help from others consists mainly of vigorous massage and pressing on the genital area, which continues until the patient stops screaming from pain. The muscles are also massaged to restore feelings in the limbs. One helper attempts to pull on the retracted penis; in dire cases, the penis is so contracted and resistant that a string is used to help pull it out. Assistance from the opposite sex is prohibited; it is said that being touched by the opposite sex may be fatal to the patient. Upon revival, the patient is immediately given a medicinal potion to drink. The potion, representing the erect penis, is concocted of "masculine" substances. Ingredients include: deer horn; bamboo chips; *lasomammelong* (*laso* = penis), the flowering shoots of the male palmyra (Borassus flabelliformis); and stalk of the arenga palm (Arenga sacchariera). These are powdered and mixed with an alcoholic beverage derived from a type of rice mash, so that the patient can "keep it down".

Prognosis and Sequela

The sickness is curable in time, but some chronic cases, due to irregular living habits, eventuate in death. The sickness, being a nervous collapse, results in sexual impotence which lasts for several days. In the informant's experience, males who suffer *koro* are mostly childless.

Prophylaxis

Koro is absent or rarely manifested among people who consume moderate amounts of alcohol. It is prohibited to eat a certain legume, *kentjoer* (Kaempferia galanga), the name of which also means "retract"; or melon because of its springy tendrils; and giant scallops because the flesh greatly shrinks when cooked. One must not step over horse hair or tortoise stool. One must avoid walking in front of a tortoise, for if the animal retracts its head, it is a negative omen; but if the head retracts in the opposite direction from a person (i.e., the tortoise and person are facing back to back), it is a positive sign.

Koro in Women

The native healer (a male) could give no information about female *koro*, since assistance by the opposite sex is prohibited. But it is generally known that *koro* does exist among women. The major symptoms are flattening of the breasts, shrinking of the nipples, and retraction of the labia, which appear to be sucked inside the body.

Other descriptions of indigenous *koro* are much less complete. Beginning with two additional reports from the Macassaran–Buginese area of Sulawesi, these studies will be grouped by geographic area. Comments on geographic and temporal variance will be relegated to a section synthesizing the data.

Contrary to the reviews of some authors, Blonk did not actually witness a *koro* attack. His main informant, a *djaksa* (native legal officer), was a *koro* sufferer who agreed to inform Blonk of the next impending attack, but the opportunity never arose. The informant mentioned no assistance other than aid in holding the penis; attacks may last for hours, leaving the patient tired and worn out (Blonk 1895). A more detailed case vignette, gathered from a Macassaran informant (not the *koro* subject) more than half a century later, ran as follows:

A man, about age 45, with wife and children, took a second wife. Afraid of the first wife's jealousy, he tried to keep the new relationship secret but in time the second marriage became known. One evening, he came home tired and fatigued. He got the shivers, broke out in a cold sweat, and felt that his penis was shrinking. At his cry for help, the neighbors came running. Only men helped him. One man tightly held the patient's penis while another went for a *sanro*, a native healer. The sanro performed one ritual and after a while the anxiety disappeared, ending the day's attack. (Chabot 1950: 165)

There are two reports, widely separated in time and space, of *koro* in Kalimantan. Vorstman (1897) reported on two cases, a native and a Chinese. Details of the former case are largely circumstantial. A Chinese patrol officer induced Vorstman to accompany him to a village in Sintang district to provide medical aid to a member of the native elite. The patient was found in bed, surrounded by a retinue and with an old man sitting at the foot of the bed. Having no information about the patient's symptoms during the preceding days, Vorstman's examination and questioning failed to yield much insight into the man's problem. Based on prior experience, Vorstman concluded that alcohol abuse, a common native habit, was the background to this case. Upon leaving the house, the Chinese official, who had served as interpreter, remarked that Vorstman was probably unsure of the nature of the patient's illness. He related that for the past eight days the patient's penis had been withdrawn into the belly; as a preventive measure the old man at the foot of the bed had been gripping his master's "obstinate limb". Vorstman found this story interesting from the ethnographic standpoint but difficult to believe, especially on anatomical grounds. Subsequently, a different government patrol officer confirmed that the natives did believe in such a disease; and the district officer of Nangapinoh informed him that in his district there was a corpse of a native who had died of this disease (Vorstman 1897: 499–500).

Not knowing the local term for the disease, Vorstman adopted *koro* from Blonk's report. As to the identity of the ethnic group, we can make an educated guess. Vorstman's use of the term "native" (Dutch, *inlandsche*), his care in identifying the patrol officer and the second patient as Chinese, and evidence of social stratification in the patient's native village, all point to the Land Dyaks, the predominant group in the area; other population groups include various Malays, Chinese, and Buginese, largely urban immigrants in Sintang, and the Ot Danum peoples in the outlying areas of Nangapinoh (i.e., along the upper Melawi River) (Kuhr 1896/97; Le Bar 1972).

A similar problem exists with the second report, a letter sent to Wulfften Palthe by a physician practicing in Kualakapuas (Koeala Kapoeas), a town at the confluence of the Kapuas and Barito River drainage systems in southeast Kalimantan. Geographic details given in the letter suggest that the identification of the ethnic group is the Ngadju peoples. Ngadju predominate along the lower courses of the rivers of southern Kalimantan, with various Malays, Chinese and Buginese immigrant groups along the coastal fringe (Mallinckrodt 1924/25; Le Bar 1972).

The physician, referring to a recent report by Wulfften Palthe (1934), supplied the following information. A man, approximately 35 years old, presented at the Kualakapuas polyclinic with the same complaint as the *koro* syndrome. In contrast to Wulfften Palthe's view that *koro* was limited to educated, upper class natives, the patient was a simple *tani* (a peasant, farmer) and, in the physician's view, a "typical neurotic". The patient had periodic feelings that the penis was shrinking into the belly, causing strong fears of imminent death. Strange sensations in the arms and legs, which strode from the trunk to the hands and feet, preceded the onset of penile sensations. The experiences lasted about an hour. According to the physician's native assistants, this was a new sickness in Kalimantan the last few years. In particular, around 1930 there were many male cases along the Katapan [2] River; by 1934 sporadic cases were still appearing. In some patients, the arms and legs became stiff during an attack. Therapy consisted of pulling on the penis and vigorous massage of the extremities. Patients alone when an attack set in wound a cord around the penis to secure it. The disease was also known among women; the labia "shoot within". A woman in Mandomai [3] village died from this; adat rules (customary law) prevented men from helping in cases relating to female genitalia (Wulfften Palthe 1935a).

The last case from Indonesia is interesting in that a *koro* attack precipitated the onset of *amok*, another culture-bound disorder. A 40-year old fisherman, of Badjavanese (Ngada in current terminology, Le Bar 1972) origin and Islamic faith, was arrested for murdering his wife during a fit of *amok*. The man was transported from his resident hamlet on the northwest coast of Flores to Ruteng, where the judge ordered a psychiatric examination. During the exam the patient stated, without prompting, that he was a *koro* sufferer. The first attack came about three years earlier when one day he entered the water to wash. A sudden cold shock ran all over his body, and he felt his penis retracting. Tightly holding the penis, he shouted for help but no one offered assistance in pulling the penis; a native healer gave him some medicine which cured the *koro* little by little. After a trip to Mecca in 1933, he had no further *koro* sensations until the night he went *amok*. On the night of the murder he awoke suddenly, cold chills shot through his body, and his penis retracted; he became "furious" with fear, everything turned yellow and he lost awareness of events. He had total amnesia of murdering his wife. The patient could ascribe no cause to this attack; he did not recall having any dream that night, and denied having problems with his wife or sexual conflicts. Physical examination proved negative: the patient had no somatic anomalies of the body and genital organs, was of good nutritional status and body constitution, calm in behavior and speech, and mentally lucid (Wulfften Palthe 1937).

The final case description comes from the unpublished field research of a medical anthropologist, Kenneth Payne. In 1974 and 1975–76, Payne studied the medical beliefs and practices of the Tagabawa Bagobo of southcentral Mindanao in the Philippines. The Bagobo believe in a shrinking penis disease called *lannuk e laso'* (*laso'* = penis, *lannuk* = "to go inside"). The disease is a product of a type of sorcery used to make one's opponent weak. The sorcery, carried out by tainting the food of the intended victim, causes shrinking penis in men and renders women "tongue-tied"; there were no female genital symptoms reported.

The detailed record of one case is the most complete of all the reports. The subject, age 35, was married to a woman aged 33; both had offspring from prior marriage, but the couple had no children together during their ten years of marriage. The husband was very traditional, a good provider for his family, and a hard worker. That his harvests were larger than his neighbors' crops created a suspicion of envy and fear of sorcery. About the time of the subject's attack, his brother, a sufferer of *lannuk e laso'*, suddenly died; the death was attributed to sorcery. The subject initially complained of milky urine; later his urine turned deep yellow, a course of events duplicating his brother's final days. He complained of intermittent pain and extreme lower back pain when the penis "went inside". During the crisis the subject's wife massaged his lower abdomen and held his penis to prevent its further contraction. The wife attributed her husband's attack to lifting heavy loads. Some time after the attack, the wife ran off with another man, claiming that her husband was "not good sex". Sexual dissatisfaction was a common complaint of Bagobo women (Payne, personal communication).

ETHNOLOGICAL CONSIDERATIONS

As with the other culture-bound syndromes of Southeast Asia, *koro* manifests with some degree of variance but, overall, is strikingly similar throughout the archipelago. For example, though sorcery per se among the Bagobo is not mentioned in the Indonesian cases, the etiological role of non-conformity with community norms (i.e., irregular work and leisure patterns) is common to both. When mentioned, cure may consist of medicinal potions, ritual incantations, or both, but therapy invariably includes pulling the penis and bodily massage. The major area of divergence in the Indonesian and Bagobo belief systems is the gender of those who may provide aid to *koro* sufferers: the opposite sex is prohibited from lending assistance in the former but permitted in the latter.

Wulfften Palthe (1936), Yap (1965a) and Ngui (1969) maintained that *koro* diffused throughout Southeast Asia with the emigration of Southern Chinese peoples, but the assumption that indigenous *koro* is an adapted variant of the

Chinese syndrome has been presented with little rigor of argument. The hypothesis rests, I believe, on several stated and unstated observations: the similarity of the Chinese and indigenous syndromes; the exoticness of the syndrome argues against polyphyletic origins; cultural interaction between the Chinese and indigenous peoples in proto-historic (circa 1200 AD) and modern (1800–present) times. Let us examine these.

The Chinese and indigenous syndromes are similar in their symptomatology. Anxiety, cold sweats, paraesthesia, localized pain, palpitation, skin pallor, visual blurring, and faintness were expressed in the indigenous cases cited earlier and are typical of Chinese cases (Gwee 1963; Yap 1965a; Rin 1963, 1968; *Koro* Study Team 1969; Ngui 1969; Edwards 1976). These symptoms are expected bio-physiological concomitants of intense, panic fear (Marks and Lader 1973) and as such I would argue indicate little cultural imprint. The antecedents to the panic fear are culturally conditioned, and in this area, the ascribed etiology, there is a major difference. In the Chinese syndrome, the ascribed etiologies are frankly sexual, and imbedded in the theory of yin-yang humoral balance (Rin 1963, 1965; Yap 1965a; Gwee 1968; Edwards 1976). Genital retraction as a consequence of improper conduct of sexual relations is mentioned in ancient Chinese medical texts (Gwee 1968; Veith 1972), a fact which incidently argues against diffusion from Southeast Asian to Chinese cultures. Chinese *suoyang* attacks are usually but not necessarily precipitated by an immediate sexual experience; other activities which occasion imblance in yin-yang harmony, such as penile exposure to cold while micturating, 'excessive' masturbation, and improper diet, are also precipitating factors but these may be relatively new features in the syndrome's evolution (Edwards 1976). Explicit sexual content as precipitating factors are absent from the indigenous *koro* cases; true, all our authorities (Brero 1896a, 1896b; Slot 1935; Wulfften Palthe 1936; Chabot 1950) have seen and stressed latent sexual content in their psychoanalytic interpretations, but that is another matter to be discussed subsequently.

In Chinese medical belief shrinking penis is a *symptom* that may occur in extreme cases of sexual varied cultural diseases (Kobler 1948; Edwards 1976). Western oriented nosological classification and interpretation have fostered the distorted concept of shrinking penis as a cultural *"disease"*. Whether shrinking genitals among Southeast Asian natives is conceived as a disease or symptom of disease(s) is unclear. Chinese treatment regimens vary according to the major disease entity, but usually consist of various yang-supplementing medicinal potions (Wong 1918; Tan 1981); massage as crisis therapy is not mentioned. The Chinese patient's penis is held either by the patient or near relative, most often the wife, mother, or grandmother, or, less frequently, by a friend. With the exception of the Bagobos case, the assistants to *koro* patients are neighbors or other non-relatives of the same sex. The Chinese, in extreme cases, anchor the penis with some type of clamping device; the tying of a cord around the penis among the indigenous cases is superficially similar, but the stated intent is more to help pull out the penis than to prevent its further retraction.

The dissimilarities in the cultural aspects of the shrinking penis complaint argue against the theory that cultural diffusion has played a major role. One may, of course, argue that the idea of penile retraction as a prodrome of death was diffused, and the cultural variance is a product of differential evolution in the cultural embellishment of the concept. Though virtually unprovable, such a possibility exists; but to argue that the exotic rarity of the syndrome impels the conclusion of monotypic origin lacks theoretical and empirical support. The theory of the psychic unity of mankind, which lies behind the Freudian psychoanalytic interpretation of Wulfften Palthe (1936) and the contemporary psychiatric interpretation of Yap (1965a) among others, itself suggests that the syndrome may and can have polytypic manifestations. The increasing dissemination of knowledge of genital retraction as a culture-bound syndrome has engendered relatively numerous reports of the penile hyperinvolution complaint among diverse ethnic groups and individuals: in the Sudan (Baasher 1963); India (Chakraborty 1982; Dutta, Phookan and Das 1982; Chakraborty, Das and Mukherji 1983); Thailand [4] (Jilek and Jilek-Aal 1977a, 1977b; Harrington 1982); two Israelis, an immigrant Yemenite and Georgian (Hes and Nassi 1977); a Frenchman (Bourgeois 1968); Britons (Yap 1965a; Barrett 1978; Constable 1979; Cremona 1981); a French Canadian (Lapierre 1972) and three Anglo Canadians (Arbitman 1975; Ede 1976; Waldenberg 1981); and a Greek American (Edwards 1970). Several of these reports stressed that the patients had no awareness of *koro* or special knowledge of Chinese culture. With the exception of the reports from India and Thailand, the penile hyperinvolution complaints were structured around fears of the supposed dangers of masturbation or excessive sex, or were drug induced; penile retraction as a prodrome of death, with the exceptions mentioned, was not reported.

An interesting feature of this series of reports is that in several the case material was drawn from records several years old; the data remained unreported until the physician became aware of the syndrome, could 'label' the case, and perceive the data as worthy of reporting. This pattern of one report drawing out other cases was evident in the earlier Indonesian material (Vorstman's cases were seen three years before the first published report, Blonk's, appeared in the medical literature). Thus, it seems unlikely that the distribution of reported cases actually reflects the true temporal and spatial incidence of *koro* [5], a conclusion which further discredits the hypothesis that *koro* in Southeast Asia can only be a result of Chinese influence.

The third factor to examine is culture contact. Presented without elaboration or substantiation, Wulfften Palthe's suggestion of culture contact and diffusion appears unduly speculative; the record is not unfavorable to his position. In precolonial times, the Chinese Empire had developed trade and political relations with Southeast Asia. These contacts were especially strong in the tenth, twelfth, and fourteenth centuries; though political relations were never firmly and consistently established, trade relations persisted throughout the centuries. Culture contact was never very extensive, but there are traces of Chinese influence, particularly in Kalimantan and Sulawesi: the extensive use of ancient Chinese pottery as prestige/wealth objects and funerary jars is a testament of this early contact. One of the major categories of trade items the Chinese sought were products which, in Chinese medicine, are used as aphrodisiacs and potency strengthening potions: rhinoceros horn and bird's nest are the most well-known examples. Perhaps Chinese ideas of medical/sexual health spread with the trade in these items.

In the nineteenth century colonial era, large-scale Chinese immigration was encouraged, with Chinese communities being established throughout the archipelago and mainland. The possibilities of cultural diffusion were certainly enhanced, but the argument that indigenous *koro* sufferers 'adopted' the Chinese syndrome during this period is not on firm ground. First, as we have seen, concepts of etiology and treatment, which differed from the Chinese syndrome, were already established. Secondly, though immigrant Chinese were known to reside in areas from which *koro* was reported, the extent of interaction between the native peoples and the Chinese, either at the community or individual level, is unspecified. We know from modern studies (c.f. Kleinman et al. 1975; Leslie 1975) that there is a great deal of pluralism in health seeking behavior in Southeast Asia, but whether this pattern held in the earlier period is uncertain.

A more likely candidate for investigation is the role of the Buginese and Macassarese peoples in disseminating the *koro* syndrome. Both peoples, especially the former, regularly voyaged throughout the archipelago and, at times, also established political control. Macassaran cultural and genetic influence was strong in the Manggarai area of Flores (Bijlmer 1929; Le Bar 1972), the locale of the *koro-amok* case report; Buginese immigrants were in the Sintang (Kuhr 1896/97; Le Bar 1972) and Kualakapuas (Mallinckrodt 1924/25; Le Bar 1972) districts of Kalimantan. Among the Bagobos, direct Chinese influence was not apparent in either the earlier or contemporary periods (Payne, personal communication), but the similarity in Bagobos and Macassarese—Buginese terms for penis is suggestive of some past, close link between these not unrelated population groups.[6] Wulfften Palthe (1937) noted that *koro* was also reported among Malays in Sumatra and Malacca but, lacking any other details, this bit of information can not be integrated.[7]

The review of indications for and against the role of cultural diffusion does not permit a definitive assessment, but tentative conclusions can be drawn. Genital retraction complaints can be polygenetic in origin, both at the cultural and individual level. If the *suoyang* and *koro* syndromes are related, it is most likely through an ancient Chinese prototype. That *koro* was reported to be a "new disease" by indigenous informants of Kualakapuas (Wulfften Palthe 1935), indicates that cultural diffusion in modern times can not be ruled out; the Buginese—Macassarese peoples, rather than the Chinese, are more likely influencing agents. *Koro*, as a panic fear, often presents in small-scale, localized epidemics: knowledge of one case precipitates attacks in other susceptible individuals. This being the case, the presence of immigrant groups among whom genital retraction is a not uncommon complaint (the Chinese, Macassarese—Buginese), may raise the incidence of the complaint among the indigenous populace and change the syndrome from one of sporadic, individual incidence to a generally distributed fear bearing greater cultural significance. The ability of one genital retraction attack to precipitate others is stronger within ethnic/cultural groups than across these lines. An example, often cited, is the major *koro* epidemic of 1967 in Singapore, which was touched off by reports of swine fever; rumour had it that eating meat from infected or innoculated animals could cause the disorder. Of the hundreds of daily patients seeking treatment at the height of the epidemic, the Chinese cases were in excess of their representation in the general population: 97.8% as opposed to 74.4% (Ngui 1969; *Koro* Study Team 1969). This finding is less conclusive than presumed, for ethnic differences in pork consumption and professional health care seeking behavior were not considered in the analysis of differential incidence. Other evidence is minimally suggestive: during ten years practice in an unidentified, predominantly Malay district one physician saw eight Malay and two Chinese cases of the genital retraction complaint (Mun 1968). The analysis presented here does not contradict the general thrust of Tan's (1981) thesis that Chinese ideas have influenced the incidence of non-Chinese cases of genital retraction in the modern-day pluralistic societies of Singapore and Malaysia.

Of critical importance in understanding both the development and incidence of *koro* are the culture traits which support the syndrome. The Freudian castration complex, as a universal feature of psychic development, comes readily to many minds. In analyzing Chinese case data and extending his observations to include indigenous manifestations, Wulfften Palthe (1936: 535) concluded: "We have here before us, therefore, a living example of Freud's castration complex". Leaving aside the controversial issue of the universality of the castration complex, at the most basic level, the syndrome lacks an attempt to disguise the castration fear with another fear, nor is the penis symbolized or displaced with another object. Kobler (1948), though finally accepting the castration fear label for Chinese cases, provides a worthy analysis of the differences in the two complexes. Moreover, though aspects of Chinese child rearing practices, e.g., threat of castration or shrinking penis as a punishment for masturbation, do support the hypothesis, this only provides part of the picture; the medico-sexual aspects of the yin-yang humoral theory may be more essential and elemental. The castration complex does little to explain the food "poisoning" epidemics of genital retraction in Singapore and Thailand. Even the modern psychiatric interpretation, which recognizes that *koro* may vary in nosological classification, e.g., as a mass hysteria in the Singapore and Thai epidemics and as a psychosis in individual, disturbed patients, can not adequately 'explain' the syndrome without reference to the wider cultural context. This aspect needs to be examined for each culture specific manifestation.

To date only minor attempts have been made to set indigenous *koro* within its wider cultural context. After reviewing the various psychological interpretations, Chabot (1950) pointed to the competitiveness of the Macassarese people as a contributing factor: men continually strived to surpass other men in all endeavors, especially sexual conquests; anxiety centering on failure or loss in power to achieving goals may have precipitated *koro* attacks. We may add that assistance by other males in holding the penis of a *koro* sufferer may serve as a symbolic statement of the patient's acceptance and integration into the male community. Slot (1935), although not precise in establishing a connection, thought that there may be a relationship between *koro* and the local prevalence of transvestite priests/healers, homosexual practice among both sexes, and pseudo-hermaphrodites. The three culture traits have been noted in ethnographics of South Sulawesi (Matthes 1872, 1875; Kennedy 1953), and in fact are so widely distributed throughout the archipelago (cf. Adriani and Kruijt 1912; Jacobs 1894; Mallinckrodt 1924/25; Riedel 1886; Schawaner, translated in Roth 1896; Scharer 1963) that, with the exception of the Iban and related peoples of Malayasian Borneo (Hose and McDougal 1912), they may be considered a common pattern. Details are rather sketchy; for example, we are only told that homosexual practice often involves ritual prostitution and ritual mockery of the opposite sex, but the theme of sexual antagonism/complementarity seems to be the central organizing feature. Scharer (1963) has even argued that the theme is the basis of Ngadju religion, the organizing principle of their society.

Several reasons can be given for suggesting that further investigation of the theme of sexual antagonism would be a productive avenue. In the wider comparative perspective, the theme is a well documented, major aspect of Melanesian culture (Meggit 1964; Herdt 1982). A shrinking penis syndrome, *tira*, caused by overindulgence in coitus, has been reported from the island of Mangaia in the Cook group (Marshall 1980), a Melanesian—Polynesian transition area. In the Indonesian archipelago and in Malaya, the soul of a woman who dies in parturition or postpartum becomes a malicious spirit which takes vengeance on males. Though the name varies (e.g., *pontianak, koklir, langsuyar*, etc.), belief in the spirit is widespread (Adriani and Kruijt 1912; Jacobs 1894; Mallinckrodt 1924/25; Matthes 1875; Riedel 1886; Roth 1896; Scharer 1963; Skeat 1900). The spirit is alternatively described as a vampire or castrator who tears off the victim's penis and/or testicles. Sather (1978), in analyzing in relation to Iban culture and psychosexual life, the *koklir* and related demons which drain sexual vitality, provides the most complete description of the spirit. Similar beliefs in incubi and succubi were reported among the Sen'oi Semai, an Austro-asiatic people of central Malaya; a class of evil spirits, the *semelit*, cause sexual disorders effecting the glands and genitals, including (my emphasis) *retraction of the genitals into the body* (Dentan 1968).

Though only brief details have been given, it seems probable that investigation of sexual opposition and malicious spirits will yield a better understanding of the genesis of indigenous *koro*. Destruction and degeneration of the genitals was found to be a common feature among non-*koro* psychiatric patients (Oesterreicher 1948), and such fantasies are sometimes translated into reality: reports of a jealous wife or mistress emasculating her paramour periodically come out of Southeast Asia. The data suggest that genital insecurity may be a basic feature of Indonesian—Malaysian psychic and cultural life.

BIOMEDICAL CONSIDERATIONS

Finally, comments on the biomedical aspects of genital retraction are in order.

Physicians and psychiatrists, as befitting their medical background, have investigated the possible role of somatic disorders in *koro* patients. Several common infectious and degenerative diseases, malaria, cholera, asthma, typhus, coronary thrombosis, among others, have symptomatologies which sufficiently resemble that claimed for *koro* and *suoyang* to raise the question of native misdiagnosis. The rare physical exams of *koro* patients have generally proved negative, but that should not mean that the role of somatic diseases should be entirely discredited; it may be that their influence is at the cultural/community, not individual, level. In a hypothetical example, as hearsay of a malaria or other epidemic disease spreads, susceptible individuals may interpret the disease symptoms as *koro* and succumb to an attack. I present this argument largely on theoretical grounds; pinpointing the co-occurrence of infectious epidemics and *koro* outbreaks would provide a substantive basis. The statement that *koro* is never accompanied by fever (Slot 1935) would seem to rule out malaria, but falciparum malaria, the most common and dangerous form in Southeast Asia, can present with 'atypical' manifestations such as non-clinical (i.e., imperceptible or non-existent) fever. Plasmodium falciparum is the pathogenic agent of the highly fatal cerebral malaria; Dr. Sujit Das (Chakraborty et al. 1983) suggested that cases of a "mysterious disease", diagnosed as cerebral malaria, may have been the precipitating factor in the recent genital retraction epidemics in India. Another report includes the fascinating statement that,

According to doctors, the intensity of the current scare is so great because the outbreak of this neurotic "epidemic" has come close on the heels of a strange strain of malaria in the Siliguri area, in which the victims' genitals suffer atrophy, resulting in permanent damage (Anonymous 1982: 139).

Debhanom Muangman (personal communication), who has investigated the "Flower Shrinking" epidemics of Thailand, has reported that most patients were suffering from hysterical fear, but some had a verified, unexplained, non-transient shrinkage of the penis.

The biomedical issues extend beyond the possible penile retraction in response to disease and the attendant cultural fears. The central symptom of *koro*, retraction of the genitals, has generally been discussed as lacking any physio-anatomical basis in reality. In fact, "reassurance" and "education" on the impossibility of genital retraction has been the mainstay of modern medical therapy for both individual and epidemic cases. After noting that both anthropologists and psychiatrists considered genital retraction complaints an impossibility bordering on delusion, Devereux (1954: 488, N5) continued:

Yet, a glance at any good textbook of urology will indicate that the luxating penis can, for all practical purposes, retract into the abdominal wall or into the inguinal tissue. The fact that none of our authorities makes any reference to this condition once more underscores the well-known fact that no amount of technical knowledge can cancel the forces of repression.

Phenomenological observations also support the anatomical potential for penile retraction; Kobler (1948: 289) noted "certain masturbatory habits of children to play with the penis by alternatingly pushing it behind preputium and skin until the penis disappears and then letting it appear again". There is no reason to suppose this facility disappears over age.[8]

But can non-manipulated retraction of the penis occur? There is some evidence on this as well. One only needs to consult the classic study of medical anomalies (Gould and Pyle 1896) to discover that physician-verified cases of genital retraction into the body, due to accidental physical trauma and inexplicable causes, were reported in the Western medical literature years before colonial physicians encountered the first non-Western cases. To my knowledge, no reviewer of *koro* has ever cited this material. Apparently the first inexplicable case of penile retraction, in a Russian peasant aged 23 with a wife and family, was reported by A. A. Ivanov in 1885; though I have not yet obtained Ivanov's report, it is summarized by Raven (1886). Raven's report of a case he witnessed highlights several of the issues I have stressed throughout:

I should have published the following singular case some two years ago had I not feared that the strange details would be received with incredulity, but since a similar but more strongly marked example of the same condition has recently been recorded by Dr. Ivanoff (sic.) in a Russian medical journal, I do not hesitate to bring my own experience forward.

A.B- - -, a healthy, steady, single man, aged twenty-seven years, shortly after he had gone to bed one night, felt a sensation of cold in the region of the penis. He was agitated to find that the organ, a fairly developed one, was rapidly shrinking, and was, he thought, finally retiring. He at once gave the alarm, and I was hastily summoned from my bed to attend him. I found him highly nervous and alarmed. The penis had almost disappeared, the glans being just perceptible under the public arch. The skin of the penis alone was visible, and looking as it does when the organ is buried in a hydrocele, or, in an extreme degree, as it does after death by drowning. I reassured him, and gave him some ammonia, and found next day that the natural state of things had returned. But he remained weak and nervous for some days. He could give no explanation of the occurrence, and the un-natural condition has never returned. (Raven 1886: 250)

Devereux's admonition applies less to the more recent writers. Some have acknowledged that *koro* attacks may be precipitated by genuine somatic changes in the genitalia — e.g., penile and testes retraction in response to sudden exposure to cold, but this is often presented in an ad passim, desultory manner. Suggestive evidence that physio-anatomical changes among such patients may be more common than previously assumed, is found in the pioneering study of Masters and Johnson (1966: 180–81):

Hyperinvolution of the penis beyond resolution-phase levels of detumescence has been observed clinically on numerous occasions. Penile involution following exposure to cold (e.g., swimming in cold water) is well established. In situations of acute exhaustion consequent to severe physical strain, the penis usually is smaller than its normal flaccid size. Advancing age or surgical castration may and frequently does produce a secondary involution of the penis which permanently reduces organ size below previously established normal states for the individual involved.

The authors further noted that penile hyperinvolution particularly became clinically obvious immediately consequent to failed attempts at sexual encounter, suggesting that penile hyperinvolution, like erection, may also respond "directly to higher cortical centers" (Masters and Johnson 1966: 181). Some case material, especially from Chinese *suoyang* subjects, seems to fit into the category of rapid penile detumescence in response to a disturbance during coital activity. Obviously, when this type of acute, transient hyperinvolution of the penis precipitates the cultural panic, the physician is unlikely to discover anatomical abnormality. Hence, some genital retraction complaints may be based on astute personal observation rather than disorganized, confused thinking. However, even if aspects of the syndrome are found to be 'normal' physiological responses, the supposed dangers of said responses may still be over-exaggerated fears conducive to pathological mental states.

What of the belief that total penile retraction is a prodrome of death? This is also partially based on reality; it is a transposition of cause and effect. In an unelaborated statement one study noted that penile retraction was "a phenomenon not uncommonly seen at death" (*Koro* Study Team 1969: 234); Raven's (1886) statement of penile appearance in death by drowning is supportive. Decreased vasocongestion, arterial pressure, and muscular tension are probable mechanisms of this finding. It should also be noted that a corpse left in its natural state rapidly undergoes hyperbloating, and the abdominal distension could cause further retraction of the penis. In living obese males and in individuals with disease engendered bloated abdomens, the penile organ, being partially subsumed within the inguinal folds, appears smaller than normal. This then is another area in which medical studies and cultural studies (e.g., of funerary practices among groups manifesting genital retraction syndromes) can be extended to provide a better understanding of the cultural beliefs.

CONCLUDING REMARKS

Deficiencies in our current understanding of *koro* have been pointed out. These center on inadequate ethnographic distribution and localization, over-reliance on psychiatric interpretation, and neglect of biomedical issues at the ecological and intrapersonal levels. Indigenous *koro* in the Indonesian archipelago is distinct from *suoyang*; at the most, it may have been derived from an ancient Chinese prototype. *Suoyang* normally appears as a product of intra- and inter-personal violations of medico-sexual regulations, while *koro* normally appears as a product of wider social transgressions against a background of sexual (gender) antagonism/complementarity.

The temporal and spatial distribution of the genital retraction complaint, within Southeast Asian and world-wide, is more diffuse than previously recognized. The diverse manifestations are commonly labelled as *koro*; though there is a legitimate need for a standard rubric, the elevation of one culture specific manifestation (Chinese *suoyang* cloaked with the Malay term) as the transcultural label/prototype creates considerable confusion and hinders full understanding. For example, upon the recent outbreaks of what was termed Jinjinia and diagnosed as *koro* in India, investigations were conducted to discover if there were recent immigrants from China or Southeast Asia; subsequent failure to uncover Chinese influence then brought attention to the need for a local socio-anthropological analysis (Dutta et al. 1982). To avoid this type of barrier to understanding, I propose the general adoption of the rubric *Genital Retraction Syndromes*, which would subsume the various culture specific manifestations: *koro* in the Indonesian archipelago (possibly including Lannuk e Laso' in Mindanao); *suoyang* among Chinese; *rok joo* in Thailand; *jinjinia* in India; *tira* in Mangaia, etc.

Each of these need to be examined from a broadly defined ecological framework, including cultural beliefs and practices, psychocultural functioning, and environmental and biomedical influences. Any one perspective alone is likely to gloss over significant details. For example, *suoyang* is typically explained from the emic perspective of medico-sexual regulations. Yet this fails to account for the peculiar distribution of reported *suoyang*: cases occur almost exclusively in individuals either from South and (to a lesser extent) Central China, or descendants of emigrants from there. In an earlier paper (Edwards 1976), variance in adherence to yin-yang beliefs was suggested as accounting for *suoyang*'s nosogeographical distribution, but there is little evidence to support the facile conjecture. Rather, the distribution may be a product of inadequate investigation and reporting, other cultural variance (e.g., in child rearing practices), or of environmental influences. The last is particularly promising since the reported prevalence of *suoyang* closely corresponds with the sub-tropical, rice growing area of China, which has had a markedly different historical experience of disease than North China.

A second example of the narrow focus of a disciplinary perspective serves to elucidate the heterogeneous case material subsumed within *koro*. A recent case in a Caucasian ran as follows. A businessman, a 38 year old Anglo Canadian of depressed mood and irritability, was started on a nightly course of 50 mg maprotiline (Ludiomil), an anti-depressant:

He was at first reluctant to take it but did so regularly for two weeks without improvement. The dose of medication was increased to 100 mg nightly and two weeks later he complained that he could not find his penis when he wanted to urinate. He said that his testicles shrank back into his body and his penis also shrank so that the foreskin prevented him easily from urinating. He had never previously had this problem and the whole thing cleared up spontaneously when he stopped the Ludiomil of his own volition. Altogether he had taken Ludiomil in the dose of 100 mg nightly for eight nights. Since discontinuing the drug there has been no further trouble of this sort. (Waldenberg 1981: 141)

In the author's brief analysis the possibility that the patient's complaint was a statement of objective conditions, rather than subjective impressions, never seems to have arisen: this was a case of *koro*, a delusion of penile shrinkage.

Similarly, in a recent review of the cross-cultural data Rubin (1982) noted that subjective impressions of genital changes were reported against a background of organic brain syndromes, depressive disorders, and schizophrenia, as well as one case of amphetamine (Benzedrine) use (Dow and Silver 1973). Apparently no effort has been made to determine if such subjective symptoms are also objective signs. In this paper I have used the term "retraction" because it is the earliest and most commonly used term. Several medical professionals have pointed out the need to distinguish between the various penile changes which, lacking precise and agreed upon definitions, are often used interchangably. Following Dr. M. L. Ng's definitions (personal communication), which generally correspond to others I have received, the various conditions are:

Shrinkage: A temporary and reversible size reduction of the penis due to decreased blood flow to the organ.

Hyperinvolution: Extreme shrinkage so that organ size is much smaller than normal.

Retraction: Withdrawal of the penis into the body by active contraction of its attached muscles; an alternate mechanism is swelling of the surrounding tissues (Dr. Terry Hensle, personal communication).

Atrophy: Size reduction due to tissue cell size reduction in response to lack of hormonal stimulation or other hormonal anomalies.

Any of these physiologic reactions may precipitate the culturally defined fear of genital disappearance into the body.

Instead of considering all cases of genital symptoms to be understandable a priori in terms of the "primacy of sexuality in human psychodynamics" (Rubin 1982: 172), might one not also consider the possibility that neurophysiological pathways may at least sometimes be involved? The growing body of literature on drug effects on brain chemistry and altered sexual response suggests that the question is not so farfetched. Raven's (1886) eye-witness confirmation of penile retraction remains a rare account not only because of the rarity (?) of the phenomenon and the technical logistics of having a physician readily available to examine an acute episode (observations of subjects and their family and friends tend to be dismissed); since an a priori explanation exists, genital examination is glossed over. This is not to say that real genital retraction occurs in all or even most cases; the physical exams of subjects during the epidemic episodes in Singapore, Thailand, and India indicates that. But to use an analogy, suppose "colds" were studied from a similarly broad perspective: a "colds" group may include people who are either aware or not aware of having a cold; a "no colds" group may include those who claim to have a cold, feel they are coming down with a cold, or take measures to prevent colds. Genital retraction (physiological, pathophysiological, and psychological) may have a similar distribution.

This raises a question which must be asked from both the emic and etic perspectives, how is a "case" to be defined? The 1967 epidemic in Singapore is typically taken as a prime illustration of the psychocultural dynamics of Chinese *suoyang* (and, derivatively, of *koro*); yet, the Chinese Physician Association (traditional practitioners) held a special conference at the time, and concluded that the epidemic was in no way similar to true *suoyang* (Gwee 1968). Would Raven's (1886) case have been diagnosed as *koro* (*suoyang*) by a traditional Indonesian (Chinese) healer? How do we tease out and select data for interpretative relevance? Falling off a horse seems immaterial or extraneous in the discussion of *koro* as a "nerve contracting" disease (Slot 1935); most readers probably glossed over the statement or assumed a symbolic significance. Reading the case of a six year old boy who fell from a cart and suffered a displaced penis (the organ was imbedded in the scrotum for nine days), and other traumatic cases (Gould and Pyle 1896) might change the reaction. A prevalent belief in Chinese culture is that semen, conceived of as a vital substance, is important in maintaining health (Edwards 1976; Haslam 1980; Kleinman 1980, 1982; Tan 1981; Wen and Wang 1981). Highly similar beliefs exist in South Asia, in Western medical history, and most probably in Southeast Asian cultures as well; "semen anxiety" has been proposed as the transcultural rubric for these culture specific manifestations (Edwards 1983). That claims of abnormalities in genital morphology and functioning are also found in all the aforementioned medical systems raises several questions: are these merely coincidental, parallel developments out of similar ethnophysiologies of sex; are semen anxiety and genital retraction pathoplastically related; and are we dealing with purely cultural material? In sum, we need a discriminative analysis before we can fully operationalize what *koro* as a culture bound syndrome may mean.

It naturally flows from these arguments that the category of genital retraction syndromes conveys little nosological significance; rather it is a heuristic rubric for drawing together diverse sets of observations to be subjected to comparative analysis. The data already suggest three broad categories of genital retraction subjects which may have as much, if not more, transcultural than intracultural relatedness: those who experience a true physiological reaction; those who experience panic fear of genital retraction in response to a real or imagined environmental insult; and chronic somatizers who portray culturally patterned illnesses. Biomedical epidemiologists may find fruitful a comparative study of genital atrophy reports in India and Thailand; the psychiatrically oriented researchers may find transculturally valid diagnostic labels for the latter two categories; and for the anthropologist, as the review of the *koro* literature indicates, the full cultural dynamics of genital retraction syndromes are awaiting analysis.

NOTES

1. Wulfften Palthe also suggested that *koro* may account for the origin of the use of *palang*, small rods or pins placed through a perforation of the glans penis and often held in place by small knobs at either end; i.e., the devices would prevent total penile retraction. This is an interesting, but unprovable, hypothesis which needs not be examined here.
2. I have not been able to locate this river on maps or in the text of ethnographies, or in standard geographical atlases; perhaps "Katapan" is a (mis)spelling of the Kahayan, or is a minor tributary of the major river systems in the Kualakapuas area.
3. Mandomai is located on the Kapuas River, about 25 km upriver from Kualakapuas (see endplate map in Scharer 1963).
4. There are also Thai language publications. Debhanom Muangman has graciously sent one which includes photographs of retracted penes; I have not yet had this translated.
5. In personal communications, Indonesian physicians (A. Marlinata and A. Adimoelja) have confirmed that *koro* cases, though rare, still occur in parts of Indonesia.

6. Respective terms for penis are: Buginese: *lasa*; Macassarese: *laso*; Bagobo: *laso'*. The standard Malay term is *butoh* or *butu* (Wilkinson 1932); proto-Malay (Iban and related peoples) terms are close cognates of the Malay terms (Roth 1896). I tentatively suggest that sexual terms may be more resistant to change than other lexical items and, if so, traces of correspondence in this lexical area would be more meaningful than a percent analysis of correspondence in a sample of the entire lexicon.

7. Similarly, Gwee (1968: 4) noted a *koro*-like condition in the Philippines, known as *Bang-utot*. The information was based on a personal communication, which Gwee was unable to verify in locally available literature or from Philippine doctors; specifics of the disease and ethnic group were not reported. I am researching the identification of *Bang-utot*.

8. In working out a semi-structured interview schedule to elicit perceptions of genitalia, I first asked a few acquaintances if they had ever or still could perform the act described by Kobler; the responses were positive. Years ago, while attending Stanford University, a pre-operative transsexual who was performing as a topless female dancer told me that one way to disguise the male genitalia was to push the penis inside the body, tape over it and pull the scrotum between the legs.

REFERENCES

Adriani, N. and A. C. Kruijt
    1912 De Bare'e-Sprekende Toradja's van Midden-Celebes. Batavia: Landsdrukkerij.
Anonymous
    1982 *Koro*, Psychological Scare. India Today October 15, 1982: 139.
Arbitman, R.
    1975 *Koro* in a Caucasian. Modern Medicine of Canada 30, 11: 970—71.
Baasher, T. A.
    1963 The Influence of Culture on Psychiatric Manifestations. Transcultural Psychiatric Research Review 15: 51—52.
Barrett, K.
    1978 *Koro* in a Londoner. The Lancet 2, 8103: 1319.
Bijlmer, H. J. T.
    1929 Outlines of the Anthropology of the Timor-Archipelago. Weltevreden, Dutch East Indies: Indisch Comite voor Wetenschappelijke Onderzoekingen.
Blonk, J. C.
    1895 *Koro*. Geneeskundig Tijdschrift voor Nederlandsch-Indië 35: 562—63.
Bourgeois, M.
    1968 Un *Koro* Charentais (Transposition Ethnopsychiatrique). Annales Medico-Psychologiques 126: 749—51.
Brero, P. C. J. Van
    1896a Naar Aanleiding van het Opstel over *Koro* van den Heer J. C. Blonk in de Vorige Aflevering van dit Tijdschrift. Geneeskundig Tijdschrift Voor Nederlandsch-Indië 36: 48—54.
    1896b *Koro*, Eine Eigenthumliche Zwangsvorstellung. Allegemeine Zeitschrift für Psychiatrie und Medicin 53: 596—73.
Chabot, H. T.
    1950 Verwantschap, Stand en Sexe In Zuid-Celebes. Djakarta: J. B. Wolters.
Chakraborty, A., S. Das and A. Mukherji
    1983 *Koro* Epidemic in India. Transcultural Psychiatric Research 20: 150—51.
Chakraborty, P. K.
    1982 *Koro*: A Peculiar Anxiety Neurosis (A Case Report). Indian Journal of Psychiatry 24: 192—94.
Constable, P. J.
    1979 *Koro* in Hertfordshire. The Lancet 1, 8108: 163.

Cremona, A.
    1981   Another Case of *Koro* in a Briton. British Journal of Psychiatry 138: 180–81.
Dentan, R. K.
    1968   Semai Response to Mental Aberration. Bijdragen Tot De Taal-, Land- en Volkenkunde
           124: 33–58.
Devereux, G.
    1954   Primitive Genital Mutilations in a Neurotic's Dream. Journal of the American Psy-
           choanalytic Association 2: 484–92.
Dow, T. and D. Silver
    1973   A Drug Induced *Koro* Syndrome. Journal of the Florida Medical Association 60:
           4: 32–33.
Dutta, D., H. R. Phookan and P. D. Das
    1982   The *Koro* Epidemic in Lower Assam. Indian Journal of Psychiatry 24: 370–74.
Ede, A.
    1976   *Koro* in an Anglo-Saxon Canadian. Canadian Psychiatric Association Journal 21:
           389–92.
Edwards, J. G.
    1970   The *Koro* Pattern of Depersonalization in an American Schizophrenic Patient.
           American Journal of Psychiatry 126: 1171–73. (Reprinted in this volume.)
Edwards, J. W.
    1976   The Concern for Health in Sexual Matters in the 'Old Society' and 'New Society'
           in China. Journal of Sex Research 12: 88–103.
    1983   Semen Anxiety in South Asian Cultures: Cultural and Transcultural Significance.
           Medical Anthropology 7: 51–67.
Gould, G. M. and W. L. Pyle
    1896   Anomalies and Curiosities of Medicine. Philadelphia: W. B. Saunders.
Gwee, A. L.
    1963   *Koro* – A Cultural Disease. Singapore Medical Journal 4: 119–22. (Reprinted in this
           volume.)
    1968   *Koro* – Its Origin and Nature as a Disease Entity. Singapore Medical Journal 9: 3–6.
Harrington, J. A.
    1982   Epidemic Psychosis. British Journal of Psychiatry 141: 98–99.
Haslam, M. T.
    1980   Medicine and the Orient: Shen-K'uei Syndrome. British Journal of Sexual Medicine
           7: 31–36.
Herdt, G. H. (Ed.)
    1982   Rituals of Manhood, Male Initiation in Papua New Guinea. Berkeley: University of
           California Press.
Hes, J. and G. Nassi
    1977   *Koro* in a Yeminite and a Georgian Jewish Immigrant. Confinia Psychiatrica 20:
           180–84.
Hose, C. and W. McDougal
    1912   The Pagan Tribes of Borneo. 1966 reprint, London: Frank Cass & Co., Ltd.
Jacobs, J.
    1894   Het Familie- en Kampongleven op Groot-Atjeh. Leiden: E. J. Brill.
Jilek, W. and L. Jilek-Aall
    1977a A *Koro* Epidemic in Thailand. Transcultural Psychiatric Research Review 15: 57–
           59.
    1977b Massenhysterie Mit *Koro*-Symptomatik in Thailand. Schweizer Archiv Für Neurologie,
           Neurochirurgie und Psychiatrie 120: 257–57.
Kennedy, R.
    1953   Field Notes on Indonesia, South Celebes 1949–1950. New Haven, Ct: Human
           Relations Area Files Press.

Kleinman, A.
    1980 Patients and Healers in the Context of Culture. Berkeley: University of California
          Press.
    1982 Neurasthenia and Depression: A Study of Somatization and Culture in China. Culture,
          Medicine and Psychiatry 6: 117—90.
Kleinman, A. et al. (Eds.)
    1975 Medicine in Chinese Cultures: Comparative Studies of Health Care in Chinese and
          Other Societies. Washington, D.C.: John E. Fogarty International Center.
Kobler, F.
    1948 Description of an Acute Castration Fear, Based on Superstition. Psychoanalytic
          Review 35: 285—89.
Koro Study Team
    1969 The *Koro* Epidemic in Singapore. Singapore Medical Journal 10: 234—42.
Kuhr, E. L. M.
    1896/7 Schetsen uit Borneo's Westerafdeeling. Bijdragen tot de Taal-, Land- en Volkenkunde
          46: 63—88, 214—39; 47: 57—82.
Lapierre, Y. D.
    1972 *Koro* in a French Canadian. Canadian Psychiatric Association Journal 17: 333—34.
Le Bar, F. M.
    1972 Ethnic Groups of Insular Southeast Asia. Volume I: Indonesia, Andaman Islands, and
          Madagascar. New Haven, Ct: Human Relations Area Files Press.
Leslie, C. (Ed.)
    1976 Asian Medical Systems: A Comparative Study. Berkeley: University of California
          Press.
Mallinckrodt, J.
    1924/5 Ethnografische Mededeelingen Over de Dajaks in de Afdeeling Koealakapoeas.
          Bijdragen tot de Taal-, Land- en Volkenkunde 80: 397—446, 521—600; 81: 62—
          115, 165—310.
Marks, I. and M. Lander
    1973 Anxiety States (Anxiety Neurosis): A Review. Journal of Nervous and Mental Disease
          157: 3—18.
Marshall, D. S.
    1980 Too Much in Mangaia. *In* C. Gordon and G. Johnson (eds.), Readings in Human
          Sexuality: Comparative Perspectives. New York: Harper & Row, pp. 236—40.
Masters, W. W. and V. E. Johnson
    1966 Human Sexual Response. Boston: Little, Brown and Company.
Matthes, B. F.
    1872 Over de Bissoe's of Heidensche Priester en Priesteressen De Boeginezen. Amsterdam:
          C. G. Vander Post.
    1875 Bijdragen tot de Ethnologie van Zuid-Celebes. 's-Gravenhage: G. Belinfante.
Meggitt, J. J.
    1964 Male—Female Relationships in the Highlands of Australian New Guinea. American
          Anthropologist 66: 204—24.
Mulder, J. G. A.
    1935 Over *Koro*. Geneeskundig Tijdschrift voor Nederlandsch-Indië 75: 837—38.
Mun C. T.
    1968 Epidemic *Koro* in Singapore. British Medical Journal 1: 640—41.
Ngui, P. W.
    1969 The *Koro* Epidemic in Singapore. Australia and New Zealand Journal of Psychiatry
          113: 263—66.
Oesterreicher, W.
    1948 Sadomasochistic Obsessions in an Indonesian. American Journal of Psychotherapy
          2: 64—81.

Raven, T.
  1886 Retraction of the Penis. The Lancet 2: 250.
Riedel, J. G. F.
  1886 De Sluik- en Kroesharige Rassen Tusschen Celebes en Papua. 's-Gravenhage: Martinus Nijhoff.
Rin, H.
  1963 *Koro*: A Consideration of Chinese Concepts of Illness and Case Illustrations. Transcultural Psychiatric Research Review 15: 23–30.
  1965 A Study of the Aetiology of *Koro* in Respect to the Chinese Concept of Illness. International Journal of Social Psychiatry 11: 7–13.
Roth, H. L.
  1896 The Natives of Sarawak and British North Borneo. London: Truslove & Hanson.
Rubin, R. T.
  1982 *Koro* (*Shook Yang*): A Culture-Bound Psychogenic Syndrome. *In* C. T. H. Friedmann and R. A. Faguet (eds.), Extraordinary Disorders of Human Behavior. New York: Plenum Press, pp. 155–172.
Sather, C.
  1978 The Malevolent Koklir: Iban Concepts of Sexual Peril and the Danger of Childbirth. Bijdragen tot de Taal-, Land- en Volkenkunde 134: 310–55.
Scharer, H.
  1963 Ngaju Religion, The Conception of God Among a South Borneo People. The Hague: Martinus Nijhoff.
Skeat, W. W.
  1900 Malay Magic. London: Frank Cass & Co., Ltd. 1965 reprint.
Slot, J. A.
  1935 *Koro* in Zuid-Celebes. Geneeskundig Tijdschrift voor Nederlandsch-Indië 75: 811–20.
Tan E. S.
  1981 Culture-Bound Syndromes Among Overseas Chinese. *In* A. Kleinman and T. Y. Lin (eds.), Normal and Abnormal Behavior in Chinese Culture. Dordrecht: D. Reidel Publ. Co., pp. 371–86.
Veith, I.
  1979 The Yellow Emperor's Classic of Internal Medicine. Berkeley: University of California Press.
Vorstman, A. H.
  1897 *Koro* in de Westerafdeeling van Borneo. Geneeskundig Tijdschrift Voor Nederlandsch-Indië 37: 499–505.
Waldenberg, S. S. A.
  1981 *Koro*. Canadian Journal of Psychiatry 26: 140–41.
Wen J. K. and C. L. Wang
  1981 Shen-K'uei Syndrome: A Culture-Specific Sexual Neurosis in Taiwan. *In* A. Kleinman and T. Y. Lin (eds.), Normal and Abnormal Behavior in Chinese Culture. Dordrecht: D. Reidel Publ. Co., pp. 357–69.
Wilkinson, R. J.
  1932 A Malay–English Dictionary. Mytilene, Greece: Salavopoulous and Kinderlis.
Wojowasito, S. and W. J. S. Poerwadarminta
  1974 Kamus Lengkap, Inggeris–Indoesia, Indonesia-Inggeris. Djarkarta: Hasta.
Wong, K. C.
  1918 An Inquiry into Some Chinese "Sexual Diseases". National Medical Journal of China 4: 26–31.
Wulfften Palthe, P. M. Van
  1934 *Koro*, Een Eigenaardige Angstneurose. Geneeskundig Tijdschrift voor Nederlandsch-Indië 74: 1713–20.

1935a Aanvulling op het Artikel "*Koro*, Een Eigenaardige Angstneurose". Geneeskundig Tijdschrift voor Nederlandsche-Indië 75: 836—37.

1935b *Koro*, Eine Merkwürdige Angsthysterie. Internationale Zeitschrift für Psychoanalyse 21: 249—57.

1936 Psychiatry and Neurology in the Tropics. *In* C. D. deLangen and A. Lichtenstein (eds.), A Clinical Textbook of Tropical Medicine. Batavia: G. Kolff & Co., pp. 325—47.

1937 Il Significato Forense del *Koro*. Archivio Di Anthropologia Criminale, Psichiatria, Medicina Legale 57: 173—82.

Yap, P. M.

1965a *Koro* — A Culture-Bound Depersonalization Syndrome. British Journal of Psychiatry 111: 43—50.

1965b *Koro* in a Briton. British Journal of Psychiatry 111: 774—75.

THE GENITAL RETRACTION TAXON
Commentary

The major symptoms and behavior displayed in cases discussed under this taxon are sufficiently striking and unusual that they probably merit the term "exotic" as much as any of the other syndromes discussed in this book. They consist of a fear of such intensity and focus that it goes beyond the typical anxiety syndrome, together with the involvement of other people to assist the victim in preventing his penis from retracting into his body.

In DSM-III terms, data in the cases reported in the preceding papers suggest a principal diagnosis of Conversion Disorder (300.11) for the most dramatic symptom, as some authors mention. But with the extreme fear and apprehensiveness displayed by victims it might also be appropriate to add Panic Disorder (300.01) as at least a secondary diagnosis (". . . sudden onset of intense apprehension, fear, or terror, often associated with feelings of impending doom"). In a given case, if the data are insufficient for further specification of the problem(s), "Atypical Somatoform Disorder" (300.70) might be appropriate: ". . . a residual category to be used when the predominant disturbance is the presentation of physical symptoms or complaints not explainable on the basis of demonstrable organic findings or a known pathophysiological mechanism and apparently linked to psychological factors" (p. 251). Finally, in a case such as that discussed by J. W. Edwards (p. 175), the element of sexual dysfunction might enter prominently, and in any situation of this type psychosocial stressors could be involved, as they appear to be in the latter case.

A fuller DSM-III formulation of data presented in the Edwards case would appear to be:

Axis I: 300.70 Atypical Somatoform Disorder (fear of penis shrinking into abdomen).
300.01 Panic Disorder (Provisional).
203.89 Psychosexual Disorder Not Elsewhere Classified (Provisional) (Wife claimed that her husband was "not good sex" and ran off with another man)

Axis II: Insufficient data

Axis III: Victim complained of milky urine; later urine turned yellow. During *koro* attack, complained of intermittent pain and extreme lower back pain.

Axis IV: *Psychosical stressors*: suspicion of envy and fear of sorcery; sudden death of brother and fear of sorcery; wife's dissatisfaction with his sexual functioning.
Severity: 5? — Severe (Operational definition: "Serious illness in self or family; major financial loss; marital separation, birth of child")

Ronald C. Simons and Charles C. Hughes (eds.), The Culture-Bound Syndromes, 193—194.
© 1985 *by D. Reidel Publishing Company.*

Axis V: *Highest level of adaptive functioning during past year*: 4 — Fair ("Moderate impairment in either social relations or occupational functioning, *or* some impairment in both." Patient is known as "a good provider for his family, and a hard worker . . ." but ". . . his harvests were larger than his neighbors' crops, created a suspicion of envy and fear of sorcery").

B. THE SUDDEN MASS ASSAULT TAXON

INTRODUCTION: *THE SUDDEN MASS ASSAULT TAXON*

The *Sudden Mass Assault taxon* is comprised of Malayo–Indonesian *amok* and the parallel instances of indiscriminate homicide reported from many parts of the world. This section contains five papers. The first is John Carr's carefully thought out and strongly presented argument for a particularistic perspective; the others are papers describing sudden mass assaults in a variety of societies written by authors who take a universalistic perspective and who see sudden mass assault as the result of a human potential which may be manifest in any society if the circumstances are right. In his paper Carr argues for a social learning model and states explicitly his view that "the notion that [sets of] culture-bound syndromes share underlying disease features is rejected".

Westermeyer, in a paper written especially for this volume, discusses sudden mass assault in a contemporary social context, and he shows how the form of sudden mass assault in Laos has changed with the availability of new means of killing. Burton-Bradley analyzes sudden mass assault with an argument which is the polar opposite of Carr's, and he describes cases he has collected in Papua, New Guinea. Taking a universalistic perspective, Burton-Bradley quotes Yap, who wrote of "a crying need for a conceptual language applicable to all cultures" (1962).

Also taking a universalistic perspective, Arboleda-Florez describes an instance he has personally studied in considerable detail, that of a Canadian, 'The Calgary Mall Sniper'. All five authors describe the relevant social circumstances, cultural context, and inferred psychodynamics in sufficient detail to allow readers of the set of papers to come to their own conclusions as to whether the geographically remote cases are only superficially similar to classic *amok* reported from Malaysia and Indonesia or whether they indeed may be culture-specific instances of the same underlying behavioral propensity.

In some of the cases reported here, the mass killing was performed by someone who, as far as is known, was otherwise psychologically healthy. In others, the killer is described as suffering from considerable previous psychopathology. Perhaps it would be useful to eliminate from the taxon those cases in which the mass killing is only part of a larger and more continuous pattern of disturbed behavior. The taxon name and the term "*amok*" could then be reserved for those instances of random mass homicide which are performed after a period of brooding on some deeply felt insult or loss by a person who has not previously shown signs of marked pathology.

Ronald C. Simons and Charles C. Hughes (eds.), The Culture-Bound Syndromes, 197.
© 1985 *by D. Reidel Publishing Company.*

JOHN E. CARR

ETHNO-BEHAVIORISM AND THE CULTURE-BOUND SYNDROMES: THE CASE OF *AMOK*

Devoting increasing attention to the role of socio-cultural factors in determining maladaptive behavior, transcultural researchers have urged the inclusion of a category of 'culture-bound reactive syndromes' in the nomenclature of mental illness. It is argued that '. . . certain systems of implicit values, social structure, and obviously shared beliefs produce unusual forms of psychopathology that are confined to special areas . . . [but] these are only atypical variations of generally distributed psychogenic disorders' (Yap 1969: 38).

The concept of culture-bound syndrome has been generally acknowledged (e.g., Denko 1964; Yap 1969; Kiev 1972; Murphy 1972; Guthrie 1973), but researchers have tended to ignore or deemphasize certain key aspects and implications of the concept. Yap's definition emphasizes the role of (1) implicit values, (2) belief systems, and (3) social structure in determining the manifest behaviors but not the *basic form* of the disorder. Thus, the concept argues strongly in favor of a *social learning process* being central to the acquisition of at least the symptomatic behaviors of such disorders, yet behavioral or social learning principles are almost totally ignored. Yap, who defined the culture-bound syndrome, appears to have been strongly opposed to the consideration of a learning role in these syndromes, arguing that somehow this would detract from the 'obvious abnormality' of disorders such as *amok* (Yap 1969: 46).

Instead a combination of descriptive psychiatry and Western psychodynamic concepts have been applied, sometimes indiscriminantly, to disorders in various cultures. Researchers have erroneously focused upon manifest symptom similarity as evidence of a commonality in underlying basic disorder. Then they draw on Western psychodynamic categories in order to explain a range of behavioral disorders world-wide, often ignoring the indigenous culture's 'implicit values, social structure, and obviously shared beliefs,' supposedly the defining criteria in the culture-bound syndromes.

An example to be considered is the phenomenon of *amok*, defined as an acute outburst of unrestrained violence associated with homicidal attack, preceded by a period of brooding, and ending with exhaustion and amnesia. While *amok* is indigenous to the Malay peoples of Southeast Asia, it has been loosely associated with *cathard* in Polynesia, *pseudonite* in the Sahara (Kiev 1972), *mal de pelea* in Puerto Rico (Yap 1969), *wihtiko* among the Cree Indians, *'jumping Frenchmen'* in Canada, *imu* in Japan (Cooper 1934), *mirachit* in

Ronald C. Simons and Charles C. Hughes (eds.), The Culture-Bound Syndromes, 199–223.
© *1978 by D. Reidel Publishing Company.*

Siberia (Lin 1953), *pibloktoq* among polar Eskimos (Kloss 1923), *'frenzied anxiety state'* in Kenya (Carother 1948), *'wild man behavior'* in New Guinea (Newman 1964), and finally, *'Whitman syndrome'* in the United States (Teoh 1972). The supposed commonality based on the shared quality of frenzied and bizarre behavior tends to ignore the complex idiosyncratic cultural determinants specific to the disorder. Similarly, a listing of the various etiological factors that have been mentioned in connection with *amok* (e.g., constitutional predisposition, mental subnormality, stress, chronic illness, infections, sleep deprivation, heat, alcohol, sexual excitement, fear, anger, repressed sexual desires, frustration, and a varied list of familiar psychodynamic mechanisms) reveals an emphasis upon Western medical and psychiatric concepts relevant to the behaviors in question. The notion of 'culture-bound,' though seemingly accepted, appears to have been understood and applied differently by different researchers, few of whom have used it in its strict sense.

ETHNO-BEHAVIORISM

The purpose of this paper is to reexamine and redefine the concept of culture-bound disorder within the context of a review of *amok*. Our consideration of this condition will be based upon a behavioral approach to cross-culture phenomena involving the following assumptions:

A. The basic principles of human learning are applicable to *all* humans regardless of race or culture. We include here the behavioral principles of positive and negative reinforcement, stimulus and response generalization, discrimination, extinction, modeling, and imitation (Bandura 1974).

B. These principles define the mechanisms by which cultural norms, beliefs, and expectations are acquired and lead to culture-specific behaviors. Thus, the learning process involves *cognitive* as well as *behavioral* dimensions. It does not necessarily follow that these principles are recognized or have conceptual equivalents in the indigenous belief systems.

C. *All* humans, regardless of race or culture, are faced by basic existential problems, such as survival, protection of young, social acceptance, the need for a sense of competence or worth; and in each of these stated areas there are goals that are culture-specific.

D. The basic principles of human learning define the mechanisms by which individuals of all races and cultures acquire (1) culturally specific goals and (2) culturally appropriate coping responses to blocked goal attainment.

E. These coping responses may be judged 'appropriate or inappropriate' based on culturally relevant criteria (indigenous or Western). It is those coping responses labeled inappropriate which constitute the phenomena of 'pathology' or 'illness.'

We shall attempt to present evidence consistent with these assumptions which contributes to an understanding of the relation between the phenomenon of *amok* and the culture of the rural Malay. Specifically, we shall attempt to outline a behavioral-cognitive model which shall have as its main premises the following:

A. The preeminent social values of Malay culture are acquired through a process of socialization largely dependent upon negative reinforcement (avoidance learning).

B. The Malay conceptual system is both precise and ambiguous in nature. This seeming inconsistency derives from identifiable, but not unique, contextual and structural aspects of the conceptual system, e.g., the centrality of a finite number of superordinate evaluative dimensions at one level and a complex array of specifically defined behavioral exemplars at another level.

C. The ambiguity of the system at one level contributes to a greater risk of interpersonal tensions while the specificity with regard to behavioral expectancies at another level decreases the likelihood of both the recognition as well as the resolution of interpersonal tensions.

D. The Malay conceptual system, like all cultural systems, has loopholes or 'escape clauses' which define specific conditions under which the culture may provide sanction for extreme exceptions or 'violations.' Like other elements of the conceptual system, loopholes are socially reinforced and have the same structural characteristics as other behavioral norms in the system.

E. Finally, these exceptions to the code are 'explained' in terms of indigenous concepts of pathology or illness which, again, are similar structurally to other concepts in the system.

AMOK: AN HISTORICAL REVIEW

In the Malay language, the term *amok* or *amuk* refers to a violent or furious charge of homicidal intent. *Mengamok* refers to the act of running *amok*, and *pengamok* to the actor who runs *amok* (Iskander 1970). It is a phenomenon that has been a source of fascination to Western travelers and scholars from early colonial days. It is believed to have had its origins in the cultural training for warfare which the early Javanese and Malays adopted from the Hindu states of India. En masse attacks by warriors, each brandishing the *keris*, a dagger or short sword, accompanied by hysterical screams of '*Amok! Amok!*' were a popular tactic among Malay warriors. They were presumably intended to terrify the enemy into believing they could expect no mercy and could save themselves only by flight. The tactic, like many other forms of the martial arts in the Orient, was highly regarded and culturally reinforced through epic poems citing examples of heroes and champions who exemplified this behavior. Warriors were encouraged to emulate the epic heroes through self-sacrificial, fanatical charges, indiscriminant slaughter, and refusal to surrender (Shaw 1972).

With the introduction of Islam into the Malay Archipelago in the fourteenth century, *amok* occasionally became an act of religious fanaticism. The faithful were induced to indiscriminately slay all infidels with no concern for their own lives. The best known of these religious fanatic bands was the *Juramentado* of the Philippines (Shaw 1972).

How these early forms of the phenomenon relate to the personal *amok* so vividly described in the journals of early European travelers to the Malay Archipelago is unclear. The latter were described as occurring without warning, although in retrospect, the *pengamok* was often noted to have manifested a sudden shift in mood. He might be sitting with friends when suddenly, he would leap up, with *keris* in hand, and attack anyone within reach. The attack might last for several hours and would continue until the *pengamok* was either himself killed, or finally overwhelmed. He would then pass into a deep sleep or stupor for several days, followed by total amnesia for the event, a morose or taciturn mood state, and an unwillingness to converse.

The personal *amok* was also culturally sanctioned as an instrument of social protest by individuals against rulers who abused their power. No ruler could afford to be oblivious to the fact that any one of his subjects could defy his rule and publicly demonstrate the ruler's inability to keep the peace. Thus, Gullick (1958) interprets the *amok* as the ultimate 'veto' which each Malay exercised over an otherwise all powerful ruler.

Early descriptions of the phenomenon agree that the *pengamok* was almost always a male, a Malay farmer or mountain dweller, of middle age or older. Early speculation that the act might be related to suicidal wishes has been discounted by some writers on the grounds that Malays, being Muslims, have an aversion to the concept of suicide. Whether or not this is a significant factor, Malays do have one of the lowest suicide rates in the world (Hassan 1970; Teoh 1974). An etiological association with alcohol has been similarly discounted since Malays, again for religious reasons, rarely drink and have a low alcoholism rate (Murphy 1959). Drug-induced states were suggested as a precipitating condition, but, again, these seemed to be the exception rather than the rule (Carr and Tan 1976; Tan and Carr 1977; Shaw 1972).

By the end of the nineteenth century, the prevailing medical opinion was that the *pengamok* was suffering from some disorder of the gastrointestinal system! By the beginning of the twentieth century, this position was revised in favor of a psychotic or other mental condition of variable etiology. It was believed the condition could be brought on by post-febrile insanity associated with diseases such as malaria, dengue, paratyphoid; while others drew an association between *amok* and leprosy, epilepsy, schizophrenia (Shaw 1970; Murphy 1972).

Current psychiatric thinking regarding *amok* was significantly influenced by the writings of the late P. M. Yap (1951; 1969). While Yap felt *amok* was similar to '. . . acute psychopathic reactions described in constitutionally predisposed or intellectually subnormal persons under stress, familiar to psychiatrists everywhere . . . ,' the unique cultural parameters of the condition made the ordinary usage of 'acute psychopathic reaction' inappropriate or inapplicable (1969: 45). Therefore, Yap suggested a new category for the standard psychiatric nomenclature, 'atypical culture-bound reactive syndrome.'

Recent reports in the literature suggest that the *amok* syndrome may be either more wide-spread or changed from its original classic form. Several writers have presented evidence that the 'disorder' is no longer limited to males or Malays, nor is it found only in the Malay Peninsula and Archipelago (Teoh 1972; Westermeyer 1972; Burton-Bradley 1968). Statistical evidence is lacking, but the impression is that the frequency of occurrence in its traditional form appears to have increased in Southeast Asia, where it is now found increasingly associated with cases of severe mental illness, e.g., schizophrenia (Tan 1965), and other psychiatric syndromes (Schmidt 1967; Murphy 1972). While in some instances this appears to be a function of a change in the defining criteria by which observers, professional and otherwise, have elected to label and explain this particular phenomenon, there is now evidence that *amok* has undergone modification in response to specific changes in the cultural context in which the phenomenon occurs (Carr and Tan 1976; Westermeyer 1973). Our research has led us to conclude that *amok* is a culturally prescribed form of violent behavior, sanctioned by tradition as an appropriate response to a highly specific set of socio-cultural conditions. It is not a disease, but rather a behavioral sequence that may be precipitated by any number of etiological factors, among them physical, psychological, as well as socio-cultural determinants (Tan and Carr 1977).

SOCIAL LEARNING AND CHILDHOOD

The classical *amok* syndrome, as originally described, was a set of beliefs and behaviors specific to the indigenous peoples of the Malay Peninsula and Archipelago. Since centuries of Hindu, Moslem, Chinese, and subsequent European influences have acted upon this original cultural system and resulted in significant modifications, especially in the urban centers, an appreciation of the nature of this indigenous Malay cultural system can only be obtained by studying the reports of field studies carried out in the rural areas and *kampongs* (villages).

These ethnographic studies uniformaly depict Malay youth (especially males) as being reared in a highly protected environment, indulged of almost every desire up to age five or six, with little or no demand that they work or develop vocational expectations up to marriageable age (Djamour 1965; Firth 1966; Wilder 1974; Wilson 1967). From a social learning perspective, this would suggest that the contingent reward of either economic- or achievement-oriented behavior is not a significant mechanism in socialization. Swift concurs with this hypothesis in stating that Malay child care reflects a '. . . tendency to see only a loose connection between reward and effort in economic affairs . . . or in life generally . . .' (1965:30). This distinctive attitude may relate to the Malay view that nothing is done for the sake of pleasure alone. Rather, '. . . a deed is done because it is proper and not because it gives one the pleasure of achievement' (Mahathir 1970). The predominant endeavor in socialization is to constrain the child from expression of aggression toward his environment or others. As a result, the Malay youth is inculcated with '. . . such total norms as dependence, obedience, submissiveness, and withdrawal which eventually reinforce him to become less active and to lack independence . . .' (Othman 1973). Children are taught to be quiet and nonemotional, never to confront others about a difference of opinion, always to be obedient, passive, and undemonstrative. The socialization process by which this behavioral effect is accomplished appears to involve a complex system of social values implemented primarily through an induced sense of shyness or embarrassed sensitivity called *mendapat malu*. Similar to our concept of shame, *malu* implies an unequal status between people, or 'put down' in Western colloquial usage. Malay values of social conduct, therefore, are acquired through the avoidance of *malu* and reflect a system of social learning based *not* upon positive reinforcement or punishment, but almost totally upon negative reinforcement (reward that comes from the avoidance of noxious conditions such as pain, criticism, guilt, etc.).

NORMS GOVERNING SOCIAL CONDUCT

Social conduct among the rural Malay, therefore, is controlled by adherence to the following principles:

A. All interpersonal relations imply an interaction between individuals of particular status and, therefore, must be accompanied by mutual respect (for the status) such that the status needs of the other ideally are anticipated.

B. A person is *halus* if he is correct in behavior, shows proper consideration, anticipates the needs of others, speaks softly, uses proper words (in accordance with status), openly displays 'sensitivity' in interpersonal relationships, and conducts himself with refinement.

C. One is *kasar* if he does not observe expected etiquette, or is insensitive, improper in languguage, or crude (Wilson 1967).

If one is *halus*, one is considered to possess greater social status (and thereby avoids *malu*), while to be *kasar* implies lower status and a greater risk of *malu*. The degree of social status implied is dependent on other factors, however, such as whether the behavior in question occurs in the private or public domain. In the privacy of one's home and family, social restraints on behavior may be relaxed; whereas public behavior, on view to others, requires that the formal code be observed.

Thus, the values of social conduct in Malay society emphasize respect, esteem, sensitivity toward others' needs, and social skill, modulated between private and public domains. Wilson suggests that the code may have been more flexible among the pre-Moslem Malays, but became rigidified and ritualistic in response to the influence of Islam.

MALAY CONSTRUCTION OF THE WORLD

We turn now to the second premise of our model, namely, that the Malay cultural system is characterized by broad and sometimes ambiguous conceptualizations of phenomena at one level and a complex array of highly differentiated behavioral exemplars at another. The structural differential between abstract concepts and concretely observable behavior is, of course, common to all cultural systems. In the case of the Malay, however, we feel there is sufficient evidence, albeit circumstantial, to warrant considering the magnitude of the disparity such that it leads to predictable consequences on both cultural and personal levels.

In describing the norms governing behavior in Malay culture, Mahathir has written that '. . . the first thing that strikes the observer is the distinct difference between the professed code and the actual practice. . . . Equally striking is the apparent failure by the Malays themselves to notice the difference' (1970:156). Mahathir is less concerned with the moral implications of the disparity than he is with the behavioral and socio-political implications of the seeming inability of the Malay to see or be concerned with these discrepancies. As in other cultures, the apparent incongruity may in part be traced to a concern with propriety and form as consistent with custom or cultural precedent. While certainly not unique, Malay culture is at least distinctive in its reputation for propriety and form. Indeed, it has been said that for the Malay, form may be preferred to the actual substance, e.g., the formality of social status being regarded as far more important than the actual authority involved. To this end, therefore, the Malay social code is remarkably differentiated and precise in defining the formal proprieties of social interactions, i.e., behavior and language appropriate to rank, status, interaction setting, situation, etc. Therefore, one can construe the result to be a society that is seemingly self-constrained, polite, harmonious, and eminently predictable. What is remarkable is that the Malay can demonstrate a propensity for precise and highly predictable behavior (the form) while tolerating an almost limitless degree of ambiguity and indefiniteness in conceptualizing the substantive reasons for that behavior. Several writers have commented on this disparity between behavior and cognition and specifically on the purported vagaries of conceptual process among the Malay peoples (Mahathir 1970; Omar 1968; Endicott 1970). The indefiniteness so described, however, may be a function more of distinctive structural characteristics of the Malay conceptual system, rather than the relative absence of structure, as I shall argue in the following paragraphs.

The Malay view of the world has been described as reflecting certain conceptual characteristics common to Eastern philosophy and phenomenology, e.g., less of a clear differentiation between the material and spiritual worlds than one finds in Western conceptualization and a 'fluidity of thought' reflecting the inherent ambiguity of many of the concepts (Cuisinier 1936). The basic orientation of the Malay World View, predating the intrusion of Indian, Arabic, Chinese, and later Western concepts, has been described as an all-pervading animism centering on the belief that all things in nature, human and otherwise, share a common vital spirit called *semangat*. *Semangat* is not analogous to the Western usage of 'soul,' but rather is conceived as both an invisible universal force and material manifestation, differentiated as well as integrated, but never individualized. Through *semangat* a person is always '. . . at one with the universe' (Skeat 1900; Cuisinier 1936; Endicott 1970). Thus, it has been argued that the early Malay should have had little difficulty in accepting the mysticism and pantheism of Hindu beliefs, and 'the cosmic unity which is God' of *Sufism*, a mystical perspective within Islam that developed in Persia, was influenced by Indian thought, and later appeared in Hindu-dominated Malaya around the midfifteenth century (Endicott 1970). Indeed, the fundamental idea of *Sufism* is quite similar to *semangat*. The universe is of a single essence which is manifested in a multiplicity of things. Thus, it becomes conceivable that *semangat* was readily translatable into Allah and the belief that 'Allah is in everything' into a pantheistic concept totally inconsistent with Orthodox Islam, but compatible with the primitive Malay belief structure (Ryan 1971; Endicott 1970). Perhaps it is not remarkable, therefore, that *Sufism* should be the form of Islam that would find some acceptance among the peoples of the Malay Archipelago (Winstedt 1947). What is notable is that Islam, as officially practiced in Malaysia, is of the *Shafi'i* school of the Orthodox *Sunni* sect, which considers the popular mysticism of the *Sufis* and animism of indigenous beliefs to be heretical. Again we see what appears to be a disparity between precise behavioral expectations and ambiguous cultural conceptualizations. That the Malay can 'resolve' or at the least tolerate these apparent major theological conflicts may be a function of the same propensity for the universal which characterizes the structure of the Malay belief system. Perhaps the Western scholars' difficulty in determining the precise nature of the concept *semangat* derives in part from this characteristic of Malay cognitive processes. An idea, like *semangat*, is defined and redefined in differing situations according to differing needs and conditions specific to those situations. Thus while this 'vital force' is universal and unitary at one level, it can only be described in terms of the highly differentiated material forms manifested along the spectrum of sensations at another level. To Westerners such characteristics may seem antagonistic, but to the Malay they represent only the varying facets of a concept that is so abstract as to allow exceptional latitude in definition.

CONCEPTUAL STRUCTURE AND LANGUAGE

In his theory of personal constructs, Kelly (1955) has argued that human conceptualization is the result of attempts to construct the world in such a way as to maximize our ability to predict and control events. Individuals within cultural groups develop unique systems of constructs for this purpose, both between and among themselves (Kiev 1972). These latter public or consensually-agreed-upon conceptual dimensions within a cultural group provide the basis for a 'shared world view,' and represent that unique system of concepts out of which social and ethical values are derived for the cultural group. The concepts are interdependent with the language of the group, defining the cognitive representations for experiential events and, in turn, being limited in their power to define by the lexical properties of the language (Bruner 1966; Whorf 1956). Thus, we should see reflected in Malay language the properties of conceptual structure described above. We have hypothesized that there is an ambiguity resulting from the application of broad evaluative dimensions at the higher conceptual level simultaneous to the existence of a greater degree of preciseness at the observable behavioral level.

Unfortunately, the testing of this hypothesis is made exceedingly difficult due to the lack of systematic and comprehensive linguistic studies of the Malay language. However, the reasons cited for this scholarly neglect would appear to indirectly confirm our hypothesis. In his study of traditional Malay literature,

Hussein (1968) traces the historical development of Malay and reminds us that it evolved as the '. . . medium of communication in [a] region of some 250 mutually unintelligible languages, whether in the Moluccas, or in New Guinea, or in Achyh' (81). Because of its intermediary role, it became a highly '. . . assimilative and flexible language . . .' and it was because of this '. . . vague characteristic of the Malay language . . . ,' according to Hussein, that it was very much neglected by linguistic scholars. Winstedt (1923) similarly has noted that the language can be vague at one level and specific at another.

The Malay language has a dozen words for 'fall,' 'hit,' 'carry' and so on, and terms for every instrument and process of agriculture, but it is destitute of words to express feelings and abstract ideas (1923:94).

Our evidence can be derived from yet another source — that having to do with the study of parallels between the structure of society (social strata) and the organization of language.

The propensity for highly specific behavioral guidelines and the role played by language in relating conceptualization and behavior are both seen in the social ranking system within Malay society. Since propriety or form is essential, the culture must provide a system for easy recognition of the appropriate status manifested in the ranking which enables the Malay to demonstrate his awareness of the proper protocol. Hence, the appropriate form for social intercourse is prescribed within the language system which provides fully distinct linguistic forms according to the rank and status of the participants in the interaction as in the following examples:

    A. Royal or Court Language — used only by and in addressing royalty;

    B. Honorific Languages — used to speak 'up' to someone of higher status with specific subforms for:

        1. rural honorific and

        2. urban honorific; and

    C. Rough or Market Language.

Setyonegora (1970) has similarly described the structural correspondence of Javanese social strata and language and how this structure may determine behavior. The Javanese are a Malay people, being derived from common indigenous ancestors of the Malay Archipelago, and this commonality is reflected, not only in similarities in customs, but also in similarities in concepts and languages (Wallace 1962).[1] Among the Javanese (and other Malays), a person is viewed as being in a perpetual struggle to maintain an equilibrium between conflicting forces within the environment and one's social relations. Thus, according to Setyonegora, the Javanese conceptualize the world in dichotomous terms, such as *old-young*, and most importantly, *appropriate-inappropriate*. What constitutes appropriate-inappropriate, however, is defined in terms of an elaborate hierarchy of exemplars, and what emerges is a complex and fluid code which defines the proper form of behavior and symbolically represents the hierarchically elaborated avenues for appropriate social inter-action within the community. A similar analysis of Malay conceptual structure has been reported by Colson (1971) in the context of devising a typology of instances of abnormal behavior in Malaysia. He obtained a matrix composed of two superordinate evaluative dimensions: usual-unusual and correct-incorrect (proper-improper). Under these superordinate concepts were subsumed a number of discrete situations defined in terms of their tolerability by the community and degree of variation from the cultural ideal (see Figure 1). Here we see the most clear and direct evidence of the relationship between illness behavior and Malay conceptual structure.

What we have hypothesized, therefore, is a conceptual system characterized by a finite number of superordinate dimensions so broadly defined as to apply to a seemingly infinite variety of behavioral exemplars depending upon nuances of time, place, situation, person involved, etc. What we are describing are dimensions that are at an abstract level, are 'central' to the conceptual system and have a wide range of convenience, i.e., relate to a broad range of phenomena. Further, they are highly 'permeable,' i.e., are sufficiently flexible as to permit the inclusion of new elements or phenomena within their range of meaning. Among the more important of these superordinate dimensions is the evaluative concept, 'appropriate-inappropriate' or 'proper-improper' (*betul-tidak betul*), which appears to be almost universally applied but the importance of which is especially manifest in evaluations of social behavior, the focal concern among Malay values.

The central role of the appropriate-inappropriate dimension and the abstract level of such evaluative dimensions in the Malay conceptual system has been independently confirmed by Osgood et al. (1975) in their comparative semantic analysis of 22 language systems throughout the world.

Starting with a diverse sample of 100 culture-common, translation-equivalent nouns, Osgood and his collaborators obtained a list of descriptive qualifiers, together with their opposites, which was then factor analyzed into its principal components. The first three factors obtained (Evaluation, Potency, Activity) proved to be qualitatively the same both intra- and interculturally.

When the same procedure was initiated within a specific culture without regard to cross-linguistic comparability, the results were essentially the same (i.e., the first three factors analyzed were still E, P and A), but the indigenous concept scales which contribute to or 'load' on these principal factors showed interesting variations between cultures.

By looking at the types of concepts which load on the principal factors in each language, Osgood was able to characterize the nature of each of the E-P-A

Fig. 1*

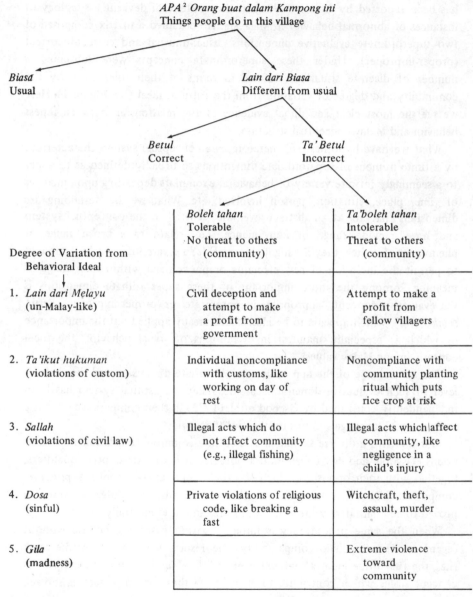

APA² *Orang buat dalam Kampong ini*
Things people do in this village

	Boleh tahan Tolerable No threat to others (community)	Ta'boleh tahan Intolerable Threat to others (community)
Degree of Variation from Behavioral Ideal ↓		
1. *Lain dari Melayu* (un-Malay-like)	Civil deception and attempt to make a profit from government	Attempt to make a profit from fellow villagers
2. *Ta'ikut hukuman* (violations of custom)	Individual noncompliance with customs, like working on day of rest	Noncompliance with community planting ritual which puts rice crop at risk
3. *Sallah* (violations of civil law)	Illegal acts which do not affect community (e.g., illegal fishing)	Illegal acts which affect community, like negligence in a child's injury
4. *Dosa* (sinful)	Private violations of religious code, like breaking a fast	Witchcraft, theft, assault, murder
5. *Gila* (madness)		Extreme violence toward community

*Adapted from Colson (1971b)

factors for various cultures and specify the indigenous conceptual dimensions which contribute most to defining the factor.

As we have predicted, in the case of the Malaysian language (Bahasa Malaysia), (1) the Evaluation factor is dominantly 'abstract' in character and more so than any other of the 22 languages studied. (2) One of the two concept dimensions which contributes most to the Evaluation factor is 'fitting (proper)-not fitting (not proper).' What is remarkable is that this dimension does not appear among the principal component concepts for any other of the 22 languages studied! Thus, Osgood's findings clearly support the hypothesized distinctive centrality of the appropriate-inappropriate dimension to the Malays.

In an attempt to bring definition into his vague conceptual world, perhaps the Malay has had to continually 'fine tune' his behavioral 'perception of the universal essence' until he has developed such an elaborately complex hierarchy of exemplars that he is able to explain everything, and nothing! That is, he can behave precisely in most established social situations, but his explanations, being universal, are not precise enough to guide him in new situations. The net result is, that on a day-to-day basis, he is faced with the constant task of discriminating appropriate from inappropriate, but the cues are complex with the inevitable consequence that there is a high risk of violation 'in the eye of the beholder.' Since Malay propriety dictates that one never confronts another, the perceived violation will seldom be mentioned. Thus, the system provides for the creation of tension through ambiguity and a block to its resolution through propriety.

LOOPHOLES AND THE QUESTION OF CONSEQUENCES

It is at this point that additional features of the Malay system of behavioral norms invite our consideration. First, it has already been suggested that despite the propensity for stringent proprietary rules, the Malay has available a wide range of behavioral options. 'There is always a loophole somewhere for his escape' (Mahathir 1970). In the case of societal sanctions against aggression and confrontation, the behavioral alternatives include a loophole option in the form of traditional sanctions for the phenomenon of *amok* — that under prescribed behavioral conditions (e.g., insult to self-esteem) there are both expectance and reinforcement for the consequent act of running *amok* (McNair 1972; Clifford 1927; Swettenham 1895). Second, consider the concept of courage which to the Malay is equated with a willingness to face up to a hopeless situation, to take on an adversary when it is beyond one's capacity (Mahathir 1970; Clifford 1927; Swettenham 1895; Vaughan 1857). Here we see a relatively greater fatalistic quality in the Malay concept of courage than is generally found in comparable Western values. The brave Malay '. . . is likely to do things without thinking of the consequences, the average Malay treats him with fear and respect' (Mahathir

1970:161). Thus we find a convergence of several aspects of the value system which we would argue contribute to the *amok* phenomenon:

A. a relative disregard for the consequences of behavior;

B. socialization of acquiescence and passivity leading to a sense of fatalism (one's fate is often in the hands of others); resulting in

C. courage being defined in terms of acquiescence to fate regardless of the consequences; combined with

D. social sanctions for exercising the loophole option in a code prohibiting aggression.

One possible result of this set of circumstances is a personality generally characterized by seemingly passive acquiescence punctuated by infrequent episodic explosions of anger. A nineteenth-century description of the Malay vividly captures this aspect of the culture to which Mahathir (1970) refers almost a century later:

Externally impassive the Malays are, as a race, but no one can long have had intimate dealings with them without being struck by their extraordinary susceptibility and peculiar sensitiveness to the influence of what we should call the accidents of every-day life . . .

No man, *pace* all Irishmen, is more 'touchy' than a Malay . . . .

It is this nervous impressionability which leads to those mysterious *Vendettas* and unaccountable *Amoks*, which so often place the European completely at fault in dealing with this otherwise charming and loveable people (O'Brian 1883:145).

Perhaps it is this 'extraordinary susceptibility and peculiar sensitiveness' that people refer to as both the impulsiveness and fatalism of the Malay. Whether it is in keeping with his penchant for the bipolar evaluative concept, or for whatever reason, the Malay has been described as thinking in all-or-none terms when it comes to social action. There is a popular notion that 'half measures are to no avail.' One will generally remain submissive and quiet, but if action is decided upon, it must be with no constraint.

In other words, if you are driven to slaughter, slay as many people as you can; the more you kill, the more you will be remembered. This is the spirit of the 'Amuck.' Caution and prudence are the very breath of life to the normal Malay; when the strength of his endurance has been strained to snapping-point, the reaction of feeling is appalling in its consequences. The man who elects 'Amuck' is beyond the canons of human reason; he is already a dead man. He even cares little if the oppressor himself is slain; the 'fat goes to others, the bones and the feathers' fall to the share of the agent of retributive justice (Wilkinson 1925:5–6).

MALAY CONSTRUCTION OF HEALTH AND ILLNESS

In the preceding sections I have attempted to show that social learning processes, the value system of the Malay, and the structure of the Malay conceptual system contribute to the predisposition to and precipitation of the behavioral events termed '*amok*.' In the sections that follow I shall attempt to show how these same factors contribute to the explanatory model used by the Malay to account for the *amok* event. Specifically, I shall show that the system of concepts used by the Malay to define the nature, etiology, and treatment of illness includes some of the same superordinate dimensions seen earlier in the Malay conceptualization of social behavior. I shall present evidence that these preeminent social evaluative dimensions play a central role in defining not only illness, but also mental illness, of which *amok* is the most severe form recognized.

As with Malay concepts of social behavior, the Malay system of constructs defining the parameters of health and illness similarly include a superordinate dimension focused upon the ethicality or 'appropriateness' of illness-related conditions or behavior. Anthony Colson's monograph (1971a) analyzing Malay illness concepts and behavior provides a sample description of this conceptual system obtained during several years of intensive field research in a rural *kampong* in peninsular Malaysia. According to Colson's informants, Malay concepts of health emphasize:

A. *health* in the sense of a positive attribute, more than just the absence of illness;

B. *strength* or vigor apppropriate to one's own (not others') norms;

C. *age*, in the sense of what is appropriate for one's age;

D. *role* performance, or the ability, or impairment thereof, to carry out appropriately one's vocation or responsibilities; and

E. *social* behavior that is normal or appropriate. Any behavior which sets one apart from other community members (e.g., social withdrawal) is generally viewed as evidence of reduced health status. This focuses especially upon the consequences of such behavior as:

– *conflict*, violence, or other forms of threat to the community (recall that avoidance of conflict or threat is among the most basic of social values), and

– *extreme economic status*, either poverty or wealth. Extreme deviations from the moderate are considered potential sources of stress.

Health so defined is viewed as impairable as a result of any one of four major causes:

A. natural causes, e.g., natural pathogens, germs, trauma;

B. supernatural causes, e.g., spirit possession;

C. punishment for unethical behavior, by witchcraft or divine intervention; or

D. inappropriate behavior, including behavior due to a 'weakened condition.'

Under each cause may be subsumed several specific agents which might operate at various levels. For example, Colson (1971) has suggested that causes may be grouped according to their origin. At one level are those causes which originate or have their effects within the individual, like 'wind,' blood, germs, trauma, or poisons.

At a second level are causes which originate from sources outside the body, such as magic, spirits, God, and natural pathogens.

At a third level are found causes which are the consequences of behavior or result from traits of the individual, e.g., unethical or inappropriate behavior.

Illness may also be caused by a weakened condition resulting from a loss of *semangat*, the 'vital force,' which, when diminished, makes the person more vulnerable to illness. As noted earlier, the Malay believes that *semangat* is possessed by all living things and even some inanimate objects, such as boats, weapons, stones, food, clothes, tools, etc. It is manifested in humans as a sense of competence, well-being, or 'goodness.' It is not synonymous with strength since a wise old man can have more *semangat* than a young militant, but it is generally assumed that adults have more than children. Any of the above causes can precipitate a loss of *semangat* by rendering the victim at risk to invasion by agents that might attack or possess the *semangat*. I shall return to this point later.

At a practical level, the dimensions of the rural Malay concept of illness are reflected in the type of questions Colson (1971) found were most commonly posed when an individual was confronted with sickness:

A. What kind of illness is it?

B. How has it been (or should it be) treated?

C. What caused the illness?

D. How serious is it?

E. Does the illness pose a threat to other people? through madness? through contagion (*jangkit*)?

F. Will the condition endure (is it chronic or acute)?

G. Was it inherited?

H. Is the condition appropriate to the individual (e.g., a young man should not have edema, an illness of old age)?

TABLE I

1. Madness	Most serious
2. Loss of consciousness	.
3. Enduring high fever	.
4. Hemorrhage	.
5. Acute abdominal pain	.
6. Paralysis	.
7. Enduring bloody diarrhea	.
8. Chronic cough	.
9. Edema	Least serious

In general, these are the types of illness-related questions that would encompass the diagnostic and prognostic concerns of an individual in Western culture. What is of special interest are the defining characteristics of the illness, its cause, severity, threat, chronicity, etc., which are culturally specific. Let us focus our attention on the Malay's view of the relative severity or seriousness of various disorders (see Table I, taken from Colson 1971). We note that 'madness,' which is defined as acting violently toward others or threatening violence, is clearly seen as the most serious of the symptoms mentioned by Colson's informants, and concurs with observations made by Cuisinier almost 40 years earlier (1936).

CONCEPTS OF MENTAL ILLNESS

As with illness concepts in general, concepts of mental disorder are invoked to explain specific forms of behavior that are regarded as inappropriate. We have hypothesized that the paradigmatic events to be explained are derived from a few superordinate evaluative dimensions. Colson's (1971b) typology of Malay perceptions of abnormality, based on field work done in the state of Pahang in 1966–68, supports our contention and is illustrated in Figure 1. As can be seen, mental illness in its extreme form, *gila* ('madness'), occupies a unique category in the typology in that it has no 'tolerable' component. Defined primarily in terms of manifest or threatened physical violence toward the community, *gila* is categorically intolerable and dealt with through banishment, i.e., turning over to civil authorities outside the village. In the particular *kampong* studied, Colson noted that 'In all recorded cases the "banishment" was permanent. Either the person was institutionalized for life, or after discharge was not allowed to return to the same village' (1971:95). Evidence of this severe sequelae has also been reported by Tan and Carr (1977). Of course, not all mental illness is '*gila*.' Further, the typology reported by Colson applies to events and does not include concepts applied to persons who manifest chronic behavior regarded as tolerable.

As with other forms of illness, loss of *semangat* is a primary predisposing condition in mental illness. Further, the Malay recognizes that severe mental stress can also predispose to mental disorder. Such stress may take varied forms such as *hati ta'senang* (anxiety), *fikiran lebeh* (excessive mental concentration), and *mengaji lebeh* (excessive study or other strenuous mental work). It is believed that the mind is unable to withstand severe emotional stress, especially in adults under age 35. The result is a weakened condition which leaves the person especially vulnerable to spirits and witchcraft, and the risk of loss of *semangat*.

Chen (1970) has provided a detailed overview of Malay concepts of mental illness based on a study of 231 households in five different *kampongs* in Malaysia. His analysis has been independently confirmed by Resner and Hartog

(1970) based on interviews and observations made in *kampongs* throughout four states in Malaysia from 1966–68. Similar concepts have also been obtained by Schmidt (1964) in his analysis of the *Iban* of Sarawak. Mental Illness is classified into three broad categories of disorders: serious threatening (to others) states, chronic nonthreatening states, and acute nonthreatening states. Included among the serious threatening states, or *gila* (insanity) are three disorders of note:

1. *Gila Kena Hantu*, a form of insanity due to evil spirits, characterized by fits of violence, superhuman ability to cause destruction, and auditory hallucinations;

2. *Gila Buatan Orang* which may be identical in symptoms but differs in cause, being attributable to witchcraft as opposed to spirits, a subtle distinction to the Westerner, but important in the Malay pantheon of supernatural beings and powers; and

3. *Gila Mengamok*, or as it is more commonly known, *amuk* or *amok*, an extreme form of *Gila Kena Hantu* and *Gila Buatan Orang*. A description of the symptoms, etiology, course, and prognosis conform to the traditional description of *amok*.

Chronic nonthreatening states include conditions such as:

1. *Gila Babi* (epileptiform disorders);
2. *Otak Miring* (senile dementia);
3. *Bodoh* (mental deficiency); and
4. *Latah*, a state of extreme involuntary behavior, characterized by echopraxia, echolalia, and other 'echo' behavior.

Acute nonthreatening states differ from *gila* only in degree, and include threats that are the consequence of illness. If threat to the community is severe, then the disorder is classed as *gila* (insanity). If nonthreatening, then it is classed as *penyakit* (illness).

I have traced the pervasive influence of the superordinate evaluative dimension, appropriate-inappropriate, from its preeminent position among Malay concepts governing social conduct, to its role as a defining dimension in health, illness, and, specifically, mental illness. I have shown that the most severe form of illness in the Malay conceptual system, *Gila Mengamok*, is defined primarily in terms of social behavior that is considered to be 'inappropriate' in the most extreme sense, i.e., homicidal assault against the community in a culture where the definition of propriety begins with the admonition that one never even confronts another, let alone expresses aggression. The inescapable logic is that in such a culture, one must be 'insane' (*gila*) to run *amok*.

Defined as insane because of the social consequences of his behavior (severe-threat to the community), and relieved of responsibility because of spirit possession and amnesia (Chen 1970; Colson 1971b), the *pengamok* is provided a conceptualization which allows for the subtle social sanction of the behavior. Insanity is viewed as the most common form of illness and is most frequently associated with 'depression' and 'persecution' (Cuisinier 1936), affective states closely associated with attacks upon self-esteem. Thus, the Malay is afforded the means by which to seek restitution for an accumulation of perceived violations of integrity and self-esteem (inappropriate treatment at the hands of others). Since the perceived insults upon self-esteem may be accumulated from a variety of individuals, it is not remarkable that the *pengamok* should vent his anger against society. Indeed, Gullick (1958) has observed that the essential elements of *amok* are (1) an intense sense of grievance and (2) indiscriminate and murderous violence against society. Clearly, *amok* is an act of social protest by an individual against his immediate social group. Under certain prescribed conditions, the cultural system can not only 'explain' it, but in so doing sanctions its continued exercise by members of the group.

CONCLUSION

Culture is not simply an organization designed for the satisfaction of sociological needs, but rather a complex system of internalized adaptation prescriptions evolved to meet the coping needs of members of the culture. Each culture develops its own unique system of beliefs, institutions, and sanctions to enable individuals to cope with the environmental stresses that impinge upon them. Of course, not all stress is external. The culture itself, evolved to reduce tensions, may contribute significantly to the stress of its members. Still, the cultural system does provide the means by which threatening phenomena can be defined and explained, corrective measures prescribed, and favorable outcomes anticipated.

What is less clear are the precise steps by which the above take place and the applicability of behavioral principles, studied and developed within the context of Western cultures, to the understanding of the evolution of the non-Western cultural system. More specifically, while it may be clear that different cultures reinforce different psychopathological patterns and the acceptable guidelines for their expression, transcultural researchers must continue to demonstrate step-by-step the contribution of mechanisms of behavioral acquisition and change to cultural specificity.

In the present paper I have tried to demonstrate that while the belief system of the Malay fulfills in large measure the principal function of cultural systems, i.e., to reduce stress by making the world more ordered and predictable, at the same time, it establishes a unique set of necessary (albeit insufficient) conditions for the precipitation of a culturally specific form of aggressive behavior. While

TABLE II
Superordinate Evaluative Constructs in the Malay Conceptual System and Their Relation to Amok

Concept	'Appropriate'	'Inappropriate'	Process of Acquisition
	↓	↓	
SOCIAL VALUES			
	Passive	Active	
	Nonemotional	Emotional	
	Nonconfronting	Confronting	
	Obedient	Disobedient	
SOCIAL STATUS	'Halus' if behavior is:	'Kasar' if:	
	↓	↓	
	Appropriate (re: rank of other language)	Inappropriate	
	Considerate	Inconsiderate	
	'Sensitive'	'Insensitive'	
	Respectful	Disrespect	
	Anticipates needs	Does not anticipate needs	
	Refined	Not refined	
CONCEPTS OF HEALTH			
	Health (positive state)	Illness	
	↓	↓	
	Strength	Weakness	
	Appropriate (re: age, role, social relations)	Inappropriate	

SOCIALIZATION, NEGATIVE REINFORCEMENT
(AVOIDANCE OF MALU)
.... SOCIAL REINFORCEMENT ....

this process adds to the stress of individuals within the culture, the conceptual system attempts to reduce this stress by providing culturally consistent explanations for the nature, causes, and treatment of the behavior in question.

The principal characteristics of the Malay conceptual system which we have argued contribute to the *amok* phenomena are schematically represented in Table II. Central to the conceptual system are a finite number of bipolar superordinate constructs which are repetitively manifest in judgmental decisions by the Malay about life events. A principal evaluative dimension throughout this structure is appropriate-inappropriate which pervades judgments regarding social status, social interaction, health in general, and mental illness in particular. Value systems and contingent behaviors are learned through a socialization process that relies heavily upon negative reinforcement (the avoidance of '*malu*'). As a result, the Malay behavioral repertoire consists of relatively little in the way of positively reinforced coping skills, but rather a negatively reinforced passive-dependent posture as the best means of avoiding *malu*. Hence, the traditional rural Malay, especially, is ill-prepared and inexperienced to cope with social stress in the form of interpersonal confrontation; social, economic, and political frustration; and psychological assault. According to social expectation, he must comply and withdraw until the conditions for exercising traditional options for retaliation (classical *amok*) and subsequent social sanctions (expectation and explanation as 'insanity') are fulfilled. In the urban Malay, by contrast, the increasing incursion upon the traditional Malay conceptual sytem of foreign concepts (not only Western) should effect an increase in complexity of both the structure as well as the content of the conceptual system (Mahathir 1970). Thus, we would anticipate a reduction in the occurrence of individual *amok* in urban centers where such influences are most prevalent, and among middle and upper classes where educational opportunities are more likely to impact upon the conceptual system. This prediction runs counter to the hypothesis that the stresses of modernization and urbanization lead to psychological conflict and, therefore, increased pathological behavior. Under that urbanization hypothesis, an *increase* in *amok* in urban centers would be predicted. Precise epidemiological data are lacking and the potential impact of a wide array of sociopolitical variables remains undetermined. However, there is a body of available evidence (Murphy 1959; Carr and Tan 1976; Tan and Carr 1977; Schmidt et al. 1976; Tan 1965; Colson 1974; Mahathir 1970) which suggests a reduction of individual *amok* in urban centers and, therefore, would appear to support the conceptual change hypothesis.

We are now able to return to the concept of the culture-bound syndrome and reconsider its definition in light of our examination of the *amok* phenomenon. I have demonstrated the important role played by implicit values, belief systems, and social structure in determining the manifest behavior of *amok*, and to this extent I must concur with Yap's definition (1969). However, I take issue with the position that the behaviors upon which culture exercises so pervasive an influence are only superficial and that underneath this facade is the 'real disease,' the basic form of which is inviolate and universal in nature. I find no support in the case of *amok* for this assumption. Further, I would argue that such a definition is nondiscriminating since the case has been made that for every instance of sickness the illness behavior, as distinct from the disease process, is always culturally determined (Kleinman et al. 1978). A reformulation of the concept of 'culture-bound syndrome,' therefore, must focus not on the universality of the underlying disease process, but rather upon the universality of the acquisition and attribution processes by which the behavior in question becomes distinctively labeled as *illness*. I would define culture-bound syndrome as a distinct repertoire of behaviors that (1) have evolved as the result of a social learning process in which the conceptual and value systems, and the social structural forms that mediate their effects, have served to define the conditions under which such behavior is an appropriate response, and (2) have been legitimated within the indigenous system as *illness* primarily in terms of extreme deviation from the behavioral norm as defined by preeminent culturally-specified conceptual dimensions governing social behavior.

The psychological mechanisms by which the content and lexical structure of the conceptual system and its related behaviors have been acquired are universal in nature and include empirically established principles of human learning governing concept formation and behavioral acquisition. Thus, the criteria by which both the manifest behavior is labeled and the cause defined are culture-specific while the mechanisms of acquisition are universal. The behavior may be precipitated by various etiological factors (e.g., including a number of psychiatric conditions observed cross-culturally), but the nosological system and criterial concepts are indigenous. That is, culture-bound syndromes are culturally sanctioned behavioral pathways which may or may not contain 'pathology.'

It follows that such 'disorders' are not universal, i.e., inter-cultural, although similarities in manifest behaviors may so suggest.

Amok, as it is conceptualized by the Malay, will be found prevalent only among people who share Malay conceptualizations and behavioral norms. Behavior similar to the *amok* phenomenon will be found in other cultures, but it will be called by other names and conceptualized and valuated in other ways.

University of Washington

NOTES

1. The pervasiveness of the Javanese language-social strata correspondence made itself felt to such an extent among the Dutch colonials that the latter soon developed Honorific and rough levels of Dutch (Indisch-Nederlandsch) throughout the East Indies.

REFERENCES

Bandura, A.
    1974   Behavior Theory and the Models of Man. American Psychologist 29: 859–869.
Bruner, J.
    1966   Studies in Cognitive Growth. New York: Wiley.
Burton-Bradley, B. G.
    1968   The *Amok* Syndrome in Papua and New Guinea. Medical Journal of Australia
           1: 252–256. (Reprinted in this volume.)
Carothers, J.
    1948   A Study of Mental Derangement in Africans and an Attempt to Explain Its
           Peculiarities, More Especially in Relation to the African Attitude to Life.
           Psychiatry 11: 47–86.
Carr, J. E., and E. K. Tan
    1976   In Search of the True *Amok: Amok* as Viewed within the Malay Culture.
           American Journal of Psychiatry 133; 11: 1295–1299.

Chen, P. C.
1970   Classification and Concepts of Causation of Mental Illness in a Rural Malay
        Community. International Journal of Social Psychiatry 16: 205–215.
Clifford, H.
1927   The *Amok* of Data Kaya Biji Derja. *In* Court and Kampong. London: Richard
        Liesh.
Colson, A. C.
1971a   The Prevention of Illness in a Malay Village: An Analysis of Concepts and
        Behavior. Medical Behavioral Science Monograph Series 2, No. 1. Winston-Salem,
        N.C.: Overseas Research Center, Wake Forest University.
1971b   The Perception of Abnormality in a Malay Village. *In* Psychological Problems and
        Treatment in Malaysia. N. Wagner and E. S. Tan, eds. Kuala Lumpur: University
        of Malaya Press.
Cooper, J.
1934   Mental Disease Situations in Certain Cultures: A New Field for Research. Journal
        of Abnormal and Social Psychology 29: 10–17.
Cuisinier, J.
1936   Danses Magiques de Kelantan. *In* Travaux et Memoires de l'Institut d'Ethnologie,
        Vol. 22. Paris: Université de Paris.
Denko, J. D.
1964   The Role of Culture in Mental Illness in Non-Western Peoples. Journal of the
        American Medical Women's Association 19: 1029–1044.
Djamour, J.
1965   Malay Kinship and Marriage in Singapore. *In* London School of Economics
        Monographs on Social Anthropology, No. 21. London: Athlone Press.
Endicott, K. M.
1970   An Analysis of Malay Magic. Oxford: Clarendon.
Firth, R.
1966   Housekeeping among Malay Peasants (Revised). *In* London School of Economics
        Monographs on Social Anthropology, No. 7. London: Athlone Press.
Gullick, J. M.
1958   Indigenous Political Systems of Western Malaya. *In* London School of Economics
        Monographs on Social Anthropology, No. 17. London: Athlone Press.
Gutherie, G. M.
1973   Culture and Mental Disorder. Module in Anthropology, No. 39. New York:
        Addison-Wesley.
Hassan, R.
1970   Some Sociological Aspects of Suicides in Singapore. *In* Mental Health Trends in
        Developing Society. M. Yap and P. Ngui, eds. Singapore: Roche Far East Research
        Foundation.
Hussein, J.
1968   The Study of Traditional Malay Literature. Asian Studies 6: 66–89.
Iskander, T.
1970   Kamus Dewan. Kuala Lumpur: Dewan Bahara dan Pustaka, Kementerian
        Pelajaran.
Kelly, G.
1955   The Psychology of Personal Constructs. New York: Norton.
Kiev, A.
1972   Transcultural Psychiatry. New York: Free Press.
Kleinman, A., L. Eisenberg, and B. Good.
1978   Culture, Illness and Care: Clinical Lessons from Anthropological and Cross-
        Cultural Research. Annals of International Medicine 88: 251–258.
Kloss, B.
1923   Arctic *Amok.* Journal of the Malayan Branch Royal Asiatic Society 1: 254.

Lin, T.
    1953   A Study of the Incidence of Mental Disorder in Chinese and Other Cultures.
            Psychiatry 16: 313–336.
Mahathir, M.
    1970   The Malay Dilemma. Singapore: Asia Pacific Press.
McNair, J.
    1972   Perak and the Malays (Revised Edition). Kuala Lumpur: Oxford University Press.
Murphy, H. B. M.
    1959   Culture and Mental Disorder in Singapore. In Culture and Mental Health. M.
            Opler, ed. New York: Macmillan.
    1972   History and the Evolution of Syndromes: The Striking Case of Latah and Amok.
            In Psychopathology: Contributions from the Social, Behavioral, and Biological
            Sciences. M. Hammer, K. Salzinger, and S. Sutton, eds. New York: Wiley.
Newman, P. L.
    1964   Wild Man Behavior in a New Guinea Community. American Anthropologist 66:
            1–19.
O'Brien, H. A.
    1883   Latah. Journal of the Straits of Branch of the Royal Asiatic Society 11:
            143–153.
Omar, A.
    1968   Interplay of Structural and Socio-Cultural Factors in the Development of the
            Malay Language. Asian Studies 6: 19–25.
Osgood, C., W. May, and M. Mison
    1975   Cross-Cultural Universals of Affective Meaning. Urbana: University of Illinois
            Press.
Othman, A.
    1973   Some Aspects of Socialization Practices among Rural Malay Children. Conference
            on Psychology and Related Disciplines in Malaysia. University Kebangsaan, Kuala
            Lumpur. Abstract.
Resner, G., and J. Hartog
    1970   Concepts and Terminology of Mental Disorder among the Malays. Journal of
            Cross-Cultural Psychology 1: 369–381.
Ryan, N. J.
    1971   The Cultural Heritage of Malaya. Singapore: Jongnan Malaysia.
Schmidt, K.
    1964   Folk Psychiatry in Sarawak: A Tentative System of Psychiatry of the Shan. In
            Magic, Faith, and Healing. A. Kiev, ed. New York: Free Press.
    1967   Mental Health Services in a Developing Country in South-East Asia (Sarawak). In
            New Aspects of the Mental Health Services. H. Freeman and J. Farndale, eds.
            London: Pergamon.
Schmidt, K., L. Hill, and G. Guthrie
    1975   Running Amok. Unpublished Manuscript.
Setyonegora, R. K.
    1970   Latah in Java: Mental Health Trends in a Developing Society. Proceedings of the
            World Federation for Mental Health Workshop. Singapore. pp. 91–95.
Shaw, W.
    1972   Amuk. Federation Museums Journal (Malaysia) 17: 1–30.
Skeat, W.
    1967   Malay Magic. New York: Dover Press. (Originally published in 1900. Malay Magic:
            An Introduction to the Folklore and Popular Religion of the Malay Peninsular
            [sic]. London: Macmillan and Co., Ltd.)
Swettenham, F.
    1967   The Real Malay. In Stories and Sketches by Sir Frank Swettenham. Kuala

Lumpur: Oxford Press. (Originally published in 1895. Malay Sketches. London: John Lane.)

Swift, M. G.
1965   Malay Peasant Society in Jelebu. *In* London School of Economics Monographs on Social Anthropology, No. 29. London: Athlone Press.

Tan, E. K., and J. E. Carr
1977   Psychiatric Sequelae of *Amok.* Culture, Medicine and Psychiatry 1: 59–67.

Tan, E. S.
1965   *Amok:* A Diagnostic Consideration. Proceedings of the Second Malaysian Congress of Medicine, Singapore.

Teoh, J. I.
1972   The Changing Psychopathology of *Amok.* Psychiatry 35: 345–351.
1974   An Analysis of Completed Suicide by Psychological Post-Mortem. Annals Academy Medicine 3: 117–124.

Vaughan, J. D.
1857   Notes on the Malays of Penang and Province Wellesley. Journal of Indian Archipelago and Eastern Asia 2: 115–175.

Wallace, A. R.
1962   The Malay Archipelago (New Edition). New York: Dover Press.

Westermeyer, J.
1972   A Comparison of *Amok* and Other Homicide in Laos. American Journal of Psychiatry 129: 703–709.
1973   On the Epidemicity of *Amok* Violence. Archives of General Psychiatry 28: 873–876.

Winstedt, R.
1923   Malaya. London: Constable and Company.
1947   The Malays: A Cultured History. London: Routledge and Kegan Paul.

Whorf, B.
1956   Language, Thought, and Reality: Selected Writings of B. L. Whorf. J. B. Carroll, ed. New York: Wiley.

Wilder, W.
1974   Socialization in a Malay Village. Unpublished Manuscript.

Wilkinson, R. J.
1925   Papers on Malay Subjects. Malay Literature. Part III. Malay Proverbs on Malay Character. Letterwriting. Kuala Lumpur: Federated Malay States Government Press.

Wilson, P. J.
1967   A Malay Village and Malaysia: Social Values and Rural Development. New Haven: Hraf Press.

Yap, P. M.
1951   Mental Diseases Peculiar to Certain Cultures: A Survey of Comparative Psychiatry. Journal of Mental Science 97: 313–327.
1969   The Culture-Bound Reactive Syndromes. *In* Mental Health Research in Asia and the Pacific. W. Caudill and Tsung-Yi Lin, eds. Honolulu: East-West Center Press.

SUDDEN MASS ASSAULT WITH GRENADE:
AN EPIDEMIC *AMOK* FORM FROM LAOS*

INTRODUCTION

Sudden mass assault (often labeled *amok*), generally with homicide and often with suicide of the perpetrator, has been reported from Malaysia, Sumatra,[1-8] Papua-New Guinea,[9] Singapore,[2] Indonesia,[10-11] Philippines,[12] and Laos.[13-15] In all of these countries cutting blades (long knives, machetes) have been the traditional weapon. Over the last half century other weapons have been used, including the rifle in Malaysia,[8] Thompson submachine gun in the Philippines,[12] and hand grenade in Laos.[13-15] Similar assaults also occur elsewhere in the world, including the United States, but they have not been so carefully studied as in these countries of Southeast Asia and the Malay Archipelago. The cause for this discrepancy is not clear, but may be due to greater incidence in these countries.

Sampling methods for most studies described above consist of locating surviving *amok* perpetrators in prisons and mental hospitals. This *per se* excludes study of those events in which the perpetrator does not survive. This is a major problem with many studies, since it is likely that the two forms of *amok* (i.e., with and without successful suicide) have important differences as well as similarities.

Data collected in most studies have consisted of psychopathological findings observed in the surviving perpetrator. One investigator has studied social context of sudden mass assault,[9] but generally this has received little attention. As one might expect from this approach, theories have focused on psychopathology and central nervous system organicity.

The study described here was undertaken for four reasons. First, sudden mass assault had not previously been described in Southeast Asia, although it was well described in the adjacent Malay Archipelago. Second, the use of the grenade as a sudden mass assault weapon had not been previously described. Third, the sampling method encompassed all cases occurring in a particular time and place, including some in which the perpetrator died and some in which he lived. And fourth, data collection included a number of social as well as psychological variables.

METHOD

Definition

In 1901 Gimlette, based on a single clinical interview, first identified these four characteristics of *amok* in Malaysia: prodromal depression, sudden impulsive homicide, absence of personal motive, and subsequent amnesia for the violent event.[3] Burton-Bradley has questioned the criteria of amnesia and lack of motivation.[9]

Ronald C. Simons and Charles C. Hughes (eds.), The Culture-Bound Syndromes, 225–235.

Langness has doubted whether the onset need be sudden or the syndrome need be transient.[16]

Pfeiffer has described *amok* as a "twilight state with indiscriminate aggression".[17] For Azguirre, *amok* is "a state of murderous frenzy in which the individual runs about through the street with a sword or dagger and slashes everyone in his way until he is either placed under control alive or killed on the spot".[12]

For purposes of this paper grendae-*amok* is the sudden wholesale killing and maiming of unsuspecting victims with one or more hand grenades. It may or may not involve suicide by the perpetrator. Two cases of solitary grenade suicide and three cases in which grenade assaults involved careful planning have been excluded. To be included in this series of cases, at least one victim had to have died.

Sample and Data Collection

During field work in Laos during 1965–1967 a pilot study of six grenade-*amok* cases was conducted. Later, in 1971, data were collected on the eighteen cases described here. Sources of information included friends, relatives and neighbors of *amok* perpetrators, village leaders, police records, Buddhist monks, hospital personnel, surviving and imprisoned *amok* perpetrators ($n = 3$) and prison officials and guards. Number of informants per case varied from three to eight people. Interviews were conducted mostly in the Lao language. Most cases took place in Vientiane province of Laos, although a few occurred in other provinces. Another dozen or so cases were reported from distant provinces, but time and logistics prevented adequate data collection.

BACKGROUND

Elderly Lao informed me that sudden mass assaults with bladed weapons had occurred throughout their lives (i.e., back to the 1910's and 1920's). Other weapons (e.g., guns) were not used in sudden mass assaults prior to the use of grenades, even though guns were the usual weapon for homicide during robbery or disputes about interpersonal problems.[13] Only two cases, from the same geographic location and time period as the other eighteen cases, did not involve grenades. Both of these *amok* persons used bladed instruments.

Grenades, mortars and artillery tended to be more popular weapons among Lao soldiers than rifles. In discussions with several soldiers about this preference, I received rather consistent reports. They felt that direct shooting of the enemy went against their Theravada Buddhist tenets to preserve all life (unless their own life was directly threatened). By contrast, if they propelled artillery or grenades into an area of Laos which happened to be occupied by the Vietnamese, it was the latters' responsibility for being where they should not be. In other words, shrapnel weapons decreased their moral sense of personal responsibility for killing another person. (Similarly, many Lao would not hunt animals because of the stricture against killing but would go fishing because "I don't kill the fish with my net or hook, but the fish only dies because it cannot live in air.")

Grenade-*amok* occurred in an epidemic pattern in Laos. The first reported case took place in Vientiane, Laos, in 1959. Over the subsequent several years, the number of cases per year gradually increased. A particularly common location was Buddhist temple festivals, or *boun*. By 1966 there were enough cases that Souvanna Phouma, prime minister of Laos, suspended all *boun* for the remainder of the Buddhist calendar year. In that one year the author collected twenty reports of *amok* cases in Laos from newspapers, radio, and informants. The number of cases gradually declined thereafter, with only seven mass slayings by grenade in police records for 1970. During my last two field research visits to Laos in 1974 and 1975, there were no reported cases.

The first reported grenade-*amok* case in Laos is of interest since, as we shall see, the perpetrator in that case differed in certain regards from other *amok* persons. Based on informant reports, the event proceeded as follows:

A few weeks prior to his *amok* outburst, a 26 year old single Lao soldier began to express fixed, rigid ideas which were not endorsed by others (in retrospect, these were probably delusions). He was notably irascible in his relations with friends and relatives. At a temple festival or *boun*, he had a public argument. This involved his being excluded from a Lao dance or *lamvong* because of disturbing behavior (i.e., frightening the female dancers, not dancing in a traditional manner). He left the *boun* in a rage. Within an hour he returned to the *boun* and threw a grenade into the *lamvong* dance circle, killing four people and wounding twenty people. He then jumped into the midst of the mayhem which he had created, yelling that he had done it and that these people deserved to die because of their insult to him. He was readily apprehended and hauled off to prison. In prison his condition gradually deteriorated. He alternated between mumbling to himself and shouting incoherently; he did not respond to efforts at conversation. After several months of incarceration he was returned to the care of his parents at home. Over the subsequent decade he remained demented and lived peaceably at home.

As we shall see in the subsequent cases, major mental illness was not common among this group. Also, most perpetrators had not engaged just before the event in threatening or frightening behavior. And relatively few were caught alive. In other respects this person is typical: he was male, young, not currently married and living with a spouse, away from home, in the military (with access to grenades), had been drinking at the *boun*, and had recently been rejected or had publicly "lost face".

THE SUDDENLY ASSAULTIVE PERSON

Demography

All eighteen subjects were young adult men, ranging from 17 to 35 years of age (median 27.0, mean 26.2, standard deviation 6.0). Nine had no formal education, and nine had between 1 and 6 years of education. Eight were single, 7 married,

2 divorced and 1 widowed. Fourteen were ethnic Lao, and 4 were tribal Hmong. Occupation included 15 soldiers, 2 farmers and 1 merchant. The latter 3 subjects were guardsmen in the militia and had access to grenades.

Social and Geographic Mobility

Residence at birth of the *amok* persons was compared with residence at the time of their violent outburst (see Table I). This showed a drift of subjects from small communities to larger communities ($P < 0.005, X_2^2 = 14.45$). In part this migration

TABLE I

Residence at birth versus residence at *amok*

Location	Number of subjects	
	At birth	At *amok*
Village	14	4
District town	3	4
Provincial capital	1	10

may have reflected the large number of soldiers in the sample. Many non-soldiers had also moved into towns for training and occupational advancement in the decade prior to the study. However, most soldiers were not currently in towns, but were located on the front, in bivouac, or visiting their home villages on leave, so that this finding may be an important one.

Fathers of all eighteen men were peasant farmers with no formal education. The *amok* men were significantly more apt to have some education than their fathers ($P < 0.0005$, Fisher exact). This upward educational mobility was a general trend throughout Laos, and absence of census data does not permit any conclusions regarding whether this finding was unusual for young Laotian men.

Premorbid States

None of the subjects was known to have suffered psychosis (*bā*), convulsions (*bā mu*), mental retardation (*khon sā*) or incapacitating physical disability prior to the assault. Six men were described by their peers as having been average, productive, responsible people. Another nine subjects were described as having problems with interpersonal relationships and/or personality problems (i.e., emotionally unstable, irresponsible, immature, and/or passively dependent). In the remaining three cases inadequate data were available to formulate an opinion about their premorbid state.

This relatively high proportion of problematic premorbid personalities may may be a retrospective reporting artifact, since their peers may have been more critical in assessing them after the violent episode. By the same token, in my other research on socially deviant behavior in Laos (e.g., narcotic addiction, mental disorder), Laotian informants tended to gloss over premorbid problems and to typify any subject as "a good person, a hard worker" (which did in fact describe most Lao villagers most of the time).

Precipitating Events

Interpersonal discord, insults, or major losses preceded the *amok* events in sixteen of the eighteen cases. While these events appeared related to the assault in time and place, the response (as is common with this syndrome) was far out of proportion to the stressful events, as in the case described above. The following is a case in which the precipitating event seemed to be even more minor:

A 26 year old single Lao soldier wanted to join a group of comrades playing cards in a barracks. He had no money and asked if someone would stake him to a hand. No one would lend him the money since he was well known to disregard obligations and debts. A heated argument ensued, and he left the group in anger. A brief time later he reappeared, tossed a grenade in the center of the players, saying "Here then, play with this". One man was killed, and ten were hospitalized with serious injuries. The perpetrator was easily apprehended and was sentenced to a long prison term.

At the other end of the spectrum, this subject had recently experienced severe loss:

A 30 year old Hmong man and his family had been forced by Vietnamese invasions to move three times in the previous two years. Each time they lost their house, household belongings and most personal items. Two of their children died during these refugee treks. Following the last flight, the wife died with fever (probably malaria). Two days after her death the husband, while sitting with his two surviving sons, discharged a grenade in their midst, killing all three of them.

Most cases were intermediate between these two extremes, as in the following case:

A 23 year old Lao soldier had courted a young woman for two years. They planned to marry, and the man approached the woman's parents to discuss marriage. Her family refused to consider the marriage, now or at any time in the future. The woman refused to go against her family or to consider elopement. The man manifested sadness and frustration, but expressed no anger or threats. Two days after the family's refusal, he discharged a grenade while attending a movie with his girlfriend. Seven other people were killed in addition to the couple; twelve wounded were admitted to the hospital.

Apparent precipitating events in these eighteen cases were categorized as follows:

public argument	4
marital problem (divorce, separation)	4
gambling losses	4
problem involving girlfriend	3
grief (death of a wife)	1
unknown	2

These precipitating events were not especially unusual, with the possible exception of public arguments, which were rare in Laos. However, a common theme of loss runs through them, including "loss of face" (*seah nā* in Lao) — an important factor in Lao and Hmong cultures. Time lag between loss and the sudden assault varied from a few minutes to two months. Note that in two cases no cause could be identified despite considerable efforts.

Alcohol Use

Thirteen out of these eighteen violent events took place in a context of social drinking, such as a temple festival, an army card game, or a family celebration. Chronic alcohol abuse was not present in any of the cases, although varying degrees of drinking had preceded the assaults. Alcohol use accompanied gambling and public arguments, but only some marital and romantic disagreements.

Outcome

Nine of these subjects killed themselves with the grenade explosion, and one person killed himself with a knife immediately afterwards. Usually anger was more evident than grief, as illustrated in this case:

A 35 year old Lao soldier had beaten his wife repeatedly during jealous rages. Two months after she eventually left him, he accosted her at a temple festival and angrily demanded that she return home with him. When she refused, he produced two grenades and pulled their pins. He then rushed at his wife and embraced her with a live grenade in each hand. They along with six others died; thirty peple were admitted to the hospital.

Four of the eight surviving prepetrators were apprehended and imprisoned. Two of them remained incarcerated, and I was able to interview them in prison. (Sixteen of the subjects could not be interviewed; data regarding them was obtained from informants, including family members, peers, village elders, monks and the police.) On interview, neither of these two men showed gross psychopathology, although one could be described as having a sociopathic personality and the other as having a passive-aggressive personality with paranoid features. A third man, described earlier as the first case of grenade-*amok*, was eventually released due to chronic psychosis, which appeared to be schizophrenia in a late chronic phase. The fourth man escaped from prison on two occasions, having been recaptured after the first escape. During the first escape he killed a guard, and on the second attempt his pursuers shot and killed him.

Four other men escaped after throwing the grenades and were not apprehended.

THE VIOLENT EVENT

Location

Eleven of these events occurred mostly in crowded public places, including temple festivals, army camps, a movie theatre and a street. Private homes were the next most common (six cases). Only one case occurred in a lonely, remote area of forest. These locations indicate that most perpetrators chose locations which favored a maximum number of victims. In a minority of cases they chose a location designed to involve only known, close associates.

Gambling losses, public arguments and heavy drinking accompanied grenade-*amok* in public locations. Marital discord, girlfriend problems and death of a spouse preceded violence in domestic settings.

Time

Eleven of these 18 cases took place between 6 : 00 PM and midnight. Next most common were the six hours between noon and 6 : 00 PM (four cases). Only three events occurred between midnight and noon. Again, these times were conducive to involving a large number of people gathered at a morning market or an evening temple festival.

Mortality and Morbidity

In the least severe episode one person died and ten went to the hospital. At the other end of the spectrum, sixteen died and twenty went to the hospital. The average number of victims killed per event was 4.9 people (excluding the *amok* person), and the average wounded was 7.5 people — a total of 13.4 victims per episode. As one might expect there were more victims in public settings and fewer in homes.

Relationship Between Victims and Perpetrator

Half of the cases (i.e., nine) involved only people known to the perpetrator. These involved mostly domestic problems and took place in home settings. One-third of the events (i.e., six) included strangers only. Most of these involved gambling or public (often drunken) arguments. In the remaining three cases some victims were strangers and some were known to the perpetrator.

COMPARISON OF AMOK AND OTHER HOMICIDE

I also collected twelve cases of more purposive, deliberate homicide in Laos at the same time that I studied these *amok* cases. These homicides were apt to involve a gun and occur in less crowded settings. No one was wounded, and the dead victims numbered either one or two (mean 1.31). *Amok* persons were several years younger than these twelve other murderers on the average, and this difference was statistically significant ($P < 0.05$, Student "t" test). Five of the twelve purposive homicides involved robbery, which did not occur in any of the grenade-*amok* cases. Half of the *amok* perpetrators committed suicide, while the greatest number of other killers went to prison. These other homicides usually took place in the perpetrator's own birthplace, rather than in another community as with *amok* ($P < 0.05$, Fisher Exact test). The perpetrators in both groups showed no difference in ethnicity, education, or premorbid personality, although the number in both groups was so small that only major differences could be demonstrated. (This comparison has been described more fully elsewhere.[13])

DISCUSSION

Semantic and Definitional Issues

Should the term *amok* be applied only to sudden assaults among Malays or Malay-Indonesians? What about cases among Chinese in Malaysia? Or among Malays in Singapore? Should similar cases in adjacent countries be included? How about cases on other continents? Purists argue that only "classical" Malay cases in Malaysia should be considered *amok*, but as indicated earlier these "classical" symptoms were based on one surviving case examined while incarcerated.[3] By traditional standards the more recent cases in Malaysia would not be considered *amok*, since they usually involve firearms (e.g., pistols, shotguns) rather than bladed weapons.

One alternative is to use the term *amok* and define carefully how it is used. Elsewhere I have suggested the term "SMASH Syndrome" for "sudden *m*ass *a*ssault-*s*uicide-*h*omicide".[18] This also has its limitations since suicide does not accompany many cases. Despite the absence of suicide in some cases, there is usually a self destructive element even among surviving perpetrators, since they are either imprisoned or flee their homes, families, work and former associates. Their previous social identity and social existence is obliterated one way or another.

As is evident from the cases reported above, there are borderline cases in which classification is not easy. Is the grieving widower who popped a grenade in the midst of his children a simple suicide-homicide case, and not an *amok* case? Does one have to assault strangers to be considered a valid *amok* case? Must a completed homicide be present to justify the label of *amok*, or merely assault with a deadly weapon? Should one begin such a study by studying a wide variety of sudden nonpurposive homicidal assaults, or by studying only a distinct, highly circumscribed case fitting a predetermined category?

Since the answers to all of these questions are not clear, my recommendation at this time is that investigators proceed as follows. First, use whatever term you prefer, but define what you mean. Secondly, define in as detailed a fashion as you can the criteria for inclusion in and exclusion from the sample. And third, be prepared to have other serious students of these phenomena disagree with you.

Sampling and Procedural Issues

It is hoped that future investigators will show more interest in perpetrators who cannot be readily interviewed in a prison or hospital — namely, those who escape or do not survive. One might investigate both groups by obtaining school records, informant interviews, demographic characteristics and so forth. This would permit better assessment of the sampling bias. Interviews of surviving perpetrators would then contribute more useful information once we know about the bias introduced by studying only those in prison or hospital. I want to emphasize that only two out of the eighteen perpetrators in this series could be interviewed.

These data from Laos and Burton-Bradley's data from Papua-New Guinea[9] demonstrate both the possibility and the utility of studying social concomitants of *amok*. Biological tests would also be welcome (e.g., neurological examination, dexamethasone suppression test, CAT scans, EEG, psychometrics and similar tests on survivors; autopsy and neurotransmitter studies on the deceased). More extensive psychological testing — cognative, personality, organic — might also prove worthwhile. The number of cases occurring in many nations on a regular basis would support such a special multidisciplinary study.

Correlates of the SMASII Syndrome

In this sample of sudden mass assaulters, 15 perpetrators were soldiers and the remaining 3 men were in the militia. All 18 of them had access to grenades. This suggests strongly that access to such violent weapons was an important component in the syndrome.

Use of the traditional bladed weapons, with their less devastating effect, remained decidedly infrequent. Similarly, these Laotions did not use rifles or automatic weapons, although these were as much or more available than grenades. Both bladed weapons and guns involved direct killing, which went strongly against local Buddhist tenets. It appears that the grenades, as a highly destructive but also as a more "moral" weapon from the Laotian perspective (i.e., the victims "were in the wrong place"), fit well into the local culture as well as with the aims of the perpetrator.

The accumulated data on *amok* over the last half century indicates a trend towards increasingly dangerous weapons. There has been an escalation from the traditional bladed weapons,[1–11] to rifles and shotguns,[8] to machine guns,[12] to grenades.[13–15] While residing in Laos in 1966 my family and I huddled under our table while bombs fell around our neighborhood during an *amok* type aerial raid. General Ma, head of the Lao Air Force, had been asked to step down from his position. Angered by this loss of his prestigious position, he responded by ordering his pilots to bomb and strafe Vientiane, the capital city. Scores of people were killed and wounded. General Ma survived his "air-attack-*amok*" by fleeing to Thailand. This violence could not serve any constructive purpose for Ma, but was simple a vengeful act of assault.

Two major social factors also seem operative in these cases. First, there was a major loss of some kind, usually loss of an important male-female relationship or public loss of face. And second, most (but not all) perpetrators were away from their home village or town. I believe that these two factors are related. Laotian people relied on the extended kin and covillagers as a resource in time of trouble or loss. They helped to resolve problems, to cope with loss, and even to obtain vengeance (although families and clans were conservative regarding revenge or feud). Bereft of their social resources, these men took the situation into their own hands. Their losses also became magnified in many cases because the men did not have a social network base which would enable them to tolerate more personal distress.

Historical concomitants may be important. This form of violence in Laos began when the Indochinese war was expanding, and it waned as the war leveled off and then wound down. Azguirre has noted that similar violence spread in the Philippines at a time of widespread civil unrest and revolutionary movements.[12]

Major psychopathology was present only infrequently. Perhaps significantly, the initiator of this new grenade-amok form in Laos was ealy in the course of chronic paranoid schizophrenia. Premorbid personality and interpersonal problems were common in this sample, but not so severe as to keep these men out of the military. Alcohol may have been a factor for many perpetrators in reducing their inhibitions against such behavior.

NOTE AND REFERENCES

* These data were collected with the help of Messrs. Moua Lia, Adul Keomahathai, and Je Xiong. Dr. Khamleck Vilay provided historical information. The study was supported in part by the International Programs Office at the University of Minnesota.

1. Ellis, W. G.: The *Amok* of the Malays, Journal of Mental Science 39: 325–342, 1893.
2. Galloway, D. J.: On *Amok*: Far Eastern Association for Tropical Medicine: Transactions of the Fifth Biennial Congress, Singapore. London: John Bale Sons and Danielson Ltd., 1923, Vol. 5, pp. 162–171.
3. Gimlette, J. D.: Notes on a Case of *Amok*. Journal of Tropical Medicine and Hygiene 4: 195–199, 1901.
4. Norris, W.: Sentence of Death upon a Malay Convicted of Running *Amuck*. Journal of the Indian Archipelego 3: 460–463, 1849.
5. Oxley, J.: Malay *Amoks*. Journal of the Indian Archipelego 3: 532–533, 1849.
6. Rasch, C.: Über '*Amok*'. Neurol. Zentr. Bl. 13: 550–554, 1894.
7. VanLoon, F. G. H.: *Amok* and *Latah*. Journal of Abnormal Social Psychology 31: 434–444, 1927.
8. VanLoon, F. G. H.: Protopathic Instinctive Phenomena in Normal and Pathological Malay Life. British Journal of Psychology 8: 254–276, 1928.
9. Burton-Bradley, B. G.: The *Amok* Syndrome in Papua and New Guinea. Medical Journal of Australia 1: 252–256, 1968. (Reprinted in this volume.)
10. Van Wulffton-Palthe, P. M.: *Amok*. Med. J. Geneesk. 77: 983–991, 1933.
11. Kline, N. S.: Psychiatry in Indonesia. American Journal of Psychiatry 119: 809–815, 1963.
12. Azguirre, J. C.: *Amuck*. J. Philippine Federation of Private Medical Practitioners 6: 1138–1149, 1957.
13. Westermeyer, J.: A Comparison of *Amok* and Other Homicide in Laos. American Journal of Psychiatry 129: 703–709, 1972.
14. Westermeyer, J.: Grenade-*amok* in Laos: A Psychosocial Perspective. International Journal of Social Psychiatry 19: 1–5, 1973.

15. Westermeyer, J.: On the Epidemicity of *Amok* Violence. Archives of General Psychiatry 28: 873–876, 1973.
16. Langness, L. L.: Hysterical Psychosis: The Cross-cultural Evidence. American Journal of Psychiatry 124: 143–151, 1967.
17. Pfeiffer, W.M.: Transkulturelle psychiatrische Ergebnisse und Probleme. Stuttgart: G. Thieme Verlag, 1970.
18. Westermeyer, J.: *Amok*. In C. Friedmann and R. Faguet (eds.), Extraordinary Disorders of Human Behavior. New York: Plenum, 1982.

B. G. BURTON-BRADLEY [1]

THE *AMOK* SYNDROME IN PAPUA AND NEW GUINEA

> Oh, East is East, and West is West, and
> never the twain shall meet,
> Till Earth and Sky stand Presently at
> God's great Judgment Seat. – Rudyard Kipling.

Kipling was perhaps a little premature, for the twain have met in more recent times with the Judgment Seat still in the offing, and nowhere is this more apparent than in the case of the exotic syndrome stripped of its mystique under the penetrating onslaught of modern behavioural science. Thus we find such entities as *latah, koro, hsieh-ping, imu*, possession syndromes, and mass hysteria with a variety of romantic-sounding names (for example, "*Vailala madness*" and "*mushroom madness*") coming down to earth with nosological statuses more in keeping with known psychiatric concepts. It is proposed here to give an account of the Papua and New Guinea version of the *amok* syndrome which to date has received little medical attention, and to produce evidence to support a sociopsychodynamic explanation of the condition.

THE LITERATURE

According to Dennys (1894), *amok* is a form of psychosis characterized by multiple violent acts and peculiar to the Malays. Gimlette (1901) gives a fascinating account of a case of *amok* which occurred at Pahang, in Malaya. A Muslim man, aged 23 years, a former member of the Perak police force, stole a Malay sword and attacked five Chinese and one Javanese, who were either sleeping or smoking opium. He succeeded in almost decapitating one, killing three and seriously wounding the others, for no reason that could be ascertained. Gimlette considers that four cardinal symptoms are necessary for the diagnosis: prodromal brooding, homicidal outburst, persistence in reckless homicide without apparent motive, and a claim of amnesia. Ellis (1904) regards the condition as a form of psychic epilepsy, a view strongly supported by Fitzgerald (1923) and many others, such was the overwhelming influence of the epistemic paradigms of the day, tending as they did to exclude from attention important new facts and ideas. Fitzgerald was overimpressed by what he considered was the pre-ictal phase with visual auras, some subjects having stated that they "saw red" or that "everything went red", followed by an ictal explosion, the result of discharge of a nerve-cell focus in the sensory cortex. This view can be traced to the influence of Hughlings Jackson (Fitzgerald 1923) and to Kraepelin (1904), who classified some variants as epileptic dream states, similar to those in Europen societies that sometimes led to acts of

237

Ronald C. Simons and Charles C. Hughes (eds.), The Culture-Bound Syndromes, 237–249.

violence. In this, as in other matters, Kraepelin has been misunderstood. His objective was an operational nosology that would lead ultimately to a precisional one. Had more notice been taken of Kraepelin in this regard, the psychiatric classifications and terminologies of today might be less muddled than they actually are, as has been noted by Glover (1939). Coriat (1915) describes an *amok* among the Fuegian tribes in male adults, who, after an initial period of brooding, rush out of the tent and attack until exhausted. He notes the crucial point that the subject in some instances is aware of the premonitory signs and may ask to be tied up to avoid the consequences. One of the best of the older accounts is that of Galloway (1923), who lays stress on the impress of the non-literate mind, in the appropriate cultural setting, as lying broad over the whole series of events, the inflated self-esteem, the overcompensating response at its wounding, and the need for the subject to rehabilitate himself in the eyes of his fellow men. Further accounts are given by Beaton (1925), Clifford (1927), van Loon (1927), Cooper (1934), De Langen and Lichtenstein (1936), Fletcher (1938) and Strong (1944) which, although intensely interesting in themselves, do not offer much more in the way of understanding. Clifford's account of the *amok* of Dato Kaya Biji Derja is probably among the most graphic on record. Malaria, pneumonia, cerebral syphilis, bhang or hashish (*Cannabis indica* or *sativa*), heatstroke, paranoid states and mania have all been implicated in the aetiology by these and other authors. Of considerable importance is the explanation given by Wulfften-Palthe (1933), for whom *amok* is a standardized form of emotional release, recognized as such by the community and, indeed, expected of the individual, who is placed in an intolerably embarrassing or shameful situation. He notes that there is no record of any case of *amok* occurring among the many Malays living in Europe. He makes it quite clear that the Malaysian social structure with its strong kinship ties and the tensions arising out of these obligations have a definite influence on the frequency of *amok*, and illustrates this point with reference to the old hospital in the Glodock district of Djakarta, Indonesia, with its typical non-literate village-type atmosphere, where *amok* was quite common. He records that, when the patients were transferred to a new, modern, fully-equipped hospital, where an entirely different atmosphere prevailed and kinship obligations were not so pressing, *amok* among the patients ceased. Amir (1939), in referring to cases of *amok* in Northern Sumatra, indicates how some of them are associated with extreme feelings of isolation often of people away from home. Ewing (1955) records how a Moro of the Philippines often first asks permission of his parents prior to running *amok*. Yap (1951, 1958, 1962, 1965) follows Wulfften-Palthe in attributing social significance to the *amok* syndrome, which he refers to as an "atypical culture-bound psychogenic psychosis". In this context he considers that it is an acute hypereredic state,[2] in which a large amount of undirected hostility is aroused, and in which suicidal behaviour is fused with homicidal *furor*.

As far as Papua-New Guinea is concerned, *amok* has seldom been reported in the past. This is not surprising, in view of the history and terrain of the country, and the paucity of pertinent records. Seligman (1929) had been overimpressed by Jung's extroversion-introversion concept, and believed that, by and large, this viewpoint could be extended to racial groups as well as to individuals. Malays, being introverted, were therefore more prone to the *amok* syndrome, and "Papuasians", being extroverted, were largely immune. In this he somewhat anticipated modern culture and personality studies, but his views have little substance in reality, as Papuans with their many cultural groups exhibit the full spectrum of personality types – a fact readily apparent to anyone who has lived with them for any length of time. Monckton (1921, 1922, 1934), in his popular writing about the early years of this century, commented on what he considered to be the high incidence of mental illness in the d'Entrecasteaux group of islands in Eastern Papua. He described three instances of observing either members of his party or villagers running *amok* while he was on patrol. He also expressed the opinion that *amok* was not uncommon in Northern Papua, where it seemed to be accepted by the rest of the village as well as by the patient himself. According to the social anthropologist Fortune (1932), *amok* was a well-known occurrence on the island of Dobu in Eastern Papua, where he observed actual instances three times within six months. In his view, *amok* was closely related to sorcery. This is not surprising, and is in line with his assessment of the culture as having strong paranoid components. Chowning (1961) describes a case which she observed among the Molima people of the d'Entrecasteaux Islands. She made the pertinent points that no "shame" was involved and that symptoms were openly discussed. Of interest is Roheim's (1946) account of the wording of war spells in the southern part of Normanby Island, which is clearly designed to make a warrior go berserk, so that he works himself up into a dissociative reaction in which he has no fear and will attack all in his path.

For differential diagnostic purposes, mention should be made of three other entities superficially similar but distinct from *amok* – namely, the "wild man behaviour" of Newman (1964), the behaviour of the male in the "collective hysteria" of Reay (1965), and the hysterical psychosis of Langness (1965). The wild man episode is distinctively different, in that the harmful component is lacking, and the rushing about and gesticulating are done in a much more permissive environment. In the recurrent "collective hysteria" or so-called "mushroom madness" of the Minj area of the middle Wahgi Valley of the Western Highlands, a man may appear to run *amok*. He takes a spear and runs around in an aggressive manner, which can be very impressive to the onlooker. However, he carefully ensures that no one is hurt. The relationship of this last mentioned pseudo-*amok* to the mushroom is somewhat doubtful. Reay and I fed alleged "long long" (insanity) mushrooms to two potential subjects, with negative results. Others also were reported to have indulged in the behavior without having eaten the mushrooms at all. A case of "hysterical psychosis", which occurred among the Bena Bena people of New Guinea, is described by Langness (1965). This example of an aggressive outburst lacked the continuing homicidal drive, and the man concerned stopped in the middle to accept a cigarette. Langness considers that the attack was in part a response to the cultural pressures that are focused on the age group of the young adult male.

CLINICAL MATERIAL

It is impossible to estimate the incidence of *amok* in Papua and New Guinea, but the condition appears to be relatively uncommon at the present time. Over the last eight years in the Territory of Papua and New Guinea, I have had the opportunity of studying the seven cases of *amok* reported in this paper. Apart from these, there have been numerous other instances which could be described either as abortive cases or as dissociated components of the condition in which some intervening situation prevented their full expression. The cases cited represent only a minute fraction of the totality of violence, including multiple violent acts, presenting for medical assessment during the period under consideration. None of the subjects exhibited evidence of epilepsy or of overt schizophrenia, or of any other form of mental disorder. All were in good physical health, although a recent history of brief exposure without food or shelter was not uncommon. All were young adult males, single or married, labourers, village gardeners or artisans. None had any schooling; all could be considered as only partially acculturated. Summarizing the cases in the form of a clinical amalgam one arrives at the following type of picture. A healthy young adult is quieter than usual or "goes bush" for a few days. There may be a history of slight or insult. He may regain his normal composure, or the condition may continue and remain unchanged (an abortive attack), or it may become worse. In this case, suddenly and without warning, without anyone expecting such an immediate response at this point of time, he jumps up, seizes an axe or some spears rushes around attacking all and sundry and even destroying inanimate objects such as yam houses or hospital property. Within a very short period of time, a number of people will be dead or wounded. He shouts "I am going to kill you", and everyone in the neighbourhood seeks safety in flight. All are now fully aware that the man is suffering from a special form of "kava kava" or "long long" (insanity), that he will not be satiated or stop of his own accord. They recognize that this, and similar types of reaction, are available methods of tension reduction, used from time to time as acts arising from despair. The man continues in this fashion until overpowered, by which time he has become exhausted. He may also be killed or wounded. The attack may be aborted at any time by anyone who is brave enough to attempt it. On the subject's recovery, it is usually claimed that there is no recollection of the events that occurred during the acute phase.

REPORTS OF CASES

Case 1. – This patient was a young adult male indigene from Mapamoiwa, Fergusson Island. On his admission to hospital, he said that he had killed an old man and a young "meri" (woman) and speared three others. He said that he must have done this because people said that that was what he had done, and therefore it must be so; but that he himself had no clear recollection of the details. He said that he did not have anything against any of these people, and that they had done him no harm. He said that he had been in the bush without food for two days prior to the offence. On further examination of the patient it was clear that his amnesia was not as absolute as he had originally said, and he indicated that at the time of the offence he was aware that his actions might lead to death and that they were wrong both in the eyes of his own people and in those of the Administration. An eye witness said that he was sitting in front of his house, with some of his relatives, at about 7 o'clock on the night of the episode, when he saw the patient standing about 25 feet away from the group. It was dusk, and there was light from the cooking fire. The patient had a spear, which he raised and threw at them, and it hit one of them in the side. The victim was carried inside, and while this was being done, another spear hit another member of the group, who withdrew the spear from her own body. Everyone ran away, and in the process some had to defend themselves. The patient said: "Where are you all? I am coming after you." The eye witness then hid until daybreak, when he found two bodies, one inside and one under the house. Then, with five other villagers, he searched for the patient, who was found in the bush, having been wounded in the chest and on the head. He had five spears stuck in the ground standing up beside him. He was overpowered. In addition to attacking and killing people while running around, he damaged and destroyed yams in the yam house. After his admission to hospital, no evidence of any other form of mental disorder was detected.

This case illustrates the full syndrome, and emphasizes the supposed lack of direction of the act.

Case 2. This patient was a healthy young adult male, who originally came from the hinterlands of Abau, Central District. At the time of the act he was working with a building gang on Fergusson Island. He was a foreigner to his workmates, one of whom called him an "Abau bush pig" – a grave insult. One night at about 6.30, the others were in their dormitory reading or lying down, when the patient came in with a 12 in. bush knife and suddenly attacked them, going from bed to bed hacking at them with the knife, mostly in the vicinity of the head and neck. Six died then or later, some with terrible wounds, their heads being almost chopped off. Finally, another man in the vicinity heard the noise and came in with a rifle and one cartridge. The amok attempted to attack him, was fired at, and still did not cease attacking. He was then put out of action by the butt of the rifle and died.

This case was aborted by killing the *amok*. It also illustrates the gravity of the insult, which he apparently considered to be intolerable.

Case 3. – This patient was a healthy, athletic young adult Orokaivan, a carpenter, who had been working in a district town. He became homesick and decided to return. He had almost reached his destination, after a long walk of some 50 miles over a number of days, when he entered a village where he was known. Suddenly he sprang up and attacked the man who had offered him a meal, shouting that he was going to kill him. He picked up an axe, and the man ran away. A village dog bit him, and he then chased the dog and some children, who were in their canoes on the river. He grabbed an empty canoe and endeavoured to chase and capture them, without success. He returned to the shore, and with an axe and spears chased anyone he could find, eventually spearing a woman in the back, and another man in the thorax with a four-pronged fishing spear. According to the village people, there had been no provocation, only friendliness. He was then hit with a stone, overpowered and handed over to the police. He refused to eat and drink, was admitted to hospital, given electroplectic treatment and tube-fed, after which he started eating, and was shortly ready for discharge from hospital. During the following 12 months he was examined frequently, and no form of mental disorder was detected. He claimed to have only a hazy memory of the acute phase.

This case illustrates prodromal isolation in the bush, explosive and continued violence and a claimed amnesia. The asymptomatic pre-*amok* and post-*amok* history points to the absence of any other mental disorder than the *amok* syndrome. His refusal to eat was related to fear of retribution on a "pay-back" basis.

Case 4. – This patient was an adult male Eastern Highlands indigene from Chuave Subdistrict. The patient was admitted to hospital after an oubturst of violence, in which he attempted to attack the men, women and children in his immediate vicinity with an axe and some spears and to destroy property without apparent cause. His kinsfolk said that he had been unusually quiet for several days before the attack. No one was killed, but several people were gravely injured. The *amok* was overpowered by his kinsmen and tied up prior to being brought to hospital. On examination, the patient denied all recollection of the occasion, and was then completely free of any signs of psychiatric illness. The patient was transferred to the rehabilitation annexe of the hospital. There was no further disturbance until one month later, when he became quiet and appeared to be brooding, and suddenly took hold of a fishing spear which was lying in the vicinity and attacked both staff and patients until he was overpowered. Again the patient denied recollection of the event. Staff members insisted that, had they not locked themselves in a building, at one stage someone would have been killed. No evidence of any other form of mental disorder was detected, and his physical health was excellent. He claimed that he was skilled as a warrior, and had killed many men in intergroup warfare.

This case illustrates the phenomenon of the war *amok* of the group reappearing in the individual on two occasions in another context.

Case 5. – This patient was an adult male indigene from Tari Subdistrict in the Southern Highlands. He was admitted to hospital with a history of suddenly having taken a knife and an axe, and having started attacking and wounding other people in his immediate vicinity, for no apparent reason. The attack was aborted by injuries inflicted on the *amok* by a man who protected himself with the aid of a bush knife. The patient subsequently denied all recollection of the occasion, other than saying that a kinsman had shown him a knife and that he remembered someone accusing him of having sexual intercourse with his mother.

A grave insult preceded this running *amok*, which was aborted in the early phases.

Case 6. – This patient was a young adult male Goilala indigene. He was employed as a painter in a newly-constructed swimming pool in Port Moresby, when he suddenly dropped his paint brush and started throwing house bricks at people in the vicinity, and continued to do so until he was overpowered by the other workers. He claimed to have no recollection of the outbrust, and his fellow workers said that there had been no provocation. It is significant, however, that in their eyes he was a foreigner. Within half an hour there was no evidence of any other abnormality.

The stereotype of the Goilala as a dangerous foreigner is a widespread belief among other people in Papua. In this instance, there may have been expectations of the employment of the *amok* tension-reducing device, or at least of hostility, which was aborted by overpowering the *amok*.

Case 7. – This patient was a young adult male Chimbu. He was brought to hospital by the police, with a history of suddenly attacking his fellow workers, chasing them with an axe in one hand and a knife in the other and saying that he was going to kill them. However, he was overpowered. It was stated that he had brooded for several days after being insulted by another worker, who said he was a "rubbish man" (a recognized form of abuse in this area, meaning somebody who is "good for nothing"), and had thrown water in his face. He claimed amnesia, and was otherwise asymptomatic.

This case exemplifies brooding after an insult, the subject being overpowered in the early stages.

PSYCHOPATHOLOGY

As the result of my discussions with those *amoks* who survived, their "one-talks" and other Papua-New Guineans, I am of the opinion that the individual's mode of thinking (inevitably expressed here in transcultural paraphrase) is somewhat as follows:

I am not an important or "big man". I possess only my sense of personal dignity. My life has been reduced to nothing by an intolerable insult. Therefore, I have nothing to lose except my life, which is nothing, so I trade my life for yours, as your life is favoured. The exchange is in my favour, so I shall not only kill you, but I shall kill many of you, and at the same time rehabilitate myself in the eyes of the group of which I am a member, even though I might be killed in the process.

The evidence suggests that the killings are envisaged as a means of deliverance from an unbearable situation. No doubt much thinking precedes the nihilistic feeling of desperation — kill and be killed. At some point, however, there is complete loss of control, when strong emotion becomes unchecked by deliberation and reflection.

FORENSIC ASPECTS

It is clear that each individual case suspected to be one of *amok* or quasi-*amok* should be assessed on its merits. Although the classical syndrome is fairly clear-cut, some cases are of dubious nature, and there will be the added problem of dealing with supposed contributing factors. The apparent lack of motive and the claimed amnesia will need special attention.

According to the M'Naghten formula, to avoid assignment of responsibility, the defendant must show that "he was labouring under such a defect of reason from disease of the mind as not to know the nature and quality of the act or, if he did know it, that he did not know he was doing what was wrong". In Papua-New Guinea, the Queensland Criminal Code has been adopted. The law relating to the excusatory effect of insanity under this code follows, but also goes beyond, the common law rules formulated in M'Naghten's case. Wrongfulness is interpreted by Australian courts to mean "wrong, having regard to the everyday standards of reasonable people". For the indigenous person, the reasonable people who make up his particular world are his own "one-talks" on the one hand and the rest of the community on the other, which includes those people who make up the Administration. In addition, this code adds a further ground of excuse —

namely, if the mental disease produces the result of depriving the sufferer of the capacity to control his actions. For the purpose of forming an opinion, the questions which must be answered are as follows:

(1) Does the person suffer from a state of mental disease or natural mental infirmity? Nosological niceties are not required, since the court will accept the fact of disease when, from whatever cause, the functions of the understanding are thrown into derangement or disorder. Such disease may be mental or physical and either temporary or permanent. In terms of this definition, classical *amoks* can be regarded as suffering from mental disease. Nonclassical *amoks* may not necessarily be so regarded.

(2) If the answer to the first question is in the affirmative, can it be regarded as more probable than not that, as a result, the supposed *amok* did not know what he was doing, or that it was wrong? Or even if he knew these things, was he unable to control his actions? Or was he under the influence of a delusion as to what he doing, so that had the delusion been true, then his act would not have been wrongful? In the examination of such a person, the first thing the doctor will do will be to determine whether in fact mental disorder or any physical disease process was present at the time of the act in question. He will carry out a full psychiatric and physical examination, including a full blood count and X-ray examination of the lung fields. In particular, he will have blood films examined for malaria parasites before administering suppressives. He will endeavour to determine whether there was knowledge at the time in question of the nature of the act — namely, that the activities would result in death. He will determine whether or not there had been knowledge (cognizance) of the harmfulness and wrongfulness of the act, both in the eyes of the people of the defendant's own culture and also in the eyes of the Administration. The question will arise whether there was an element of premeditation. Psychiatric examination may be able to reveal whether the defendant was able to form an intent. Usually there have been several days of brooding when this has been possible, but these days have often been spent in the bush without food and shelter. In short, the defendant may have suffered from exposure and hunger, with possible impairment of ability to form conscious intent. Confronted with the claim of amnesia for the period of the killings, the examiner will remember that there are a number of other possibilities — namely, malingering, hysterical reaction, other forms of psychosis, epilepsy, drug intoxication and head injury. When the prospect of a feigned amnesia is under consideration, an exact note should be made of what the defendant says about the events of the killing. He may know more than he says and may reveal this fact unintentionally, or he may say "everything went red", or "everything went black", or "I remember nothing, I see that I am in gaol and if you say I killed these people, then that must be so". The diagnosis of malingering will be made only if the other possibilities are excluded, and if there is, in addition, positive evidence of malingering apart from such an exclusion. Malingering may be defined as a deliberate feigning of illness in order to avoid an obligation or to gain a privilege. The examiner should be sensitive to, and make allowances for,

his own subjective responses and prejudices derived from the current social values of the group from which he (the examiner) comes, in assessing a supposed instance of malingering. A feigned amnesia has a patchy and self-serving quality not present in genuine amnesia. To implicate hysterical reactions, it is necessary to demonstrate the previous occurrence of episodes of this kind or the presence of a known hysterical personality, as well as showing that the outburst is consistent with a coexistent trance or fugue.

The formal psychiatric examination may have established the presence of a previous psychosis and, if so, it would be necessary to show, on the presumption of its continuity, that it was operative at the time in question. Epilepsy has often been alleged to be associated with an attack of *amok*, and the examiner needs objective evidence of the presence of ictal phenomena. In practice, this usually means the direct observation of a *petit mal* or *grand mal* seizure by a trained person on this or some previous occasion. The observations of untrained persons in respect of epilepsy in the jungle context are virtually useless.[3] The presence of large burn scars on a Highlands subject is almost diagnostic. Betel chewing is widespread, and the defendant may have been chewing at the time. Its pharmacological action is that of producing euphoria; there is clarity of consciousness with an increased capacity for work (Burton-Bradley 1966), so that its value as a defence at law is unlikely to be very great. Very rarely betel chewing is associated with a psychosis, in which case it would be necessary to demonstrate, for example, the presence of hallucinations or delusions. Head injury needs special attention, as the *amok* often becomes injured during the course of the attack.

The apportionment of responsibility in the case of the individual supposed to be *amok* is always difficult. The examiner should look at the totality of the situation. The more the symptomatology and total picture correspond to the classical description, the less likely is the individual to be legally responsible for his actions. If the cardinal symptoms — namely, prodromal brooding, outburst with homicidal intent, persistence in this fashion without apparent reason and claimed amnesia — are present, and the *amok* is committed without any possible motive at the time of the offence, without profit to the subject or others, without premeditation immediately prior to the explosion, although it may have existed earlier and is unlike any other form of criminality or psychosis, then it is unlikely that the *amok* could be reasonably considered criminally responsible for any death, injury and/or destruction of property that may ensue.

DISCUSSION

The fully developed cases cited support Gimlette's (1901) four cardinal postulates, except that one would doubt whether the action is as motiveless, or the amnesia as absolute, as is held by some authors. It is not enough to be satisfied when someone says that he cannot remember, nor is a motive necessarily absent when it cannot be demonstrated. In some accounts the action is said to be undirected. An explosive reation may well involve every animate or inanimate thing in its path. Nevertheless, the notion should not be taken too literally, since the subject places himself in a situation where an appropriate series of objects is present, and what he actually does clearly symbolizes his case against the group. Another view stresses the supposed exotic and culture-bound nature of *amok*, and this certainly highlights the fact that it is rather concentrated in and around Malaysia. This is understandable for two reasons: (i) the expectation of such behaviour is greater with the established *amok* tradition; and (ii) the religion and social structure are favourable to the employment of this type of tension-reducing device. It should be remembered, however, that cases fulfilling all the necessary criteria have been reported from many countries. It has been reported from Trinidad, India and Liberia (Masters 1920), from Africa (Carothers 1948) and from Siberia and Polynesia (Adams 1951). There is no doubt also that cases identical on all cardinal points occur in European countries. Yap (1958) considers that *amok* is not seen in the Chinese people, and it mey well be that this culture does not greatly favour the employment of such a technique. However, this is no universal proposition, at least as far as migrants or their descendants are concerned. In Singapore, in 1958, I examined two *amok* patients who were both ethnically and culturally Chinese. One was the subject in a notorious case which received wide publicity, and the other was in gaol, having performed the act some years previously. In all essential respects, the incidents were identical with the classical Malay *amok*. Galloway (1923) and De Langen and Lichtenstein (1936) also refer to odd cases occurring among the Chinese. Kline (1963), in his survey of psychiatry in Indonesia, states that the incidence there is as high in individuals of Chinese origin as among the Indonesians. Wulfften-Palthe (1933) stresses that Chinese have been observed to "use" *amok* in Indonesia, and states that it occurs among the Dutch in that country as well. I have also observed *amok* expectancies among Tamil labourers in Singapore. They would anticipate a potential danger and take one of their members to the doctor if they thought that he was brooding too much, with the request that he be locked up to avoid an *amok* episode.

Whatever the virtue or otherwise of the foregoing considerations, it is clear that the so-called *amok* syndrome has a very widespread distribution indeed, including Papua-New Guinea. One cannot help agreeing with Yap (1962), who states that there is "a crying need for a common conceptual language applicable to all cultures". The time is long overdue for the elimination of the exotic element in our thinking. Faergeman's (1963) suggestion of the use of the term "reactive psychosis" has much to commend it.

The indigenous person of Papua-New Guinea has his own *Weltanschauung*, the product of his views of the cosmic order, of life and death united functionally into one comprehensive system, of his cognizance of the attitude to murder of the group of which he is a member, and of his own individual idiosyncrasies derived from life experiences, physical health and genetic endowment. Whether he be a potential *amok* or an ordinary group member, these are the elements brought to the conflict situation. If the expectancies of the group are such that the *amok* response is an institutionalized form of tension reduction, then there will always be individuals who will act in this way, as is shown in the cases cited. This is clearly shown in the case of Fergusson Island and other islands of the d'Entrecasteaux group in Eastern Papua, where there is an *amok* tradition known to all the people.

SUMMARY

(1) Psychiatric aspects of the Papua-New Guinea version of the *amok* syndrome are described for the first time, with seven illustrative cases, and the literature is reviewed.

(2) The local medico-legal situation is discussed, and suggestions are made concerning the examination of the suspected *amok* from this point of view.

(3) Although the condition is heavily concentrated in Malaysia, certain cultural elements favourable to the *amok* response have a much wider distribution, and the supposed exotic nature receives little support from the present study.

(4) A socio-psychodynamic explanation of the condition based on individual idiosyncrasy, a psychogenic precipitating factor and group expectancies is supported.

ACKNOWLEDGEMENTS

This paper is published with the permission of the Acting Director of Public Health, Territory of Papua-New Guinea, Dr. W. D. Symes. I am indebted to Professor J. E. Cawte, School of Psychiatry, University of New South Wales, and to Professor R. H. Black, School of Public Health and Tropical Medicine, University of Sydney, for their stimulating comments. The assistance with the Dutch literature of Dr. Robert J. Wolff, Associate Professor of Public Health, University of Hawaii, is greatfully acknowledged.

NOTES

1. Assistant Director, Publis Health Department, Mental Health Division, T.P.N.G.: Adviser in Ethnopsychiatry, South Pacific Commission.
2. Hypereredism is defined by Lindemann (1950) as a morbid state of hostile tension, following continued provocation, sometimes leading to explosive behaviour out of proportion to the circumstances.
3. Hoskin et al. (1967) have also pointed out how convulsive body language, a common form of emotional expression in New Guinea, may be confused with epilepsy.

REFERENCES

Adams, A. R. D.
     1951 *Amok. In* British Encyclopaedia of Medical Practice. London: Butterworth, 2nd edition, Vol. 8, p. 6.
Amir, M.
     1939 Over Eenige Gevallen van *Amok* uit Noord Sumatra. Geneeskundig Tijdschrift voor Nederlandsch-Indië 79: 2786.

Beaton, T.
    1925 Review of Articles by Fitzgerald, Van Loon and Galloway. Tropical Disease Bulletin
          22: 70.
Burton-Bradley, B. G.
    1966 Papua and New Guinea Transcultural Psychiatry: Some Implications of Betel
          Chewing. Medical Journal of Australia 2: 744.
Carothers, J. C.
    1948 A Study of Mental Derangement in Africans and an Attempt to Explain Its Peculiari-
          ties, More Especially in Relation to African Attitudes to Life. Psychiatry 11: 47.
Chowning, A.
    1961 *Amok* and Agression in the d'Entre-casteaux. *In* Proceedings of the Annual Spring
          Meeting of the American Ethnological Society. University of Washington Press.
Clifford, H.
    1927 The *Amok* of Dato Kaya Biji Derja. *In* Court and Kampong. London: Richards, p.
          78.
Cooper, J. M.
    1934 Mental Disease Situations in Certain Cultures. Journal of Abnormal Social Psychology
          29: 10.
Coriat, I. H.
    1915 Psychoneuroses Among Primitive Tribes. Journal of Abnormal Social Psychology
          10: 201.
De Langen, C. D. and A. Lichtenstein
    1936 A Clinical Textbook of Tropical Medicine. Amsterdam: Kolf, p. 529.
Dennys, N. B.
    1894 A Descriptive Dictionary of British Malaya. London: London and China Telegraph
          Office.
Ellis, W. G.
    1901 Some Remarks on Asylum Practice in Singapore. Journal of Tropical Medicine
          and Hygiene 4: 411.
Ewing, J. F.
    1955 Juramentado: Institutionalised Suicide Among the Moros of the Philippines. An-
          thropological Quarterly 28: 148.
Faergeman, P.
    1963 Review of Schipkowensky's 'Pathologische Reaktionen der Persönlichkeit'. Acta
          Psychiatrica Scandinavica 39: 516.
Fitzgerald, R. D.
    1923 A Thesis on Two Tropical Neuroses (*Amok* and *Latah*) Peculiar to Malaya. Far
          Eastern Association for Tropical Medicine: Transactions of the Fifth Biennial Con-
          gress, Singapore, p. 148.
Fletcher, W.
    1938 *Latah* and *Amok*. *In* British Encyclopaedia of Medical Practice, 1st Edition. London:
          Butterworth, Vol. 7, p. 641.
Fortune, R.
    1932 The Sorcerers of Dobu. London: Routledge.
Galloway, D. J.
    1923 On *Amok*. Far Eastern Association for Tropical Medicine: Transactions of the
          Fifth Biennial Congress, Singapore, p. 162.
Gimlette, J. D.
    1901 Notes on a Case of *Amok*. Journal of Tropical Medicine and Hygiene 4: 195.
Glover, E.
    1939 Psychoanalysis. London: Staples.
Hoskin, J. O., L. G. Kiloh, and J. E. Cawte
    1967 Guria and Epilepsy: The Convulsive Body Language of New Guinea. In preparation.

Kline, N. S.
    1963 Psychiatry in Indonesia. American Journal of Psychiatry 119: 809.
Kraepelin, E.
    1904 Vergleichende Psychiatrie. Zentralblatt für die gesamte Neurologie und Psychiatrie 27: 433.
Langness, L. L.
    1965 Hysterical Psychosis in the New Guinea Highlands: A Bena Bena Example. Psychiatry 28: 258.
Lindemann, E.
    1950 Epidemiology of Mental Disorder. New York: Millbank Memorial Fund.
Masters, W. E.
    1920 Essentials of Tropical Medicine. London: John Bale & Danielsson, p. 407.
Monckton, C. A. W.
    1921 Experiences of a New Guinea Resident Magistrate. London: Lane, Bodley Head.
    1922 Last Days in New Guinea. London: Lane, Bodley Head.
    1934 New Guinea Recollections. London: Lane, Bodley Head.
Newman, P. L.
    1964 Wild Man Behaviour in a New Guinea Community. American Anthropologist 66: 1.
Reay, M.
    1965 Mushrooms and Collective Hysteria. Australian Territories 5: 18.
Roheim, G.
    1946 Yaboaine, a War God of Normanby Island. Oceania 16: 210.
Seligman, C. G.
    1929 Temperament, Conflict and Psychosis in a Stone Age Population. British Journal of Medical Psychology 9: 187.
Strong, R. P.
    1944 *In* Stitt's Diagnosis, Prevention and Treatment of Tropical Diseases, 7th Edition. Philadelphia: Blakiston, p. 1143.
Van Loon, F. G. H.
    1927 *Amok* and *Latah*. Journal of Abnormal and Social Psychology 21: 434.
Van Wulfften-Palthe, P. M.
    1933 *Amok*. Nederlandsch Tijdschrift voor Geneeskunde 7: 983.
Yap, P. M.
    1951 Mental Diseases Peculiar to Certain Cultures: A Survey of Comparative Psychiatry. Journal of Mental Science 97: 313.
    1958 Hypereredism and Attempted Suicide in Chinese. Journal of Nervous and Mental Disease 127: 34.
    1962 Words and Things in Comparative Psychiatry, with Special Reference to the Exotic Psychoses. Acta Psychiatrica Scandinavica 38: 163.
    1965 Affective Disorders in Chinese Culture. *In* A. V. S. de Reuck and R. Porter (eds.), Ciba Foundation Symposium on Transcultural Psychiatry. London: Churchill.

J. ARBOLEDA-FLOREZ

AMOK

Violence has become a way of life. Newspapers, magazines and the daily news feed us a steady ration of assaults and murders. The peacefulness of domestic life is broken by the bangs on the television sets, where life is cheap and murder is a ritual and an expected outcome of human affairs. Murderers play God, as powerful snuffers-out of Nature's most perfect creation.

We are assured that murder is a family affair (Tanay 1972) and we understand intuitively that our emotions may be more powerful than our reason, and that rage may make us dispose of even those we love. The power of our loins to create life is matched only by the power of our hands to destroy it. But these passions we understand. They do not baffle us, for in one degree or another, at one time or another, we all have experienced them. The killings in a war, the excesses of political and social struggles, or even the hired gun, we understand too; for glory, prejudice, intolerance, ambition, avarice or pettiness are all too common human frailties. Mass murder, however, the kind involving an individual who suddenly breaks into the public life wreaking destruction in his path, is violence that strikes us as alien, murder that is out of tune with our feelings and beyond our understanding. This murderer is different from the one who through months or years kills off his contacts, methodically and carefully, to avoid detection. He is also different from the psychotic individual who, in the depth of his illness, murders his family. This type of murder is not the same as military or political massacres, where there is more than one perpetrator and where whole populations, usually hapless civilians, are slaughtered as dehumanized and worthless objects of contempt (Nevit and Craig 1971). The mass murderer referred to in this paper is the Madman in the Tower (*Time* 1966), the mall sniper, or the deranged amoker.

This paper will review some of the characteristics of this individual, looking at him through what we know about *amok*, a peculiar mass murder phenomenon said to be found only in the remote lands of Malay.

THE CALGARY MALL SNIPER

On June 16, 1977, at 20.40 hours, J. — 25 years old and single, dressed in army fatigues and carrying several guns, one of them a Magnum rifle with a scope — emerged from his home shooting at cars passing by. He swiftly moved to the shopping mall across the street, zigzagged, knelt down, got up and ran, all the while aiming and shooting at anybody who moved in his field of vision. In a few minutes several shoppers had been moved down and were bleeding on the pavement of the parking lot. The gunman then turned his attention to the policemen and held their fire while running across the mall; two officers went down. After

251

Ronald C. Simons and Charles C. Hughes (eds.), The Culture-Bound Syndromes, 251–262.
© 1979 by the American Academy of Psychiatry and the Law.

exiting on the other side of the mall, he ran and zigzagged to a nearby field, threw himself down and made military rolls over the grass while intermittently slowing down to aim and fire. He was finally cut down by a fusillade coming from different points. Severely wounded, as were several of his victims, he was charged with attempted murder (8 counts).

Background: J. was the fourth of five children. The mother was the disciplinarian, and the father was usually away working. The three oldest children were sisters, and J. was "the baby" for ten years until his brother came along. By then J. had already been described as hyperactive and restless. His sisters teased him and he saw himself as "the shadow or afterthought" of his youngest sister. At school J. was the butt of jokes, teased and pushed around. He did not fit, felt rejected and frustrated and turned into a lonesome and withdrawn youngster. He was a dreamer; in his active fantasy life he saw himself as "Conon", a literary character who rebelled against society. J.'s feelings of alienation grew worse when his family moved from the farm to the city. He was not only afraid of mixing, but also afraid of his own feelings; he had almost killed a playmate who was teasing him. He realized that his anger would know no bounds if he left it unleashed. Externally he was passive and unassertive, and felt that others abused his kindness. His few acquaintances tended to unload their troubles on him, but he never confided his to anyone. He had high moral standards and abhorred dishonesty, rapaciousness, cheating, bigotry and the many other evils of society. He was a crusader and would tell his "honest opinion" to anybody regardless of whether it antagonized others or made him more unpopular. He despised double standards, hated society in general and had a fantasy of going back to the bush where he could live his life away from people. He used to belong to the militia and claimed that the only time he had felt at ease and had had some measure of self-respect and worth was during militia practices. Then he felt his own man, had a purpose in mind, and enjoyed the sense of rectitude and the military discipline. Those years were terminated, however, when he resigned following a conviction on an indecent assault charge. The victim was a relative, a girl whose father was a policeman. J. felt bitter because he believed the court had dealt with him harshly and unfairly to appease the police department. From his militia years J. kept a small arsenal in his basement, where he would spend hours taking care of his guns. He was a good marksman. After he left the militia J. wanted to join the fire department, but was turned down without a satisfactory explanation, he felt. J. was a student tradesman, but he had an overriding sense of unfulfillment and lack of purpose. He was always resentful and convinced that he had no place in society.

Immediate Circumstances: The day of the shooting J. left his school in the afternoon and went with the group for some beers, of which he had four. On his way back home he had a minor automobile accident due to brake failure. The police arrived while he was checking his car, and when they noticed his smell he was asked for a breathalizer sample. He submitted accordingly, convinced that he would not blow over the limit. He was in a good mood and boisterous at the police station, but his mood changed radically once he was advised that his reading was over the 0.8% mark and he was served with a summons. A policeman at the station remarked that he became very despondent. J.'s mood darkened as he went home. He felt angry because he could not prepare for an exam he had the following day, and he felt that the breathalizer had not been operated properly. He grew more resentful and bitter at the police. At home he did some marijuana and he brooded about his problems. He felt trapped, a total failure, unable to take it any more, and depressed. He thought suicide was the only decent alternative. He wrote two suicide notes, one to his friends and the other to his mother. The first one could be considered as a capsulized description of his state of mind:

Dear Friends:
I know and love all of you, tried to help as much as possible, but something go wrong and know that is what happen. I could have done any thing, stay and live with it or do what I am doing. I've worked in this world and see good and bad, fair and unfair, but when the world works against the people, and kills all their dreams, etc., it is time to fight back. I am fighting to my last because it is only for that I go that way. I love the family very much and will miss them, but the world they live in! Too many people that don't care to make it good here [*sic*].

J.'s memory became hazy and he remembered only "going downstairs" and having "big pockets" (possibly a reference to his army fatigues). Somewhere in his mind he wanted "just to drive away and disappear in the bushes". He remembered going outside and feeling that cars and people were closing on him, and that he had to shoot his way through. He felt they were "his real enemies", that he had to have it our with them once and for all, and to make his last stand against the world. He felt he was out of himself, saw lights and colours and heard a boom. His memory went blank.

Diagnosis: Psychiatric assessment determined that J. had a personality disorder, schizoid with paranoid features, and a tendency to remain aloof and to avoid close or prolonged relationships. There was no evidence of organicity. He was described as sensitive to social rejection, misunderstood, and an outsider in the normal activities of his peer group. He carried a sense of alienation and detachment. He was suspicious of the intentions of others, and although feeling inferior and inadequate, he cut himself off from the rest of humanity in an act of defiant grandiosity. He brooded about past hurts and made up in fantasy what the world failed to provide him.

A complex mood state, a mixture of depressive feelings, suicidal thoughts, frustration, suspicion, histility and anger and a dissociative reaction brought about by his mood state, and the possible interaction of the tetrahydrocannabinol and alcohol were present at the time of the shooting. His condition was not considered to be severe enough to make him fall within the Canadian Test of Insanity (Section 16 of the Canadian Criminal Code).

AMOK

Gimlette (1901) gave four cardinal symptoms as necessary for the diagnosis of *amok*: prodromal brooding, homicidal outburst, persistence of reckless homicide without apparent motive, and a claim of amnesia. Johnson-Abraham (1912) described the *amok* attack thus:

The first symptom is an acute depression which deepens, darkening everything around him. Then follows the premonitory aura. The blackness disappears, he sees colours, usually red, and the attack of maniacal fury follows immediately. His memory becomes a blank. He rushes out among his fellow men, armed with a 'kris' or 'chopper', and assaults with homicidal fury every living person he meets – friend or foe, man, woman, or child. The violence of the attack lasts for a few hours only, memory during the period is a blank. The patient is sleepy and stuporous for some days after. Apparently then he becomes quite normal again.

Westermeyer (1972) described *amok* as "those instances in which a person suddenly and unexpectedly begins an indiscriminate assault on those about him". His *amokers* had the following characteristics: personality disorder, a precipitating event, use of alcohol, use of most destructive weapons, choice of a most crowded location, and outcome usually suicide. Although traditionally bladed weapons have been used, rifles and even Thompson submachine guns have been reported (Van Loon 1928; Zaquirre 1957). Of Westermeyer's twenty *amokers*, eighteen used grenades.

AMOK ONLY AMONG MALAYS?

"A furious assault" or "to engage furiously in battle" (*amok* in Malay) is, according to Dennys (1894) a form of psychosis characterized by multiple violent acts peculiar to the Malays. Ellis (1833) stated that "a Malay that runs *amok* is always in a state of furious homicidal passion". He cited Oxley, who in 1845 wrote that

Amoks result from an idiosyncrasy or peculiar temperament common among Malays . . . , a proneness to common disease of feeling resulting from a want of moral elasticity, which leaves the mind a prey to the pain of grief, until it is filled with a malignant gloom and despair, and this whole horizon of existence is overcast with blackness.

Ellis (1893) concluded that the *amoker* "undoubtedly suffers from some form of impulsive insanity generally of a most transient character". He was struck by the fact that his *amokers* suffered from *sakit hati* (literally liver sickness), an ailment understood by Gimlette (1901) as "spite, envy, or being affronted".

Wittkower (1969) classified *amok* within the "special group of unusual symptom patterns which constitute [the] so called culture-bound syndrome". Phenomenologically he considered *amok* to be a dissociation state. Yap (1969) also classified *amok* within the culture-bound reactive syndromes which he described as related to "certain systems of implicit values, social structures, and obviously shared beliefs [which] produce unusual forms of psychopathology that are confined to special areas". As recently as 1976 Carr and Tan (1976) agreed with Yap and stated that "*Amok* is a culture-bound reactive syndrome. It is a culturally specific, complex pattern of behaviors with identifiable antecedent and consequent conditions and is defined as psychopathology within the indigenous culture". Murphy (1973) ascertained that "*latah* and *amok* are found almost exclusively in a single person and culture".

It is controversial, however, whether *amok* is entirely a Malaysian phenomenon, or whether, given certain conditions, it could be found in other cultures. Burton-Bradley (1968), in his discussion of *amok* among the Papua-New Guinea groups, suggested that "certain cultural elements favorable to the *amok* response have a much wider distribution". He gave a complex socio-psychodynamic explanation based on individual idiosyncrasy, a psychogenic precipitating factor, and the presence of group expectancies. Other authors have described *amok* in Trinidad, India, Liberia, (Masters 1920), Africa, (Carothers 1948), and Siberia and Polynesia (Adam 1951).

TWO OTHER NORTH AMERICAN CASES?

Cheng (1972), in his discussion of Westermeyer's (1972) paper stated that "the only instance in which Americans behaved somewhat similarly to running *amok* was the Mai Lai Masacre". It was already mentioned, however, that military or political massacres respond to different sociodynamic circumstances (Nevit 1971). In making his statements, Cheng apparently forgot Charles Whitman (*Time* 1966) who, only six years before, had killed thirteen and wounded thirty-one during a ninety-six-minute murderous rampage from the tower of the University of Texas in Austin. Cheng also forgot Unruh's twenty-minute death spin in 1949, during which he killed thirteen. And in the same year of 1972 when Cheng made his remark, on Memorial Day, a twenty-two-year-old, nicely dressed man, entered, at noon time, a crowded metropolitan shopping center in North Carolina and started shooting, carefully aiming towards the entrance. Five died and seven others were wounded during the spree. The gunman shot himself in the head when he heard the police sirens (Gallemore 1976). Personal and family characteristics of two of these men, the Madman in the Tower and the Memorial Day Man, are similar to those of the Calgary Mall Sniper. Characteristics of the three different events are also similar, as could be noticed from Tables I—III.

DISCUSSION

Westermeyer's (1972) twenty Laotian *amokers* were all men, with a mean age of 26.2, equally likely to be married or single, with occupations different from their fathers' and most of them living away from their original birthplace. Seventeen of them had an immediate precipitating factor or a "recent loss". The seven cases presented by Burton-Bradley (1968) were all men, five described as "healthy young adults", and most of them living away from home and in professions

TABLE I
Personal characteristics

	The Madman in the Tower	The Memorial Day Man	The Calgary Mail Sniper
Sex	M	M	M
Age	25	22	25
Profession	Student	No definite trade	Student
Military service	Yes	No	Yes
Experience with guns	Marksman	Unknown	Marksman
Previous difficulties controlling aggression	Yes	Yes	Yes
Felt picked on	Yes	Yes	Yes
Seen as good natured and pleasant by others	Yes	Yes	Yes
Quiet, restricted social life	Yes	Yes	Yes
Criminal record	No	Yes	Yes

TABLE II
Family characteristics

Family breakdown	Yes	Yes	Yes
Psychiatric history	Yes	Yes	Yes
History of Violence	Yes	Yes	Yes
Job different from father's	Yes	Yes	Yes
Away from birthplace	Yes	Yes	Yes

TABLE III
Characteristics of the events

	The Madman in the Tower	The Memorial Day Man	The Calgary Mall Sniper
Precipitating event	Yes	Yes	Yes
Weapons used	Rifle	Rifle	Rifle
Place chosen	Crowded public place	Crowded public place	Crowded public place
Brooding period	Yes	Yes	Yes
Homicidal outbursts	Yes	Yes	Yes
Persistence of reckless homicidal behavior	Yes	Yes	Yes
Contact with police shortly before incident	No	Yes	Yes
Amnesia	–	–	Yes

different from those of their fathers. The cases described by Ellis (1893) were all men, apparently in early adulthood and away from home.

The three North American cases discussed above had three of Gimlette's (1901) four cardinal symptoms necessary for the diagnosis of *amok*. Also the Calgary Mall Sniper, the only surviving case, had the fourth of Gimlette's symptoms:

that is, amnesia for the episode. In addition, the three cases followed the demo-graphic characteristics of *amok* cases described by other authors, and as well, the actual homicidal events were similar to the other *amok* cases found in the literature.

These three North American cases followed, with exception made of the educational level, Westermeyer's (1972) cross-cultural psychosocial profile of *amok*:

A young or middle aged adult male, from peasant or lower class origins and with little formal education, has moved away from his birthplace to work at a job different from that of his father. While he has not had previous mental aberration, his past behavior pattern has evidenced immaturity, impulsivity, poorly controlled emotionally or social irresponsibility. . . . Following the loss of wife or girlfriend, a large sum of money, social prestige (or rarely, for no apparent reason) he suddenly and unexpectedly strews death and injury about himself.

The ingredients necessary to make up this profile could come together within any culture, anywhere and at any time, depending apparently on the presence of three factors: a social one, that is a society in transition or in the midst of change; and two personal ones, a feeling of alienation and a need for assertiveness.

A Society in Transition: According to Murphy (1973), *amok* is not an off-shoot of Malaysian cultural tradition but a transitional product of an interaction between that tradition and certain modernizing influences. The first reports of *amok* (*amouco* in Portugese), from the sixteenth century, originated not from the Malay peninsula but from India, where exceptional warriors burnt their properties, including their wives and children, and swore to die in their fight against the Portugese. Later similar behavior was reported among slaves in the Malaysian region, where some of them, preferring death to slavery, would suddenly attack others with their swords. Other political situations, such as cooperation with invaders, led some cooperators to murderous attacks. As Wallace (1898) put it *amok* was associated with slavery, warfare or politics and was considered "the national and therefore honorable way of committing suicide". The culture allowed and may have even fostered this sort of rebellion against the foreigners. It was some time later that *amok* became also an honorable means of solving personal crisis as well. Thus, as pointed out by Murphy (1973) in his extensive review of *amok*, it was used first to defend the country, later to defend personal freedom, and subsequently to remedy personal loss of self-esteem. He concluded that epide-miologically the syndrome shifted from a conscious form of behavior to a dis-sociation reaction in individuals who found themselves in the middle of intolerable situations in their respective social groups. "*Amokers* are", stated Burton-Bradley (1968), "methods of tension reduction, used from time to time as acts arising from despair".

The three North American cases presented above were also acts of despair. They revealed an inability of the individual to come to terms with a particular social situation. One, the Madman in the Tower (*Time* 1966) could not master the final breakdown of his family; and of the other two, one, the Memorial Day Man (Gallemore 1976) stated that he was "through talking to people", and the

Calgary Mall Sniper indicated in his farewell notes how much he felt let down by his social group.

The reasons for social change in North America are different from those that wrought change in Malay: The change, however, is none the less drastic in its impact upon and disruption of individual patterns of adaptation. Its driving forces include a socio-economical imperative, that is, the over-riding need to succeed regardless of who gets trampled in the process; the measuring of success in terms of economic power, and the need to flaunt it, even at the expense of other basic needs, to prove it; and a sense of transience that pervades all transactions with people, places and things. Distance and time have lost their binding character; there is built-in obsolescence in material goods; and there is a lack of commitment in interpersonal relationships that reaches as deep as the very family core. Accelerated changes produce an inability to act rationally. Toffler (1971) calls it "confusional breakdown", and gives as signs "the spreading use of drugs, the rise of mysticism, [and] the recurrent outbursts of vandalism and undirected violence". In his opinion "social rationality presupposes individual rationality, and this, in turn depends not only on certain biological equipment, but on continuity, order and regularity in the environment. It is premised on some correlation between the pace and complexity of change and man's decisional capacity". When the channels of adaptation become overloaded there follows confusion, and a need to introduce order, even if it entails destruction.

A Feeling of Alienation: Erickson (1974) defines identity as "a sense of being at one with oneself as one grows and develops; and it means, at the same time, a sense of affinity with a community's sense of being at one with its future as well as its history or mythology". The more the community becomes fragmented, with the constant moving away of individual members and the arrival of new ones, and the anonymity in his own neighborhood and his lack of commitment to a place increases, the less is the individual able to keep up with Erickson's second component for a wholesome sense of identity; his sense of history and mythology becomes irrelevant and his sense of future dims among the cacophony of new places and new faces. Rootlessness and fragmentation of interpersonal relationships, and the stultifying influences of modern labor that make the individual feel like a marionette at the mercy of external circumstances, all lead to alienation. Much like his Malay counterpart lost in a sea of "foreigners", modern man, as posited by Fromm (1971), is "an impoverished 'thing' dependent on powers outside of himself".

Weiss (1971) mentions that estrangement from environment and others leads to inner dissociation and emotional withdrawal. Alienation leads to severance of ties, a lack of communion with the purposes of the community, and unresponsiveness to its strength and needs. In turn, the individual feels that the community has failed him, and a paranoid resentment against the community as a whole develops. A personal sense of failure is converted into a social sense of failure; that is, it is society that has failed to give the individual a better and deserved share of recognition and reward.

Yap (1958) considers *amok* as an acute hypereredic state in which there is an arousal of large amounts of undirected hostility and a mixture of suicidal behavior with homicidal furor. During the *amok*, however, the victims are not strangers senselessly murdered or maimed, but highly personalized and cathected persecutors, the real enemy against whom a desperate and last homicidal-suicidal stand is necessary.

Need for Assertiveness: In Malaysia, as in other cultures, *amokers* have been described as quiet, well-mannered and withdrawn young men. These individuals may be able to express aggression in direct ways, and they may even be afraid to becoming angry for fear of losing their controls. On the other hand they feel constrained in displaying their aggression in more socially acceptable and constructive ways. They blame the social group; it aggravates their sense of personal failure and feelings of worthlessness and depression. A paranoid rationalization develops.

Cultural disorganization leads to pressure for change. As described above, it introduces personal disorganizations which may occasionally be absorbed by the culture in general. Fortes and Mayer (1966) explained, for example, that among the Tallensi the ones that adapted best to cultural change were those holding semi-communal beliefs concerning factors leading to success or failure. They utilized traditional dissociative techniques (possession state) but substituted imagined spirits of the European Governor or other Western symbols for the traditional spirits. Murphy (1967) ascertained that simple schizophrenia with few or no delusions is observed considerably more frequently among Asian schizophrenics than among European ones, but that the latter are prone to produce more paranoid reactions than the former. They suggest that this is due to the emphasis in European cultures upon explaining experiences more rationally. Murphy (1967) goes further and suggests that a culture may call on individual members to sacrifice their mental helath by the development of individual delusions which relieve communal anxieties. The lack of major irrational themes in a culture would then prevent the development of socially acceptable delusional beliefs that could be utilized as delusional safety-valves for society in general. The culture, however, would need ways to relieve the tension.

Mahathir (1970) considers *amok* as representing "the external physical expression of the conflict within the Malay . . . an overflowing of his inner bitterness". This would result from the Malay's traditional courtesy and self-effacing behavior, which is interpreted by others as weakness and leads them to take advantage of him. The Malay gives way until he can give no more. Mahathir feels that this generalized "unassertiveness" and the overflowing of the capacity to take any more may have been the reason for the riots of May 13, 1969, which he interpreted as a grand *amok*, a desperate act of defiance by the embittered people. Similarly in the Western world culture change is felt by everybody alike. A great number of individuals experience alienation and suffer from lack of identification with the purposes of the community at large. Many feel outside the main stream of social rewards. Like the Malay, it may be that the unassertive individual, "the failure", with his pent-up reservoir of resentment and his already developed paranoid position, is the one chosen by the undercurrent of the alienated to vest their frustrations and to act as a safety valve that could prevent a total blow-up.

CONCLUSIONS

Based on Gimlette's four cardinal symptoms of *amok*, this syndrome has been reviewed both as it is known among the Malays, and in relation to broader socio-cultural issues in Western cultures. The author presented one North American *amok* case worked upon by him in his practice, and reviewed from the literature two others which, while not previously classified as *amok*, presented the same characteristics as the author's case. The author contends that *amok* is not a culture-bound syndrome, but one that could be found in any culture, depending on the presence of three factors, a social one, a society in change, and two individual ones, a feeling of alienation and a need for assertiveness. It is possible that, ultimately, the amoker acts as the unwitting aggregate of the collective frustrations, releasing pent-up cultural resentments in his scapegoating act.

NOTE

*   Dr. Arboleda-Florez is Director, Forensic Services, Calgary General Hospital, and Associate Professor of Psychiatry, University of Calgary, Calgary, Alberta, Canada.

REFERENCES

Adam, A. R. D.
    1951   *Amok. In* British Encyclopaedia of Medical Practice 3: 6, 2nd Edition. London: Butterworth.
Burton-Bradley, B. C.
    1968   The *Amok* Syndrome in Papua and New Guinea. The Medical Journal of Australia, February 17: 252–256. (Reprinted in this volume.)
Carothers, J. C.
    1948   A Study of Mental Derangement in Africans, and an Attempt to Explain Its Peculi-arities, More Especially in Relation to African Attitudes and Life. Psychiatry 11: 47.
Carr, T. E. and E. K. Tan
    1976   In Search of the True *Amok: Amok* as Viewed Within the Malay Culture. American Journal of Psychiatry 133: 11: 1295–1299.
Cheng, L. Y.
    1972   Discussion. American Journal of Psychiatry 129: 6: 708–709.
Dennys, N. B.
    1894   A Descriptive Dictionary of British Malay. London: London and China Telegraph Office.
Ellis, G. W.
    1893   The *Amok* of the Malays. Part One – Original Articles. The Journal of Mental Sciences XXXIX, No. 116.

Erickson, E. H.
   1974 Dimensions of a New Identity. New York: W. W. Norton & Co., Inc.
Fortes, M. and D. Mayer
   1966 Psychosis and Social Change Among the Tallensi and Northern Ghana. Cahiers
          d'Etudes Africaines 6: 21: 5—40.
Fromm, E.
   1971 Alienation Under Capitalism. *In* Eric and Mary Josephson (eds.), Man Alone —
          Alienation in Modern Society. New York: Dell Publishing Co. Inc.
Gallemore, J. L. and J. A. Panton
   1976 "Motiveless" Public Assassins. The Bulletin of the American Academy of Psychiatry
          and the Law IV: 1: 51—57.
Gimlette, J. D.
   1901 Notes on a Case of *Amok*. Journal of Tropical Medicine and Hygiene 4: 195.
Johnston-Abraham, J.
   1912 *Latah* and *Amok: Nova et vetera*. The British Medical Journal, February 24: 438—
          439.
Mahathir, M.
   1970 The Malay Dilemma. Singapore: Asia Pacific Press.
Masters, W. E.
   1920 Essentials of Tropical Medicine. London: John Bale & Danielson.
Murphy, H. B. M.
   1967 Cultural Aspects of Delusion. Sudium Generale 20: 11: 684—692.
   1973 Chapter 2: History and the Evolution of Syndromes: The Sticking Case of *Latah*
          and *Amok*. *In* Hammer, Salzinger and Sutton (eds.), Psychopathology: Contribu-
          tions from the Social, Behavioural and Biological Sciences. Toronto: John Wiley
          and Sons.
Murphy, H. B. M., E. Wittkower, J. Fried, and H. Ellenberger
   1963 A Cross-Cultural Survey of Schizophrenic Symptomatology. Journal of Social Psy-
          chiatry IX: 4: 237—249.
Nevit, S. and C. Craig
   1971 Sanctions for Evil. San Francisco: Jessey-Bass, Inc., Publishers.
Tanay, E.
   1972 Psychiatric Aspects of Homicide Prevention. American Journal of Psychiatry 128:
          815—818.
Time
   1966 The Madman in the Tower. Time, August 12.
Toffler, A.
   1971 Future Shock. Toronto: Bantam Books of Canada Ltd.
Van Loon, F. G. H.
   1928 Protopathic Instinctive Phenomena in Normal and Pathologic Malay Life. British
          Journal of Medical Psychology 8: 264—276.
Wallace, A. R.
   1898 The Malay Archipelago, the Land of the Orang-utan and the Bird of Paradise, A
          Narrative of Travel, with Studies of Man and Nature. London: Macmillan.
Weiss, F. A.
   1971 Self-Alienation — Dynamics and Therapy. *In* Eric and Mary Josephson (eds.), Man
          Alone — Alienation in Modern Society. New York: Dell Publishing Co. Inc.
Westermeyer, J.
   1972 A Comparison of *Amok* and Other Homicide in Laos. American Journal of Psychiatry
          129: 6: 703—709.
Witthower, E. D.
   1969 Perspectives of Transcultural Psychiatry. International Journal of Psychiatry 8:
          5: 811—824.

Yap, P. M.
   1958   Hydereredism and Attempted Suicide in Chinese. Journal of Nervous and Mental
          Disease 127: 34.
   1969   The Culture-Bound Reactive Syndromes. In Caudill and Li-T-y (eds.), Mental Health
          Research in Asia and the Pacific. Honolulu: East-West Center Press.
Zaguirre, J. C.
   1957   Amuck. Journal of the Philippine Federation of Private Medical Practitioners 6:
          1138–1149.

CHARLES C. HUGHES

SUDDEN MASS ASSAULT TAXON

Commentary

The principal *symptoms* of cases reported under this taxon are not confined to any particular cultural area of the world, although indigenous explanations and specific behavioral forms by which they are expressed in any given place obviously are localized. Indeed, the term by which such a disorder was first discussed (*amok*) has now crept into common usage in the English language (as well as others?) to describe those wild, out-of-mind sprees of killing and mayhem in the industrialized world as well, episodes that usually end in the death of the perpetrator. Such episodes of random killing are to be differentiated from the well-planned and focussed acts of terroristic killing that is becoming commonplace.

Depending upon the specifics of a given case, a first approximation of a principal diagnosis might be either Brief Reactive Psychosis (298.80) or Isolated Explosive Disorder (312.35). As noted in the commentary to the *Startle Matching Taxon*, in the Brief Reactive Psychosis the

... essential feature is the sudden onset of a psychotic disorder of at least a few hours' but no more than two weeks' duration, with eventual return to pre-morbid level of functioning. The psychotic symptoms appear immediately following a recognizable psychosocial stressor that would evoke significant symptoms of stress in almost anyone [in that particular culture! CCH].... Invariably there is emotional turmoil, manifested by rapid shifts from one dysphoric affect to another without the persistence of any one affect. (p. 200)

Moreover, an associated feature is "suicidal or aggressive behavior", and "disorientation and impairment in recent memory often occur". DSM-III also notes that "... usually the psychotic symptoms clear in a day or two ..." and "... transient secondary effects, such as loss of self-esteem and mild depression, may persist beyond the two weeks, but there is eventually a full return to the preborbid level of functioning" (p. 200).

Note that the Brief Reactive Psychosis diagnosis specifically includes a significant role for psychosocial stress in predisposing the afflicted person to such behavior; and in the discussions presented by the authors of papers included here it is clear that stress in the form of a grave insult or harsh social embarrassment frequently was the precipitant.

In the Isolated Explosive Disorder (312.35) the essential feature is ... a single, violent, externally directed act, which had a catastrophic impact on others and for which the available information does not justify the diagnosis of Schizophrenia, Antisocial Personality Disorder, or Conduct Disorder. An example would be an individual who for no apparent reason suddenly began shooting at total strangers in a fit of rage and then shot himself. In the past this disorder was referred to as "catathymic crisis". (p. 297)

Ronald C. Simons and Charles C. Hughes (eds.), The Culture-Bound Syndromes, 263–264.
© *1985 by D. Reidel Publishing Company.*

In view of victims' purported amnesia for the event reported in several of the cases discussed, it might also be appropriate to list Psychogenic Amnesia (300.12), and perhaps also (as in Burton-Bradley's case #1), Factitious Disorder with Psychological Symptoms (300.16), based on the clinician's inference that the patient's amnesia was not as absolute as claimed.

Continuing with that Case #1 as an example (see p. 240), the DSM-III formulation might look like this:

Axis I: 312.35 Isolated Explosive Disorder
            298.80 Brief Reactive Psychosis
            300.16 Factitious Disorder with Psychological Symptoms
Axis II: No diagnosis
Axis III: No food for two days prior to the episode
Axis IV: *Psychosocial stressors*: in another account of this same case, Burton-
            Bradley (1972: 300) mentions that the patient had been "brooding
            over an insult".
            Severity: 5 or 6 — Severe or Extreme (to infer from the consequences)
Axis V: Highest level of adaptive functioning during past year: no data

REFERENCE

Burton-Bradley, B. G.
   1972 The *Amok* Runner in Cross-Cultural Perspective. Indian Journal of Psychiatry 14:
         299–305.

C. THE RUNNING TAXON

INTRODUCTION: *THE RUNNING TAXON*

The papers included in this section amply illustrate both the desirability of a better descriptive classification and the difficulty of achieving it. The first paper by Zachary Gussow is a classic descriptive analysis of *pibloktoq*, sometimes called *arctic hysteria*, among the Polar Eskimo. This paper emphasizes the importance of separating descriptions of symptoms from inferences about etiology and from descriptions of locally specific curing practices. There is an exemplary sorting of cases in terms of most frequent to least frequent descriptive symptoms. Gussow points out that the term *"arctic hysteria"* has sometimes been used to refer to what may be a specific syndrome but a other times has been used as "a rubric under which every form of mental disorder observed in the arctic has been subsumed". Reading his cases and his careful sorting of descriptive features, most readers will, I think, derive some idea of a core syndrome which includes the tearing off of clothing, speaking irrationally "in tongues" or in unfamiliar languages, fleeing, nude or clothed and a series of "senseless" often mildly to strongly aggressive or threatening acts not including actual physical injury to other persons. Gussow describes typical prodromal symptoms and notes that "invariably individuals are thoroughly exhausted after an attack and may ... sleep for as long as fifteen hours". Between attacks individuals appear otherwise normal and are so accepted by their peers. Gussow reports and tabulates the symptoms of thirteen specific cases and some collective accounts.

The second paper, written especially for this volume, is by Philip Dennis who describes *grisi siknis* a condition found among Miskito Indians in Nicaragua and Honduras, previously only very incompletely reported. The resemblance of some of his cases to *arctic hysteria* (and to "wild man" behavior in New Guinea) (Newman 1964) has not escaped him. It is interesting to re-read Gussow's first two cases after reading the Dennis paper. Is there an underlying unitary phenomenon with different cultural glosses in the tropical and the arctic sites or is the resemblance trivial and coincidental? The answer does not depend on similarities or dissimilarities in the local cultural construction of the event but rather in its microdetail, particularly the microdetail which is not specified culturally. Good audio-visual records of attacks of both the running form of *pibloktoq* and of *grisi siknis* would be very helpful, but the logistics involved are formidable, and such records are not available. In their absence, the case for a unitary phenomenon is not conclusive.

Dennis' paper describes variations in the syndrome by locality and also at a single site over time, and he notes that indigenously or locally attributed causes range from "poisoned fish" to "sorcery". Dennis explicitly describes "irrational anger with those around them" and a modulation of this anger so that other persons are not actually injured. He describes an epidemic of the syndrome; apparently

Ronald C. Simons and Charles C. Hughes (eds.), The Culture-Bound Syndromes, 267–269.

grisi siknis can spread from one individual to another much as *koro* has been described to have spread by Gwee and co-workers (*Koro* Study Team 1969) and by Jilek and Jilek-Aall (1977). Dennis explains *grisi siknis* as a form of social drama and points out that social structural features, especially those having to do with the status of women, are relevant to its understanding. Interestingly, he notes that Miskito informants see *grisi siknis* as worthy of research and are desirous of some means of prevention and more effective treatment.

In the last paper Foulks also describes *pibloktoq*. He presents more extensive case descriptions, with family histories and accounts of the course of the lives of persons experiencing a syndrome he refers to as *arctic hysteria* over several years. Foulks has been studying in the arctic for several decades, and he points out how the introduction of alcohol and alcoholism have altered older behavior patterns.

The juxtaposition of the three papers and their order was a deliberate one, and it is suggested that they be read in order. Doing so raises the question of whether Dennis' case in Nicaragua are more like Gussow's than are Foulks'. One striking difference between Foulks' cases and those of both other authors is that Foulks describes life-long debilitating conditions which interfere with normal functioning and which are recognized as such by members of the sufferer's society. Foulks' Case 1 Amos, is mocked, ostracized, and lives the life of a failure. Case 2 is of an eight year old girl who suffers from an organic seizure disorder and "occasionally without warning throws violent fits". In neither case are symptoms of fleeing prominent.

Foulks' paper contains some excerpts from the literature on *arctic hysteria* which are worthy of mention. Especially interesting is Nachman's report, e.g., "one typical kind of account is of a teenage girl who has sudden outbursts of excited behavior, sometimes with convulsions or paralysis or anesthesias for which no organic basis can be found, who yells and tears her clothes and performs some bizarre acts then becomes drowsy and later is amnesiac for the experience". This report appears much like the cases described by Dennis. Foulks also discusses Wallace's physiologic hypothesis, which is interesting not only in and of itself but which also raises the larger question of the possible relevance of *any* physiologic factor, not only the specific one posited in this case (calcium deficiency). Wallace, quoted by Foulks, puts it eloquently: "incipient neurological dysfunction is susceptible to different interpretations by the victim and his associates and therefore precipitates different overresponses depending upon particular customs of the individual and group".

I firmly believe that the *latah* of Malayo-Indonesia, *imu* of the Ainu and the variously named forms of startle-precipitated naughty talk, obedience and matching which occur around the world are examples of a single syndrome. I likewise believe that the evidence for sleep paralysis's being elaborated in the form of local culturally-specific named phenomena is very strong. I do not have the same confidence that the disturbed behavior of the teenagers described by Nachman, Cases 1 and 2 of Gussow and the majority of Dennis' cases share significant etiologic as well as descriptive features. Evidence that Running is a valid taxon is as yet very weak and inconclusive, yet the resemblances are too strong, it seems to me, to dismiss out of hand.

REFERENCES

Newman, Philip L.
    1964 "Wild Man" Behavior in a New Guinea Community. American Anthropologist
        66: 1–19.
Koro Study Team
    1969 The *Koro* Epidemic in Singapore. Singapore Medical Journal 10: 234–42.
Jilek, Wolfgang and Louise Jilek-Aall
    1977 A *Koro* Epidemic in Thailand. Transcultural Psychiatric Research Review 15: 57–59.

ZACHARY GUSSOW

PIBLOKTOQ (HYSTERIA) AMONG THE POLAR ESKIMO*

An Ethnopsychiatric Study

The cross-fertilization of the sciences of culture and psychiatry has, in recent years, led to significant modifications of thinking concerning the relative nature of mental illness. Recent studies in culture and psychopathology negate the view that there are "bizarre native psychoses", that mental illnesses are "unique" to the society in which they occur, and emphasize instead cross-cultural parallelism in the structure and process of mental disorders.[1] It is the specific content of mental disorders which is held to be related to a given society at a given time, a factor which accounts for the variety of detailed symptomatology from one culture to another, reflecting differences in prevailing beliefs, customs, traditions, interests and conflicts.

The present paper is a contribution to the field of ethnopsychiatry. It presents data on a mental disorder found among, though not confined to, the Polar Eskimo of Northwestern Greenland, and referred to in the literature as *pibloktoq*.[2] In 1913, when A. A. Brill published the first account of this disorder in the psychiatric literature, drawing on the works of Admiral Robert E. Peary and conversations with Donald B. Macmillan for his material, he drew attention to the underlying similarities between this native Eskimo illness and certain psychiatric manifestations present in modern Western society.

The present paper extends the efforts of Brill. It brings to the study of this ethnic disorder a considerable body of new data. This material will be used to provide a clinical-anthropological picture of *pibloktoq*, and will relate this disorder to concrete situations in the lives of the Polar Eskimo. Data on the precipitating causes of this condition will be used to criticize the common and labored view that *pibloktoq* and other Eskimo and arctic mental derangements are brought on by the "depressing", "melancholy", "monotonous", etc., effects of the arctic winter climate on the Eskimo mind. And finally, an exploratory section on the psychodynamics of this disorder will be offered.

THE *PIBLOKTOQ* SYNDROME

In the literature the term *pibloktoq* (arctic hysteria, polar hysteria, transitional madness, etc.) has become the designation for a group of "hysterical" symptoms which may afflict adult Eskimo men and women at any time.

In *pibloktoq* there are no single and recurring symptoms to be found in each case. The syndrome is composed of a series of reactive patterns, any number of which may combine with other symptoms in each seizure performance. Thus, features found in case A may be totally reproduced in case B, but only partially present in case C. B may then share features of its own with C, but not with A, and

271

Ronald C. Simons and Charles C. Hughes (eds.), The Culture-Bound Syndromes, 271–287.
© 1960 *by the International University Press, Inc.*

so on. In other words, the total repertoire of symptoms does not necessarily appear in each instance, but each seizure will, as it were, draw its symptoms from among the "pool" of reactive patterns.

CASE MATERIAL

It is the purpose of this section to present the available case material and to draw up an inventory of symptoms for the attack proper. Prodromal and terminal symptoms will be listed separately. Some of these data — the personal observations and comments of Niels Rasmussen — are new, never having been published before.[3] The material is organized into (1) discrete cases, (2) composite cases, general ideas or comments about *pibloktoq* and (3) one story or tale of a past occurrence of this disorder.

Discrete Cases

(1) "Tukshu began suddenly to rave upon leaving the boat. He tore off every stitch of clothing he had on, and would have thrown himself into the water of the Sound but for the restraint of the Eskimos. He seemed possessed of supernatural strength, and it was all four men could do to hold him" (Whitney 1911: 67).

(2) "We were on the threshold of the long dismal night at last. They [Eskimo women] were affected not only by the natural depression that impresses itself upon all with the vanishing of the day, but an increasing apprehension had sprung up for the safety of the hunters. A rapid driving of the ice pack . . . had raised a fear that the men had gone adrift on it. . . . I dropped into [one of the igloos] one evening and amused the woman . . . presently Kudlar's kooner [wife] came in and the two women began to cry and moan . . . (Give me my man! Give me my man!). At half-past one that [same] night I was awakened . . . by a woman shouting at the top of her voice — shrill and startling, like one gone mad. I knew at once what it meant — someone had gone *problocto*. Far away on the driving ice of the Sound a lone figure was running and raving. The boatswain and Billy joined me, and as fast as we could struggle through three feet of snow, with drifts often to the waist, we gave pursuit. At length I reached her, and to my astonishment discovered it was Tongwe [Kudlar's wife]. She struggled desperately, and it required the combined strength of the three of us to get her back to the shack, where she was found to be in bad shape — one hand was slightly frozen, and part of one breast. After a half hour of quiet she became rational again, but the attack left her very weak" (Whitney 1911: 82–84).

(3) "On the evening after the hunters returned . . . Tongwe [see case 2] was again attacked by *problocto*. She rushed out of the igloo, tore her clothing off and threw herself into a snow-drift. I ran to [her husband's] assistance, but the woman was as strong as a lion, and we had all we could do to hold her. A strong north wind was blowing, with a temperature eight degrees below zero, and I thought she would surely be severely frozen . . . but in some miraculous manner

she escaped even the slightest frost-bite. After getting her into the igloo she grew weak as a kitten, and it was several hours before she became quite herself. In connection with this woman's case, it is ... interesting to note that, previous to the attack which she had suffered the day before the return of the hunting party, she had never shown any symptoms of *problokto*" (Whitney, 1911, pp. 87–88).

(4) "In July 1909 I was witness of such an attack in the woman Inadtliak. It lasted 25 minutes. She sat on the ground with the legs stretched out, swaying her body to and fro, sometimes rapidly sometimes more slowly, from side to side and tortuously, whilst she kept her hands comparatively still and only now and then moved her elbows in to her sides. She stared out in front of her quite regardless of the surroundings, and sang and screamed occasionally, changing the tone, iah-iah-iaha-ha ... , now and then she interjected a sentence, e.g., that the Danish had at last come to them, and again the great happiness this gave her now in the glad summer-time and so on. Her two small children sat and played about her, whilst the members of the tribe scarcely looked at her during the attacks; they seemed to be very well acquainted with such things. She recovered quite suddenly and only some hectic, red spots on her cheeks indicated anything unusual. Without so much as looking about her or betraying a sign of anything unusual she began, literally with the same movement, to give her youngest child milk and then went quickly on to chew a skin" (Steensby 1910: 377–378).

(5) "In one case NR [Niels Rasmussen] was a passenger on a sled driven by a very simple, friendly not too bright young man; always friendly, untalkative, but reliable fellow. They had had some trouble on the land before they got to the ice cap, very tough going, no snow and very tough work. Finally reached the ice cap which meant safety and then they had some smooth going of course, and they would be home in a day or two. NR thought that everything was all right with him. Had his back towards him; he was standing in front of the sled and disentangling the dogs. He heard him talk very strangely; didn't understand a word of it.[4] Suddenly he began to kick the dogs, one or two of them. Then systematically he started to kick them all, talking louder and louder until he was screaming unintelligibly. He warmed up for about a minute or so that way and after about a minute or so he was in full swing screaming all the time. He tore all the stuff off the sleds, skins, boxes, stoves, and hurled them at the dogs. It lasted about ten minutes. . . . It didn't do much harm to the dogs, in fact nothing at all, couldn't hit them actually. All of a sudden it was over. He sat down on the sled completely exhausted. A short attack. Later, days later when they got back to the village, he had a lot of fun about it. The other companions on the trip kidded the fellow about his behavior and the young boy himself always asked NR whether he had been scared; it is not disgrace that these things happen. It can happen to anybody. It's a natural incident. Usually turns it into a funny story . . ." (Steed 1947–48: 205–206).

(6) "NR has seen another 'bird' [man] rolling in the snow without any clothes on, completely naked, for about a half hour. That is what usually happens: KR [Knud Rasmussen] described it that way too, they tear off all their clothes. NR

saw only one instance of this; but it's supposed to be a common characteristic" (Steed 1947—48: 207).

(7) "One was a girl who suddenly decided she wanted a piece of sea-weed and without a stitch waded into the sea; still open water and it was bitter cold, way below freezing point. She waded out dangerously — she had hardly any foothold she was out so far; got the seaweed, came back triumphantly and with great dignity and with the same dignity she suddenly threw it away again. All of a sudden her dignity broke — completely — she started screaming and made a continual somersault. Could not have done that in a sober state. Must have been a couple of hundred feet. She was so exhausted that she slept for 15 hours or so" (Steed 1947—48: 207—208).

(8) "Knud Rasmussen tells an incident, reported by NR, of a man who had had more than one [inebriation]. He suddenly climbed up a steep cliff; bluffs outside the village; completely vertical. Climbed up to top of those although obviously humanly impossible to do it; but he did it somehow. There is no doubt . . . that he could not have possibly done it under normal circumstances. The he grabbed the knife and went into a tent where three little children were sleeping; they were alone there but the father of the children followed the man, quietly took the knife out of the hand and at that moment the man collapsed" (Steed 1947—48: 208).

(9) "In 1898 while the Windward was in winter quarters off Cape D'Urville, a married woman was taken with one of these fits in the middle of the night. In a state of perfect nudity she walked the deck of the ship; then, seeking still greater freedom, jumped the rail, on to the frozen snow and ice. It was some time before we missed her, and when she was finally discovered, it was at a distance of half-a-mile, where she was still pawing, and shouting to the best of her abilities. She was captured and brought back to the ship; and then there commenced a wonderful performance of mimicry in which every conceivable cry of local bird and mammal was reproduced in the throat of Inahloo.

"This same woman at other times attempts to walk the ceiling of her igloo . . ." (Peary 1907: p. 384).

Macmillan (Brill 1913: 515—516) also describes the attacks of this woman: "Inahloo, woman of 45 years, was very violent during her attacks. She did not know what she was doing, she appeared crazy and demented, and would bite when an attempt was made to restrain her. Her specialty was to imitate the call of birds and to try to walk on the ceiling. She also put ice on her chest. Her face was very congested, her eyes were bloodshot during the attack, and . . . she foamed at the mouth."

(10) "Whenever Elkiahsha, nicknamed Bill, had an attack she would walk around the deck of the Roosevelt and pick up everything lying loose and throw it up in the air. She also climbed up the rigging and foresheet and stuck her head under the sail" (Brill 1913: 515—516).

(11) "Inahwaho showed her attacks by walking on the ice, singing and beating her hands together."

According to Macmillan, this woman also feigned attacks. Macmillan was told that "Inawaho was running around on the ice having an attack. He got his camera and went out to take some pictures of her while in this state. He saw her running on the ice and beating her hands, but as soon as she noticed him her whole attitude changed, she became very excited, grabbed big chunks of ice and hurled them at him. The following day she told him that she did not have *piblokto*, that she was only shamming, and asked him not to use her pictures because she was naked. Whether or not she was fully conscious during the attack is difficult to say" (Brill 1913: 516).

(12) "Alnaha, nicknamed Buster, 25 years old, was the only woman who jumped into the water during her attacks." She "was the only unmarried woman in the north". No one wanted her "not because she had no charms but because she was a very poor seamstress. She had more attacks than any one else" (Brill 1913: 515–516, 518).

(13) "Macmillan also witnessed an attack of *piblokto* in an Eskimo woman immediately following a rebuff by a White man who just showed her some favor" (Brill 1913: 518).

Composite Cases, General Ideas, Comments

(14) *Niels Rasmussen*: "Certain things are common to all people as NR has observed it; they are always completely oblivious to their surroundings; they are always . . . strongly agitated, have a feverish light in their eyes, talk very fast but completely unintelligibly; and their speech makes no sense, 'speaking in tongues' so to say, just jabbering away but not in the Eskimo language. There is no way of telling where and when it may come. Some people can feel it coming. In . . . severe cases, they become completely exhausted and go to sleep for 12 hours; completely drained of all strength. Do most fantastic things, completely idiotic. Picking up all kinds of junk outside the house, carrying it into the house as if they had found some great treasure. Or the person in question may decide that he wants a little stone that he sees way up on top of the mountain. He will go and get it naked sometimes. Nudity won't keep him or her from running way up on top of the mountain. Women don't behave differently from men. Eskimos believe it is an absolutely natural phenomenon. They don't fear it" (Steed 1947–48: 204–205, 207, 209).

(15) *Peary*: ". . . women, more frequently than men, are afflicted. During these spells, the maniac removes all clothing and prances about like a broncho. A case of *piblocto* lasts from five minutes to half-an-hour or more. When it occurs under cover of a hut, no apparent concern is felt by other inmates, nor is any attention paid to the antics of the mad one. It is only when an attempt is made to run abroad, that the cords of restraint are felt" (Peary 1907: 384–385).

"I have never known a child to have *piblokto*; but some one among the adult Eskimos would have an attack every day or two, and one day there were five cases. The immediate cause of this affection is hard to trace, though sometimes it seems to be the result of a brooding over absent or dead relatives, or a fear of the future. The patient, usually a woman, begins to scream and tear off and destroy her clothing. If on the ship, she will walk up and down the deck, screaming and gesticulating, and generally in a state of nudity, though the thermometer may be in the minus forties. As the intensity of the attack increases, she will sometimes leap over the rail upon the ice, running perhaps a half a mile. The attack may last from a few minutes, an hour, or even more, and some sufferers become so wild that they would continue running about on the ice perfectly naked until they freeze to death, if they were not forcibly brought back ... nobody pays much attention, unless the suffers should reach for a knife or attempt to injure someone. The attack usually ends in a fit of weeping, and when the patient quiets down, the eyes are bloodshot, the pulse high, and the whole body trembles for an hour or so afterward" (Peary 1910: 166–167).

(16) *Macmillan*: "A woman will be heard softly singing and accompanying herself by striking the fist of one hand with the palm of the second, making three sounds, one long followed by two short ones. The rhythm and motion continues to increase for some time, during which she usually tears off her clothing, and ends in a fit of crying or screaming in which the woman may imitate the cry of some familiar animal or bird. No two women act alike; there is a certain individuality to every attack. Some drop down on their hands and knees and crawl around barking like a dog. One woman used to lie on her back on the snow and place some ice on her breasts. Some jump into the water and wade among the ice cakes, all the time singing and yelling. Others wander away from the houses into the hills, beating their hands as if demented." According to Brill, "Macmillan was certain that all of them showed a loss of consciousness; he thought they were all in a confused state. I asked Professor Macmillan whether he formed any idea as to the causation of this malady, and his answer was as follows: 'I believe that the attacks are caused by abuse. Most of the Eskimo women who had this disease were of a jealous disposition. They either imagined themselves ill treated or they actually suffered abuse at the hands of their husbands, who often beat them with their fists' " (Brill 1913: 515–517).

(17) *A Tale*: "This is a 'very old story'. It must have happened about November. ... A whole family had met to pass the winter. ... Everything appeared all right — good hunting during the summer. In August the sky had been full of birds. ... There had been so many ... [seakings] that they had caught hundreds and hundreds. A little before September the streams ... were boiling with salmon. Foxes, good gracious, they were everywhere not to mention walruses and seals. 'We're rich', said the father. But with the winter misfortune was to fall on them. For some days, now that the sun was low on the horizon, the mother had changed. She who used to work from morning till evening, who could be heard laughing from the time she got up, now remained for hours doing nothing in the igloo, silent, her expression vague. They weren't worried because ... [they] know that people are generally a little out of sorts at this time. Once or twice, however, she had said strange things. One evening when the father and one of his sons went

to eat seal with some neighbours, the mother remained lying down, saying that she was tired. Suddenly, towards midnight, they heard the dogs howl. 'Let's go back', said the father. 'Something is wrong over there. I feel it here', and he pointed to his skull. They could see the igloo light, which seemed to shine and then go out. One would have said that somebody was passing backwards and forwards ceaselessly. . . . When the father and son opened the door they saw a horrible sight. The house was upside-down. Torn caribou skins were strewn on the floor in the midst of seal-meat and streams of blood. The mother, her face black and congested, was running backwards and forwards, with her clothes in disorder, and an *oulou* (round woman's knife) in her hand. The children were trembling in the corner. The sound of the door made her jump. Suddenly she leapt, but the father was on her before she had taken three steps. The unhappy woman broke free and ran off, with hardly any clothes, towards the sea-ice in spite of the cold. She still held her knife, and without stopping picked up everything that seemed solid – pebbles, wood and so on. When she felt the men coming too close she threw everything at them over her shoulder. If she saw dog's droppings she smelt at them, rubbed her face with them and then gluttonously devoured the rest. The men pursued her to an iceberg. She tried to haul herself up, but she was badly shod and slid down. But she hung on to a spur, and finally managed to sit astride an ice-ridge. From here she managed to get away. Running toward the sea-ice . . . she leapt from ice-floe to ice-floe and defied her pursuers. Her situation was terrible. Every moment she almost fell into the water. Fortunately her strength suddenly failed, and the *Inouit* managed to reach her not far from the camp. The woman was exhausted by then. They tied her on the sledge, and, trembling with fever, she was taken back to the . . . igloo. Her face was pale. She had lost consciousness and rapidly fell into a heavy agitated sleep. When she woke some hours later she remembered nothing.

"The cases of *piblocta* (hysteria) were frequent among women, said the Eskimo. But one no longer saw such serious ones. And these hysterias have never killed anybody as far as I know" (Malaurie 1956: 75, 78–80).

Symptomatology

Loss or disturbance of consciousness during the seizure and amnesia for the attack appear as the central clinical features in the *pibloktoq* performance. Attacks are short-lived episodes, lasting from a few minutes to, in a few cases, a little over an hour, and terminate in complete remission afterwards.

Behavioral symptoms – motor and verbal – present in the *pibloktoq* seizures are listed below, roughly, in order of their frequency of appearance. These symptom categories have been delineated on the basis of fourteen seizure performances (discrete cases and one tale; data from composite cases, general ideas and comments re *pibloktoq* have been omitted from this frequency count).

(A) Tearing off of clothing; achieving partial or complete nudity. This is frequently one of the first behavioral signs of an attack. Niels Rasmussen speaks of it as a "common characteristic", as does Peary. *References*: 7: 5 women (case 3, 7, 9, 11, 17); 2 men (case 1, 6).

(B) Glossolalia and related phenomena. Two types appear here: *phonations frustes* (a miscellaneous group describing mutterings that vary from gurglings to meaningless syllables; see Carlyle May 1956: 79), which forms our main group; and animal language. *References*: 7: 5 women (*phonations frustes*: cases 2, 4, 7, 11; animal language: case 9); 2 men (*phonations frustes*: cases 1, 5).

(C) Fleeing, nude or clothed. Running across ice or snow. Wandering into hills or mountains. If indoors, afflicted persons may run back and forth in an agitated state. If aboard ship, they may pace the deck ceaselessly, climb the rigging, and so forth. *References*: 6: 5 women (cases 2, 9, 10, 11, 17); 1 man (case 8).

(D) Rolling in snow. Jumping into water. Throwing self into snow drift. Placing ice on exposed breasts. These actions may be performed either in a clothed or nude state. *References*: 5: 3 women (cases 3, 9, 12); 2 men (cases 1, 6).

(E) Performing acts of slightly bizarre but harmless nature, viz., attempting to walk on ceiling, picking up and cherishing all sorts of odd objects, etc. *References*: 3: 3 women (cases 7, 9, 10); no men.

(F) Throwing everything handy around, creating disordered scene. *References*: 3: 2 women (cases 10, 17); 1 man (case 5).

(G) Performing mimetic acts, engaging in choreiform movements, accompanied by vocalization. *References*: 2: 2 women (cases 4, 9); no men.

(H) Coprophagia (feces eating). *References*: 1 woman (case 17).

Supernatural Strength, Restraint and Capture

During attacks *pibloktoq* individuals are possessed of supernatural strength which (1) enables them to perform the difficult and exhausting feats described above, and (2) abets them in forcibly resisting restraint and capture. We suggest, however, that the *pibloktoq's* desire for escape is not altogether a genuine one, but rather represents a dramatic invitation to be pursued and overtaken. This point will be discussed more fully later.

Prodromal and Terminal Symptoms

Prodromal symptoms — tiredness, depressive silences, vagueness of expression, confusion — have been reported. These symptoms may precede the attack by several days.

Weeping, body tremors, feverishness, bloodshot eyes, high pulse are frequent terminal symptoms.

Invariably, individuals are thoroughly exhausted after an attack and may, in some instances, sleep for as long as fifteen hours. Rational behavior is resumed immediately once an attack has terminated.

Sex and Age Factors

Previous writers have characterized *pibloktoq* principally as a female disorder. Peary (Brill 1913: p. 517) is quoted as saying that in twenty years he saw only one man who had what was thought to be *pibloktoq*. According to our data, on the basis of 14 seizures (discrete cases and one tale), we observe ten instances in women and four in men. This sample suggests that although occurring predominantly in women, *pibloktoq* is also far from infrequent among men.

Although reliable testimony (Niels Rasmussen) states there are no sex differences in symptomatology, our data suggest that *pibloktoq* is more florid in women: for example, no instances of symptoms E (slightly bizarre, harmless acts), G (mimetic acts, choreiform movements, etc.) or H (feces eating) appear in men. Symptom C (fleeing, nude or clothed) is represented by only one male example (case 8) – and that, a doubtful one.

No instances of *pibloktoq* have been reported for children. Age and marital status data are too incomplete for generalization. All persons, however, are described as adult; the youngest age mentioned is twenty-five, the oldest forty-five. Four women are mentioned as married, one unmarried. For four other women and the four men no data are available.

ALLEGED HARMFULNESS OF *PIBLOKTOQ*

Various writers (Knud Rasmussen in Steensby 1910: 377–378; Kloss 1923: 254; Ackerknecht 1948: 917; Mowat 1952: 189–190; among others) refer to the potential harmfulness of *pibloktoq*, while others (see cases 8, 17) cite instances of acts which appear to be the beginnings of real violence, but which, significantly, are never carried through. We have already cited Malaurie's informant to this effect. According to the available evidence, there are no recorded instances of afflicted individuals ever causing harm to others. Personal injury, with the exception of occasional frostbite, is also unknown; this despite the terrifying risks undertaken. Damage to property, yes; to persons, no. Thus, Ackerknecht's (1948: 917) and Kloss's (1923: 254) comparison of *pibloktoq* with *amok* is not affirmed by our examination of the data. Unlike true *amok*, the *pseudo-amok* like behavior present in some of the *pibloktoq* cases, with no aggressive, harmful intentions, is a well-known feature of agitated hysteria and has been reported by Dembovitz (1945) to occur among West African troops and by Dobrizhoffer (1822) for the primitive Abipones of Paraguay. According to Dembovitz (p. 73):

Running *amok* is a popularly known form of abnormal behavior. The picture is one of a man suddenly seizing a hatchet or a tommy-gun or a rifle and rushing around slaying all he meets. These cases usually have a rapid and fatal ending. . . . Pseudo running *amok* is seen in excited hysterics. They are always careful not to injure anybody and, when cornered, they go quietly, in sharp distinction to the true berserk who fights to the end.

Among the Abipones, according to Dobrizhoffer (1822), the agitated *Loaparaika* – men as well as women – "rave and storm like madmen", threaten the villagers with armed violence, "strike the roof and mats of every tent again and again with their sticks", etc., but do not actually cause injury to any of the inhabitants (p. 233ff).

In this connection, it is important to distinguish *pibloktoq*, as described in this paper, from "psychotic" episodes which terminate in maniacal, murderous acts. Such acts are not uncommon among the Eskimo. However, there is no evidence of similarity in symptomatology or behavior between these two manifestations. They appear as distinct phenomena. The confusion seems to stem from the term "arctic hysteria", which has been used as if it were a unit phenomenon, a rubric under which every form of mental disorder observed in the arctic has been subsumed (Czaplicka 1914: 307–325; Aberle 1952: 294–295).

The calmness with which Eskimo culture receives *pibloktoq* is further evidence of its nondangerous nature. The Eskimo accept *pibloktoq* as a natural phenomenon, as something that can happen to anyone. This suggests that the *pibloktoq* reaction does not arise from any special difficulties of adjustment to particular situations on the part of abnormal individuals, but rather that it is a manifestation of aspects of the personality and ego organization common to the individuals comprising the group. Yap (1952: 552) reaches the same conclusion with respect to the *latah* reaction among Malays. The tolerant attitude displayed by the Polar Eskimo toward *pibloktoq*, combined with their failure to view *pibloktoq* as a "disease", supports the inference that we are dealing more with an aspect of the basic ethnic personality than, strictly speaking with a mental illness.

It is important, as this point, to note that Eskimo culture institutionalizes "hysteroid" behavior that is directly related to those events, happenings, anxieties, etc., perceived as ego and culturally dystonic. Briefly, at the onset of winter, women, singly and in small groups, weep disconsolately, wail, cry and groan. Some frantically writhe to and fro in expressions of mournful anguish. At other moments they dance about with "emotions of madness". The men take part in similar, though separate, displays. In emotive dances and chants which terminate in bouts of uncontrollable weeping and "hysterical laughter" the men give vent to their emotionality. When these "mourning" rites, which may last a number of days, are over, the Eskimo lapse into a brief period of lethargy and melancholy from which they soon recover (Cook 1911: 92–97).

A careful examination of this group "hysteroid" behavior — which represents a memorialization of all misfortunes and hardships of the past year, but at which time individuals also express their grief for events which transpired many years ago — reveals the major axes of stress and trauma embedded in Eskimo culture: threat of starvation, insufficiencies of food, loss of members through hunting and other accidents, as well as the physical discomforts and dangers ever present in their lives. In a later section, we will see that these identical anxieties recur as precipitating causes of *pibloktoq*.

CLIMATE AS CAUSE OF *PIBLOKTOQ*

The arctic winter climate has frequently been cited as a cause of Eskimo mental derangements (Steensby 1910: 377–378; Novakovsky 1924: 113–127; Jenness

1928: 52; Weyer 1932: 386; Birket-Smith 1936: pp. 54–55; etc.). The Polar winter, which lasts from about the beginning of November to the middle of February, has been termed "depressing", monotonous", "melancholy", and for these reasons seen as productive of morbid reactions on the part of the Eskimo.

The deficiencies of the climatological point of view as causation of mental disorder are considerable, and in this connection. Aberle's (1952: 295) findings of the negative relationship between Siberian *latah* and the arctic winter are pertinent. The writings of long-experienced arctic explorers offer telling evidence that the Eskimo are not morosely affected by the arctic winter climate as such, that they do not, as a group, become depressed and morbid once winter sets in. According to Knud Rasmussen (1908: 79–80):

The first dark evenings are hailed with the same glee as the first daylight, after the Polar night. Up there, as here, people like change. When, a whole summer through, your eyes have been bathed in light, day and night, you long to see the land vanish softly into the darkness again. ... And with the idea of change they associate the thought of all the good things the winter will bring with it: the frozen sea, and the hunting on the ice, and the swift sledge-drives, far from the sweltering houses, after bears.

Stefansson (1922), writing of the Mackenzie Delta Eskimo, says:

In the books I had read about the Eskimos I had always been impressed with how lonesome and depressing it must be to spend the several weeks of midwinter without one ray of sunlight. This had been worrying me a great deal even before the sun disappeared, but Roxy [an Eskimo] had told me that he had never heard of any Eskimos who minded the absence of the sun, and had added that all white men got used to it after a year or two. Sten had confirmed this and, altogether, I had gathered from his and the Eskimo that in the Arctic the period of the sun's absence is looked forward to by everybody and is the jolliest time of the year [p. 130].

Niels Rasmussen (Steed 1947–48) states:

Dark time for whites is depressing, irritating more than in other times. But Eskimos have a gay time during that period. Not so for the whites. There are other whites who get very temperamental about it. Trader and parsons don't have this trouble. When one knows what to expect of the dark time, it is not a strain, especially if one has work. NR didn't feel it the first two years because he had plenty of work; but the third year when he was a weather observer, felt excessively sleepy, depressive, no interest in the future; lived alone and if he had had a companion he would have acted quite irritably he believes [p. 209].

Bertelsen (1929) sums up the effect of the arctic winter on Europeans:

Of the greatest importance in respect of health, is, however, the influence of the country on the nervous system of those who come to live here. The long distance from the Mother-country, the forced association with the same people or the absolute loneliness, the lack of suitable variety, the comparative inactivity, the monotony which often makes life feel curiously unreal and shadowy, an existence essentially limited to the daily metabolic process, the journeys, frequently with a distinct element of danger, the close contact with the forces of nature, the illimitable space, the stillness and the darkness, operate strongly on the mind. During the first part of the stay all of these factors not infrequently result in an increased irritability and a morbid distrust of the surroundings; later on a certain dulling of the initiative and a coarsening of the whole mental life are the most conspicuous symptoms. In certain cases, with special mental predispositions, the reaction may set in far more strongly, terminating in pronounced insanity [p. 382].

On the basis of the above, and other similar statements, we suggest, therefore, that the theory of the arctic winter climate as a cause of *pibloktoq* or other Eskimo or Siberian mental derangements represents nothing more than a projection of what the European in the Arctic may experience, and in no way accounts for Eskimo psychopathology.

PRECIPITATING CAUSES OF *PIBLOKTOQ*

Our data show little that is specific about the precipitating causes of *pibloktoq*. *Pibloktoq* may occur at any time of the year and may be precipitated by a sudden fright, unusual mental shock, brooding over absent or dead relatives, fear of the future, imagined or actual abuse, and so forth. Earlier, we suggested that *pibloktoq* did not arise from the difficulties of adjustment on the part of abnormal persons to specific situations, but rather that such reactions were a manifestation of the basic Eskimo personality. To this will now be added the fact that *pibloktoq* represents reactions of the Polar Eskimo to situations of unusually intense, but culturally typical, stress. Certain "triggering situations" are generally recognized as traumatic. The knowledge that Eskimos are prone[5] to panic when out of sight of land and in unfamiliar waters was, according to Frederick Cook[6] (1911: 11–12) used by him to *prevent* panic among his Eskimo by deliberately creating among them the delusion that the mirages and low-lying clouds they saw from his ship were signs of land. The abnormally high rate of *pibloktoq* among the Eskimo accompanying Peary — "some one among the adult Eskimos would have an attack every day or two, and one day there were five cases" (Peary 1910: 166–167, 230) — may, we suggest, be attributed to panic at being so far from home, in unfamiliar surroundings and fearful of whether they would, in fact, ever return. Peary's Eskimo, unlike Cook's, became *pibloktoq*, we suggest, because no defenses against this trauma were provided. Cook supported his Eskimo into believing what they could not help knowing to be false; they were willing to be deceived as a defense against panic.[7] Peary, on the other hand, employed no such therapeutic measures, and in fact did the opposite, forcibly encouraging them to accept reality, thus "feeding" their panic (Peary 1910: 230; Cook 1911: 11–12).

Writers stressing climatological factors in the etiology of *pibloktoq* point to its prevalence in winter. We have already noted that consciously the Eskimo look forward to winter as a relatively happy time of year. We suggest, however, that *unconsciously* winter is perceived by the Eskimo traumatically, not for reasons of darkness, oppressiveness of environment, etc., but rather that winter, more than other seasons, intensifies Eskimo insecurity and hence their proneness to derangement, because increased threats of starvation, high accident rates, etc., are inherent, though perhaps psychologically denied, features of the Polar winter.

Case 17, a legend, and therefore a culturally selected synthesis, dramatically calls attention to the close relationship between *pibloktoq* and repressed winter starvation anxieties by overemphasizing the amount of food on hand *prior* to winter.

CULTURAL MATRICES AND *PIBLOKTOQ*

The *pibloktoq* syndrome, bizarre and incomprehensible as it may appear at first glance, is nevertheless composed of elements, many of which appear regularly in Eskimo culture but in a variety of different matrices.[8] In the *pibloktoq* performance these behaviors are lifted out of their cultural context and fitted into new patterns.

Nudity, one of the more statistically prevalent symptoms and often one of the first to appear in an attack, is not an uncommon feature among Eskimos. Partial or complete nudity is a frequent state of dress indoors. Following a sweatbath, Eskimos will emerge and roll naked in snowbanks or have snow thrown on them. Glossolalia and mimetic animal behavior are well known standard features of Eskimo medicoreligious functionaries. Shouting and singing are features which also appear in verbal duels (drum fights). A number of the "mourning"-rite features described above — weeping, wailing, crying, groaning, etc. — are also repeated in *pibloktoq*. In another part of the world, Korea, behavior in exact duplication of Eskimo *pibloktoq* is found in connection with the initiation rites of sorcerers (May 1956: 82).

The "individuality" of *pibloktoq* would seem to stem from a fusion of culturally linked symptoms either with idiosyncratic features (representations of the individual unconscious), or else with subjectivized elaborations or modifications of cultural behavior. We suggest, further, that there exists a "fitting" of the individual ethnic neurosis pattern to particular situations; that is, there is an unconscious relationship between precipitating contexts and the specific symptoms chosen. Unfortunately, there are at present insufficient data upon which to test this assumption.

PSYCHODYNAMICS

The principal psychopathological element in *pibloktoq* is some basic underlying anxiety, "triggered off" by severe, culturally typical, stress: fear of certain concrete or impending situations; fear of, or experience of, loss, especially of emotional support, including the sense of being within safe, solid, familiar land, etc. The *pibloktoq* performance represents a culturally patterned panic reaction to such trauma. It is apparent that afflicted persons face a double danger: a threatening real world and unconscious material stirred up by the traumatic experience. The *pibloktoq* seizure aims at restoring the ego balance through the instrumentation of various defense mechanisms.

Regressive features play an important role in *pibloktoq*. Such features dramatize the underlying psychodynamic element, namely the *infantile* need for love and emotional support in the disturbed individual. One of the chief characteristics of *pibloktoq* is the childlike and naïve quality of the performance. This quality did not escape the perceptive eye of Macmillan: "It [*pibloktoq*] reminded me of a little child discouraged and unhappy because it imagines that no one loves it or cares for it and therefore runs away" (Brill 1913: 517).

Earlier we cast doubt upon the genuineness of the *pibloktoq's* desire for escape. We suggest that the flight reaction represents a regressive act, a dramatic, though thoroughly unconscious, invitation to be pursued, i.e., to be attended to, taken care of. It is noteworthy that attacks tend to occur under favorable circumstances,[9] at times when their occurrence will not put into jeopardy the lives of other members of the group and when other persons are available to render assistance. Furthermore, there is no evidence that attacks ever take place while an individual is alone. The dread of attacks occurring under unfavorable conditions probably lies behind the fact that seizures may be delayed until it is safe to have one (see case 5). Whitney (1911: 67) commenting on Tukshu's attack (case 1) remarks that it "would have been a very serious matter . . . had Tukshu been attacked while in the boat". As it was, he had his attack while *leaving* the boat.

Furthermore, *pibloktoq* demonstrates important denial and compensatory features. The individual experiencing deep anxiety and fear attempts via *pibloktoq* to deny these feelings and compensate for these emotions by dramatically engaging in antithetical behavior which stresses mobility, dangerous and strenuous feats, etc. In other words, *pibloktoq* represents an expression of control over, denial of, and compensation for, feelings of helplessness and deep anxiety.

To sum up: it would appear that afflicted individuals experience acute helplessness and deep anxiety. In *pibloktoq* the traumatized ego reacts in a psychologically primitive and infantile, but characteristically Eskimo, manner. In other words, though the psychological mode is ontogenetically primitive, much of the behavior is congruent with adult Eskimo ethnic personality.

The interpretation of helplessness may, in part, help explain why women are both more prone to *pibloktoq* and why their symptomatology tends to be more florid. The dependence of Eskimo women on the male hunters for food and, more particularly, their added helplessness in the face of culturally typical traumatic experiences increases their vulnerability. In case 2 and 3, for example, Tongwe had no alternative but to sit and await the return of the hunters.

DIAGNOSIS

Finally, we come to the question of diagnosis. Forty-six years ago, upon reviewing the Peary and Macmillan material, Brill (1913) wrote:

And yet is there really so much difference between the hysterical mechanisms as evidenced in piblokto and the grande hysterie or other modern hysterical manifestations? We may assume unhesitatingly that the difference is more apparent than real. The deeper determinants as we have seen are the same in both. With due apologies to Mr. Kipling we may say that the modern lady and Eskimo Julia O'Grady are the same under the skin [p. 520].

Nothing in the cases cited in this paper seems to warrant any substantial change in Brill's original diagnosis of hysteria. Certainly, schizophrenia is ruled out, despite feces eating in one case, on the grounds of the brevity of attacks and their complete remission afterwards.

NOTES

* An earlier version of this paper was read at the Annual Meeting of the American Anthropological Association, 1958. Materials for this paper were gathered by the author while assisting Dr. George Devereux on a study of mental disorder in primitive society. Funds for research, granted to Dr. Devereux, were supplied, in part, by the National Institute of Mental Health (M-1669), and the Society for the Investigation of Human Ecology. The author is deeply indebted to Dr. Devereux for his guidance and constructive criticism of the research and for his clarification of a number of methodological and diagnostic problems.

Credit is also due Mrs. Gitel P. Steed for allowing the author access to her unpublished interviews with Niels Rasmussen, and to Mr. Samuel Moskowitz for valuable criticism.

1. Yap (1951; 1952), Joseph and Murray (1951), Teicher (1954), Devereux (1956). Among earlier writers, see Seligman (1932), Zilboorg (1938).
2. *Pibloktoq*, as described in this paper, bears a striking, if not identical, resemblance to one form of the so-called "arctic hysterias", found among a number of Paleo-Siberian peoples, and referred to in the literature as *menerik* (Czaplicka 1914). Scattered references to *pibloktoq*-like performances have also been reported for a number of Indian groups in the Yukon-Mackenzie area of Alaska (Aronson 1940: 33; Dall 1870: 171–172; Honigmann 1949: 239–240), and in Korea (May 1956: 82).
3. Steed's interviews with Niels Rasmussen, son of the famed arctic explorer, Knud Rasmussen. Niels Rasmussen was in Greenland from 1939 to 1945. Three years of this period were spent among the Polar Eskimo near Etah. The Rasmussen interviews were taken in 1947–48 as part of a larger study, *Directed Culture Change in the Far North*; Gitel P. Steed, Director. Interviews consist of data on Rasmussen's own observations and personal experience, his knowledge of his father's life among the Eskimo, and his critical comments and discussion of the available arctic literature. In this paper, materials from the Rasmussen interviews are quoted verbatim.
4. According to Steed, Niels Rasmussen understood enough of the Eskimo language at this time to know that the individual in question was not speaking "ordinary" Eskimo.
5. Panic and desertion by Eskimo from the ships of European exploring parties was not an uncommon occurrence. For some accounts, see Melville (1896: 464).
6. The merits of the Cook-Peary controversy have no bearing upon the validity of Cook's Eskimo observations.
7. I am indebted to Dr. George Devereux for this insight.
8. For a discussion of matrices in anthropology and psychoanalysis, see Devereux (1957).
9. Whitney (1911: 67) mentions that attacks may also take place under unfavorable conditions, but cites no cases.

REFERENCES

Aberle, D. F.
    1952 *Arctic Hysteria* and *Latah* in Mongolia. Transactions of the New York Academy of Sciences, Series II, 14: 291–297.
Ackerknecht, E. H.
    1948 Medicine and Disease among Eskimos. Ciba Symposia 10: 916–921.

Aronson, J. D.
  1940 The History of Disease among the Natives of Alaska. Transactions and Studies of
        the College of Physicians of Philadelphia, 4th Series, Vol. 8.
Bertelsen, A.
  1929 Sanitation and Health Conditions in Greenland. *In* Greenland 3: 363–386. London:
        Humphrey Milford.
Birket-Smith, K.
  1936 The Eskimos. W. E. Calvert (tr.). London: Methuen.
Brill, A. A.
  1913 *Pibloktoq* or Hysteria among Peary's Eskimos. Journal of Nervous and Mental Disease
        40: 514–520.
Cook, F. A.
  1911 My Attainment of the Pole. New York: Polar Publishing Co.
Czaplicka, M. A.
  1914 Aboriginal Siberia. Oxford: Clarendon Press.
Dall, W. H.
  1870 Alaska and Its Resources. Boston: Lee & Shepard.
Dembovitz, N.
  1945 Psychiatry amongst West African Troops. Journal of the Royal Army Medical Corps
        84: 70–74.
Devereux, G.
  1956 Normal and Abnormal: The Key Problem of Psychiatric Anthropology. *In* Some
        Uses of Anthropology: Theoretical and Applied. Washington, D.C.: Anthropological
        Society of Washington.
  1957 Psychoanalysis as Anthropological Field Work: Data and Theoretical Implications.
        Transactions of the New York Academy of Sciences, Series II, 19: 457–472.
Dobrizhoffer, M.
  1822 An Account of the Abipones, 2. London: John Murray.
Honigmann, J. J.
  1949 Culture and Ethos of Kaska Society. Yale University Publications in Anthropology,
        No. 40.
Jenness, D.
  1928 The People of the Twilight. New York: Macmillan.
Joseph, A. and V. F. Murray
  1951 Chamorros and Carolinians of Saipan. Cambridge, Mass.: Harvard University Press.
Kloss, C. B.
  1923 *Arctic Amok*. Journal of the Royal Asiatic Society, Malayan Branch 1: 254.
Malaurie, J.
  1956 The Last Kings of Thule: A Year among the Polar Eskimos of Greenland. G. Freeman
        (tr.). London: George Allen & Unwin.
May, L. C.
  1956 A Survey of Glossolalia and Related Phenomena in Non-Christian Religions. American
        Anthropologist 58: 75–96.
Melville, G. W.
  1896 In the Lena Delta. Boston: Houghton, Mifflin.
Mowat, F.
  1952 People of the Deer. Boston: Little, Brown.
Novakovsky, S.
  1924 Arctic or Siberian Hysteria as a Reflex of the Geographic Environment. Ecology
        5: 113–127.
Peary, R. E.
  1907 Nearest the Pole. New York: Doubleday, Page.
  1910 The North Pole. New York: Frederick A. Stokes.

Rasmussen, K.
   1908 The People of the Polar North. G. Herring (ed.). London: Kegan Paul, Trench, Trubner.
Seligman, C. G.
   1932 Anthropological Perspective and Psychological Theory. Journal of the Royal Anthropological Institute 62: 193–228.
Steed, G. P.
   1947–Unpublished Interviews with Niels Rasmussen.
Steensby, H. P.
   1910 Contributions to the Ethnology and Anthropogeography of the Polar Eskimo. Meddelelser om Gronland 54.
Stefansson, V.
   1922 Hunters of the Great North. New York: Harcourt, Brace.
Teicher, M. I.
   1954 Three Cases of Psychoses among the Eskimos. Journal of Mental Science 100: 527–535.
Weyer, E. M.
   1932 The Eskimos: Their Environment and Folkways. New Haven: Yale University Press.
Whitney, H.
   1911 Hunting with Eskimos. New York: Century Co.
Yap, P. M.
   1951 Mental Diseases Peculiar to Certain Cultures: A Survey of Comparative Psychiatry. Journal of Mental Science 97: 313–327.
   1952 The *Latah* Reaction: Its Pathodynamics and Nosological Position. Journal of Mental Science 98: 515–564.
Zilboorg, G.
   1938 Critique: Section Meeting on Culture and Personality. American Journal of Orthopsychiatry 8: 596–601.

PHILIP A. DENNIS

GRISI SIKNIS IN MISKITO CULTURE

Miskito villages line the Atlantic coasts of Nicaragua and Honduras. Nietschmann (1973: 47) estimated the number of Miskito speakers in Nicaragua at 35,000 in the early 1970s, and the population has been increasing. "Miskito" is a cultural category more than a racial one. Long contact with outsiders has resulted in racial mixture with Europeans, creole blacks from the Caribbean, and Chinese merchants. As a result, a wide variety of physical types are found among the modern Miskito. Culturally, however, all those people identified as Miskito share such common core elements as a matrilocal residence pattern and a strong kinship ethic, a Miskito variety of Christianity, belief in the world of Miskito supernaturals, and use of the Miskito language itself.

As we will see, the history of the Miskito is reflected to some extent in the *grisi siknis* experience, a dramatic culture-bound syndrome, unreported in either the medical or the anthropological literature, which occurs among the Miskito. Victims of the condition lose consciousness, believe that devils beat them and have sexual relations with them, and run off through the village and into the bush. The condition may also involve violent, aggressive behavior such as threatening others with machetes and broken bottles. It affects mainly young women, and is epidemic and contagious in form.

FIELDWORK

I first became aware of *grisi siknis* from typewritten reports by Rubel (1976) and Cross (1975), who had both worked very briefly among the Miskito. These reports indicated an as yet undescribed culture-bound syndrome, similar in some ways to *piblokto* among the Inuit (Foulks 1972) or wild-man behavior in New Guinea (Newman 1964). I hoped field research on the syndrome would contribute to our general understanding of the culture-bound syndromes.

One perplexing problem with study of such syndromes, particularly *piblokto*, has been the lack of complete and accurate data. Interesting theories about their causes, such as Foulks' calcium deficiency hypothesis, remain inconclusive because the data on *piblokto* are so scarce. One purpose of my research, then, was to gather as complete and accurate data as possible.

During a year of postdoctoral research at Michigan State University, I studied the Miskito language, read the available ethnographic and medical literature, and prepared for fieldwork. In 1978–79 I travelled to the Miskito coast, and eventually chose as the site of my fieldwork the village of Awastara, which had been the center of a major *grisi siknis* epidemic. I lived in Awastara for eight months, studying *grisi siknis* and collecting general ethnographic information on the Miskito.

289

Ronald C. Simons and Charles C. Hughes (eds.), The Culture-Bound Syndromes, 289–306.
© 1985 by D. Reidel Publishing Company.

I recorded the history and course of the epidemic and interviewed nearly one hundred victims in Awastara and the surrounding villages. All my interviews were conducted in Miskito, in which I acquired reasonable fluency. I also interviewed local medical personnel and worked with several indigenous curers who treat *grisi siknis*. I also observed four actual attacks and managed to photograph one of them. This research produced a large body of data on *grisi siknis*, recently published in more detail elsewhere (Dennis 1981a).

In medical anthropology, the culture-bound syndromes have been a classic research problem. They represent the point of intersection of culture, biology, and psychology, manifested in particular types of illness behavior. As papers in this volume show, they challenge us to understand the causes of illness in more sophisticated ways, and they seem to offer the potential for deeper insight into the nature of illness itself. Comparison of *grisi siknis* with the other culture-bound syndromes should help provide such understandings. In this paper I will briefly describe *grisi siknis*, and then try to place it within its Miskito cultural context. I will suggest that it is a patterned response to stress, related to other, similar kinds of behavior common among the Miskito.

GRISI SIKNIS: THE DATA

Interviews with victims produced many interesting descriptions of attacks.

(1) A person comes, you lose your senses. If you're a man, a woman comes for you. If you're a woman, a man comes.

(2) People, men come for you, they do it to women [giggles]. We get afraid when other people are looking at us and laughing at us.

(3) A handsome man comes from a big ship. He does like your husband would to you.

(4) A white woman comes to me in a taxi and says, "Let's go!" She takes me to a fine place, a town like Puerto Cabezas to travel around (*kirbaia*). She has sex with me, but sometimes she cuts me with a knife. I don't like it! [male victim speaking]

(5) He is a handsome man, he wants to carry you away to his own country. He comes and lays down between me and my husband. "The machete is there! The bottle is there! Grab it!" he says.

(6) Something like a man comes, a white man, a Spaniard, riding a horse. He carried me away down the beach, six hours or more I was gone and people didn't know where I was. He took me to a big saloon, gave me food, and wanted to dance with me. He was a handsome man, he didn't hit me. Yes, he did it to me!

As they run from their houses during attacks, victims shriek and whoop and speak with the devil. They often use English or Spanish, languages which may be spoken only with great hesitation in ordinary daily life. Since the devils who appear are often non-Miskito, it seems logical that the language spoken with them is English or Spanish.

Victims reported several symptoms which indicated an attack was likely: head-aches, *bla*, and general anxiety and fear. The headaches were said to be sharp, stabbing pains in the head (in Miskito, *won lal klauisa* or *won lal sabisa*). *Bla* is a general Miskito category which includes dizziness drunkenness, and seasickness as well. Some victims also reported an irrational anger with all those around them. Such symptoms were said to alert an individual and her family that an actual attack was imminent, and that herbal medicine should be done to prevent it.

An attack begins when the devil appears to carry his chosen victim away. The individual loses consciousness (*auya lap tiwan*) and is not aware of what she does. She may perceive other people in the area as devils, for example, and have complete anesthesia for injuries suffered during an attack. When an attack begins, the victim falls to the ground, but soon gets to her feet and attempts to run away through the village or off into the bush. This running away is perhaps the most distinctive defining characteristic of *grisi siknis* behavior.

Catching and Restraining the Victim

When a *grisi siknis* attack occurs, groups of men and boys run after the victim, catch her, disarm her if necessary, and bring her back to the house. If she is not restrained, she may run off into the bush and be lost there for a day or more until she returns to her senses. Some victims who had not been restrained found their own way back through the savannah and mangrove swamps, after their attacks had ended. Some mentioned catching snakes with their hands and performing other remarkable feats. These feats, like the ability to speak in other languages, are regarded as proof of supernatural possession. Back inside their houses, victims are often tied with ropes to keep them from breaking loose and running away again.

Attacks are exciting, dramatic occurrences, certainly one of the major social dramas that occur in Miskito villages. The young men laugh and shout to each other as they run after the girls, and the element of danger (the girl may be armed and may injure someone) adds to the excitement. However, it is also regarded as a serious responsibility to restrain the girl and prevent her from running into the lagoon or the river, where, it is believed, she would drown herself. Running after a *grisi* woman may be exciting, but it is also a serious male responsibility.

Aggressive Behavior

In Awastara, deliberate aggressive behavior has become a part of *grisi siknis*. Since the early 1960s victims there have grabbed machetes and knives and waved these weapons in a threatening manner as they run. Dealing with these women is dan-gerous, and several serious accidents have occurred. In the attacks I observed, however, the victims did not attempt to harm bystanders who did not interfere with them. They seemed to be swinging the machetes at individuals they see in their minds, not deliberately aiming at the people around them. Even so, they are regarded as extremely dangerous and are feared accordingly. The women sometimes seem to enjoy this fear they inspire. Before one attack, the neighbor woman who was staying with the victim quietly gathered up the various machetes and knives in the house and sent her little girl to carry them away and hide them. Relatives attempt to keep all such weapons hidden from women who are currently having attacks, but the victims are said to be very clever about finding them again.

In swinging machetes, knives, and broken bottles, *grisi siknis* victims sometimes cut themselves badly. A number of women in Awastara have multiple scars from self-inflicted injuries. The most serious injury was a deep cut in the breast which required hospital attention. The Miskito regard such self-mutilation during attacks as a terrible, unfortunate consequence of devil possession. They discuss it in connection with running away and drowning in the river or lagoon, and argue that victims are quite likely to kill themselves through such acts. Actually, in all the case material collected I found no instance of victims drowning, or of them cutting themselves deeply enough to bleed to death, although many had the opportunity to do both. The Miskito say that this good safety record so far is a result of carefully watching the victims to prevent fatal accidents. To me, however, it seems that in spite of their apparent loss of self-control, the victims, like patients suffering related varieties of conversion hysteria (Weintraub 1977), were exercising some degree of self-restraint.

Sexual Aspects of Attacks

The *grisi* attacks have a frankly sexual basis, according to the Miskito. The devils who appear want young women for sex, and they come particularly for the ones they find most attractive. The Miskito phrase, *mairen nanira laik*, used to explain attacks, can be translated, "He wants women!" The native explanation for why some individuals are affected and others are not is simply that the devil likes some young women better than others.

Although most victims of *grisi siknis* are women, some men are affected as well. Five out of sixty-two victims in Awastara were male. They reported experiences generally similar to those of women, except the devils who possess them and who have sexual relations with them are female. This is especially interesting in light of the fact that four of the five male victims were effeminate and were regarded as homosexuals by the rest of the community. None of them reported sexual relations with male devils during *grisi siknis* attacks, however, even when questioned closely about this possibility.

During interviews, women who had experienced attacks often giggled and acted embarrassed at questions concerning sex with the devil. To some extent this is the normal reaction of young women in Miskito society: they find the discussion of sex embarrassing, especially with older people or high status visitors. In addition, though, they regarded the sexual nature of their *grisi siknis* experiences as funny and titillating. Informants would readily admit that the devil has sex with them, but most emphasized other aspects, such as being taken to eat and dance in a fine saloon, or negative experiences, such as being frightened to death by ugly dogs or the horrible appearance of the devil.

Another dimension of sexuality in attacks is that girls having attacks have sometimes been gang-raped by the young men who ran after them to subdue them. One reason the parents of *grisi* girls have been anxious to keep them inside the house and tied up, if necessary, was simply to prevent any possibility of their being raped.

The converse of the gang rape possibility is that attacks were sometimes used to seduce young men. Some of the Awastara *grisi siknis* victims would call out that only a certain young man could catch them, and then run off into the bush waving a machete. The young man indicated would follow her into the bush and bring her back later, and they would presumably have an opportunity for sexual relations.

Attacks in Individual Lives

Interviews with many victims showed that *grisi siknis* is highly patterned. First attacks begin suddenly after a period of severe headaches and episodes of *bla*, and occur very frequently for several weeks. Attacks may occur every day or even several times a day. This puts the family under great stress, since someone must stay home with the victim all day and accompany her everywhere, in case an attack should occur. The mother usually has the major responsibility for watching over her daughter, but nearby men are called to subdue her once an attack has started. During the initial stage of the illness the victim usually has little appetite and may lose weight. If Miskito herbal medicine is done, the attacks may be quickly brought to an end. Even if it is not done, the attacks begin occurring less and less frequently, and eventually end by themselves.

Apparently first attacks do not occur among older persons. The average age of onset reported by Awastara victims was about fifteen, and by Dakura victims about eighteen. If one has escaped *grisi siknis* as a teenager, it is very unlikely it will strike later in life. On the other hand, if one has had it early in life, it is quite likely to occur again periodically. Previous victims often have recurrences later on in life. In fact, all the attacks I witnessed in late 1978 were recurrences. These attacks follow the same pattern as first ones, occurring very frequently for a few days or weeks, then slowing down or stopping altogether. However, they are usually less severe than the original attacks. Any sort of emotional problem, or seeing someone else have a *grisi* attack, may bring on a recurrence, even years later. The case material shows quarrels with a husband, the death of a close relative, and physical illness as among the precipitating events. Getting very angry and upset about any personal problem in itself may provoke a recurrence, and *grisi siknis* victims also try to stay away from girls currently having attacks, since they consider themselves at risk. As the Miskito phrase it, "Once you have seen the devil there is a good chance he will come back again, especially when you are upset". From a clinical point of view, having had an initial attack as a young person seems to provide the option of responding to stress with subsequent attacks later in life.

Most *grisi siknis* victims recover and lead normal lives. There is no special stigma to having had it in the past, since it is regarded as a disease for which one is not responsible. For a few individuals, however, attacks continue to occur in spite of efforts to stop them, or begin recurring in an alarming way. For these people attacks become closely associated with a variety of other physical and emotional problems.

Contagious Nature of the Disease

The Miskito regard *grisi siknis* as highly contagious. Some informants said it was "like a magnet" or "like electricity". Young women are the most susceptible to the condition, and simply seeing or being around other girls who are having the attacks is dangerous. Church meetings and other places where a number of young women are congregated are thus likely places for an outbreak to occur.

There is also a specific mechanism of contagion: victims having attacks may call out the names of others (usually other young women), who later contract the disease and begin having attacks themselves. In Miskito thought, the devil wants more "workers", more victims to possess sexually and carry away, and he forces the person having an attack to give him other names. Calling out the names is selling those individuals to the devil. It seems to serve to some extent as a rationalization of why individuals have attacks, even months later: their names have been called and so they are likely to get the disease.

Since it is contagious, a number of victims often contract the disease at the same time, and large-scale epidemics occasionally result. During epidemics victims "work together" for the devil, and may create a serious social problem, as whole groups of people run through the village, shouting and threatening others.

The Awastara Epidemic

Grisi siknis in Awastara clearly reached epidemic proportions during the last twenty years. I identified sixty-two victims during this period, in a village whose population in 1978 was 664. Prevalence figures were also collected from the other villages affected.

The epidemic actually began in the nearby village of Krukira in 1956. The first woman to have it still lives there and was interviewed. She reported that before her attacks began, her head hurt, she felt very angry with everybody around her and didn't want to listen to them, and then she saw white-skinned people, coming towards her from the lagoon and from the graveyard. She interprets these creatures as *liwa*, a traditional kind of Miskito devil. She lost consciousness and then ran away with the devils who had come for her, much like later victims. Her son-in-law quickly contracted the disease, followed by about a dozen other poeple, mostly young women. At this stage in the epidemic there was no violent, aggressive behavior, no threatening of others and no self-mutilation. This aspect of the epidemic developed only later in Awastara.

The epidemic in Krukira quickly gained outside attention. A detachment of National Guardsmen came to investigate, and a Nicaraguan doctor apparently made some cursory investigation. According to informants, he thought perhaps eating poisoned fish was the cause of the strange behavior, and questioned victims about their diet. Within Krukira, there was suspicion that some individual was causing the problem, through poison or some other sorcery technique.

The epidemic arrived in Awastara about two years later, in 1958. It came through contact with Krukira; there is frequent travel back and forth between the two villages, and the Awastara people had been aware of the epidemic in Krukira from its beginning. From Awastara it was to spread to other neighboring villages. Awastara residents believe it is still spreading, and they interpret distant reports of possession and crazy behavior as involving the same epidemic.

There seemed to be three broad phases in the Awastara epidemic. In the first phase, there were seven victims. Three of these people were available to interview, and none of their accounts were much different from those of subsequent victims. Like the Krukira group, they had attacks as a group and ran away together, shouting and screaming, and defending each other from those who tried to restrain them. At this point, there was still no self-mutilation or waving of machetes.

The epidemic began growing in proportions in Awastara in the early 1960s. During this second phase most of the first group's attacks had ceased, but a second, much larger group of people began having attacks. I identified forty individuals who had attacks during the period from about 1960–1975. At some points, ten or more of these people were having attacks simultaneously, running through the village together and "working for the devil". It was during this period that groups of *grisi* women ran into the schoolhouse (as children jumped out the windows and hid under desks), burst into the church where services were being held, and in general, thoroughly disrupted the usual pattern of daily life. People barred their doors tightly in the evenings to prevent the *grisi* women from entering. Even during the attacks I witnessed in 1978, the boys who chased the victims ran through town shouting, "Shut your doors! They're coming!" It must have been a dramatic and frightening spectacle during the height of the epidemic to see a dozen possessed women running through the village, brandishing machetes and bottles, and terrorizing the local inhabitants. During this period the village headman assigned groups of men to watch through the night, and Awastara became known as the center of the *grisi siknis* phenomenon along the whole coast.

The third phase of the epidemic began about 1975. By this time most of the earlier victims had stopped having attacks and many had moved away. The climax of the epidemic had evidently passed, but a group of "stragglers" continued to have attacks up through April, 1979, when I left Awastara. During the attacks which I witnessed, several people expressed fears that a major epidemic was beginning all over again.

It is interesting that in terms of its temporal and spatial dimensions, *grisi siknis* seems to follow the classic model for contagious disease (see, for example Dubos 1965: 165–95), even though I could find no indication of an organic cause. In Krukira it began at one particular point, and grew out of a set of related, endemic conditions in a local population. The new devil became as virulent compared to the older devils as a new strain of bacteria which evolves from an endemic but less potent older strain. Introduced into a new area, Awastara, it first affected a small group of susceptible people, then built to a climax as a larger second generation of victims were exposed. Since the climax of the epidemic, it has affected a steadily decreasing number of people. It appears as if a new disease had struck a population with no immunity, built to a climax in the second generation as more individuals were exposed, and then declined as some immunity was built up in the population.

As the illness spread from village to village and increased in frequency, it seemed to grow richer in its repertoire of expressed symptoms. The traditional devils, called *liwa*, were replaced by newer devils as the epidemic progressed. Also, instead of simply running away, victims began to grab machetes and bottles and threaten others, as well as cut themselves. New developments continue to occur. For example, recent victims in Dakura generally reported more positive kinds of experiences with devils than did the earlier Awastara victims. The last person to have *grisi siknis* in Awastara during my fieldwork had an attack during labor preceding childbirth, something which had never occurred before. An important aspect of epidemics, then, seems to be that as they spread, the behavior involved changes, develops, and becomes more elaborate.

GRISI SIKNIS IN MISKITO SOCIETY AND CULTURE

Grisi siknis, like the other culture-bound syndromes, must be understood within its own cultural context. On the Miskito coast, the rich ethnohistorical literature allows us to piece together information from contemporary Miskito culture with accounts from the past, thus giving historical depth to the phenomenon. In the 1850s Charles Napier Bell observed what was apparently a case of *grisi siknis*.

I have seen a young girl, who was shrieking hysterically in a dreadful manner, carried in a canoe a long distance to consult a celebrated *sookia*. All that the *sookia* did was erect round her painted sticks with charms tied to them, to blow tobacco-smoke over her while muttering strange words, to make a bubling with a tobacco-pipe in a calabash of water, which she was then made to drink and to tie a knotted string around her neck, on every knot of which was a drop of blood from his tongue. For as many days as there were knots she must not eat the meat of certain animals, must suffer no one to pass to windward of her, and must not see a woman with child (Bell 1899: 97).

Bell grew up on the coast, spoke Miskito fluently, and was a careful and accurate observer. He is the most reliable of the early commentators on the Miskito. In this case, the symptoms described and the curing system applied to them are similar to those of *grisi siknis* today.

Curing

As in Bell's time, there is today a well worked-out system of remedies with which *grisi siknis* is treated. These remedies seem to be effective in stopping attacks and are part of the larger system of Miskito herbal medicine. Among the Miskito, knowledge of particular medicinal plants is individual property. Most people know a few plants, but individuals who specialize in curing ("bush doctors") know a great many. Knowledge of herbal medicine must be purchased from someone else, often at a considerable price. The plants used also seem to vary a good deal between different practicioners. *Grisi siknis*, snakebite, or other problems may be treated with a variety of different plants, and each curer usually claims that his/hers are the most effective.

I observed one cure for *grisi siknis*. The girl involved had had attacks for several days when the curer and I arrived. She had come back from Managua, where she had complained of *bla* and headaches. When the curer and I arrived at the girl's house she was having an attack, thrashing on the floor as her father and mother held her down. Her attack stopped as we arrived, and she climbed onto the bed and lay there quietly. The curer questioned the family about whether any woman in the house was pregnant. He then asked for a pot with a cover and put seven coins in the bottom. This is the *sika mana*, or price of the medicine, which must be paid when the plant is picked and again when it is boiled for steam. After the cure the coins can be taken back out of the pot and pocketed.

Next, the curer produced the brown paper packets of herbs he had brought, put them in the pot with the coins and some water, and went outside to boil them on a small fire which had been made outside. When the water in the pot was boiling, he brought it inside and set it on the floor, and called to the patient. She quickly sat down on a small stool on the floor directly over the pot, and covered up with a blanket. The steaming lasted about a minute in this direction, then the pot was taken outside and boiled again, brought back in and given to her in each of the four directions.

The crucial elements in the cure seem to be: using packets of secret herbs, paying the *sika mana*, steaming the patient in each of the four directions, and careful attention to those things which will make the medicine ineffective.

Each medicine not only has its price (*mana*), but its counteragents (*waila*), which will destroy its effectiveness (*sika slingwisa*). Three basic counteragents seem to be common to all medicines:

(1) seeing or being around a dead person

(2) being around a pregnant or menstruating woman

(3) eating certain kinds of fish or meat, especially hawksbill turtle, tarpon, jack, and lobster.

The common element in these things, according to Miskito theory, is that they all have a strong or bad smell (*kia saura*). The "bad smell" of the fish or menstruating woman counteracts the medicine, which has also been introduced into the body through the sense of smell (steam containing the essence of the plant). Because of their odor, fish may not be cooked upwind of the patient, nor may anyone walk upwind of her after she has taken medicine (as Bell accurately recorded). The reasoning is that causal passersby might be pregnant or menstruating women, or someone who had recently eaten some kind of prohibited fish.

It is interesting that the success of such treatments is attributed to the magical efficacy of the plants themselves, and that the curer, or bush doctor, simply acts as a herbal technician applying superpotent substances. He is not respected because of his sensitivity to other people's problems or insight into their lives; indeed, the curer with whom I worked most closely was remarkable for his insensitivity in this regard. Miskito bush doctors obviously operate very differently from the Ndembu doctor in the well-known article by Victor Turner (1967), who carefully investigates the patient's psycho-social background.

The Miskito theory of curing seems to be very mechanistic: the correct herbal medicine, properly administered, whose counteragents are carefully avoided, will cure the disease. The herbal medicine seems to act in an analogous way to the ropes sometimes used to tie up victims: it acts as a restraint, and when a counteragent breaks its potency, it is much as if the restraining ropes had broken, allowing the devil to come again and take away the victim.

Malevolent Supernaturals

For the Miskito, many kinds of health problems, including *grisi siknis*, are attributable to devils. The natural world is believed to be full of malevolent supernaturals who cause illness, have illicit sexual relations with humans, and in general cause mischief. These devils include the *swinta*, a short figure in a broad-brimmed hat who is the "owner of the deer"; and the *liwa*, who lives in streams, lagoons, and the ocean, and whose female form is said to appear like the European mermaid.

The *liwa*, in particular, are closely related to *grisi siknis*. They occur in both male and female form, and appear at night to sexually molest people of the opposite sex. Women sometimes report visits from male *liwa*, who may beat them as well as have sexual relations with them. It is said that the morning after, one can see the prominent bruises left by the *liwa*. Albino and deformed children are believed to be *liwa* offspring, and individuals without spouses, who do not have children, or whose sexual life is in some other way abnormal, are suspected of having sexual liasons with a *liwa*.

The *liwa* and the *swinta* and the other supernaturals are the agents traditionally responsible for *grisi siknis*. When the epidemic first began, in Krukira, it was attributed to *liwa* who came from the lagoon. Only later did other devils begin to appear. As the epidemic progressed, these devils became increasingly prominent, replacing the *liwa* as the causative agents.

Miskito History

Many characteristics of the devils reflect the historical experiences of the Miskito. Helms, an authority on the Miskito, describes them as a tribal people who have prospered and spread as a result of contact with Europeans (Helms 1971: 16—23). After acquiring muskets from the early English traders and buccaneers, they subjugated surrounding groups, spread up and down the coast, and began functioning as middlemen in the trade with the English (Helms 1969, 1983). Early English visitors to the coast were careful to stay on good terms with their Miskito hosts, from whom they got provisions, lumber and skins, and sexual access to Miskito women. The Miskito pattern of accepting outside men into the community, and of Miskito men frequently working away from home, dates at least from these early times.

Another major historical influence has been the work of Christian missionaries. The Moravian missionaries arrived in 1849, but their first real success came in 1881 with the mass conversions known as the Great Awakening. The missionaries learned the Miskito language and translated the Bible, and by the turn of the century were living in many of the coastal villages. They vigorously opposed Miskito practices they found immoral: in particular, shamanism, polygyny, and ceremonial beer feasts.

Today each Miskito village has its own Miskito Moravian lay pastor. The few foreign missionaries who remain, as well as the creole missionaries, regard *grisi siknis* as another silly Miskito superstition, but it is interesting to note that it also occurs among the families of the Miskito lay pastors, in spite of their religious training. The lay pastors' explanation for *grisi siknis* usually involves Biblical references: the Bible shows that people suffered from the same kind of affliction in ancient times, Jesus cast out devils who possessed people, and faith in God will help. The lay pastors I knew were not averse to trying bush medicine (which is on the borderline of Christian acceptability), but they were firmly opposed to *sukias*, shamans who go into trance to exorcise evil spirits.

An important historical event for the Miskito has been the employment of Miskito men by the various foreign companies which have worked on the coast, mining, lumbering, raising bananas, prospecting for oil, and most recently, fishing for turtles and lobsters (see Helms 1971: 27—33, and Nietschmann 1973). The Miskito also share the coast with the creole, or black, English-speaking population, which is centered in the area around Bluefields. Long contact with creole people has brought many items of Caribbean creole culture, including English loan words, to the Miskito. In the larger towns there are also Spanish-speaking people, more recently arrived from the west. Thus, *grisi siknis* victims who reported seeing a black man on a big ship, a white woman in a taxi, a white man with a pistol in khaki pants, are describing real life experiences the Miskito have had. White men in khaki probably represent the lumber company managers and other company personnel of the recent past, and the references to black men reflect the continuing Miskito contact with the creole population.

Since 1981, the Miskito have been involved in a bloody and destructive civil war in eastern Nicaragua, in which counter-revolutionary forces supported by the United States, allied with local Miskito villagers, have opposed the Sandinista government. The background of this tragic conflict is recounted in Dennis (1981b). How these tragic events may be reflected in *grisi siknis* behavior remains a subject for future research.

In the multi-ethnic situation in which the Miskito live, *grisi siknis* seems to be a truly culture-bound phenomenon. Barrio El Muelle in Puerto Cabezas provided interesting data in this regard. Barrio El Muelle contains both creole and poor Spanish-speaking families interspersed with the majority Miskito population. However, the nine cases of *grisi siknis* I was able to locate in the barrio were all Miskito girls. A creole woman living next door to one of the Miskito girls suffering attacks laughed when we asked if her daughters were likely to get it, explaining that it was something that only happened to Miskito girls. According to her, the Miskito *grisi siknis* victims had called the names of creole young people many times during their attacks, but no one named had ever been affected. Being culturally Miskito, and believing in the Miskito devils, seems to be necessary to contract *grisi siknis*.

The common element in all the Miskito devils, traditional or modern, seems to be their desire to sexually possess their victims, and their generally evil intentions (to harm one or make one harm someone else). The Miskito clearly state that their own attitudes towards the evils are a mixture of pleasure/desire for sex and new experiences, and fear of what the devils may do to them.

The devils also fit well into the Christian Miskito belief system, as different manifestations of Satan. Theologically sophisticated Miskito explain that when God expelled Satan from heaven, his various forms went to live in refuge areas: the ocean, the deep forest, and the rivers, where they continue to live today. In this way they account for the *liwa* and the other traditional Miskito devils who live in the natural surroundings.

All these devils seem to be supernatural representations of preoccupations and fears the Miskito face in such daily situations as hunting and gardening, interacting with powerful and unknown outsiders, and dealing with unsatisfied sexual impulses. Sometimes the personification of these problems is ingenuous, as in the case of a widower I knew who lived alone, and complained that every night a *liwa* in the form of a beautiful young woman came to torment him and prevent him from sleeping. Stress, whose source may be worries about interpersonal relations, sex, or the dangers of the bush (which are real enough), presents itself to the Miskito as a personified devil, thus provoking some behavioral response from the individual affected. Illness, or wild, hysterical behavior are two common responses. Since the devil is regarded as responsible, curing efforts are directed at him, not at the original stress which caused the problem. And, although curing efforts may be quite successful for individuals, they presumably do not alter the underlying patterns of stress.

The Hysterical Miskito

Fieldwork revealed many kinds of extreme emotional expressiveness among the Miskito. Crying, pulling one's hair, talking loudly, and dramatic gesticulation all occur in a variety of circumstances. The following kinds of behavior seem to provide the cultural foundation for *grisi siknis*.

(1) *Grief reactions to sickness and death*. At the funeral of a Dakura girl which I attended, the girl's mother cried, sobbed, and chanted a loud funeral dirge. Early reports on the Miskito describe even more emotional grief reactions:

... [the relatives of the dead person] try to injure themselves by knocking the head against the house posts, or by inflicting wounds on themselves with the aid of arms, rocks, or other objects, but the guests intercede and prevent them from harming themselves in a serious way. At a *sikro* on Río Platano I was witness when an old woman made a deep cut in her arm with the aid of an old, rusty machete. (Conzemius 1932: 162)

The grief displayed by the women is most passionate: they dash themselves to the earth till they are covered with blood, cast themselves into the river or the fire, and frequently steal away and hang themselves. (Bell 1862: 255)

Suicide was apparently rather common as an extreme grief reaction. Interestingly, hysterical grief reactions, like *grisi siknis*, were apparently expected more of women than they were of men.

(2) *Religious experience*. *Sukias* traditionally went into trance as part of religious and curing rituals.

Through the use of narcotics, especially the excessive use of tobacco, the sukya throws himself in a condition of wild ecstasy, and goes into trances and hypnotic states. During such an abnormal condition he is supposed to be in relation with friendly spirits who he had invoked previously ... (Conzemius 1932: 123)

Bush doctors also contact another reality directly through dreams. Spirit beings in dreams show them the correct diagnosis and the appropriate herbal medicines to use. These kinds of experiences do not provide a direct model for *grisi* type behavior, but they do validate the existence of another reality, peopled by various kinds of spirits, which is the precondition for possession by the *grisi siknis* devils.

Some aspects of Christian religious experience provide more direct models. During the "Great Awakening" of the 1880s, the Moravian missionaries reported widespread revelations, falling to the ground and reacting with other frenzied, trance-like behavior.

The Lord is at present engaged in "purging His floor", and in deepening and strengthening the movement which has spread to so large an extent. Many hidden sins are being brought to light. ... Others still imagine that they receive direct and wonderful revelations from the Lord. One man, since his awakening, is said to have spoken occasionally in a strange and unintelligible tongue. Others are at times overcome with a sort of paroxym, when their whole frame is convulsed, and they seem to lose entire control over themselves. These phenomena were especially frequent at the commencement of the revival. (Moravian Church 1883: 545–546)

The missionaries optimistically interpreted this behavior as an outpouring of the spirit, but it is clear that it represented a direct continuation of Miskito methods of contacting the supernatural and of "hysterical" behavior which demonstrated that contact with the spirit world.

(3) *Drunkenness*. In premissionary days, huge drunken feasts occurred periodically, especially at funeral celebrations. A large amount of *mishla*, or cassava beer, was brewed and entirely consumed in a spree which sometimes lasted several days. Wild, unrestrained behavior, with fighting and sexual license, was characteristic of these *mishla* feasts.

Missionaries have generally been successful in stamping out the *mishla* feasts per se, but contemporary Christmas celebrations in many Miskito villages retain the essence of the *mishla* feast: days of drinking, dancing, loud and boisterous singing, fist fights, and sexual promiscuity.

An interesting difference between aggressive drinking situations and *grisi siknis* has to do with sex roles. Women do drink, but the Miskito mention female drunkenness with disapproval. Normally it is men who become inebriated and are then cared for by women, whereas *grisi siknis* primarily affects women, who are then chased and restrained by men. To some extent drunkenness and *grisi siknis* seem to provide equivalent male and female roles for "crazy behavior". The sex not involved meanwhile plays the role of caretaker.

(4) *Child-raising*. From my observations in Awastara, yelling at children, ordering them brusquely to do this or that, and shrieking at them for misbehavior are all common child-raising techniques. In my experience Miskito adults often try to coerce children into doing what the adults want, through both physical punishment and loud scolding. A typical response on the part of the child is to ignore the adult, however, thus provoking a contest of wills. One general consequence of these kinds of child-raising techniques is probably to produce individuals who are used to screaming, shrieking, and similar behavior used to influence others. *Grisi siknis*, then, is an extreme kind of emotional behavior, but the general pattern of using such behaviors in interpersonal relations is well-established.

Relevant Miskito Concepts

Several Miskito concepts are closely related to emotionally expressive behavior. One is the verb *palaia*, to fly into a rage or to scold. Parents are expected to *palaia* at their children, and headmen at their villagers. It is a legitimate response of authority figures to misbehavior on the part of those beneath them.

Taibi briaia means to restrict, or to have another person under one's control. Literally, it can refer to holding down and tying up a person having *grisi siknis* attacks. Less literally, it can refer to the restriction implied in subordinate relationships — for example, children as restricted by their parents. It is *palaia* sort of behavior that keeps subordinates properly *tabi briaia*; scolding children, for example, keeps them from misbehaving.

Grisi munaia means to act crazy or go out of one's mind. To the outside observer, *grisi munaia* seems to be just an extreme form of *palaia*. Both force other people to respond, to take note of one's own feelings and desires. In fact a great deal of Miskito behavior seems aimed at forcing such responses from other people. Interestingly enough, the reaction of those around is often to disregard the flamboyant display, or to laugh at it, which in turn provokes even more extreme displays. I interpret *grisi munaia* type behavior as a demand for attention and response, which has escalated beyond the *palaia* stage. I have seen children walk away when their parents began to *palaia* at them, but it is impossible to disregard *grisi siknis* victims, who are hysterical, armed, and apparently dangerous.

Miskito children growing up are thus exposed to hysterical behavior in a number of different contexts. They learn that such behavior is the normal way to express frustration and stress. They also learn that there are supernaturals who cause *grisi* behavior, thus relieving the individual of responsibility. Although "ordinary" hysterical behavior is tolerated and even encouraged, "extraordinary" hysterical behavior is attributed to devils, which legitimates it as a disease in Miskito eyes.

Stress, Women's Role and Grisi Siknis

It is clear that *grisi siknis* is related to emotional upset, worry, fear and general anxiety. Severe headaches and irrational anger with those around precede attacks, and informants say they are "terribly afraid" (*uba si brin daukisa*) when they know an attack is imminent. Devils also reappear later in life at periods of personal trauma, such as the death of a spouse or a serious physical illness. The Miskito themselves identify such stresses, and regard previous victims as being at special risk later on during periods of emotional disturbance. They cannot identify the stresses which presumably cause first attacks in young women, however.

Young women do face special problems. They must find a husband and establish a household of their own, since women are dependent on men for financial support and for certain kinds of work in the village. Without a man, who will clear and burn her fields, and who will build her house? say the Miskito. Women realize they must use their charm and sexual appeal to attract a man, but they are also keenly aware of men's unreliability. When a man finds a pretty younger woman, or a job somewhere away from the village, he is likely to leave, women say. Marriages are brittle and the Miskito Christian ideal of a lifelong marriage commitment is rarely attained.

Women are closely attached to their mothers emotionally and would like to remain close physically, but realize their husbands may want them to move away. Adolescence is a time when such a choice is close at hand. When relationships do end in fact, women move back to be close to their mothers. Household relationships are still based around groups of mothers and their grown daughters. Helms (1968) interprets this Miskito matrilocal residence pattern as being responsible for the preservation of Miskito language and culture, and at least in Awastara, the pattern is still strong.

On the other hand, young women also want to leave, to have new experiences and romantic relationships with men. They are strictly chaperoned by their mothers and other relatives while they are living at home. They are not allowed to wander through the village in the evening looking for entertainment (*kirbaia*) as do young men, and they look forward to jobs away from the village as a way of escaping these restrictions. Going dancing, going to the movies, having boyfriends, are all pleasures which one can have in Puerto Cabezas or Bluefields. The security young women find at home contrasts with the excitement and attraction of relationships with men which they imagine away from home.

The general picture painted by Helms of adolescence as a stressful time for Miskito girls from Asang, also seems accurate to me from my observations in Awastara.

It [adolescence] is also a period of insecurity, especially for girls. This is observed in the need for close physical contact between *tiaras* [young, unmarried women]. When several go walking in the evening, for example, they inevitably hold hands, link arms, or put their arms around each other's waists. This close physical contact . . . may be understood as a seeking of reas-surance among young women who soon expect to marry and hope for the best, but who are aware of the subordinate position and often difficult life accorded to wives in this society, and who regard men in general as potentially untrustworthy. (Helms 1971: 61).

These kinds of adolescent stresses are of course not unique to the Miskito, nor are the "hysterical" behavior and sexual fantasies with which they respond. The uniqueness lies in the degree to which they have been institutionalized and channelled into recognized "illness" behavior.

Grisi Siknis Attacks as Social Dramas

Having attacks seems to guarantee a great deal of attention to the young victims, and attacks are "scheduled" to allow their full potential as dramatic events to be realized. Most attacks take place at *saiwan*, the late afternoon hours after work and before sunset. This is the traditional time for visiting and relaxation. Most people are on their front porches, sitting and talking. Young men stroll through the village, playing guitars and lounging in small groups. On Wednesdays and Sundays, evening church services attract other people. Of these *saiwan* time activi-ties, *grisi siknis* attacks are by far the most dramatic and interesting.

Analyzing attacks as a demand for attention and response suggests a further look at their message content. Young Miskito women are expected to be relatively passive and subordinate to their parents and later to their husbands. In having an attack, a woman seems to be saying something like:

I may be young and subordinate but I am also a sexual, aggressive, self-assertive person! I can have sex with the devil! I can grab a machete and scare everyone to death! I am even stronger physically than you are! Catch me if you can, but at your own risk!

It is interesting that the social response to this assertiveness is additional re-straint: young men catch the *grisi* girl, subdue her, and bring her back to the house where she may even be tied up. The girl has a chance to deliver her "message", but it is society that seems to win in the confrontation. The subordination and passivity against which the girls seems to be reacting is again forced upon them. Going beyond the bounds of proper behavior evokes a counter-response, which reestablishes the subordinate position of the *grisi siknis* victims. I think it is for this reason that the young "victims" laugh and giggle when questioned about their illness. If only for a short time, they have been able to behave in a forbidden and improper manner: threatening others with dangerous weapons, having sex with the devil, and accompanying him to wild and exciting places.

Grisi siknis, like other related behavior among the Miskito, appears to the observer as an uninhibited expression of emotions, a flood of repressed libidinal feelings pouring out at once. *Grisi siknis*, like the earlier *mishla* feasts, seems to be a wild, orgiastic rite of sex and violence. Miskito culture has institutionalized periodic outbursts of violent emotions, and turned them into social events like the *mishla* feast, or "diseases" like *grisi siknis*.

CONCLUSIONS

From my research it seems clear that *grisi siknis* is a culture-bound condition occurring only among the Miskito, and that it has a long history in Miskito society. Furthermore, "hysterical" type behavior occurs frequently in other contexts. *Grisi siknis* seems to be an institutionalized form of the extreme emotional expressiveness which characterizes Miskito culture in general. There is a traditional system of herbal curing for the condition, and a complex set of beliefs about its causes and treatment.

The epidemic form of *grisi siknis* which occurred in the Awastara area seems to be an elaboration on the traditional folk illness. New devils began to appear, possessing people and causing them to run away. The condition was contagious and involved groups of people "working together for the devil". In this situation groups periodically became possessed and ran through the village shouting and threatening others. To villagers, such epidemics are major public health problems and they genuinely desire help in dealing with them.

I think it is clear that *grisi siknis* is stress related. Victims having recurrent attacks identify specific stresses as the cause, and all victims talk about severe headaches, dizziness, worry, and anxiety as preceding attacks. This evidence seems to point to *grisi siknis* as a Miskito response to stress in life situations, although more work needs to be done to identity and understand those stresses, particularly in the case of first attacks. Miskito informants also indicated they would welcome further research into the condition, which might result in better means of prevention and treatment.

ACKNOWLEDGEMENTS

Support for this research was provided by an NIMH Postdoctoral Traineeship in Medical Anthropology, through the Department of Anthropology, Michigan State University. Special thanks are due to my friend and colleague Arthur J. Rubel, who directed my research on *grisi siknis*. I would also like to thank the medical anthropology group at Michigan State, particularly Drs. Geb Blom, Norman Hayner, and Ronald C. Simons. In Nicaragua I would like to thank Dra. Myrna Cunningham and Dr. Tom Shea, as well as Napoleón Chow, Jaime Incer, Lucy Lau, Ramsley Thomas, and Ali Webster.

REFERENCES

Bell, Charles Napier
  1862 Remarks on the Mosquito Territory, Its Climate, People, Productions. . . . Journal of the Royal Geographical Society 32: 242–268.
  1899 Tangweera: Life and Adventures Among Gentle Savages. London: Edward Arnold.
Conzemius, Edward
  1932 Ethnographical Survey of the Miskito and Sumu Indians of Honduras and Nicaragua. Bureau of American Ethnology Bulletin No. 106. Washington, D.C.: U.S. Government Printing Office.
Cross, Shelly Ann
  1975 Investigation of Cultural Beliefs and Practices Concerning Health and Illness: Northeastern Nicaragua. Report submitted to the Office of International Health Affairs, University of Wisconsin.
Dennis, Philip A.
  1981a *Grisi siknis* among the Miskito. Medical Anthropology 5: 445–505.
  1981b The Costeños and the Revolution in Nicaragua. Journal of Interamerican Studies and World Affairs 23: 271–296.
Dubos, René
  1965 Man Adapting. New Haven and London: Yale University Press.
Foulks, Edward F.
  1972 The Arctic Hysterias of the North Alaskan Eskimo. Anthropological Studies No. 10. American Anthropological Association.
Helms, Mary W.
  1968 Matrilocality and the Maintenance of Ethnic Identity: The Miskito of Eastern Nicaragua and Honduras. Verhandlungen des XXXVIII Internationalen Amerikanisten Kongresses. Stuttgart-München.
  1969 The Cultural Ecology of a Colonial Tribe. Ethnology 8: 76–84.
  1971 Asang: Adaptions to Culture Contact in a Miskito Community. Gainesville: University of Florida Press.
  1983 Miskito Slaving and Culture Contact: Ethnicity and Opportunity in an Expanding Population. Journal of Anthropological Research 39: 179–197.
Moravian Church
  1893 Periodical Accounts Relating to the Missions of the Church of the United Brethren Established Among the Heathen. "From H. Peper", December, 1883, pp. 545–546. Moravian College Library, Bethlehem, PA.
Newman, Philip L.
  1964 "Wild Man" Behavior in a New Guinea Community. American Anthropologist 66: 1–19.
Nietschmann, Bernard
  1973 Between Land and Water: The Subsistence Ecology of the Miskito Indians, Eastern Nicaragua. New York and London: Seminar Press.
Rubel, Arthur J.
  1976 Medical Anthropology Reconnaissance of the Miskito Coast of Nicaragua. Mimeograph.
Turner, Victor W.
  1967 A Ndembu Doctor in Practice. In The Forest of Symbols, pp. 359–393. Ithaca and London: Cornell University Press.
Weintraub, Michael I.
  1977 Hysteria: A Clinical Guide to Diagnosis. Clinical Symposia Vol. 29, No. 6. CIBA Pharmacentical Co.

EDWARD F. FOULKS

THE TRANSFORMATION OF *ARCTIC HYSTERIA*

As has been the case with other culture-bound syndromes, the subject of *Arctic hysteria* has been much debated for well over a century. Arctic explorers and adventurers returned from expeditions with many romanticized versions of native life which often included tales of how Eskimos behaved when they became upset. Their descriptions of Eskimos having bizarre tantrums reminded many of the hysterical fits so commonly observed among psychiatric patients studied by Freud and his colleagues at the turn of the century. The outbursts were thus termed the *Arctic hysterias*, and were understood according to prevailing psycho-analytic theories which argued that human psychology was the same worldwide, and that the Eskimo disorder was basically no different than those seen in the clinics of Charcot and Freud.

On the other hand, there were many features of *Arctic hysteria* which appeared to be specifically related to Eskimo life and beliefs. The dramatic descriptions of early explorers provided many colorful examples of the unique mental disorders manifested by these people whose culture differed so much from our own. In the context of a developing tradition of cultural relativism in American anthropology, *Arctic hysteria* was considered a mental disorder specific to the Eskimo, and took its place among other culture-bound syndromes.

The research discussed in this paper indicates that *Arctic hysteria* behavior is culturally patterned, and for centuries has represented stylized Eskimo expressions of overwhelming affect usually generated by interpersonal conflicts. While *Arctic hysteria* can be partially understood in universal psychological terms, a more complete understanding is offered by considerations of the unique framework of Eskimo culture. The ritualized patterns of *Arctic hysteria* behavior repeat themselves and become manifest in various cultural contexts; in the trances and soul trips of the Eskimo shaman; in collective seances; in modern collective charismatic religious services; in expressions of personal distress; and in modern patterns of drinking alcohol. *Arctic hysteria* behavior has meaning to the Eskimo and communicates and confirms a system of beliefs concerning the nature of the human soul.

Many travelers in the Arctic including Cranz (1820), Rink (1875), Bertelsen (1905), R. Peary (1907), Steensby (1910), Whitney (1911), and Rasmussen (1927) reported frequent trance-like episodes of acute onset and short duration which Eskimos called *pibloktoq*. A more recent study conducted by Ehrstrom in Greenland (1951) included a series of 1,073 Eskimos whom he examined for medical and emotional disorders. Of these, he found twenty cases of pure hysteria, presumably of the dissociative or conversion types, twenty-six cases of "kayak phobia" (fear of being alone in the kayak at sea) and eighty-one cases of psychophysiological

307

Ronald C. Simons and Charles C. Hughes (eds.), The Culture-Bound Syndromes, 307–324.
© 1985 *by D. Reidel Publishing Company.*

disorders. He concluded that the incidence of hysterical neurosis was higher, and psychophysiological disorders lower, than among peoples in more intense contact with Western civilization. On the basis of this finding, Parker (1962: 78) speculated that in the past the dramatic forms of *Arctic hysteria* were more common, and that psychophysiological disorders are now becoming increasingly prevalent as more and more contact is maintained with the Western world.

Hysteria has been observed among the Eskimo in other areas of the Arctic as well. The Eskimos of the Hudson Bay region still distinguish hysterial behavior from other forms of behavioral disturbance, such as epilepsy, acute melancholic withdrawal, and depression with paranoid hostility (Vallee 1966). Several cases which Jane Hughes (1960) felt resembled *pibloktoq* were observed among the Eskimos of St. Lawrence Island, Alaska. Her informant related:

Once and awhile X does acting, slapping faces, screwed around. . . . I thought at first she was partly shaman out of mind a little bit I think . . . I've heard something . . . hollering behind me, it was X. I seen her a little bit, she was making faces like that with wrinkled eye, she was winking her one eye so tight and seems to me that part of her face was shrinking. I didn't look, I hates to keep looking at her like this, scared me so much. I think she was out of mind. . . . But few minutes afterwards, she is become Okay (Hughes 1960: 68).

In her survey of the inhabitants of Sivokok, Alaska, she found forty-six individuals neurotic and thirty-five with psychophysiological disorders, which roughly corresponds to the frequencies of these disorders cited by Ehrstrom in Greenland. In addition, there were twenty people with organic brain syndromes, nineteen mentally defectives, and six psychotics. Interestingly, she discovered eighteen who manifested seizures (Hughes 1960).

Regarding *Arctic hysteria* in Alaska, Nachman, a psychologist with the US Public Health Service, reported,

We do not have at present any accurate record of the incidence of hysterical spells which might be closely related to (*Arctic hysteria*), but our clinical experience suggests that they are not infrequent. One typical kind of account is of a teenage girl who has sudden outbursts of excited behavior, sometimes with convulsions or paralysis or anesthesias for which no organic basis can be found, who yells and tears her clothes and performs some bizarre acts, then becomes drowsy, and is later amnesic for the experience. Another is of the man in his 20's or 30's who had spells (again sometimes giving rise to suspicions of convulsive disorders which remain unconfirmed) of sudden violence in which he will tear up the house, shoot up the town, or take off onto the tundra ill-clothed in severe weather.

The documentation of the meaning of such episodes has usually been too fragmentary to permit any definitive statements about them. The fragments, however, suggest that they often serve in the case of the girls, as protests about sexual threats and temptations which cannot safely be acknowledged and in the case of the men, as escapes from humiliations around the inability to meet the responsibilities of married life.

There is still another set of behaviors . . . child beatings which also show many of these characteristics . . . (they have not been studied in Alaska though their occurrence in both white and "native" populations is reported to be high). The essential dynamic here, as in the other kinds of episodes we have considered – is a sudden loss of control in an otherwise reasonable person – frequently with either denial or genuine amnesia for the act afterward –

and in a person who, because of the severe deprivations he has himself suffered and the influx of demands that he cannot meet – reacts with rage and violence at the childishness of the child and its requirement that he himself be a responsible adult (Nachman 1969: 7–11).

On the basis of some of these reports, a number of documentary researchers have proposed several interesting theories to account for the *Arctic hysteria* syndrome. First among these was the noted psychoanalyst and translator of Freud, A. A. Brill. Brill interviewed Peary's lieutenant, Donald MacMillan, regarding his observations of the Eskimos and *pibloktoq* during the attainment of the North Pole. MacMillan remarked that *pibloktoq* reminded him of a little child discouraged and unhappy because he imagined that no one loved him or cared for him and therefore runs away (Brill, 1913: 517). Brill built on this theme in generating his hypothesis and concluded that,

this plainly shows that just as in civilized people, it is love that plays the great part in the causation of the malady . . . the greatest determinant of *pibloktoq* is sex in all its broad ramifications. This, too, corresponds with our psychoanalytic experiences gained among our own women, where contrary to the prevailing opinion of some, the gross sexual (heterosexual intercourse) does not necessarily play the great role in the determination of the hysterical symptoms (Brill, 1913: 518).

Brill concluded that like a child, the Eskimo has not as yet acquired the necessary ego mechanisms for repression of impulses, and therefore no definite line of demarcation between conscious and unconscious exists. Their neuroses are correspondingly not as complicated and hidden as those of "grown-up and intelligent adults".

They may evince themselves in crying spells, screaming spells, or some simple manifestations. . . . There is hardly anything more childish than the imitation of the dog or bird, or the running away into the hills singing or crying. And yet, is there really so much difference between the hysterical mechanisms as evidenced in *pibloktoq* and the grande hysterie or other modern hysterical manifestations? We may answer unhesitatingly that the difference is more apparent than real (Brill, 1913: 519–520).

In a more recent documentary study, Gussow (1960) attempted to define *pibloktoq* and formulate its etiology phenomenologically. Based on many of the cases cited previously in this paper, he summarized the symptomatology into the following categories according to the frequency of their occurrence:

(1) Tearing off of clothing, achieving partial or complete nudity. This was frequently one of the first behavioral signs of the attack.
(2) Glossolalia, "speaking in tongues", making animal sounds.
(3) Fleeing across the tundra, wandering into hills, if outdoors, running back and forth in an agitated state.
(4) Rolling into the snow, placing ice on oneself, jumping into water.
(5) Acts such as attempting to walk on ceiling, hoarding old objects, etc.
(6) Throwing things and thrashing about.
(7) Mimetic acts (Gussow 1960: 226).

Most significant is the fact that during these attacks the individual appears to be in a daze, out of conscious contact with those around him. The episodes last from several minutes to several hours, and are often accompanied or terminated with epileptotetanoid seizures. Carpo-pedal spasms resulting from simultaneous tonic contractions of the flexor and extensor muscles of the forearms and feet are an obvious part of these seizures in photos of a woman going *pibloktoq* which were taken by MacMillan and which are now preserved at the American Museum of Natural History.

The attack is often preceded by irritability, photophobia, confusion and inactive depression for several hours or days. After the episode, the individual is apparently exhausted and often falls off into sleep. Following this, he is again normal mentally and in contact with his surroundings. Routine activities are resumed. There is reportedly amnesia for the event.

Gussow (1960) felt that *pibloktoq* does not represent the behavior of mentally disordered individuals. Instead, he believed it to be the basic way Eskimos in general reacted to situations of intense stress. Food supplies in the winter often were very low or depleted, and Gussow suggested that the Eskimo unconsciously perceived this season as a most insecure and stressful time; thus, the emphasis on rituals such as "The Messenger Feast" during this time of year. Winter was also the time of the shamans, and not unexpectedly the time of going *pibloktoq*.

Like Brill, Gussow emphasized the Eskimo's psychological ability to regress and act out his "infantile" needs for love and emotional support. The frequently reported running off on the ice or tundra was analyzed as the afflicted individual's desire to be pursued and attended to. In other words, the Eskimo is here seen to respond to stress and feelings of helplessness, by resorting to the same expressions of frustration often utilized in our own society, i.e., the temper tantrum.

In a later paper on this subject, Parker (1962) lumped *pibloktoq* with hysterical disorders reported from other societies. He concluded that there were certain practices and beliefs which rendered some societies more hysterogenic than others. He found that hysterical behavior tended to prevail in societies:

(a) Where early socialization experiences are not severe and involve minimal repression of dependency needs and sexual drives. In such societies, where there is relatively high gratification of dependency needs, the modal superego structure will not be severe or rigid.

(b) Where there is an emphasis on communalistic values, a relatively great amount of face-to-face cooperative patterns, and high expectations of mutual aid.

(c) Where the female role involves considerable disadvantages and lower self-esteem compared to the role of the male.

(d) Where the religious system involves beliefs in supernatural possession, and where "hysterical-like" behavior models are provided in the institutionalized religious practices (Parker 1962: 81).

In addition, Parker points out that the shamanistic practices of the Eskimo provide socially-sanctioned outlets for hostility, and in fact, the very role-model for hysterical behavior. Combining this proposition with the notion that *pibloktoq* is a behavior basic to the psychology of the shaman himself, suggests a self-rein-forcing model of basic personality interacting with a social institution.

Wallace (1960) proposed that the *Arctic hysterias* might profitably be investi-gated from still another direction. In discussing the etiology of this mental disorder, he turned attention to the obvious, but for the most part, long overlooked ecologi-cal determinants of psychological functioning. He cited earlier investigators such as Novakovsky (1924), who felt the *Arctic hysterias* were precipitated by such en-vironmental factors as the extreme cold and the "long Polar night" during the win-ter months. A more credible hypothesis was later suggested by two Scandinavian investigators, who studied nutritional deficiencies in Greenland. During a health survey among the Angmaggsalik in 1936–37, Hoygaard (1941: 72) found dietary deficiencies in calcium and also noted the extreme proclivity of these people for "hysterical fits". Baashuus-Jessen (1935) reported epileptotetanoid behavior in dogs (also termed *pibloktoq* by the Eskimos) which he felt was caused by dietary vitamin and mineral deficiencies, principal among these, calcium. Wallace con-sidered that the low calcium diet plus the low vitamin D_3 synthesis during the dark winter months possibly rendered the Eskimo hypocalcemic at this time. Anxiety from chronic stress or sudden fright frequently leads an individual to hyperventilate, which may further lower the levels of ionized serum calcium by raising the pH of the serum. The interaction of these physiological factors was hypothesized to lower serum calcium to levels which could impair the functioning of the central nervous system. In such a state of nervous excitability, normal cognitive functions would become distorted and *pibloktoq* behaviors would ensue. Seizures, and especially tetany which have been reported as terminating the *pibloktoq* episodes, are also commonly associated with symptoms of hypocalcemia.

Wallace's main contribution to this subject was not the mere suggestion of a hypocalcemic diagnosis for *pibloktoq*. It was more far-reaching in nature. It focused for the first time on possible physiological factors involved in mental disorders in non-Western societies, and implied future models of interaction between phy-siological, psychological, cultural, and environmental systems. He rightly recognized that certain diseases and environmental perturbations can affect the functioning of the central nervous system, and thus psychology and behavior itself.

It should be emphasized that such organic formulations by no means negate psychological and historo-cultural determinants of behavior. In fact, Wallace pointed to their articulation by stating that such

incipient neurological dysfunction is susceptible to different interpretations by the victim and his associates and can therefore precipitate different overresponses, depending on parti-cular customs of the individual and group (Wallace 1961: 270).

NORTH ALASKA – 1969

Following Wallace's model, research was conducted in North Alaska during 1969–70. As consulting psychiatrist, I was responsible for administering psychiatric care to communities north of Fairbanks, which included almost all Innuit Eskimos living in Alaska. Also included were Athabascan Indians and whites who were also settled in the northern regions. The position enabled me to review directly cases of mental disorders which occurred among the Innuit from July 1969 through June 1970. Cases were often initially referred from the village health aide who was Eskimo, or from the local school teacher, public health worker, or minister.

Several cases are illustrative of how *Arctic hysteria* behavior is used to express individual distress which resulted from disease and conflicting social events.

Case 1 – Amos

Amos, an Eskimo in his mid-twenties, experienced periodic "spells" since the time of his puberty. Amos' mother was not married at the time of his birth. She had had two previous children, the eldest a boy, and the second child, a girl, four years older than Amos. When Amos was three weeks old, his mother abandoned the three children and went to live in another town. The three children were immediately adopted by a kindly, childless couple. Villagers remarked that the adopting parents were too indulgent and "spoiled" the children by giving in to their every wish. One of the old midwives who was present at Amos' birth remembers that while Amos' mother was in the last three months of her pregnancy, she was "behaving very strangely; she would stare into space". After his birth, however, she was again quite normal. There was no other history on his mother's side of disturbed behavior or supernatural experiences. The situation on his father's side, however, was quite different.

Many of the older people of the village still remember Amos' paternal grandfather. They still speak about "his great power; sometimes he went and acted real crazy; he always talked to the spirits; sometimes he got real wild and would beat his family". Amos' father was said "not to be as powerful as the grandfather, but he was real crazy too. He was real jealous, he'd run after people and fly into a fury; sometimes he'd stay out on the tundra by himself long time." Amos' father also left the village shortly after his son was born. Many people in the city where he eventually settled remember this man and his frequent attacks of "fury". During these times he was said to be fantastically destructive, breaking windows, smashing furniture, at times running out into the street screaming. He was jailed and hospitalized a number of times. Amos never knew either one of his parents personally. He had never met them, although he knew he was adopted and had heard stories about his grandfather and his father's behavior.

Amos' adoptive father was a kind gentleman, who took great interest in his adopted children. He was a religious man of the Presbyterian faith and every night before bed would read a portion of the scripture to the children before they went to sleep. Amos was always a serious youth, very interested in religion; and, for this reason, was said to be his adoptive father's favorite child. Most significant during the period of Amos' latency was the fact that he shared a room with a very old granduncle who had been infirm and confined to bed for many years. Amos would spend hours with this old man, "That man taught me a lot about old-fashioned ways; he told me where power comes from; he told me how to get it; then he died". Amos states that shortly after the death of this old man, supernatural things began to happen to him:

Things that I can't explain, that nobody really believes. When I was ten years old my father told me to fill a can with gasoline. I went out and looked at the gasoline drum; it was big; it was too heavy; I couldn't budge it. I knew my father wanted me to do that, so I got down on my hands and knees and prayed to God. Suddenly a spirit entered my body and I felt strong all over; it was a miracle; I could pick up the whole drum overy my head (he demonstrated with his arms); and I was only a boy. Ever since that time supernatural things happen to me; when I'm alone, out on the tundra, hunting for caribou, sometimes my mind leaves me, I become strong; this has happened two or three times a year, since I've been ten years old.

As a youth, Amos had severe otitis media. Pus drained chronically from both ears; however, in adulthood the condition subsided. When he was twelve or thirteen years old he was hit on the head by a chunk of ice and knocked unconscious. He went to school to the eighth grade and was then separated from his family and sent to a boarding school to continue his education. While there he experienced, "communications in my mind, which tell me to go to preach the Scriptures to all the people. The communications told me where to go and where to preach; it was like a voice, but it was in my mind."

While a student at the boarding school he experienced a severe fall from a bicycle. A witness mentioned that he thought he had a seizure when he fell and that he was "crazy like and real sick" after he fell. He returned to the village and resumed hunting caribou, seal and whale, and trapping. One day in 1966, Amos was on a boat trip with a number of other men. While at sea in a skin boat (umiak) Amos "became unmanageable, throwing his arms and legs around and frothing at the mouth". The crew members restrained him and started to take him back to the village. After a while Amos started feeling better and persuaded the men to continue the trip. Amos had no memory whatsoever for this episode.

Amos had heard so much about his father that during the summer of 1967 he decided to go to the city and find him. When he arrived he was told that several weeks previously his father had gone into a rage, and had been throwing furniture around his small home. Something had happened to ignite a fire and his father had burned to death and the house had burned down. Amos returned immediately to the village; there he became even more engrossed in the Presbyterian Church. He developed a very close attachment to an Eskimo man who was an ordained minister of the Church. He was around the Church constantly. During this time Amos also became enamored of a young woman named Lilly. She was a very immature woman, afraid to go outside, preferring to be with her parents constantly. Amos and Lilly became very close to one another, and developed such an intense dependency that mutual jealousy was a constant issue even if one of them casually glanced or conversed with another person. They slept together and Lilly became pregnant.

After an illness, the Eskimo minister died. Amos did not grieve, however; instead one evening, when discussing hunting with his wife and her family, he made some veiled comments about what it would be like to freeze on the tundra. The family did not take him seriously, as he had always been a good hunter and knew his way around. As it is dark most of the time during that period of the year, villagers do not remember just what time of day he set out. Several hours later, however, his dog team returned to the village with an empty sled. They thought little of it, as it was common to have dog teams get away and return home on their own. But, after he did not return to the village within several hours, search parties were organized. He was finally found in the dark walking away from the lights of the village. He seemed to be in a daze; they had difficulty in convincing him to return home. He remarked that "I was called by God". He felt called by God, and since the Eskimo minister died, he felt that it was he who should be the spiritual leader of his people.

In June his daughter was born. People say that Amos was in a disgruntled mood most of the day. Apparently his mother-in-law early one morning insisted that he cut ice so that it could be melted for water. He did not respond, so she began to nag him to get busy and to make jokes about his masculinity. Finally, he went to his adoptive father to borrow the snowmobile; he said "these Pentecostal people are so bossy". Several hours later he returned with the river ice. He was obviously quite agitated. After unloading the ice he entered the house and with a scream grabbed his throat with both hands and tried to strangle himself. After being stopped, he dashed out of the house and went to his adoptive parents' home. He returned that evening apparently in his full senses. He stated that he remembered what happened quite well and goes on to tell:

About 12:00 a.m., I was lying in bed with my wife and had a vision. I don't know whether anyone can understand this, but here's the way it went. I walking through a town that looked a lot like our village, there was a church and a graveyard nearby. All the people in town were out drunk, drinking whiskey and fighting with each other and doing all kinds of things and I was watching this; and there were also some people running around on top of the graves who came from the town. Then I saw other people coming up from the graves, rising from the dead; this was a vision. I saw them drinking and fighting. At first I didn't feel anything at all; I felt like I was right there, but I wasn't doing what they were doing. I had no feeling about it at all. Then I felt that all these people were evil.

He got out of bed and began to ask others in the household why they did not get up. By this time it was 12:00 a.m. He ran to his adoptive father's house and asked them to get up. His father thought that he was acting like he was drunk; but he could smell no liquor on his breath. Amos began praying and rocking; he then got up and began to beat his wife and his father on the head. His brother-in-law came in, and the family was able to restrain him. They said, "He had foam in his mouth". They held him until 7:00 in the morning when he finally went to sleep. While he slept people sat with him and watched him. They took turns until the next day. At about one o'clock the village health aide attempted to arouse him. He responded only with nods or shakes of his head. About five minutes later he suddenly "came to" fighting, and had a seizure with lots of foaming and saliva coming out of his mouth. After being subdued he went back to sleep.

He spent the following five months at the Alaska Psychiatric Institute. During that time staff noted that he had "spells" on three occasions. Apparently, when he became annoyed or angry "he would suddenly fall backwards on to the bed or floor. His body would become rigid, with his arms outstretched and he was biting as hard as he could". There was no loss of consciousness or incontinence; there were no clonic convulsive movements. During one of these spells he was given intravenous valium (a tranquilizer). He believed it to be truth serum and soon began to talk about how to beat his wife "because she really loves others and not me". He was returned to the village in December. At that time he was described by villagers as being extremely "docile". He had been away from his wife and child and family. It was noted that after his return from the hospital "he no longer acted like a man".

He never again went out hunting or trapping, but perferred to stay at home or walk about the village. He was cajoled and nagged constantly to act "like a man". He was always friendly and communicative, but seemingly had lost all confidence in himself to act independently. He became even more dependent upon his wife and his mother-in-law, and moved his things into his mother-in-law's house. He openly expressed his desire to be taken care of by his mother-in-law. She and a number of other people in the village began to jest and make fun of him, making jokes about "Amos is now a woman; he acts like a woman". Then he said, "I am going to get a place of my own; I'm going to take my wife and baby to live in my own house; there's a place I know that's going to be empty soon; maybe I can rent it. I'm going to get a job and make money and then become a minister." One night soon afterward, Amos was seen coming out of his room carrying an ulu (an Eskimo knife). He appeared dazed and would not respond to his father's inquiries. He walked "like a zombie" out the door, heading for his mother-in-law's house. His father grabbed him and called for help. A number of men were aroused and came to his aid. All said that Amos "had the strength of ten men; he had supernatural strength". When he awoke he said, "My wife doesn't want me any more; she wants someone else; I know she loves someone else. I don't know who it is. Everyone in the village hates me. They all want to get rid of me; no one wants me." For several days Amos had episodes of sitting up in bed with a fixed stare on his face, or rocking back and forth on his hands and knees. He was unable to communicate during these episodes. While in this state he would often tie his pajama tops around his neck and pull them tight. This would usually result in some rapid breathing and a red face on his part. He was not restrained during any of these spells and they would characteristically last only thirty to forty-five minutes.

Soon, in addition to his mother-in-law's calling him a "woman", many of the villagers would mock him in his presence. They would discuss lurid details of what Amos looked like during his convulsions. Amos isolated himself more and more from village life. Many people began to make obtuse statements along the

lines of "maybe next time you go out into the tundra alone, we won't find you". He
was psychologically ostracized; no one would have much to do with him. However,
they did talk to Lilly. He was torn between leaving the security of the village of his
boyhood where he was now obviously unwanted, or staying and enduring the mock-
ing and derision of family and village members. His wife and her mother joined in,
and berated Amos for having the "thoughts of a woman". He expressed to me, as
each day went by, an increasing shame about his wife, his mother-in-law, and other
people in the village talking about him behind his back, talking about the fact that
he is no longer a hunter and that he has "the thoughts of a woman."

He finally separated from his wife and child and his mother-in-law and went
to live with his adoptive father. He remained alone in his room most of the time
and did not bother to communicate with others. Several weeks later, he took
an ice pick and carved two long lacerations down the palmar surface of his left
forearm. He bled profusely, but he called for no help. Instead, several days later
he showed me his arm and said that "It was sort of a suicide attempt; God has
required that I suffer in this world". His again retreated into his room and became
uncommunicative. One month later, just before Christmas, he left a note with
his father, addressed to his wife. It read, "I am going for a long, long walk". Following this, he went down to the beach winter trail, heading for another village
about one hundred miles distant. He was found about an hour later, heading
back toward the village along the well-traveled winter path. When he returned
to the village he was noticeably agitated. He exhibited gross tremor of both hands
and he stammered a great deal during the conversation. He told me that he had
been bothered a long time by thoughts that while he was away from his house
his wife was spending time with her alleged boyfriend. He had no one in particular
in mind to accuse of consorting with his wife, but said that they must be "teenagers.
Even they are more manly than me." He said:

Since Lilly and I been married we never been alone; we've always lived with her mother or
my father. They watched me and they watched her. There is a house here which is owned
by a relative who might rent it to us. I think it would be in the right direction if we moved
in there. I feel I've never been a good trapper or hunter, anyway, this kind of work sometimes
leaves a woman and her family unprovided for. If I could become a missionary, I'd have a job
in the village that would give me steady pay and keep me busy.

One might speculate that in times past Amos' power may have been accepted
and confirmed by his fellow villagers. Today, his academic inabilities to achieve
formal missionary status in the church are a painful demonstration of his personal
inadequacies and lack of power. Because of this, he is not accepted as a church
leader whereas, in times past, he may very well have been accepted as a powerful
shaman. This poses an obvious dilemma to the observer in delineating the sources
of Amos' psychological difficulties. Is Amos' sense of superiority and grandiostiy
since childhood years in itself psychopathological? Seemingly, in times past, Amos
may have experienced no incongruence between the way he saw himself and the
way others saw him. In today's society, however, there is no room for a shaman.

Psychological testing was done on Amos at the University of Alaska and the profiles of the Minnesota Multiphasic Personality Inventory were analyzed. His profiles indicated superficial friendliness, but fear of close emotional involvement with others, and a tendency to keep psychological distance between himself and others. They indicated his sensitivity to environmental demands and his avoidance of any situation where his performance would not be considered better than the performance of others. There was also indication that under stress he has the tendency to lose control and act out in "circumscribed" paranoid episodes.

Case 2 – Akek

Akek is an eight-year-old North Alaskan Eskimo girl who occasionally without warning throws violent fits. She shouts, she strikes out at others, falls to the floor screaming and kicking, then has trembling and contracting of her arms and legs. The episodes last about five minutes and have occurred several times a year usually during November and January for the past several years.

Akek's family is "very old-fashioned". Her parents are first cousins and speak only Inupiat. They live in a two-room plywood shack. This household is very crowded; the parents sleep on the floor. The family is subjected to much gossip and derisive joking because of their poor economic status. Akek's father cannot provide for his family the meat and clothing considered adequate by most other villagers. Akek is very shy and retiring; even with her peers she says almost nothing, prefers not to be seen; in school she never says a word. Because of joking and mockery from others, the family stay to themselves inside the house. In fact, the parents are said to be afraid of people and they do not allow their children out of the house often.

This family's poor economic condition is generally reflected in their state of poor health. Akek's mother has borne ten children; four of them died in early childhood from respiratory infections. The remaining six children have also been ravaged by respiratory infections and all have long medical histories of chronic drainage from the ears.

School teachers have observed that several of Akek's attacks have occurred after what they assumed was an episode of extreme shyness and embarrassment at being called upon to recite in class. She is so shy and retiring that is difficult to gain any impression of her capabilities. Her art work and design copy, however, indicate perceptual abilities and motor abilities which do not differ from peers and the content and execution of figures on the drawings are age appropriate (Gesell et al. 1940).

Akek suffers from epilepsy. Her seizures have gained her the care and special attention of a white missionary and a Bureau of Indian Affairs teacher who have taken a special interest in "praying that Jesus will take away her affliction". Akek's relation with her siblings is much the same as with her peers. She is scapegoated because she is shy, passive, and retiring. She is easily made the brunt of many jokes and is pushed around by the older, more aggressive children. She is frequently hurt, and cries.

Akek has felt rather neglected and inadequately provided for by parents who have endured many hardships themselves. Furthermore, she is frequently ashamed, put upon, pushed around, and bullied by siblings and peers. This further substantiates basic feelings of inferiority and inadequacy. When confronted by older people whom she considers overwhelmingly powerful and adequate, especially white people, her own smallness, insignificance, and ineptitudes are further emphasized. She withdraws for fear that her weaknesses will be exposed, that she will be asked a question she cannot answer, that the white doctor will find her wanting, and that others will find her stupid. Inwardly she resents being pushed around, yet she can do little to stop this cycle of events. Her seizures afford her some care, concern, and attention she would otherwise not receive, and to a certain extent, give her a supernatural or religious countenance, since many of the religious Eskimos and white people pray to Jesus for the removal of this symptom. The symptom also affords her an escape from the anxiety and conflict-ridden situation of the classroom. While in a "lapsed state" she is beyond the torments and mockery of others.

Eight additional cases of individuals who experienced *Arctic hysteria* behavior were also studied during fieldwork in 1969, and events in their lives are summarized with Amos' and Akek's in Table I.

The most consistently occurring events in the life histories of the ten North Alaskan Eskimos who manifested *Arctic hysteria*-like behavior were: (1) being raised by tradition-oriented elders who in many cases related experiences of past human powers or shamanism; (2) having themselves felt religiously or supernaturally inspired; (3) having been shamed and ridiculed by elders and peers which frequently resulted in a shy, retiring, suspicious characterological position. Many wished to escape from the village, yet felt too strange and insecure going anywhere else. They were essentially double-bound in a conflict-ridden social situation. Most felt alone in facing their social difficulties after the death or illness of, or abandonment by, close relatives.

There are many differences among our ten subjects. They vary greatly in age. Both sexes are represented. Some have demonstrable, underlying cerebral impairments. A few sustained their attacks at the real or threatened loss of a loved one. Others demonstrated psychopathology which transcended their seemingly isolated attacks of *Arctic hysteria*-like behavior. All of them, however, were threatened or were actually unable to maintain a way of life that was gratifying socially. Case 3 (Kajat) faced the possibility of having to give up a traditional way of life he had known for so long by the removal and near fatal illness of his wife. Case 1 (Amos) unsuccessfully sought an identity as a religious leader; in doing so he failed to follow the ways of the village hunters and whalers and was considered a "woman". Case 8 (Sautak) withdrew into himself and likewise was not considered a participating, external member of the community. Case 9 (Tesogat) withdrew to an equal degree from the mainstream of his society, perhaps because of the

TABLE I
Life history events

	Case number									
	1	2	3	4	5	6	7	8	9	10
Adopted or abandoned by parents	X	0	0	0	X	0	X	0	0	X
Influenced by "old-fashioned" elders	X	X	X	X	X	0	X	?	X	X
Shamanistic associations	X	?	X	?	?	0	X	?	?	?
Religious or supernatural experiences	X	?	?	X	?	0	X	0	X	X
Sexual or spouse jealousy	X	–	0	0	–	X	0	0	0	0
Shamed by peers	X	X	0	X	X	X	X	X	X	X
Shy and suspicious of peers	X	X	0	X	X	X	X	X	X	X
Loss of significant support of wife, etc.	X	0	X	0	X	X	X	0	0	0
Family ridiculed and ostracized from village	0	X	0	0	X	0	0	X	X	0
Family history of hysterical behavior	X	0	0	0	0	0	0	X	0	0

X = presence of event in life history of individual.
0 = absence of event.

liabilities of hearing loss. Case 7 (Montak) and Case 6 (Sanraq) were attracted to modern Western ways, yet could not feel wholly comfortable away from their village. They fit into neither way of life. Case 10 (Nirik) could not behave as a normal Eskimo girl because of her fear of sexual contact. Case 2 (Akek), Case 4 (Matamuk), and Case 5 (Kalagik) could not maintain a normal Eskimo way of life because of organic difficulties. All of these individuals at some point experienced the anxiety of being inadequate and helpless in maintaining a way of life that others in their village would find acceptable and admirable. They were insecure as to their identity and place in their society. They felt their inadequacies intensely, and feared others would also see their weaknesses. They were shameful at not being able to live up to a "meaningful" way of life. The gossip, ridicule, and joking that followed many of these individuals from childhood on could do nothing but reinforce their shameful feelings. None had the feeling he had sinned or had transgressed. There was nothing to be guilty about even for Case 4 (Montak), who had tried to eat her baby. Instead, all felt impaired, weak, or inadequate, and were ashamed of their "lack of manliness", or their being "different", or not "fitting in". They felt inadequate in their own eyes, and in the eyes of others. Many constantly feared being seen and exposed.

They wished for escape, somewhere to hid, from themselves and others.

ANALYSIS: THE CULTURAL MEANINGS OF *ARCTIC HYSTERIA*

The traditional Eskimo way of life was highly specialized and adaptive to living in the Arctic. Deviance from those time-tested ways perhaps realistically endangered a group's survival. Adherence to these ways ensured food, shelter, and cooperative relations with others most of the time. No society, however, is able to meet all the needs, or solve all the conflicts of its members. In Eskimo society, personal expression outside the prescribed channels was usually met with ridicule and joking. Eskimos, however, did recognize "soul trips" or mental dissociations as legitimate behaviors which did solve many practical and personal problems through magical beliefs. These soul trips were recognized as being beyond the personal control and responsibility of the individual. The prototype for this dissociative behavior was present throughout the life of the growing Eskimo child in the personage of the shaman.

Before Christianity, soul trips took place collectively during the Bladder Festival, the Messenger Feast, and at the whaling festivals. These were not only occasions for night-long chanting and expressive dancing, but were also occasions where one could vent himself personally against another through an established traditional ritual, such as a song contest, or a contest of muscular strength and coordination. Such outlets were also provided collectively and individually during times of psychological or social stress through the shaman's seance. The Eskimos generally considered that everyone had a bit of shamanistic power, some having more than others. Power was the basis for being formally initiated into the ancient arts of shamanism. In addition to various devices, skills, and tricks in the shaman's repertoire, he was also an individual who was able to completely "lose his soul". During such a performance, a shaman would appear to lose control of his senses, scream the sounds of animals, dash about quite wildly, and even proceed to convulsions. The cathartic value of such an outburst, whether experienced directly or vicariously, would obviously have considerable emotional value to a people bound by their roles to proper Eskimo behavior, unable to otherwise release frustrations, dissatisfactions, and angry feelings to one another. The behavior manifest by the shaman, by the Eskimo with epilepsy, and by the Eskimo with *Arctic hysteria* is often quite similar. Mutual relationships may exist between them. This is not to say that shamans are epileptics, or shamans have *Arctic hysteria*, or *Arctic hysteria* is epilepsy, but that shamanistic performances during times of group stress provided a model for the participants. This model could be used in times of personal stress. Since the near demise of shamanism, transformed versions of these behaviors have persisted although often unconnected consciously to their original source.

THE SHAMAN'S BEHAVIOR: TRADITIONAL PATTERNS OF BEHAVIOR UNDER STRESS

Shamanistic behavior serves as a model and is central to understanding *Arctic hysteria* and its recent transformations. The social contexts and cultural meanings attributed to the shaman's soul-loss provide the Eskimo with a hypothesis regarding the nature of his own experience of distress as well as a mechanism for expressing his conflict to others.

Shamans became most active in holding seances to demonstrate their power during the dark winter months of November, December, and January. Today the month of November in Eskimo is called Uvluilaq Taatquq, the moon of short days. In the past this period was known as Kiyeevilwik, the time when the shamans get busy (Spencer 1959: 304). The shaman would summon the community when illness, food shortage, bad weather, or other mishaps occurred. Often the meeting would result in a seance which commenced with the shaman beating his drum and chanting his own powerful songs in an intense rhythmic fashion. With the darkness, the heat and stuffiness of the crowded situation in the house, and the rising tempo of drumming and chanting, the group would often become spellbound and somewhat fearfully in awe of what was to happen. At such a point, the shaman often stopped his frenzied beats and lapsed into trance-like silence. Voices of spirits would be heard at this time calling from doorways and the roof, often in the tones of his tunraq, a wolf or bear growl. Such a trance might continue for many hours. When the shaman was seen to move again, it was thought that his soul was returning. Often the performances became extremely frenzied, with the shaman wildly dancing about, his eyes rolling back, his clothes ripped off and his body sweating profusely. Intimidated audiences agreed, "he was a devil", he acted like crazy" (Spencer 1959: 307).

Today, people in North Alaska profess to be Christians and generally will say little about shamans. As late as the mid 1950s, however, it was said that there was an old woman at Wainwright who practiced shamanism (Spencer 1959: 381). Milan's informant, Iqaaq, told him about a tunraq of a dead shaman who lived near the village of Atanik, who would cry out when people went past during the winter. He was felt to be dangerous. He also told of a large stone at Tutulivik, three miles from Wainwright, that once had been a shaman. People would bring offerings of meat and blubber to gain good luck in hunting (Milan 1964: 69). It is well known that many people have had considerable experience with shamans in the recent past.

The psychological realities experienced by the shaman formed an Eskimo theory of how the world and how human beings work. As Kroeber long ago observed:

The traditional person may "not really fail to discriminate the objective from the subjective, the normally natural from the supernatural. He distinguishes them much as we do. He merely weights or favors the supernatural, as we disfavor and try to exclude it. The voice of the dead, the dream, and the magic act stand out from him from the run of commonplace experience of reality much as they do for us; but he endows them with a quality of special superreality and desirability, we of unreality and undesirability. The values have changed, rather than the perception. And values are cultural facts." (Kroeber 1952: 313).

NORTH ALASKA, 1979: MODERN TRANSFORMATIONS

The last decade has brought many dramatic changes to Eskimo life in North Alaska. Oil production commenced in their land at Prudoe Bay, and a road and pipeline

were constructed linking their territory to the industrial south, and bringing shifts
from a subsistence to a cash economy for the majority of Eskimos. Parallel with
these developments has been a major introduction of technology, consumer goods,
and complex financial institutions with the consequent bureaucratization of
Eskimo life.

We continued our research in North Alaska in 1979, and discovered an emerging
pattern of behavior under stress, this time associated with alcohol. We found
that a traditional segment of Eskimo society adhered to a transformed version
of *Arctic hysteria* behaviors in their use of alcohol, whereas another segment,
more prepared for social change, has acquired an alcohol use pattern similar to
that of the urban U.S.

Drinking alcohol for the traditional group involves an attempt by many to
reach a state of intoxication as rapidly as possible, wherein they occasionally
become frenzied, get into fights with others, and at times go outside improperly
clothed to run away over the frozen tundra. Traumatic injury and sometimes
death results from these intensely intoxicated episodes. For survivors, there is
often loss of memory regarding the event and the explanation that, "I must have
been out of my mind", or "the spirits got to me".

Leach (1971) likens the persistence of traditional microstructures, in the face
of change in social macrostructures, to an image on a piece of rubber which when
stretched distorts the picture, while the elements of the pattern remain in a consistent relationship. The original patterns of soul loss are now stretched and distorted, but are still recognizable in the state of intoxication. Many Eskimos have
consciously and unconsciously persisted in conforming to traditional cultural
patterns and social relations. The seasonal migrations of animal life were expressed
in beliefs about transmigrations and transformations of the human soul. Psychological, rather than chemical, methods were used to obtain the altered state
of consciousness associated with these transformations. Against this traditional
background, we can now interpret the social and symbolic meanings inherent
in the particular manner in which alcohol is used by Eskimos today. The patterns
of behavior associated with *Arctic hysteria* persist in modern transformations
of traditional shamanistic behaviors now expressed in alcoholism, but continuing
to manifest the anxieties of Eskimo life.

REFERENCES

Aberle, D.
   1952 *Arctic Hysteria* and *Latah* in Mongolia. Transactions of the New York Academy
         of Science 14: 7: 294–297.
Ackerknecht, E.
   1943 Psychopathology, Primitive Medicine and Primitive Culture. Bulletin of the History
         of Medicine 14.
Banhuus-Jessen, J.
   1935 Arctic Nervous Diseases. Veterinary Journal 91: 339–350, 379–390.

Bertelsen, A.
  1905 Neuro. Patologiske Mendelelser fra Grønland. Copenhagen: Bibliotak for Laeger
        6: 109–135, 280–335.
Brill, A.
  1913 *Pibloktoq* or Hysteria among Peary's Eskimos. Journal of Nervous and Mental Disease
        40: 514–520.
Burch, E. S., Jr.
  1975 Eskimo Kinsmen: Changing Family Relationships in Northwest Alaska. New York:
        West Publishing Company.
Cranz, D.
  1829 History of Greenland. London: Longman, Hurst, Reis, Olme, and Brown.
Ehrstrom, M.
  1951 Medical Investigations in North Greenland, 1948–1949. Acta Medica Scandanavia
        140: 11: 254–264.
Gubser, N.
  1965 Nunamiut Eskimos: Hunters of Caribou. New Haven: Yale University Press.
Gussow, Z.
  1960 *Pibloktoq* (Hysteria) among the Polar Eskimo: An Ethno-Psychiatric Study. *In*
        I. W. Muensterberger and S. Axelrod (eds.), Psychoanalysis and the Social Sciences.
        New York: International Universities Press.
Hall, II.
  1918 A Siberian Wilderness: Native Life and the Lower Yanisei. Geographical Review
        5(a): 1–21.
Hoygaard, A.
  1941 Studies on the Nutrition and Physiopathology of Eskimos. Skrifter Utgitt Av Det
        Norske Videnskaps-Akademi I Oslo: Mat.-Naturv. Klasse No. 9.
Hughes, J.
  1960 An Epidemiological Study of Psychopathology in an Eskimo Village. Ph.D. disserta-
        tion, Cornell University.
Katz, S.
  1972 Genealogy and Historical Demography of the North Slope. Data collected from the
        Naval Arctic Research Laboratory and Census Information, unpublished.
Kroeber, A.
  1952 Psychosis or Social Sanction. *In* The Nature of Culture. Chicago: University of
        Chicago Press.
Laubscher, B.
  1937 Sex, Custom and Psychopathology, A Study of South African Pagan Natives. London:
        Routledge & Kegan Paul Ltd.
Leach, E. R.
  1971 Rethinking Anthropology. New York: Humanities Press.
Milan, F.
  1964 The Acculturation of the Contemporary Eskimo of Wainwright Alaska. Anthropo-
        logical Papers of the University of Alaska 11: 2: 1–97.
Murphy, J.
  1964 Psychotherapeutic Aspects of Shamanism on St. Lawrence Island, Alaska. *In* A. Kiev
        (ed.), Magic, Faith and Healing: Studies in Primitive Psychiatry Today. New York:
        Free Press of Glencoe.
Nachman, B.
  1969 Fits, Suicides, Beatings and Time-Out. Anchorage, Alaska: Alaska Native Service,
        U.S. Public Health Service.
Parker, S.
  1962 Eskimo Psychopathology. American Anthropologist 64: 76–96.

Peary, R.
   1907 Nearest the Pole. New York: Doubleday.
Rasmussen, K.
   1927 Across Arctic America: Narrative of the Fifth Thule Expedition. New York: G. P.
        Putnam's Sons.
Rink, H.
   1875 Tales and Traditions of the Eskimos. Edinburgh & London: Wm. Blackwood &
        Sons.
Spencer, R. F.
   1959 The North Alaskan Eskimo: A Study in Ecology and Society. Bureau of American
        Ethnology, Bulletin 171. Washington, D.C.: Smithsonian Institution Press.
Steensby, H.
   1910 Contributions to the Ethnology and Anthropology of the Polar Eskimo. Medelelser
        on Grønland.
Turner, V.
   1977 The Ritual Process: Structure and Anti-Structure. Ithaca, New York: Cornell
        University Press.
Vallee, F.
   1966 Eskimo Theories of Mental Illness in the Hudson Bay Region. Anthropologica N.S.
        8: 53–84.
Wallace, A. F. C.
   1960 An Interdisciplinary Approach to Mental Disorder Among the Polar Eskimo of
        Northwest Greenland. Anthropologica 11: 2: 1–12.
Whitney, H.
   1911 Hunting with the Eskimo. New York: Century Press.

CHARLES C. HUGHES

THE RUNNING TAXON

Commentary

The central and most dramatic symptom of this taxonic grouping of behaviors is that the victim breaks out of his world of normal social routines and expectations with a sudden flight into a dissociated world. Sometimes it is a literal running off, sometimes simply a mental withdrawal (as in Foulks's cases). But regardless of which type is chosen, there is a period of retreat, of "time out" from reality and short while in which the person performs bizarre acts (e.g., tearing off clothing) and utters phrases not normally permitted or usually heard. Occasionally violence will occur, seemingly directed at those nearby. During the attack the person is oblivious to events and other persons around him and afterwards, collapsing from exhaustion, does not remember (ostensibly at least) what happened.

Several diagnostic categories appear potentially relevant to any given case, for example, Atypical Dissociative Disorder, which as indicated earlier includes ". . . those individuals who appear to have a Dissociative Disorder but do not satisfy the criteria for a specific Dissociative Disorder. Examples include trance-like states, derealization unaccompanied by depersonalization . . ." (p. 260). With some of the cases of this type of "culture-bound syndrome" reported in the literature (usually under the label of *pibloktoq*) another seemingly relevant diagnostic category is Intermittent Explosive Disorder:

. . . several discrete episodes of loss of control of aggressive impulses that result in serious assault or destruction of property. For example, with no or little provocation the individual may suddenly start to hit strangers or throw furniture. The degree of aggressivity expressed during an episode is grossly out of proportion to any precipitating psychosocial stressor. The individual may describe the episodes as "spells" or "attacks". The symptoms appear within minutes or hours and, regardless of duration, remit almost as quickly. Genuine regret or self-reproach at the consequences of the action and the inability to control the aggressive impulse may follow each episode. There are no signs of generalized impulsivity or aggressiveness between the episodes (pp. 295–296).

In addition, again with a given case, the victim's purported inability to recall events might be registered with Psychogenic Amnesia (300.12) or Factitious Disorders with Psychological Symptoms (300.16).

But let us look at an instance from what is perhaps the prototypic example of disorders of this type in the culture-bound literature, *pibloktoq*. Case #5 from Gussow's article (p. 273 above) might be framed in the DSM-III format as follows:

Axis I: 312.35 Intermittent Explosive Disorder ("Suddenly he began to kick the dogs. . . . He tore all the stuff off the sleds, skins, boxes, stoves, and hurled them at the dogs. It lasted about ten minutes. . . . It didn't

325

Ronald C. Simons and Charles C. Hughes (eds.), The Culture-Bound Syndromes, 325–326.
© 1985 *by D. Reidel Publishing Company.*

do much harm to the dogs, in fact, nothing at all. . . . All of a sudden
it was over." (Provisional)

(*Note*: the data given here do not suggest one way or the other whether
this was a single episode in the person's life or a characteristic feature
(which it is usually reported to be). If the latter, the above diagnosis
might be the more applicable one. If it was a single episode, however,
the diagnosis Isolated Explosive Disorder might be the more appropriate
one, even though its behavioral definition does not closely enough
correspond to the data presented here to make one comfortable in
using it. See the discussion of Isolated Explosive Disorder under commentary to the "Sudden Mass Assault" taxon.)

Axis II: Insufficient data
Axis III: None
Axis IV: *Psychosocial stressors*: insufficient data
            Severity: 0
Axis V: *Highest level of adaptive functioning past year*: 2 − Very Good (Opera-
            tional definition: Better than average functioning in social relations,
            occupational functioning, and use of leisure time. The person in the
            case report was ". . . always friendly, untalkative, but reliable fellow".)

PART III

FOLK ILLNESSES USUALLY LISTED AS CULTURE-BOUND PSYCHIATRIC SYNDROMES WHICH SHOULD PROBABLY NO LONGER BE SO CONSIDERED

A. THE FRIGHT ILLNESS TAXON

INTRODUCTION: *THE FRIGHT ILLNESS TAXON*

Much of the confusion about culture-bound psychiatric syndromes is attributable
to the fact that, as traditionally used, the category is too heterogenous to say
anything meaningful about. Thus, for example, though most of the entities here
grouped into the *Fright Illness Taxon* have at one time or another been listed
with the culture-bound psychiatric syndromes, they appear to be phenomena of
a radically different order.

The papers in this section describe folk illnesses which, unlike the members
of other taxa, do not include either a specific alteration of experienced reality
or any specific altered behavior. The paper by Rubel, O'Nell, and Collado describes
the well-known folk illness, *susto*, widespread in one or another form in Latin
America. It is a summary of a series of studies which is reported more extensively in their recent book.[1] As the authors point out, the unifying characteristic
responsible for the folk grouping is the attribution of a variety of illnesses and
misfortunes to a previous frightening or startling experience. It is not necessarily
the person who suffered the fright or startle who develops *susto*; it may be a
relative or close acquaintance. And as they mention in a footnote, in one case
the experience considered to be the cause of an illness occurred some thirty
years before its onset! The authors find a wide variety of somatic illnesses to
be indigenously attributed to previous frightening or startling experiences and
they note that *susto* does not represent any form of psychological disfunction,
"thus it is totally unwarranted to explain the susto illness as evidence of emotional
pathology". A reading of their cases bears this out, some of them strikingly. For
example, in case one a sleep disturbance in a 15 day old infant was attributed
to the fact that while pregnant, her mother rescued a companion who had fallen
into a stream. In another of their cases, a discharge from the ear is attributed to
a fright: "that was how the ear condition appeared; it came from the fright".
Reviewing the *susto* literature, Rubel et al. note that some previous authors as
well have suggested that "*susto* may be an indigenous label applied to physical
diseases unrecognized by those using the label". About half of their own study
population used the history of an antecedent fright to account for a variety of
illness states.

Dobkin de Rios, who worked in the Peruvian Amazon, comes to a similar
conclusion about *saladera*: "This syndrome is perceived by patients to take the
form of constant and continuing misfortune and bad luck". Reading the "presenting symptom" in the ten cases she tabulated, one does not find anything
suggestive of a psychiatric syndrome, even chronic anxiety or depression. Rather,
like *susto*, *saladera* appears to be an indigenous explanation for a heterogeny of
misfortunes. That *saladera* patients visit a healer reflects the fact that in many

Ronald C. Simons and Charles C. Hughes (eds.), The Culture-Bound Syndromes, 329–331.

societies physical, psychological, and other types of misfortune are not parceled out to specialized helpers. Unlike *susto, lanti*, and *mogo laya, saladera* (the spelling with one "r" is correct [personal is communication, M.D.d.R., 1984]) is not actually a *Fright Illness*, since the antecedent to which *saladera* is attributed is not a fright or startle. Dr. de Rios's paper is included in this section of the present volume because like the other folk illnesses described here, it is defined by its attribution rather than by its symptoms. It is especially interesting to compare and contrast it with *susto* because of the many features shared by their host cultures.

The late Donn Hart's description of *lanti* in the Philippines is strikingly similar. He introduces his paper with a description of an illness in a two-year-old girl which was attributed to her father's having been frightened or startled two days earlier when he almost stepped on a snake. The little girl was not with him. Hart gives the most frequent symptoms of *lanti* as high fever, boils and skin eruptions rather than any experiential or behavioral alteration. As in the Latin American cases reported by Rubel et al., what unifies his cases is their indigenous attribution to an antecedent fright or startle. As in the Latin American cases, the sufferer need not be the person experiencing the frightening or startling stimulus. Hart describes culture-specific rules explaining who can and who cannot acquire the illness as a result of someone else's experience. The bulk of the paper concerns such issues as preventative measures and traditional cures, especially the later. Hart makes the revealing comment, "traumatic emotional experience (fright or fear (or startle)) is also given as the reason for some skin aliments and boils, fever, convulsions, measles or digestive upsets". The relationship of the indigenous explanatory system to the more generally pervasive belief in imitative magic is well described, as is its use for social control.

The last paper, an edited extract from Stephen Frankel's doctoral dissertation, describes *mogo laya*, a folk illness of the Huli people of Papua, New Guinea. The Huli also attribute a variety of illness states to an antecedent frightening experience; "mogo laya" is the Huli word for startle. How this belief about illness causation is imbedded in the Huli social context is well described. Frankel's analysis is that though similar "fright illnesses are conventionally included amongst the culture-bound syndromes, . . . they differ from such florid syndromes as *latah* and *amok* in that the diagnosis in a fright illness commonly depends *upon the interpretation of the symptoms which are not in themselves pathognomic of the diagnosis*" (italics added). In his sample, exemplars are usually children suffering from common childhood complaints such as diarrhea and respiratory infections.

Extreme fright (and startle especially) is a noteworthy event, and except in specialized humorous contexts is likely to be perceived as unfortunate and distressing. In much the same way that exposure to material objects culturally believed to be polluting, taboo or otherwise dangerous may be considered responsible for a variety of illnesses, fright and startle are also available as attributional resources. The papers in this section testify to the widespread use of this resource.[2] This selection of papers describing illnesses attributed to fright and startle has been included in this volume because they are so often classed with culture-bound psychiatric syndromes. However, since their symptoms are neither a specifiable alteration of behavior or of experience I believe that there is no justification for continuing to so list them. Thus I disagree on this point with Hughes who suggests anxiety as a unifying characteristic (see his commentary). I do not see in any of the papers evidence that would suggest that anxiety is regularly manifested or necessary for the indigenous diagnosis, particularly anxiety of a pathological extent as opposed to the worry which may accompany any misfortune or somatic illness.

NOTES

1. Rubel, A., C. O'Nell, and R. Collado
   1984 *Susto*, A Folk Illness. Berkeley and Los Angeles: University of California Press.
2. Another exemplar is well described in a previous volume in this series: Byron and Mary-Jo Delvechio Good's 'Toward a Meaning Centered Analysis of Popular Illness Categories: "Fright Illness" and "Heart Distress" in Iran', *In* A. J. Marsella and G. M. White (eds.), Cultural Conceptions of Mental Health and Therapy. Dordrecht: Reidel, 1982.

ARTHUR J. RUBEL, CARL W. O'NELL, AND ROLANDO COLLADO

THE FOLK ILLNESS CALLED *SUSTO*

FOLK ASPECTS OF THE ILLNESS

Susto is a condition which, though unrecognized by cosmopolitan medicine, is remarkably widespread throughout many societies in Latin America. *Susto* has been reported from Guatemala (Adams and Rubel 1967; Gillin 1956; Logan 1979); Colombia (Leon 1963; Seijas 1972); Argentina (Palma 1973; Palma and Torres Vildoza 1974); Peru (Bolton 1981; Chiappe Costa 1979; Gillin 1947; Salby Rosas 1958; Stein 1981); Mexico (Adams and Rubel 1967; Alvarez and Lavana 1977; Kearney 1969; O'Nell and Selby 1968; Uzzell 1974; Vogt 1969); and from Mexican-Americans residing in the United States (Clark 1959; Kiev 1968; Madsen 1964; Rubel 1960; Saunders 1954 and Trotter and Chavira 1981, 83).

Furthermore *susto* bears striking similarities to conditions reported from other areas of the world such as India, the Philippines, Taiwan, and among American Jews of Sephardic background (Hart 1969; Firestone 1962). The wide distribution of *susto* across many different cultural groups and even sectors of complex national societies distinguish it from most of the other so-called culture-bound syndromes such as *witiko, arctic hysteria, amok, suo-yang, koro, latah*, and *grisi siknis*, which appear to be restricted either to one ethnic group or to some particular sector of a complex national society. It is unwarranted to label a condition culture-bound when it is marked by distribution across broad and diverse socio-cultural spectra.

The folk interpretation of *susto* (as a health problem) is predicated upon the understanding that a person is comprised of two elements, one spiritual and the other organic, and that the spiritual element is detachable from the host organism. Characteristically, two conditions can lead to the detachment, one relating to unsettling experiences which disturb the normally existing equilibrium assumed to exist within a healthy organism (or between the organism and its spiritual counterpart), the second resulting from the spirit beings or forces associated with features of the natural environment which may seize and control the detached or unsettled spirit. The spiritual element may be a unitary, indivisible substance, or (in some belief systems) a conglomerate of units with hierarchical functions in serving vital needs and maintaining health.[1] Except for their broader implications as sustainers of health and vitality in human beings, these spiritual and organic components are viewed in somewhat different ways across cultural groups recognizing the *susto* condition. These differences are essentially variations on a common theme, however, and are always demonstrably related to concepts in the broader based belief systems of each society. The differences in their net effect demonstrate the differential emphasis societies place on the two conditions commonly conceived as etiologically significant.

333

Ronald C. Simons and Charles C. Hughes (eds.), The Culture-Bound Syndromes, 333–350.
© 1985 *by D. Reidel Publishing Company.*

The following exemplifies the point we are making. Typically, among Indian groups of Latin America the spiritual component is captured from the body of an individual frightened by spirits or spirit forces residing in the environment — spirits deemed to be lords of the air, the mountains, the fields, the earth, or the rivers. As the result of this capture the frightened person suffers *susto*. For recovery the captured spirit must be retrieved from its captor, ransomed in the folk treatment process, and "led back" to be reincorporated into the victim's body. Among non-Indian cultural groups, however, very little or no emphasis is placed on externally residing spirit forces. In those groups *susto* illness is simply perceived as the result of a person's spiritual element becoming separated from the body as the result of fright; hence the frequent use of the Spanish word *susto* to label the condition.[2] The recovery of the individual is dependent upon inducing the spirit to return to his body. Though soul-loss is significant in both Indian and Mestizo etiologies, in this latter instance there is no element of expiation or ransom owed to a spiritual being.

The separation of the spiritual and organic components in an individual is manifested in loss of appetite, weight, and strength; restlessness in sleep; listlessness when awake; and depression and introversion, often characterized by loss of the motivation to carry out even the most ordinary tasks (Rubel 1964: 70: Salby Rosas 1958: 170, cf. Fabrega 1970). Other symptoms such as pains and generalized or localized fevers are not infrequently reported by those afflicted with *susto*. While not all cases of the illness are perceived as equally serious, afflicted individuals usually receive treatment. If one is not sufficiently motivated to obtain treatment for oneself, then one's family will usually see that treatment is provided. Virtually all groups concur in the opinion that the affliction, if allowed to persist untreated, will culminate in the victim's death.

Indians always, and non-Indians nearly always, seek treatment from a folk specialist, since physicians do not claim expertise in the retrieval of souls. Nevertheless, especially stubborn or difficult cases are often brought to the attention of physicians, it being commonly recognized that cosmopolitan medicine can be efficacious in treating severe physical disabilities, even those not occasioned by physical causes. In the treatment of *susto* the powers of native practitioners are felt to be paramount, and absolutely necessary in the all important task of spirit recovery. The powers of medical doctors are secondary, since they are limited to natural media such as antibiotics, vitamins and assistance to debilitated bodies.[3]

ILLUSTRATIVE CASES

Brief reports follow of some cases of *susto* and how they are perceived to have developed by those reporting them. We have selected these reports from diverse cultural groups to highlight similarities across folk etiologies and systems of understanding.

Case one, Doña Modesta from Morelos, Mexico. Five months pregnant, she was washing clothes in a stream when a companion fell into the water. The pregnant woman immediately going to her aid succeeded in rescuing her. The good samaritan related, "I felt no fear at the time, only a desire to rescue her. I gave no thought to the possibility that my action might prove harmful to me. Nevertheless, after my child was born, when it was 15 days old, it was unable to sleep." (Alvarez and Lavana 1977: 459).

A physician prescribed vitamins and a sleep medicine for the ailing infant, who he said suffered from rickets. Another woman suggested that the little girl be taken to a specialist in recovering souls, i.e., a *curandera*, a suggestion with which Doña Modesta complied. Using traditional diagnostic methods the *curandera* concluded that the child had lost her *sombra* (shadow) to spirits of the air and water where Dona Modesta had rescued her companion. The curer determined that the spirits of two persons who had died on the spot were detaining the soul of the child by playing with it in the water where the woman had been washing clothes at the time of the accident.

Case two, a Chinantec Indian woman traveling with her father, Domingo. As they forded a swift river, Domingo was swept off his feet by the current. He extricated himself only by grasping a vine stretched across the river. The daughter standing on the bank watched in alarm, powerless to help. Despite this ordeal and the threat it posed to him, Domingo emerged from the incident unscathed. Within fifteen days, however, when the daughter became ill, her illness was diagnosed as that of *susto*, attributed to the severe fright she had experienced.

Domingo marveled at the enigma posed by the incident of his near-drowning. "In fifteen days she was very sick with *susto*", he noted, "but I didn't suffer anything. It . . . is very interesting: some people become ill with *susto* and others do not, even when they suffer the same experience." (Rubel et al., 1984). According to Domingo, a being of the water, a powerful spirit of nature, stole strength from his daughter, resulting in her illness.

While *un susto* (a frightening incident) is a necessary factor in the etiology of the *susto* condition, it is only when a fright results in loss of the person's spiritual element that the *susto* illness results. The daughter's soul was captured by a spirit; Domingo's soul was not. She suffered *susto*; he did not.

A third case concerns a young boy from Peru whose chief symptom was a physical complaint for which his father requested help from a medical clinic. Only on direct questioning was it revealed that a fright and soul-loss were implicated as causal elements of the condition in the perception of the boy's father.

Reported by Abner Montalvo,

Luciano Sanchez brought Pablo, his son, to the clinic to have him treated for a discharge from his ear. When I asked him if this ear condition had a name he told me it did not. Then he reported that Pablo once fell to the ground from a height and took fright. "That was how the ear condition appeared, it came from the fright. The ground, i.e., lords of the ground, took hold of him and then: Mantzahasmi (he has taken fright)." (Stein 1981: 59)

In this case, as with many reported cases of *susto*, there appears to be some delay between the occurrence of fright and the emergence of discernable symptoms.

The lapse of time between fright and symptom emergence is rarely perceived as etiologically relevant in indigenous explanatory systems, although it would certainly seem to be important enough to merit attention from researchers (O'Nell 1975).

Case four is that of a young man named Antonio, about twenty-five years of age, married and with a family (Rubel 1964). Although a native-born American living in south Texas, he spoke only Spanish. A farm laborer, he helped harvest cotton and vegetables in Texas in season and migrated north to other states in spring and summer to engage in similar agricultural tasks.

Extremely poor, Antonio lived with his family in a small, flimsy shack with an earthen floor, a tin roof, corrugated paper walls and no indoor plumbing. Seriouly ill on one occasion with a diagnosis of double pneumonia, Antonio was sent to a hospital for treatment. He responded well and when his fever was controlled he was assigned to a recuperative ward. One night, noticing a deterioration in the condition of one of his ward mates, Antonio desperately tried to communicate his alarm to attendants and other hospital personnel, but to no avail; the ward mate died. When belatedly discovered by the attendants the corpse was removed from the ward.

The incident was very upsetting to Antonio, whose progress toward health was hampered by new symptoms. He slept poorly, his appetite deteriorated, he became fretful and he felt his body involuntarily "jump" as he reclined in bed. After recovering from his pneumonia he was discharged from the hospital but went home with his newly acquired symptoms. At home he continued to feel poorly, and requested his mother to come to his aid. On hearing his account of his companion's death, she diagnosed his problem as *susto* and began a traditional cure to coax her son's wandering soul back into his afflicted body.

Antonio's frustration in not being able to communicate a distressing problem to those who might have been able to do something about it, plus the fright of his "encounter" with a corpse, were sufficient to bring about *susto*. His cure was aimed at recovering his soul and reuniting it to his body.

Finally, we recount the case of a Zapotec wife and mother who reported an intractable case of *susto* following a dramatic and fearful episode in her home (Rubel et al., 1984). The woman, upset with her husband's constant criticism of her for failing to be responsive to his needs and negligent in household tasks, vowed to do whatever seemed necessary to prove her wifely industry. As her husband left their modest house of reeds one evening, she resolved to wait up for his sure-to-be-late return.

The hours wore on and when it became dark she lit a kerosene lamp to keep herself awake and light her husband's path into the yard. The lamp burned low and she became sleepy. Finally the lamp went out just as she was about to doze. Refilling the lamp she decided to hang it from a hook near the ceiling where it would shed more light and better serve its intended function.

Ultimately weary and bored with her vigil, she leaned against one of the reed walls and, despite her best intentions, soon fell asleep. Probably within minutes the lamp shifted against the wall where she rested. She awoke horrified, flames ignited by the lamp simultaneously engulfing her clothing and one wall of the house. Just at that moment, her husband returned. They somehow managed to beat out the flames, preventing her from being burned and saving the house from total destruction.

The fright she experienced was so unsettling to her that it immediately precipitated *susto*. Several months later when interviewed by the ethnographer she was still undergoing treatment for *susto* and was showing little promise of cure. She was adamantly convinced, as was the curer attending her, that her *susto* was due to the activity of powerful and malevolent spirits associated with darkness and the night — spirits unwilling to release her spirit.

In each of the cases reported, the victim of the condition, or someone attending the victim, ultimately identifies a frightening event in the victim's earlier life experience. When an experience uncovered is deemed sufficient to explain the emergence of symptoms, the explanatory requirements of the folk system are satisfied. This is so even when considerable time has elapsed between the fright and the emergence of sysmptoms.[4]

In helping to explain why some persons and not others succumb to fright and the pernicious attack of the spirits, naturalistic explanations are also sometimes cited. Individuals are considered to vary considerably in their relative susceptibility: persons debilitated by age or other infirmities are considered more susceptible than those not so debilitated. Generally speaking women are considered to be physically weaker than men, and consequently more likely candidates to fall ill. Sex differences in the frequencies with which *susto* is reported are consistent with this interpretation (cf. O'Nell and Selby 1968).

BIOMEDICAL PERSPECTIVES ON *SUSTO*

The *susto* illness, as has generally been true of folk illnesses, has not up to now been a focus of research in Western medicine. Physicians attending patients comolaining of *susto* have treated them within the diagnositc paradigms established by the Western, urbanized, techno-scientifically oriented medical community. In effect this has meant the de facto rejection of the complaint as superstition.

The cultural and linguistic gulf between *susto* patient and physician is normally considerable by virtue of the physician's education and urbanized life style. The more pronounced the cultural differences are between the patient and physician, the more likely it is that a treating physician will dismiss the complaint of *susto* as irrelevant (Rubel and O'Nell 1979).[5]

For the most part anthropologists have emphasized the descriptive aspects of the condition: its symptoms, beliefs, and treatments. Indeed, some contributions are almost completely descriptive, usually contained within the contexts of broad ethnographic accounts or more focused accounts of beliefs, magicoreligious practices or health related issues (Carrasco 1960; Guiteras Holmes 1961; Kelly 1965; Stein 1981; Trotter and Chavira 1981).

However, a few anthropological accounts of *susto* do attempt some degree of explanation beyond that provided by the folk systems under study (Crandon 1983; Uzzell 1974). Such explanations explicitly or implicitly invoke concepts of illness types or functions specified in biomedicine. Occasionally the effort is designed to approximate a diagnosis that could be supplied by scientifically oriented practitioners who hypothetically might confront the phenomena observed by the anthropologist (Bolton 1981). Non-folk explanatory statements of *susto* by anthropologists have rarely been tightly analytic, since the investigator usually lacks the clinical experience to carefully collect data required for such analytic statements. Similarly, explanations by non-anthropologists often ignore significant aspects of cultural context and may attribute greater relevance to reported symptomatology than may be warranted.

Not surprisingly, given the symptoms commonly reported for the folk illness, many investigators have suggested some neuro-psychological or psychiatric interpretation of the symptoms of *susto*, as exemplified in the following:

It is my tentative opinion that *susto* is somewhat similar to the "nervous break-down" among North Americans. Both phrases may cover, in their respective cultural contexts, a variety of psychopathic and physically pathological conditions, considered from the strictly diagnostic point of view. Both, however, are culturally defined escapes for the individual from the pressures and tensions of life. When a North American "can't take it any longer", he has a "nervous break-down"; when a Peruvian cholo "can't take it", he gets *susto*. Actually depending on the configuration of the case, one patient may have hysteria, another a depression, a third possibly an anxiety attack. Susto also becomes a mechanism for calling the group's attention to the individual by his assumption of a culturally patterned configuration of "symptoms". At all events it seems to represent at least a temporary collapse of the psychic organization of the individual and consequently of his ability to deal normally with his life problems. (Gillin 1945: 131–2)

Other writers have been specific in linking *susto* to serious functional psychiatric disorders (Leon 1963: 211), even schizophrenia (Pages Larraya 1967: 18, 23, 71). Even when *susto* is not explicitly equated with psychiatric categories of illness, reports may carry the implication that such an equation is justified.

Not all observers have equated *susto* with psychiatric disorder, however. Implicit in some of the literature is the idea that *susto* may be an indigenous label applied to physical diseases unrecognized by those using the label. Although certain earlier authors have left open the possibility that *susto* might be due both to biological and psychological factors possibly impinging on one another (e.g., Gillin 1945; Salby Rosas 1958), several more recent authors have attempted to explain *susto* in biomedical terms. Amont these authors, Bolton (1980, 1981) suggests a close relationship between hypoglycemia and reported cases of *susto* (or of *tierra*, an alternate term used in the highlands of southern Peru). Bolton's thesis is that *susto* should not be labeled as a folk illness at all since it represents a syndrome of physically recognizable disease. Crandon has suggested that several disease categories underlie the rubric *susto*, arguing ". . . that there are innumerable diseases that can account exactly for all the symptoms of *susto*, for its usual pattern of symptomatic progression and for its extremes of variation". (1983: 158)

Susto has also been considered evidence of social strain in the face of rapidly changing social conditions commonly brought about through migration and urbanization (e.g., Gobeil 1973), traditional pressures to conformity controlled through *brujeria* (witchcraft) (e.g., Kelly 1965), the establishment of a "strategic role" affording a socially respectable role outlet to persons requiring it (e.g., Uzzell 1974), and a symbol reflecting group perceptions of the social environment (e.g., Kearney 1972: 54–8).

One of the clearer statements implicating social factors in the life experiences of *asustados* (those suffering from susto) in Mexican American culture was that of Clark, who interpreted the folk illness to be a means of adjusting social wrongs, permitting escape for unsanctioned behavior, and allowing sufferers a degree of respite from carrying out normal social responsibilities (1959: 198–200).

In his study of Mexican American understandings of health problems, Rubel (1960) went further in explaining the social significance of *susto*. On the one hand, he contended that these conditions "function to sustain some of the dominant values of Mexican-American culture, those which prescribe the appropriate role behavior of males and females, of older and younger individuals". On the other hand, he asserted that, ". . . social stress *is* a necessary . . . condition of loss of soul". (1960: 813)

In still a later statement, Rubel (1964) made even more explicit the involvement of the social system in the *susto* illness. He presented an epidemiological model interconnecting one's social role performance, biological state of health, and personality system. He integrated the interplay between these systems around the concept of stress, operationalized as self-perceived deficiencies in social role performance. Rubel derived four hypotheses from the model, proposing that the "susto illness in societies of Hispanic America may be understood as a product of a complex interaction between an individual's state of health and the role expectations which his society provides, mediated by aspects of that individuals's personality." (1964: 281) Factors in the social system were made the core element for understanding the meaning of the *susto* illness.

Rubel's hypotheses offered an opportunity to test his explanation of the illness. Responding to Rubel's challenge, and inferring from their work in two Zapotec pueblos that women would be more likely than men to experience social stress (due to self perceived role failure), O'Nell and Selby (1968) predicted that women would be more likely than men to suffer the *susto* condition in those communities. In effect, their work was an empirical test of one of Rubel's hypotheses, a test which in fact was supported by the data gathered in their two independent samples. The relevance of the O'Nell and Selby study lies not so much in its confirmatory result as in the empirical stance it took toward verification of the explanation of a folk illness. The issue had finally shifted from an explanatory one to one requiring an effort to substantiate an explanatory claim.

However, the O'Nell and Selby study was hampered by a methodological approach which emphasized grouped data at the expense of measurement of the individual's susceptibility to *susto*. In short, while O'Nell and Selby could demonstrate *susto* to be associated with higher levels of social stress assumed to be experienced by groups of people based on sex related role expectations, their results did not permit them to demonstrate that individual *asustados(as)* experienced higher levels of social stress than did those who did not suffer the condition. Nor did their study permit any assesment of *asustados'* biological and psychological health.

A STUDY TESTING COMPETING HYPOTHESES

Here we describe and discuss an empirical study (Rubel et al. 1984), undertaken to test three major hypotheses explanatory of *susto* which in one form or another have emerged from scientific efforts to understand the condition as noted in the previous section. At their most general level these hypotheses address explanations relating *susto* to issues of social, psycho-emotional, and physical health. The research was an anthropological-medical team effort, shaped by the interests and expertise of the principal participants. Scientific hypotheses emerging and methods chosen to test them resulted from the efforts of the investigators to bring their divergent interests into a single, unified study. Each aspect of the research is dealt with separately in the ensuing discussion. Findings are assessed for each set of hypotheses as are the relationships between the findings.

The study area was the state of Oaxaca, Mexico. One community from each of three ethnically divergent groups, Chinantec, Zapotec, and Mestizo was chosen for study. Divided by distinct cultural identities, speaking unrelated languages, and oriented somewhat differently toward nationally dominant Mexican cultural values, each maintains a somewhat different style of life. There is no direct and customary interchange between any of the communities. The communities were roughly comparable by size, population per kilometer and rural industry. Beliefs in the supernatural related to the *susto* illness, its causuality and cure were also similar across the three groups.

The samples were comprised of 38 Chinantec, 26 Zapotec and 36 Mestizo individuals. By design, all those included in the samples were people who compplained of being ill at the time of the study, the majority of them being selected from a larger number of people who sought medical assistance from free medical clinics provided by the investigators. Only adults (i.e., individuals over 18 years of age) were included in the samples. One half of the people in the samples attributed their ill health to the susto illness[6] (the experimentals). The other half, who were paired by the investigators on the bases of sex, age, and place of residence, attributed their illnesses to other causes (controls). If more than one potential control matched an experimental person in sex and age, the final matching was randomized to eliminate bias as much as possible in the sample selection process. Thus data could be analyzed not only between groups but also for matched pairs within ethnic groups.

The first hypothesis concerned the social dimension, which predicted that the *susto* illness would be positively associated with "self-perceived inadequacy ... to meet adequately the society's role expectations". (Rubel 1964: 281) Self-perceived inadequacy was assumed to be stressful; therefore this "inadequacy" was translated into a measure called social stress.

The instrument developed to measure social stress and to facilitate tests of the hypothesis that the *susto* illness is positively related to social stress was composed of three parts and is referred to as the Social Stress Gauge.[7] The first part, called the Social Factors Questionnaire, consisted of a form for recording field data in response to a set questionnaire designed to elicit stress-related data from individual respondents. Item sets in the field instrument were designed to tap perceived role requirements and perceived level of role performance indicated by the respondents. A second part of the instrument consisted of coding and scoring instructions for responses collected in the Social Factors Questionnaire. The third part was a score sheet on which judgements were recorded and finally tabulated into a social stress measure for each respondent.

The social stress measure indicated social inadequacy as perceived by respondents; stress was inferred from that measure. Measurement of the perceptions for any set of items in the questionnaire was scored as follows: an absence of discrepancy between items dealing with perceived role requirements and self-perceived levels of role performance was scored 0, a moderate discrepancy 1, and a maximum discrepancy 2. Scores for each of the item sets cumulatively contributed to a total stress score for each individual in the sample. Because the questionnaire covered fewer items for the men than for women, ratio scores were computed to render social stress measures comparable for certain statistical tests between the sexes and when scores for men and women were combined. (There were forty-four items for women and forty-two items for men). Scores were scaled in ordinal form so that higher scores on the social stress measure connoted higher levels of self-perceived social stress than did lower scores.

The anthropologists in this study predicted that there would be a strong, positive association between their operationalized measure of social stress and the reported experience of the *susto* illness. This predictive hypothesis derived from Rubel's epidemiological model (1964) and from the supportive work of O'Nell and Selby (1968). The results of the tests of this prediction are found in Tables I and II.[8]

The results reported in Tables I and II support the prediction of a positive association between measured social stress and suffering the *susto* illness. These results reflect tests of the base hypothesis under three types of control conditions: when the total sample is controlled for culture; when it is controlled for sex; and when it is controlled for culture, sex, and age. In the tests controlled for culture, the findings reveal both positive and significant results for the Zapotec and Mestizo parts of the total sample. Although not statistically significant, the result in the Chinantec part of the sample also reveals the expected positive association between the *susto* illness and higher levels of measured social stress.

In tests controlled for sex, findings reveal positive and statistically significant

TABLE I

Results of comparing social stress scores between groups of Asustados and Controls[a]

	U	z	p levels
A. SAMPLE CONTROLLED BY CULTURE			
Chinantec	154.5	1.22	> 0.05 (ns)
Zapotec	33.5	–	< 0.025[b]
Mestizo	106.5	1.75	< 0.04[b]
B. SAMPLE CONTROLLED BY SEX			
All males	42.5	–	< 0.025[b]
All females	537.0	1.60	< 0.05[b]

[a] Mann Whitney U Test
[b] Statistically significant at $p \leqslant 0.05$. Because of the directionality in our hypotheses one-tailed tests were used.

TABLE II

Results of comparing social stress scores between each Asustado
and his or her Control[a]

SAMPLE CONTROLLED BY CULTURE, SEX & AGE	T	p levels
Chinantec		
matched pairs	68	> 0.05 (ns)
Zapotec		
matched pairs	10	< 0.01[b]
Mestizo		
matched pairs	19	< 0.005[b]

[a] Wilcoxon Matched-pairs Signed-ranks test.
[b] Statistically significant at $p \leqslant 0.05$. Because of the directionality in our hypotheses one-tailed tests were used.

results both for all males and all females in the sample. For those tests controlled for culture, sex and age, the results are both positive and significant for matched pairs of individuals among the Zapotec and Mestizo sample segments. While not statistically significant for the Chinantec segment, the result none the less suggests a positive association between perceived social stress and the *susto* illness.

Although the central interest of the study was to test the relationship between how people perceived their relative adequacy or inadequacy in meeting their own standards of role performance and reports of their suffering the *susto* illness, the investigators, as previously noted, also selected competing hypotheses for study. One hypothesis concerned with the possible relationship of organic diseases to *susto*, and the other dealt with the possible relationship between psycho-emotional illness and *susto*.

In order to test the first of these competing hypotheses, instrumentation was developed to measure organic illness. Medical data from these samples were arranged into four categories. One focused on the current complaints of patients and their signs and symptoms. Another focused on medical histories. A third focused on the results of physical examinations performed on the samples by physicians. The fourth data category dealt with laboratory analyses of blood and stool samples.

The medical data protocols taken together provided three kinds of measures used in the investigation. One measure was called the *severity* of illness measure, construed as the extent to which a condition impeded a person from carrying out ordinary tasks but which is not life threatening to the patient. A second measure was called the *gravity* of illness measure, construed as the extent to which a condition endangered the life of the individual, although it might produce little or no evidence of behavioral debilitation. A third measure constituted a clinical assessment of the classifications of morbidity for the diagnoses of each patient in the sample according to the *International Classification of Disease*, World Health Organization, 8th Edition.

The severity and gravity of illness measures were scored according to measures developed by the physician investigator for the study. Referring to the medical protocols, it is possible for a physician using the scoring system to make categorical judgements about the medical conditions of patients. Cumulative scores for both the severity and gravity of organic illnesses were derived by summing categorical scores for each classificatory measure. The agreement by a panel of two physicians working independently in producing these scores was high (Rubel et al. 1984).[9] Because of this high level of physician agreement, averages were made of their scores for each respondent, which then constituted the severity and gravity of illness scores used in computations.

Briefly, statistical tests of the association between severity of illness and *susto* reveal significant positive associations only for the Zapotec group and for males across the sample. Tests of the gravity of illness measure reveal significant positive associations for the Zapotec group and for both males and females irrespective of cultural affiliation across the sample.

The indication in general in these findings is that organic disease is implicated in the *susto* illness, but that its implication is not clear in terms of the medical measures devised for this study. Nor is organic disease implicated as strongly in the *susto* illness as social stress.

Conceived and developed as independent meausres of organic illness for the study, severity and gravity measures were not related for controls, but were for the *asustados* (Table III). This suggests that although everyone in the sample complained of being ill at the time of the study, the *asustados* were sicker than the controls.

Because of the generality of these measures, a more precisely clinical approach was also taken toward the medical data, referred to above as the third measure. This approach replaced the question, "How severely or gravely ill are these people?" with "From what categories of disease (morbidity) are these people suffering?"

TABLE III
Correlation between severity and gravity of illness

Culture	Controls		Austados	
	rs	*p* levels	*rs*	*p* levels
Chinantec	0.4	$0.05 < p < 0.10$	0.9	≤ 0.001[a]
Zapotec	0.6	$0.05 < p < 0.10$	0.9	≤ 0.001[a]
Mestizo	0.4	$0.5 < p < 0.10$	0.5	≤ 0.05[a]

Spearman Rho Test
[a] Statistically significant at ≤ 0.05.

The most unequivolcal finding was that *susto* is in no way equatable with any single biomedically diagnosed disease. For example, the findings do not warrant equating susto with anemia, cancer, rheumatism, or any other specific disease entity familiar to biomedicine. *Asustados* are not unique in the diseases from which they suffer. They share with their fellows the burden of endemic diseases, but not equitably. For some examples, among the Chinantec, onchocerciasis (river blindness) was endemic but found more frequently among *asustados*. In all three populations anemia was widely distributed, but was more prevalent among those with *susto*. Pterygium (fleshiness of the ocular conjunctiva) was a common disorder, but it was more frequently identified in those complaining of *susto*. Whereas 80% of *asustados* were found to be infested with one or more kinds of parasite, only 68% of the control sample was found to be so infested.

After the seven year study period it was possible to collect mortality data from 47 of the 50 experimentals (*asustados*), and 48 of the 50 controls. Eight deaths had occurred among the *asustados*, but no deaths had occurred among the controls. The probability of this occurrence is $0.01 < p < 0.02$, statistically significant within the predictive parameters established for all statistical tests in the study. Taken in conjunction with the other medical measures used, the mortality measure lends weight to the conclusion that *asustados* as a group are more endangered than controls. Among those in the sample who died, a generalized tendency was noted for them to have higher gravity of illness scores, providing evidence of validity for the gravity measure.

The second competing hypothesis related to psycho-emotional illness and its possible relation to the *susto* condition. Psycho-emotional illness was primarily operationalized as psychiatric impairment, and the 'Twenty-Two Item Screening Score for Psychiatric Impairment' (Langner 1962, 1965) was adopted to measure it. The modification and use of this instrument is discussed in detail in Rubel et al. (1984).[10] The psychiatric screening measure yields a cumulative score assumed to be indicative of poor emotional health at its upper reaches. As with the social stress instrument and the severity and gravity measures, scores from the Twenty-Two Item Test were treated as ordinal scale measures.

Tests were made of the hypothesis that if the *susto* illness reflects poor emotional health, as has been maintained by some (Billig et al. 1948; Gillin 1945; Leon 1963), then there would be a strong positive association between being *austado* and registering a high score on the Twenty-Two Item Test.

The results of these tests were essentially negative. When for each of the cultural groups in the sample, scores of the *asustados* were compared with those of the controls, not one difference emerged as statistically significant. This was also the case when tests were run for all the males and all the females in the sample, grouped without cultural distinctions.

Two interesting observations were made, however, with respect to the psychiatric impairment measure. One of these was that despite the fact that none of the statistical tests showed a significant positive association between the measures and the *susto* illness, a tendency was apparent in these data for *asustados* as a group to exhibit somewhat higher scores than did the controls. The second observation is that women showed a tendency to score higher than men across the sample. This was especially apparent when the number of persons scoring above 11.5 on the test was compared with the number scoring below that level, a finding consistent with others who have used this measure (Crandell and Dohrenwend 1967; Gaitz and Scott 1972; Robers et al. 1973).

The medical protocols also collected data relative to psychiatric-emotional illness. These data were diagnostically evaluated by the physicians who did the clinical assessment of the classifications of morbidity. The findings were essentially two: (1) Both physicians scoring the medical data diagnosed more emotional difficulties among *asustados* than among the controls, though there was great disparity in the conditions diagnosed, and (2) The quantitative dimensions of psycho-emotional morbidity were low as compared to total pathology. For those across the samples who reported themselves as suffering *susto* illness, 6.1% of total pathology was identified as psycho-emotional and 93.9 percent as organic. Among controls, 2.4% of total pathology was identified as psycho-emotional, while 97.6% was diagnosed as organic. Thus it is totally unwarranted to explain the *susto* illness as evidence of emotional pathology.

When the investigators tested relationships between the measures used, a positive but not significant correlation was found between the social stress measure and the modified Twenty-Two Item Test. Though the results illustrate the independence of the two measures, a weak positive relationship between them suggests that there might exist something of a "psychological overlap" which is not readily discernable by the instruments on which the measures are based.

Correlations between the social stress and severity illness measures demonstrated no significant relationship between them. Because the severity measure had failed to distinguish between experimentals and controls, this finding is not surprising.

However, because both the social stress and gravity of illness measures reported robust differences between *asustados* and controls, the researchers expected to find strong correlations *between* them. None were found in any of the communities

sampled (O'Nell, Rubel and Collado 1978). Nonetheless, we caution against drawing the conclusion that there is no possible linkage between these phenomena.
Why the social stress and gravity of illness measures do not reveal a relationship
with one another when each is demonstrably strongly associated with *susto* is
not clear.

A BALANCED PERSPECTIVE FOR THE PRESENT

It should be obvious that any simple explanation of *susto* is unwarranted at this
time. While further research may be expected to clarify certain ambiguities which
now exist, such effort should not be expected to reduce the complexity of the
interrelated phenomena which produce the condition. It should be evident from
all the work that has thus far been done on this folk illness, especially that involving tests of the major competing hypotheses, that further research must take
into consideration a multiplicity of interrelated factors contributing to the condition. Moreover, sophisticated assestments must be made not only of individual
factors, but especially of the way in which they are interrelated.

While the validity of the initial 1964 Rubel model may not as yet be completely
demonstrated, its continued utility in research appears affirmed. The *susto* illness
is formed by socio-cultural understandings which help mold individual experience
as modified by the effects of those organic diseases endemic to a population.
Together, these forces construct a malady which is meaningful to members of
these societies (see Kleinman 1973).

All members of these societies are plagued by the "diseases of poverty" (Laurell,
A. C. et al. 1977). They live on the delicate balance between life and death. However, the *asustados* carry a double burden. One results from social stresses incurred
in self-perceived failure to meet and discharge critical role expectations; the other
is a consequence of organic disease. For the *asustados* to know themselves to be
inadequately performing their important social roles in addition to suffering from
the rampant diseases tips that delicate balance towards early death.

NOTES

1. For a good discussion of some of the problems which exist in understanding a folk analysis
   of the spiritual essence of a person and of the complexity of that essence see Chapter 3
   in M. Esther Hermitte, *Poder Sobrenatural y Control Social*.
2. In both Indian and Ladino explanatory systems, the separation of the human spiritual
   component from its body is understood to result from a frightening experience. The Spanish
   word *susto* literaly translates into the English word "fright". Spanish speakers most often
   use the word *susto* to label this folk illness, which they attribute to a fright. However,
   alternate labels are also used to identify the condition. Examples are *espanto*, also meaning
   fright, *espasmo* (horror), *pasmo* (astonishment), and *miedo* (timidity implying fright).
   Pérdida de la sombra, a phrase commonly used in Mexico, emphasizes soul (shadow) loss,
   with the loss caused by a fright. In those regions of Hispanic-America where Indian languages constitute a primary or dominant idiom of the inhabitants, indigenous terms indicative of experienced fright are used to label the illness.

3. Physicians may or may not be aware that a given patient thinks himself/herself to suffer from *susto*. Attitudes of attending physicians range from bemused tolerance to officious intolerance of *susto* complaints. Patients who have been rebuked by physicians for their ignorance or superstition in complaining of folk afflictions quickly learn to report symptoms only. They refrain from offering physicians their own opinions, a practice encouraged by folk practitioners.

4. From a case familiar to himself, Rubel (Rubel et al., 1984) reports a period of approximately thirty years between the development of symptoms and the experience of the causal fright. This is uncommon, since few cases betray such a long time lapse. O'Nell (1975) reports that a time lapse between fright and symptom formation may be a function of cognitive qualities in experienced stress relating to the condition, a shorter period of time reflecting a clearer perception by the sufferer of stress associated with the frightful experience culminating in the *susto* illness.

5. The general disinterest of the medical profession in researching the *susto* illness has not markedly changed since one early investigator declared, "The present tendency of the medical profession seems to be to pooh-pooh the business because it does not fit neatly into the textbook definitions of diagnostic symptoms." (Gillin 1945: 131)

6. *Asustados* in this sample tended not to seek help from medical professionals. When they did, they rarely complained of *susto*. The identity of *asustados* in each of the communities was detected primarily through ethnographic investigation, facilitated by the aid of curers and information gathered from other informants. Once discovered by anthropologists, *asustados* were encouraged to visit the medical clinics, resulting in a high rate of compliance.

7. The development of the Social Stress Gauge is described elsewhere in greater detail (O'Nell and Rubel 1980). The gauge has been presented in its entirety in Rubel et al. (1984). The field instrument was tape-recorded for administration to all three groups. It was translated into the appropriate Chinantec and Zapotec dialects. Responses from all respondents were recorded on printed Spanish language versions of the field questionnaire. These responses were recorded by bilingual field assistants in the two Indian communities and by the ethnographer in the Mestizo community.

8. These findings have previously been discussed in O'Nell and Rubel (1980), and are more fully discussed in Rubel et al. (in press).

9. The physicians who scored the organic disease signs and symptoms had not been involved in construction of the data gathering instruments. They worked within a diagnostic frame work designed by Dr. Collado to yield scorable data; they remained unaware of which patients were experimentals or controls.

10. Langner's Spanish language version of this instrument was pre-tested among peasants living in the state of Mexico with the assistance of Dr. Raymundo Macias, a Mexican psychologist. The pre-test was to clarify the adequacy of communication in the instrument and to modify it as necessary to ensure effectiveness. Efforts were made to preserve the original meaning of each item. The modified Spanish language version was then translated into colloquial Chinantec, Zapotec, and Oaxacan Spanish by persons from each of the sampled groups. Despite our efforts to preserve the integrity of the original instrument, one item was discovered to be invalid for Chinantec respondents. To ensure comparability of results across the three cultural groups that item was deleted in the subsequent scoring procedures.

BIBLIOGRAPHY

Adams, R. N. and A. J. Rubel
  1967 Sickness and Social Relations. *In* M. Nash (ed.), Social Anthropology. Vol. 6, Handbook of Middle American Indians. Austin: U. of Texas Press, pp. 333–57.

Alvarez, Laurencia and Modesta Lavana
  1977 Un Caso de Pérdida de la Sombra. América Indígena XXXVII: 2: 457–463.
Billig, O., J. Gillin, and W. Davidson
  1948 Aspects of Personality and Culture in a Guatemalan Community: Ethnological
       and Rorschach Approaches. Journal of Personality 16: 153–87, 326–368.
Bolton, Ralph
  1980 *Susto*: The Myth of a Folk Illness. Paper presented at the 79th annual meeting of
       the American Anthropological Association. Washington, D.C.
Bolton, Ralph
  1981 *Susto*, Hostility, and Hypoglycemia. Ethnology XX: 4: 261–76.
Carrasco, P.
  1960 Pagan Rituals and Beliefs Among the Chontal Indians of Oaxaca. Anthropological
       Records 20: 87–117.
Chiappe Costa, M.
  1979 Nosografia Curanderil. *In* C. A. Seguin (ed.), Psiciatria Folklórica: Shamanes y
       Curanderos. Lima: Ediciones Ermar, pp. 76–91.
Clark, M.
  1959 Health in the Mexican-American Community. Berkeley and Los Angeles: University
       of California Press.
Collado Ardon, R., A. J. Rubel, and C. W. O'Nell
  1979 Algunas Diferencias Entre Enfermos con y sin *Susto*. Memorias, IV Jornadas Internas
       de Salud Escolar y Universitaria. Mexico: Direccion General de Servicios Médicos,
       Universidad Nacional Autónoma de México, pp. 264–274.
Crandell, D. L. and B. P. Dohrenwend
  1967 Some Relations Among Psychiatric Symptoms, Organic Illness, and Social Class.
       American Journal of Psychiatry 123: 1527–38.
Crandon, Libbet
  1983 Why *Susto*. Ethnology XXII: 2: 153–167.
Fabrega, H. Jr.
  1970 On the Specificity of Folk Illnesses. Southwestern Journal of Anthropology 26:
       305–14.
Firestone, Melvin M.
  1962 Sephardic Folk-Curing in Seattle. Journal of American Folklore 75: 301–310.
Gaitz, C. M. and J. Scott
  1972 Age and the Measurement of Mental Health. Journal of Health and Social Behavior
       13: 55–67.
Gillin, J.
  1945 Magical Fright. Psychiatry 11: 387–400.
Gillin, J.
  1947 Moche: A Peruvian Coastal Community. Washington, D.C.: (Institute of Social
       Anthropology), Smithsonian Institution.
Gobeil, Ovila
  1973 El *Susto*: A Descriptive Analysis. International Journal of Social Psychiatry.
Guiteras Holmes, Calixta
  1961 Perils of the Soul. Glencoe: The Free Press.
Hart, D. V.
  1969 Bisayan Filipino and Malayan Humoral Pathologies: Folk Medicine and Ethno-
       history in Southeast Asia. Southeast Asia Data Paper 76. Ithaca: Cornell University
       Press.
Hermitte, M. Esther
  1970 Poder Sobernatural y Control Social. (Ediciones Especiales 57.) Mexico: Instituto
       Indigenista Interamericano.

Kearney Michael
  1972 The Winds of Ixtepeji: World View and Society in a Zapotec Town. NY: Holt,
       Rinehart and Winston.
Kelley, Isabel
  1965 Folk Practices of Northern Mexico. Austin and London: University of Texas
       Press.
Kennedy, J. G.
  1978 Tarahumara of the Sierra Madre. Arlington Heights, Ill.: AHM Publishing Co.
Kiev, A.
  1968 Curanderismo, N.Y.: Free Press.
Kleinman, A.
  1973 Medicine's Symbolic Reality. Inquiry 16: 206–13.
Langner, T. S.
  1962 A Twenty-Two Item Screening Score of Psychiatric Symptoms Indicating Impair-
       ment. Journal of Health and Human Behavior 3: 269–76.
Langner, T. S.
  1965 Psychophysiological Symptoms and the Status of Women in Two Mexican Communi-
       ties. *In* Murphy, J. M. and A. H. Leighton (eds.), Approaches to Cross-Cultural
       Psychiatry Ithaca: Cornell University Press, pp. 360–92.
Laurell, Asa Cristina et al.
  1977 Disease and Rural Development: A Sociological Analysis of Morbidity in Two Mexican
       Villages. International Journal of Health Services 7: 3: 401–423.
León, C.
  1963 "El Espanto": Sus Implicaciones Psiquiatricas. Acta Psiquiatria y Psicologia de
       America Latina 9: 207–15.
Logan, M. H.
  1979 Variations Regarding *Susto* Causality Among the Cakchiquel of Guatemala. Culture,
       Medicine and Psychiatry 3: 153–66.
Madsen, William
  1964 The Mexican-Americans of South Texas. New York: Holt, Rinehart and Winston.
O'Nell, C. W.
  1975 An Investigation of Reported "Fright" as a Factor in the Etiology of *Susto*, "Magical
       Fright". Ethos 3: 41–63.
O'Nell, C. W. and A. J. Rubel
  1980 The Development and Use of a Gauge to Measure Social Stress in Three Meso-
       American Communities. Ethnology 19: 111–127.
O'Nell, C. W. and H. A. Selby
  1968 Sex Differences in the Incidence of *Susto* in Two Zapotec Pueblos: An Analysis
       of the Relationship Between Sex Role Expectations and a Folk Illness. Ethnology
       7: 95–105.
Pages Larraya, F.
  1967 La Esquizofrenia en Tierra Aymaras y Quechuas. Buenos Aires: Ediciones Drusa.
Palma, N. H.
  1973 Estudio Antropológico de la Medicina Popular de la Puna Argentina, Buenos Aires:
       Editorial Cabargon.
Palma, N. H. and G. Torres Vildoza
  1974 Propuesta de Criterio Antropológico para una Sistematización de las Componentes
       "Teóricas" de la Medicina Popular, a Propósito de la Enfermedad del *Susto*. Re-
       laciones de la Sociedad Argentina de Antropologia VIII: 161–171.
Roberts, R. E. et al.
  1973 Social Factors and Responses to a Mental Health Questionnaire. Presented at the
       American Sociological Association Meetings, New York City.

Rubel, A. J.
1960 Concepts of Disease in Mexican-American Culture. American Anthropologist 62: 79–814.
Rubel, A. J.
1964 The Epidemiology of a Folk Illness: *Susto* in Hispanic America. Ethnology 3: 268–283.
Rubel, A. J., C. W. O'Nell, and R. Collado
1984 *Susto*, A Folk Illness. Berkeley and Los Angeles: University of California Press.
Salby Rosas, F.
1958 El Mito del Jani o *Susto* de la Medicina Indígena del Peru. Revista de La Sanidad de Policia 18: 167–210.
Saunders, L.
1954 Cultural Differences and Medical Care. N.Y.: Russell Sage Foundation.
Seijas, H.
1972 El *Susto* Como Categoria Etiológica. Científica Venezolana 23 (Supl. 3): 176–78.
Stein, William W.
1981 The Folk Illness: Entity or Nonentity? An Essay on Vicos Disease Ideology. *In* Joseph W. Bastien and John M. Donahue (eds.), Special Publications 12. American Anthropological Association, Washington, D.C.: 50–67.
Trotter, Robert T. III and Juan Antonio Chavira
1981 Curanderismo: Mexican American Folk Healing. Athens: University of Georgia Press.
Uzzell, D.
1974 *Susto* Revisited: Illness as Strategic Role. American Ethnologist 1: 369–78.
Vogt, E. Z.
1969 Zinacantan. Cambridge: The Belknap Press.

MARLENE DOBKIN DE RIOS

SALADERA – A CULTURE-BOUND MISFORTUNE SYNDROME IN THE PERUVIAN AMAZON

INTRODUCTION

The culture-reactive syndromes, or culture-bound disorders, have long been discussed in the transcultural psychiatric literature (see Aberle 1952; Rubel 1964; Van Brero 1895; etc.). Early discussions by physicians, missionaries and visitors to diverse regions of the world who brought forth descriptions and analyses of psychiatric syndromes, different from those known to Europeans and Americans, stimualted both medical and anthropological interest. Such accounts continue to fill the pages of numerous journals, as one syndrome after another is subject to scrutiny. Recent examples include Lebra (1976), Yap (1969), Carr (1978), Simons (1980) and Manschreck and Petri (1978).

In Latin America, a large number of such syndromes have been reported (see for example, Rubel 1964). Additionally, there is a growing literature on urban folk healing in Third World countries, as well as a focus on mental health problems concomitant with acculturation, urbanization and modernization (see for example, Kantor 1969; Verdonk 1979; Danna 1980). This paper will review an Amazonian stress response to urban life, especially social disorganization, among recent and long-standing migrants to the northwest and central Amazon cities of Iquitos and Pucallpa, Peru. The culture-specific syndrome, *saladera* (derived from the Spanish word, *sal*, salt), will be examined in terms of the case history method. The author will present data based on a study of the clientele of one urban folk healer in the central Peruvian city of Pucallpa, where 10% of a total population of 95 patients ($N = 10$) presented with this syndrome during one months's time. what is of interest in regard to *saladera* as a culture-bound syndrome is the strong lack of somatization, either psychosomatic disorders or other types of physical complaints. Rather, *saladera* appears to be an anxiety reponse to stress engendered by the difficulties of dealing with and managing the complexities of a fast-moving urban milieu. It contrasts dramatically with *daño*, another Latin American culture-bound disorder, in which bodily complaints or other physical dysfunctions can be easily ascertained.

During a decade of research on Amazonian folk healing focusing on the use of plant hallucinogens, the author was able to establish contact in 1969 with one urban healer, don Hilde, in Pucallpa. Subsequently related to him through her marriage to his eldest son, the author maintained close contact with her father-in-law over a ten-year period, during which time she returned to Pucallpa in 1977 on sabbatical leave to tape his biography. In 1978–9, as director of an American overseas student college group, she spent the year in Lima, working with a mystical organization, *Septrionismo de la Amazonia*, to which don Hilde belonged. In

351

Ronald C. Simons and Charles C. Hughes (eds.), The Culture-Bound Syndromes, 351–369.
© 1981 *by D. Reidel Publishing Company.*

February, 1979, the author, with the help of a student assistant, administered a structured, 25-minute interview in Spanish with the healer's full cooperation to the total population of patients who visited don Hilde's clinic (see Appendix). During the month of February, don Hilde was visited by 95 patients, who generally made three visits each. Children under the age of seven comprised 52% of the population. Nosology included various somatic disorders, culture-bound syndromes associated with withchcraft beliefs and psychological problem (see Dobkin de Rios 1981).

In this paper *saladera* is described in two urban settings in the Peruvian Amazon, based on the author's fieldwork experience in Iquitos in 1968–1969 (see Dobkin de Rios 1972, 1973) and the recent study of one urban Amazonian clinic in Pucallpa in 1979. Some background material on Pucallpa and the region, focusing on urban-related stress, also is presented. Data on the healer and his treatment of *saladera* are discussed, and detailed information on the sample of patients suffering from *saladera* is reported in tabular form, with a view to understanding the psychological effects of cultural change on a cross-section of urban Amazonians (see Table I). By examining the data on one stress-related syndrome in the Peruvian Amazon, we gain insight into a process of coping by rural peasants in cities who are faced with rapid culture change. While the anxiety neurosis, *saladera*, which develops in this area is idiosyncratic in its cultural symptomatic expression, it is important to see how cultural elements can be marshalled as a response to the stress engendered by urbanization and industrialization.

We also see how traditional therapeutic elements are transformed as folk healers, such as don Hilde, are quick to incorporate new treatment and diagnostic modalities into the more traditional techniques they use. This creates a perspective that needs to be emphasized as it frequently slips from the view of many trained anthropologists and cultural psychiatrists. The data presented in this paper argue against the Rousseauian notion of the "noble savage" and the need of Westerners to find in unfettered form, an 'authentic' (read unchanged) tradition, especially in arenas such as healing. Throughout time, shamanic healers faced with the dire stresses of culture change, either forced or otherwise, have been among the first to incorporate new elements into their therapeutic systems and beliefs. The healer to be described in this paper is an excellent example *in vivo* of the syntheses of symbols and belief that are probably part of most world-wide healing traditions. In particular, don Hilde is heir to a number of traditions: those of Amazonian Indians, Christianity, European metaphysical beliefs introduced into Peru from medieval Masonic rites and from the nineteenth century spiritualist philosophy of Kardec in France. Most recently, don Hilde has been influenced by a spiritualist philosophy present in Pucallpa, derived from a mystical group in the capital, called *Septrionismo de la Amazonia* (see Dobkin de Rios and Joan Koss n.d.) itself influenced by Hindu-Tibetan tradition.

CLINICAL DESCRIPTION OF *SALADERA*

Among tropical rain forest peasants living in cities, the consistent experience of "bad luck" or generalized misfortune is viewed as a non-chance occurrence. Rather,

TABLE I
Characteristics of patients reporting *saladera*

	Case 1	Case 2	Case 3
Sex	F	F	M
Age	28	23	42
Marital status	Single	Single	Married
Occupation	Market vendor	Sells used clothing	Wholesale/grocery, dry goods
Education	High School (H.S.) completed	H.S. – 4 years	H.S. completed
No. of visits	Various	3 times	Frequent
Presenting symptoms	Things gone wrong at work and personally, sleeps a lot	Headaches, sick to stomach, liver hurts	Enemies harrass; insomnia, neighbors want him dead
Patient's opinion of Doctors	They don't know about *saladera*	No confidence; seldom uses them	They kill you
Prior use of doctors	Yes	No	No
Length of illness	Recent	6–7 months	6–8 months
Spouse/friends know of visit	Yes	No	No
Healer's diagnosis/ treatment	Suffer *amor cochinado*, body isn't well. Herbal baths and teas	Friend is envious patient took her boyfriend away	Patient's business associates envous, remedies and baths
Prior use of *Ayahuasca*	No	No	No
Patient's knowledge of treatment	Vague, herbal baths	Wants baths	None
Patient's comments	Healer will tell her who bewitched her	Believes witchcraft exists in Bible; must have faith in God	Very anxious

Table I (continued)

	Case 4	Case 5	Case 6
Sex	F	F	F
Age	22	44	30
Marital status	Married	Separated	Married
Occupation	Market vendor	Market Vendor	Market vendor
Education	Primary School completed	Primary School completed	1st year, primary
No. of visits	First	First	Various
Presenting symptoms	Business going badly; work colleague hates her; marriage going badly, weight loss	Sick, *saladera*, everything going badly at work	Suffering from *saladera*; things not going well; money was robbed several times
Patient's opinion of doctors	They are fine	They are fine	They are fine, but they don't know about *saladera*
Prior use of doctors	No	Yes	Yes
Length of illness	1½ months	1 year	1 year
Spouse/friends know of visit	No	No, one doesn't speak of it	Spouse — Yes Friends — No
Healer's diagnosis/ treatment	Husband's lover responsible for her illness	Not available	Work colleagues are envious of patient
Prior use of *Ayahuasca*	No	No	No
Patient's knowledge of treatment	None	None	Expects herbal baths and teas
Patient's comments	Healer advises her to separate from husband	Not available	Healer sees evil-doer in vision

Table I (continued)

	Case 7	Case 8	Case 9
Sex	M	M	M
Age	23	38	36
Marital status	Separated	Married	Married
Occupation	Laborer	Vendor, dry goods/grocery	Unemployed
Education	5th year H.S.	3rd year, H.S.	5th year H.S.
No. of visits	First	Various	First
Presenting symptoms	*Saladera*; things going badly in love. Ex-live-in girl friend bewitched him	Business going badly economic reverses Disequilibrium in his life.	Drinks too much, head hurts
Patient's opinion of doctors	None	Poor	None
Prior use of doctors	No	No	None
Length of illness	4 months	Recent	1½ months
Spouse/friends know of visit	No, one doesn't talk of it	Yes	Yes
Healer's diagnosis/	Special diet, healer agrees with patient	Lover is bewitching patient	Man suffers alcoholism caused by *pusangas*; healer will use vomitive-aversion therapy
Prior use of *Ayahuasca*	No	Yes	Yes
Patient's knowledge of treatment	None	Expects baths	None
Patient's comments	He attends meditation ceremony	He attends meditation ceremony	None

Table I (continued)

	Case 10
Sex	M
Age	38
Marital status	Married
Occupation	Small business sales
Education	3rd year H.S.
No. of visits	Frequent
Presenting symptoms	*Saladera* in business; no physical illness; bad luck preoccupies him all the time
Patient's opinion of doctors	They don't help
Prior use of doctors	Yes
Length of illness	1 year
Spouse/friends know of visit	Yes
Healer's diagnosis/ treatment	Mother-in-law bewitched him, wants son-in-law to leave her daughter. Intense dislike of son-in-law. Healer will use herbal baths and vomitives
Prior use of *Ayahuasca*	No
Patient's knowledge of treatment	None
Patient's comments	He attends meditation ceremonies

projections outward lead to the view that the malice of either significant others in one's life, or envious, malevolent neighbors or work colleagues is the source and responsibility for such happenings. Constant aggravation or persistent difficulties in finding a job may not be attributed to individual inadequacies or even abstracted to economic causes, but are attributed to the malice of others.

From a clinical perspective, the ten adult patients who visited don Hilde in 1979, complaining of *saladera* were distinct from the other patients in the sample (see Table II). All were highly anxious. Women frequently burst into tears and

TABLE II
Diagnosis of adult patients[a]
(Age 15–75, N = 46)

Natural illnesses	13	28.3%
Culture-bound disorders	22	47.8%
Saladera 10		
Daño 12		
Psychological illnesses[b]	11	23.9%

[a] These are the diagnoses of don Hilde.
[b] These comprise cases such as marital counseling and alcohol and drug abuse counseling.

our interviewing had to be delayed on occasion until they could compose themselves. Several of the patients volunteered the information that they were unable to perform their work tasks, that they had poor concentration or were fearful of the future. Unlike other patients also preoccupied with the outcome of their visit (e.g., mothers of sick children, N = 49), patients presenting with *saladera* had difficulty remaining seated for the duration of the interview. While these patients exhibited signs of anxiety to the observer, they did not say they were anxious. Disturbed breathing and sighing were common, which no doubt the healer would subsequently detect when he pulsed his patients. Some men and women were trembling, and despite the general lack of sweating in this sub-tropical climate, they perspired freely.

When asked why they came to see don Hilde, all patients responded that they were bewitched with *saladera*. As in many Third World countries where witchcraft beliefs exist linking illness or misfortune to the evil of others or spirit forces in nature, patients who suffer from these culture-bound disorders generally have made self-diagnoses prior to seeking help. Table III shows the congruence of the patients' presenting symptomatology compared to the healer's diagnosis which is statistically significant at the 0.001 level (Dobkin de Rios 1981: 5).

Saladera differs from another major Amazonian syndrome, *daño*, in one important way. *Daño* is an illness that people believe to be caused by the evil willing of others who harbor malice toward a patient. They seek out a witch to cause their enemy harm. *Daño* can be associated with a large number of somatic complaints including hemorrhaging, muscular pain, loss of consciousness, arthritis, etc. *Daño* differs from *saladera* on two dimensions. First, somatic complaints in the former case contrast dramatically with misfortune as the primary symptom of the latter. While in both cases healers believe they must seek out the cause of the illness before they engage in any therapeutic activity, *daño* is further distinguished from *saladera* in that *daño* is seen to be provoked by the action of a witch who is brought in to bewitch one's enemy. *Saladera*, on the other hand, often occurs through the direct act of a man or woman who is not a witch per

TABLE III
Patients' symptomatology and healer's diagnosis

	Healer's diagnosis: natural illness	Healer's diagnosis: non-natural illness	
Oresenting complaints of somatic dysfunction	58	12	70
Presenting bad luck or misfortune	1	24	25
	59	36	N = 95

$x^2 = 48.46$ $P = < 0.001$

se but who nonetheless may insinuate a *pusanga* (potion) into someone's drink or throw a noxious substance across his threshhold.

In order to fully understand the significance of the cultural expression of this anxiety neurosis, it is important to look at the folklore connected to salt usage in the Amazon.

THE FOLKLORE OF SALT

When salt is placed on living plants, it destroys them. This contrasts to the vital role that such a substance has for maintaining health, especially in tropical climates. Thus, salt is both vital, yet feared. It can make life possible, but at the same time is a potentially destructive force.

Prehistorically, Campa forest Indians of the Central Amazon either obtained salt by trade or made long and perilous journeys to the salt mountain in Chanchamayo to mine salt, until they were forcibly stopped by the Peruvian colonists in the nineteenth century (Varese 1968: 106). Interestingly enough, salt taboos exist among individuals who take the plant hallucinogen, *ayahuasca*, in order to obtain a vision that enables them to fix the source of witchcraft attribution on an evil other. Throughout the world salt taboos tend to be found among traditional users of plant hallucinogens to heighten the effects of drug substances.

Saladera disorders were first described by the author in 1972. It is difficult to estimate the incidence of this disorder in rural settings in the northwest and central Amazon. Nonetheless, there is sufficient folklore that provides a clue to the derivation of the syndrome both historically and prehistorically.

Salt plays an important role in the preservation of meats and fish, and to this day salted foods are an important part of preservation techniques among farmers and city dwellers for whom electricity and refrigeration are still something of a novelty. Game animals and fish, often retrieved at distances from campsites or urban areas, were easily transported to centers of consumption after being salted for preservation. The word for salary, or *salario* in Spanish, derives from the Latin, *salarium*, for the money given to Roman soliders to buy salt, attesting to the important role of this substance in trade and barter worldwide.

Amazonian folklore concerning salt is of interest here. Soils that yield poor produce are often referred to as *salado*, indicating a negative attribution to the substance, *sal*. The linkage of salt and bad luck can probably be traced to periods of commerce during the Colonial period, when the chemical action of salt on containers caused their decay and corroded steel on transport boats. From this period, salt became incorporated into the nefarious ingredients in popular witch-craft hexes, mixed with earth from cementeries or inorganic remains, which were used to bewitch individuals. Even today, when an unwelcomed visitor is in a house, it is believed that throwing salt on the fire will hasten his departure. Another form of witchcraft in rural areas consists of throwing salt on top of or around the plants grown by one's enemies in order to destroy them. To "salt" a person is generally seen to induce by means of witchcraft the spirit of salt (within the animistic framework of beliefs common to Amazonian residents) to cause the person, as well as those around him, bad luck. Many individuals believed to be salted are avoided, for fear their witchcraft-induced bad luck would rub off on others.

In Pucallpa, many patients interviewed also cited another way in which *saladera* could be caused. That entailed the collection of menstrual blood and other noxious substances, which were secretly introduced into a drink, called a *pusanga*, by a woman of dubious morality who wished to break up a marriage and lure a man away from his wife and family. This recurring theme is found in an area of the world, Amazonia, where menstrual taboos were widespresd in prehistoric tribal life. The power of menstrual blood is quite important and still restrains the activi-ties of women on a day-to-day basis, especially their entry into forests to gather plant materials, to weed gardens, or to travel on the rivers surrounding Pucallpa or Iquitos. The drink is often viewed as the primary way in which an evil person can cause *saladera*.

Pusangas can also play a role in live magic. Informants distinguish views about love and its persistence through time. One type of affect is natural and spontaneous, but is believed not to endure. It is only *amor cochinado* – love due to the in-troduction of potions, charms and nefarious witchcraft in *pusanga* form that is believed to be most durable.

Vultures' feces mixed with water and dropped at one's doorstep are believed to be one way to cause misfortunes to occur. Salt, when thrown across a neighbor's threshhold or placed on a window still, is enough provocation for a person to change his residence, where it is believed that adversities or death will occur.

THE INCIDENCE OF *SALADERA* IN THE PERUVIAN AMAZON

During a study of plant hallucinogenic healing in Iquitos, the author interviewed ten *ayahuasca* healers and several hundred patients. At that time (1968–69), numerous female patients reported that they suffered from *saladera*. In general, these women were heads of households, abandoned by their spouses or common-law consorts and were seeking magical help from a healer so that their spouse would return to them. In the 1979 study of don Hilde's clientele, it was estimated that the healer saw 460 new clients a year or roughly 0.39% of Pucallpa's total population of 120,000. During the course of one average month when we surveyed the total clientele visiting his clinic, we found that ten out of 46 adults presenting with a variety of symptoms suffered from *saladera*. Four of these patients were there for the first time. From this information, it can be estimated that don Hilde sees about 50 new cases of *saladera* a year, or 0.04% of the population of Pucallpa. Census figures stratified by age and sex are not available to aid in any epidemiological analysis, nor was a control group available for study at this time.

URBANIZATION AND STRESS IN PUCALLPA

Pucallpa is located on the banks of the Ucayali River in the Peruvian tropical rain forest. Connected to the capital city, Lima, by a 500 mile long highway that traverses the Andean highlands and foothills, the city was founded in 1883 as a small settlement and is the home of Shipibo and Cashibo Indians. The Portuguese colonized the area in the nineteenth century and early part of the twentieth century, and were followed by Mestizo colonizers and highland Quechua speakers, as well as acculturated natives from the northern province of San Martin. During the Rubber Epoch in the latter part of the nineteenth century, there was an immense movement of people in and out of Pucallpa as a jumping off point into the forests to gather rubber. In this period, internal and foreign migration to exploit the "black gold" was widespread, and female-headed households were commonplace. Men would travel from place to place, seeking their fortunes, establishing menages for a few years before moving on.

Today, Pucallpa is a sprawling urban agglomerate of mud-baked and muddy streets. Only recently has it been partially paved, with the large majority of housing sub-standard with wood slate construction and calamine roofing. It is fundamentally a commercial center, with both a tradition-oriented economy of trade and barter among its river's edge peasantry and acculturated native tribal peoples. There are numerous extractive industries linked to Amazonian natural resources such as lumber and oil. The surrounding countryside is filled with subsistence-oriented, small-scale farmers who bring their meager surpluses to the three urban markets. Pucallpa is probably the largest and principal industrial center in the tropical rain forest, with all levels of industry represented. In the mid 1970s, petroleum exploration created over 15,000 jobs overnight, causing a major rift in the agricultural activities of the region. While petroleum workers relocated to camps often situated in virgin forest, their families migrated en masse to cities like Pucallpa and Iquitos, and squatter settlements with large numbers of female-headed households mushroomed overnight.

In the last five years, both petroleum and lumber activities have exacerbated the stresses of modernization overtaking Pucallpa (see Rumrrill 1976). Deforestation resulting from lumber exploitation is so extreme in Iquitos, for example, that the entire ecological balance of the region is fast changing (Gentry and Lopez-Parodi 1980). Over the last ten years, long time residents of Pucallpa as well as the more recent migrants have seen dramatic changes in the city. Traditional social supports and extended family networks have become of lesser and lesser help to individuals. As the city has grown and spread over a large land area, run-away inflation in general and rising real estate prices in particular have forced the transposed, poverty-striken peasantry into more and more marginal areas of the city – the Amazonian squatments, lacking easy access to farm lands or public markets. Such ecological disruptions set the stage for real and perceived stress for old and new urbanites alike. It may be that *saladera*, rather than *daño*, has increased in frequency. New migrants to Pucallpa, with inadequate training or sills that do not equip them for jobs in an urban environment, are correct in their perceptions that bad luck, indeed, pursues them.

Almost half of our sample of don Hilde's patients ($N = 43$) came from squat-ments, or the so-called new towns, which have sprung up among the urban poor and are found throughout Latin America. These settlements are marked by mal nutrition, chronic unemployment, underemployment, lack of adequate water and sewage, and many types of endemic and chronic illnesses.

MIGRATION AND MENTAL ILLNESS

As Danna (1980) summarizes the literature on migration and mental illness, rapid and dislocating culture change accompnaying migration and industrialization is associated with higher rates of psychopathology. Categories of migrants particularly susceptible to psychocultural stress include rural dwellers in traditional communi-ties like those of the Amazon, where their traditional world view, work skills and patterns of social interaction in industrial urban communities are inadequate for successful achievement (1980: 25). Verdonk, too, points out that illusions of bewitchment are not uncommon in migrant patients, and psychosomatic com-plaints reflect the expression of migrants' difficulties (1979: 297). Favazza cate-gorizes a major form of coping behavior connected to culture changes related to modernization changes in society (1980: 101). In Press' judgment, folk healing practices in general are a response to acculturation, especially guilt displacement resulting from failure to achieve. While Press argues that folk healing practices are shifting in general to adjunct functions of healing under pressure from effective modern medical and welfare systems (1978), this does not seem to be the case in Pucallpa, where healers like don Hilde find their case loads increasing, not decreasing.

TYPES OF HEALING IN PUCALLPA

Modern health facilities in Pucallpa include one large foreign-run hospital in a neighboring town, a large but poorly staffed public hospital and several private clinics. Private medical care is available, but few specialists choose to work or live in Pucallpa, and middle-class men and women often travel to Lima for treatment of health problems.

Traditional therapeutics are varied in number and reflect a diverse number of influences stemming from the history and ethnicity of the region. The dominant population consists of an urban and rural Mestizo peasantry, which has developed over several hundred years of European and native American race mixture. Further ethnic influences include African Blacks who came to Brazil in the 18th century as slaves and found their way to Peru after emancipation, and populations of Chinese and Japanese in lesser numbers.

One encounters folk healing that represents an interesting amalgam of prehistoric traditions syncretized and changed by direct and indirect borrowing. Examples that can be cited include on-going Mestizo *ayahuasca* drug healing (which uses various *Banisteriopsis* sps.), both in urban and rural domains of the Peruvian, Colombian, Ecuadorian and Brazilian Amazon basin. Adventist and other evangelical Christian healing, poorly studied, is found intermittently throughout the area. Fortune-tellers and *curiosos* routinely diagnose illnesses and prescribe herbs. Mestizo men, generally trained during their period of army conscription as paramedics, function as *sanitarios* who dispense injections and suggest easy-to-obtain medications for a host of ailments. Biomedicine is represented as well in the form of practitioners in public hospitals and clinics or private practice, and Peruvian or foreign-trained physicians are available, generally at high cost, to the local peasantry. Finally, idiosyncratic healers such as don Hilde function in urban areas, utilizing a number of unique techniques. The range of healers includes magicians who diagnose illness, *ayahuasqueros* who use the plant hallucinogen almost exclusively among their clients, local pharmacists who are consulted for medicines for various ailments, or *vegetalistas* who are herbally knowledgeable. This latter group, a generic term for many folk healers, particularly tend to be consulted as part of a dual-medical system, especially in urban centers like Iquitos and Pucallpa (see Press 1980) for their knowledge of plant medicines, their horticultural skills in growing medicinal plants and their ability to cure witchcraft-related diseases, generally viewed by Amazonian residents as non-responsive to medicial intervention by physicians.

Treatment of illness is set within a matrix of magical beliefs concerning disease etiology. Many of the illnesses marking the urban populations of the rain forest can be classified as psychological in orgin, and their therapeutic outcome corresponds to the general success that other folk healers around the world appear to have in treating such illnesses (e.g., Kleinman 1979, Kiev 1964). Illness is believed to be caused by the capricious whim of offended spirits of nature, or else attributed to the evil of people, who for motives of envy, revenge or plain meanness, pay a witch to cause horrendous damage to another person. The main purpose of the powerful plant hallucinogen, *ayahuasca*, when used in healing, is diagnostic and revelatory. During the course of the therapeutic session, a patient is given a drink to induce visions which will permit him to see just what force or individual is deemed responsible for evildoing. It is only then that the evil magic causing illness is believed to be deflected or neutralized by the healer and returned to its perpetrator (Dobkin de Rios 1971).

Don Hilde differs from the ten other healers whom the author previously studied in one major aspect. His roots derive more directly from a Christian influence rather than a tribal one. Moreover, he is proud of his ability to entertain personal visionary experiences, generally not accessible to others around him, since his adolescent years, and is closer to a seer than an *ayahuasquero* found in surrounding rain forest communities. While most urban *ayahuasqueros* depend upon their plant hallucinogenic potions to "see", don Hilde's well-touted abilities as a visionary preempt his dependency upon the *ayahuasca* potion.

BACKGROUND INFORMATION: DON HILDE

A 63-year-old Mestizo, don Hilde was born in a small hamlet near Pucallpa and obtained only a few years primary education in the city. He served in the Peruvian army in the mid 1930s, and worked as a construction hand in building the Basadre highway connecting Pucallpa with the Andean highlands and the industrializing coastal region in the period 1937–1939. He married and settled down in Pucallpa, had three children and worked as a carpenter. As the result of a series of visions of Christian saints which originated in his adolescence, he realized his abilities to heal, and at this time he began to receive a few patients in his home, while simultaneously maintaining his carpentry shop. As his reputation spread over the years, he devoted more time to his practice, occasionally using the plant hallucinogen, *ayahuasca*, as did many other curers in the region. At this time, he also began to read about hypnosis and to induce trance-like states in himself. In 1974, he was put in contact with members of the mystical order, *Septrionismo de la Amazonia* in Pucallpa and was accepted as a member. In 1976, he moved his clinic to the outskirts of Pucallpa and a large sign on the front of his house announces his relationship with the mystical-philosophical organization.

Drawing upon the constant and continuing help of the spirit guide under whose protection he was placed when accepted into the group, he resorted less and less to the use of *ayahuasca* in his healing. To a greater degree, he now pulses his patients when he first interviews them; he does not question them about their symptoms. Rather, his diagnostic method is one of intense concentration as he passes his hand over the patient's head to obtain what he terms a reading of their electromagnetic energies. This enables him to understand if the illness is natural or related to witchcraft. Spontaneously, he enters into an altered state of consciousness. Additionally, he supplements his diagnostic intuitions concerning his patient's illness from other visions he obtains during meditation ceremonies he holds every Tuesday; further diagnostic insights come from the occasional *ayahuasca* session he conducts three or four times a month, when he ingests the *Banisteriopsis* drink.

By means of a number of exercises including yogic-like breathing exercises and the displacement of energies which he learned from his Septrionic confreres, he practices a form of "spritualist" healing. Although disclaiming religious cate-gorization, the Order acknowledges the existence of a Father Creator and sees its mission as one of serving mankind. Don Hilde grows a number of medicinal plants in his garden and is no stranger to pharmaceutical medicines that he instructs patients to bring with them from city pharmacies on subsequent visits. He generally prepares his medicines in accordance with the demands of each case, picking the plants from his garden, or on occasion, gathering such herbs in the outskirts of Pucallpa. He cooks or seeps the herbs in his kitchen, while his patients patiently wait in the clinic to be medicated, all for the same low consultation fee. On occa-sion, a difficult or chronic case might require inpatient care, and several small rooms are available in his clinic to house such clients. Don Hilde does not hesitate to refer cases to the city hospital when he feels that surgery is indicated, and he maintains a good relationship with several medical doctors in the city.

Case studies of the ten patients who presented with the anxiety neurosis are examined in detail in the following pages.

CASE STUDIES OF *SALADERA*

Of the 95 patients interviewed during February, 1979, ten patients said they were suffering from *saladera* (see Table I for a summary of patient characteristics). When asked what motivated them to see the healer, they often used the term, *saladera*, to describe their state, and related to the interviewer a series of mis-fortunes or bad luck that had pursued them either recently or as long as a year and half before and had persisted to the present time. Both men and women suffered from this syndrome in equal number. Their ages ranged from 22–44 years, with the mean age 32. Two patients finished high school, five had three or more years of high school, two finished elementary school and one had had a year of elementary school. All in all, the education profile of the patients suf-fering from *saladera* was not significantly different from that of the other adults in the sample (see Table IV).

Eight clients were married, two were single and two were separated from their spouse. All individuals can be characterized as members of the urban poor, that is, vendors, laborers, small-scale businessmen or unemployed. Forty percent came to see don Hilde for the first time, while the remainder had made several visits. All were recommended by a former satisfied client who had been treated by the healer. In all cases except one, the presenting complaints were bad luck or mis-fortune. Clinical observations, as mentioned earlier, indicated a high level of patient anxiety. Insomnia was one of the few somaticized symptoms among the group. One patient said he suffered from headaches and pain in his liver. Of the ten clients, four had seen physicians in the past, but six had not. This contrasted with the sample as a whole, in which 71% of the clientele, or 68 persons, had had access to medical care prior to seeing don Hilde. This may indicate a conservative sub-set within the client population, although the number is insufficient in this case to make generalizations. *Saladera* is perceived generally as a witchcraft-related

TABLE IV
Educational level of *saladera* patients

	Saladera patients	Other adult patients	
Primary school completed or less	17	3	20
High school completed or less	19	7	26
	36	10	$N = 46$

$X^2_{NS} = 0.373$

syndrome and believed amenable only to therapeutic intervention by a *vegetalista* and not a physician. It may be that those individuals who presented with *saladera* are more likely to believe themselves sufferers of witchcraft-related illnesses overall, and tend not to seek medical help for any types of ailments they may suffer. Thus, such a group might be more prone to explain illness by recourse to supernatural explanations of causal factors in contrast to the dual-use pattern exhibited by the sample as a whole.

With regard to the length of illness, three patients suffered for a year or so, another three suffered between four to eight months, while four were recently ill for a month or less. Most of the patients did not tell their friends about their illness. Without doubt, this is related to the fear of ostracism mentioned earlier as part of beliefs about *saladera*. When asked about the probable treatment they would receive, almost all had some expectation of herbal baths and medicines which they would be obliged to take. Three had gone to Tuesday evening meditation rituals conducted by don Hilde, although none had any substantive information about the doctrines of *Septrionismo* that don Hilde followed.

Don Hilde's diagnosis for *saladera* was similar to that of that non-natural or witchcraft-derived illnesses. Once diagnosed, he would consult with the patient and prescribe a series of herbal baths for them, generally to be taken on his premises in the evening. The patient was instructed to remain in his clothing for a 24-hour-period, and was reassured about the efficacy of the treatment. Don Hilde has a good reputation in Pucallpa. He is well respected and his low fees and simple life style, along with the recommendations of other satisfied clients, create a climate in which patients expect that he will be able to neutralize the negative forces affecting their well-being.

Needless to say, belief in the efficacy of any treatment is a necessary element in the individual's perception of changes forthcoming in his life's circumstances. Outcome measures in anthropological studies of folk therapy are meager, due in part to difficulties of funding long-term studies of this sort (see however, Finkler 1980). Block et al. (1976) pointed out that patients' expectations of therapeutic improvement do influence outcomes. Most studies rely on patient self-report alone rather than any independent assessment, and self reports are vulnerable to the bias of the patient. Bloch's study concluded that expectations are related to outcome only when the latter is assessed by the patients themselves. If we generalize these findings in American society to a Third World therapeutic milieu such as don Hilde's clinic, we find that in all cases, individuals learned about don Hilde's activities on the personal recommendation of a satisfied former client, which would raise their levels of expectation.

Followups of patients suffering from *saladera* were not made due to problems of time, adequate funds and manpower. Patients were quick to point out to me that *saladera* was not amenable to medical attention and few if any patients who believed they suffered from *saladera* would spend their time and meager resources approaching a physician. Without any individual stating it as such, the materialistic focus of medical science compared to the preternatural etiology of misfortune was clear in the minds of Pucallpinos. Economic factors, too, had played a part in the general reticence to approach physicians if one was believed to suffer from *saladera*. In general, the minimum wage for a laborer at the time of the study was 385 Peruvian soles a day (at the time of the study, US $1 = 195 soles). The average cost for a physician's visit, without any medicine, at the same time was 500 to 1,000 soles, which was out of the reach of most urban poor. Don Hilde generally did not charge a specific sum for his consultations, but accepted donations, which averaged about 100 soles a visit. This fee included herbal medicines which he prepared from his garden while the patient waited.

CONCLUSION

Far too little attention has been given to the psychological consequences of rapid acculturation among Third World urbanizing peasantry, who may respond with anxiety and despair to events occurring all around them over which they seem to have little control. Things do go wrong when one is poor, when one has insufficient capital to work, or little if any education to prepare oneself for a secure job in an urban setting. The culture-bound syndrome, *saladera*, treated widely by Amazonian folk healers like don Hilde, is an interesting response to the stress of modernization in a society where witchcraft beliefs may be invoked to explain the etiology of illness. Don Hilde, whose life has been described briefly in this paper, is a good example of how traditional healers themselves widen their repertoire of therapeutic techniques in light of changing social conditions. The culture-bound syndrome *saladera* can be viewed as a coping strategy called upon by Amazonian urbanizing peasantry to enable them to deal with change. Belief in *saladera* permits them access to a traditional healer, knowledgeable about plant remedies, sanctified as a person and with personal power believed derived from pretematural realms, so that reassurance can be gained to help ease the burden of daily discomfort.

APPENDIX

QUESTIONNAIRE

(English Translation)

Date _____ Sex _____ M _____ F   Age _____
Name _____ Married _____ yes _____ no
Do you live together? _____ yes _____ no
Address _____
Name of patient _____
Occupation _____
(If housewife) spouse's occupation _____
Education: _____ public school   _____ technical school
           _____ public school completed   _____ college
           _____ high school   _____ other
           _____ high school completed
Why did you come to see don Hilde? _____
_____

How many times have you come here? _____ first time _____ twice _____ several times
_____ frequently
What are the patient's symptoms? _____
_____

How did you first learn about don Hilde? _____
_____

What is your opinion about the quality of medical doctors practicing in Pucallpa?
_____
_____

Have you ever been seen before by a medical doctor? _____ yes _____ no
(If answer is yes) Have you seen a medical doctor in the last six months?
_____ yes _____ no
What were your average expenditures during your last illness? _____
_____

How much does don Hilde charge? _____
Does your spouse know that you came here today? _____ yes _____ no
What do your friends think about your visit(s) to don Hilde? _____

When did the patient begin to suffer? _____
What Church do you attend? _____ none , _____ Roman Catholic _____ Evangelic
_____ Adventist _____ *Espiritisa* _____ other
How frequently do you attend? _____ never _____ at times _____ frequently
_____ several times/wk.
Does your family attend too? _____ yes _____ no
People here have told me a lot about witchcraft in the rain forest. Can you tell me a little bit
about that too? _____
_____

Have you ever used *ayahuasca*? _____ yes _____ no
How many times have you taken it? _____ Why did you take it?
_____

Do you attend Tuesday night meditation ceremonies? _____ yes _____ no
How frequently? _____ never _____ once _____ several times _____ very frequently

(If the answer is yes) Can you describe your experiences after the meditation?

Would you explain to me something about the doctrine of Brahamanism-Lamism, also known as Septrionism?

*   *   *   *   *   *   *   *   *   *   *

Don Hilde's Diagnosis:

Don Hilde's plan for treatment:

REFERENCES

Aberle, David
  1952 Arctic hysteria and Latah in Mongolia. Transactions of the New York Academy of Sciences 5: 14: 291–7.
Block, Sidney et al.
  1976 Patients' Expectations of Therapeutic Improvement and Their Outcomes. American Journal of Psychiatry 133: 12: 1457–60.
Carr, J.
  1978 Ethno-behaviorism and the Culture-Bound Syndromes: The Case of Amok. Culture, Medicine and Psychiatry 2: 269–293. (Reprinted in this volume.)
Danna, Josephine J.
  1980 Migration and Mental Illness: What Role do Traditional Childhood Socialization Practices Play? Culture, Medicine and Psychiatry 4: 24–42.
Dobkin de Rios, Marlene
  1981 Socio-economic Characteristics of an Amazon Urban Healer's Clientele. Social Science and Medicine 15B: 51–63.
Dobkin de Rios, Marlene
  1972 Visionary Vine: Psychedelic Healing in the Peruvian Amazon. San Francisco: Chandler Press.
Dobkin de Rios, Marlene
  1971 Ayahuasca, the Healing Vine. International Journal of Social Psychiatry 17: 4: 256–269.
Dobkin de Rios, Marlene and Joan Koss
  n.d.   Lifeworld of the Spirit: A Comparison of Spiritist and Spiritual Healing in Latin America. (Book in Preparation.)
Finkler, Kaja
  1980 Non-Medical Treatments and Their Outcomes. Culture, Medicine and Psychiatry 4: 271–310.
Gentry, A. H. and J. Lopez-Parodi
  1980 Deforestation and Increased Flooding of the Upper Amazon. Science 210: 4476: 1354–1355.
Kantor, Mildred B.
  1969 Internal Migration and Mental Illness. In S. Plog and R. B. Edgerton (eds.), Changing Perspective in Mental Illness, New York, Holt Rinehart and Winston.
Kiev, Ari (ed.)
  1964 Magic, Faith and Healing. Studies in Primitive Psychiatry. Glencoe, Free Press.
Kleinman, Arthur
  1980 Patients and Healers in the Context of Culture. Berkeley, University of California Press.
Lebra, W. (ed.)
  1976 Culture Bound Syndromes, Ethnopsychiatry and Alternative Therapies. Honolulu, University of Hawaii Press.

Manschreck, T. and M. Petri
  1978 The Atypical Psychoses. Culture, Medicine and Psychiatry 233–268.
Press, I.
  1980 Problems in the Definition and Classification of Mendical Systems. Social Science and Medicine, 4: 1: 1–13.
Press, I.
  1978 Urban Folk Medicine: A Functional Overview. American Anthropologist, 80: 71–84.
Rubel, A.
  1964 The Epidemiology of a Folk Illness: *Susto* in Hispanic America. Ethnology 3: 268–283.
Rumrrill, Roget
  1976 Los Condenados de la Selva. Lima: Editorial Horizonte.
Simons, R. C.
  1980 The Resolution of the *Latah* Paradox. Journal of Nervous and Mental Disease 4: 195–206. (Reprinted in this volume.)
Van Brero, P. C. Z.
  1895 *Latah*. Journal of Mental Science 41: 537–38.
Varese, Stefano
  1968 La Sal de los Cerros. Lima, Peru, Ediciones de la Universidad de San Marcos.
Verdonk, A.
  1979 Migration and Mental Illness. International Journal of Social Psychiatry 25: 295–305.
Yap, P. M.
  1969 The Culture-Bound Reactive Syndromes. *In* W. Caudill and Tsung-Yi Lin (eds.), Mental Health Research in Asia and the Pacific. Honolulu, East-West Center Press.

†DONN V. HART[1]

LANTI, ILLNESS BY FRIGHT AMONG BISAYAN FILIPINOS

INTRODUCTION

One rainy morning in a small village (Lalawigan) in eastern Samar I visited a family where the two-year old daughter was sick.

"What caused her illness?," I inquired.

"Her father", answered the mother.

"How did he make her sick?"

"Two days ago he almost stepped on a big snake in the forest. He was alarmed for the snake was poisonous."

"Was his daughter with him at this time?"

"No. This is not necessary with *lanti*."

It was this incident that led me to investigate this illness in the Philippines.

Canon (1942) recognized early how fear can initiate interlocking physiological processes resulting in either sickness or death. Pathogenic causes include the terror that may result from violating a taboo the dread of witchcraft and sorcery, or frightening experiences that dislodge an insecure soul from its body (Howells 1950: 100; Norbeck 1961: 217–18). However, illness from fright among Bisayan Filipinos is not the result of breaking a taboo, witchcraft or sorcery: soul loss is not a cause as in *susto* and *espanto*, similar illnesses from fright in Hispanic America (Rubel 1964). *Lanti* results when one is either directly or indirectly frightened. The patient may be startled or another member of the family is frightened. In the latter instance, since a mystical bond connects these two persons, the emotional shock of this experience is transferred to the child, resulting in sickness.

On the basis of a world sample of 139 societies selected from his *Ethnographic Atlas* (1967), George Murdock (1980) identified thirteen theories of the natural and supernatural causation of illness. One theory of the natural causation of sickness is labelled *Stress* and is defined

... as exposure of the victim to either physical or psychic strain, such as overexertion, prolonged hunger or thirst, debilitating extremes of heat or cold, worry, fear, or the emotional disturbances which constitute the province of modern psychiatry (Murdock 1980: 9).

In other other words, the illness is perceived as a natural consequence of the precipitating event. This theory is most applicable to *lanti*, an illness traced to frightening experiences directly or indirectly experienced by the victim, while awake or asleep.

† deceased

Ronald C. Simons and Charles C. Hughes (eds.), The Culture-Bound Syndromes, 371–397.
© 1985 *by D. Reidel Publishing Company.*

When other illnesses attributed to fright, aside from *lanti*, are examined, they must be classified under the theory of the *supernatural* causation of sickness that Murdock defined as ". . . the direct hostile, arbitrary, or punitive action of some malevolent or affronted supernatural being" (1980: 20). Murdock explains that this ". . . most common and widespread of all the types of supernatural causation", the predominant cause of illness in seventy-eight of the sample societies, is understandable since ". . . it represents the most direct and obvious projection from overt human aggression" (1980: 20).

If the supernatural causative agents are the environmental spirits, this second theory poses no problems in classifying many Bisayan etiologies. However, many Bisayans consider illness traced to God and the saints (and in Lalawigan, to the souls) as having a *natural* etiology. To fit some illnesses caused by fright, Murdock's theory of spirit aggression must be further modified, for the souls may be neither hostile nor punitive yet the victim falls ill.

Illness attributed to God and the saints has a natural etiology since everything God does is considered natural for he was the Creator of the world. For example, it is natural for God to punnish sinners with sickness. Since saints are the selected ones of God from whom they receive their power, illness traced to them is also classified as natural. This classification of etiologies is not unique to Bisayan Filipinos. Lambek found that the residents of a Malagasy village he investigated considered sickness caused by God a "natural disease" (1981: 43). Among the BaKongo of Lower Zaire, sickness attributed to God is differentiated from unnatural illness blamed on humans (Janzen 1978: 8).

Souls usually cause illness to punish kinsmen for failure to honor them with various folk Catholic rituals or one's refusal to accept a call to heal from a deceased relative who once was a healer. However, souls also *unintentionally* cause illness. For example, they may visit a new child to welcome its addition to the family. Their presence (visible only to the child) and "affectionate" pinches terrorize the child who does not realize their visitation is meant to be friendly, not punitive.

This limited segment of Bisayan Filipino ethnomedicine also furnishes new data on emotional experiences that often are sickness pathogens or which explain etiologies. For example, in *lanti* the victim may be sickened when another person experiences fright, and that fright is transferred by a magical affinity between the two persons.

The central focus of this chapter is the pathogenesis, etiologies, preventive and curative measures associated with *lanti* as investigated in one Samarnon village, Lalawigan. This syndrome has been meagerly and apparently incompletely documented elsewhere in the Bisayas. Similar illnesses (and deaths) caused by fright are integrated into this account of *lanti*. Finally, this ethnographic survey is used to illustrate how the etiologies, diagnoses and treatment of these illnesses reflect basic Bisayan Filipino beliefs and values.

Medical anthropology is a neglected field of inquiry in the Philippines. Most published sources on Philippine medical anthropology focus primarily on the problems of the introduction and diffusion of non-Western (or Cosmopolitan) medical concepts and practices at the rural level (Saito 1972). Some excellent studies have exposed the underlying logic of how certain Filipino groups define illness, make diagnoses, classify etiologies, and provide therapy (Franke 1961; Gieser and Grimes 1972). Commenting on this approach, in general, Rubel believes that most of these sources ". . . do not inform us what components of the population do in fact become ill, nor under what circumstances illness occurs, nor what courses the illness follows when it does manifest itself" (1964: 268–69). Finally, the most extensive body of literature on Philippine ethnomedicine exists for the Bisayas, as often unpublished theses or dissertation (such as Magos 1978; Montepio 1978; Ponteras 1980; Tiston 1978; and Gaabucayan 1969).

RESEARCH SETTING

While the Philippines was discovered for Europe and the New World in 1521 by Ferdinand Magellan, the archipelago was known earlier by seafaring Arabs, Chinese, and other Southeast Asians. Spain's greatest impact on the Philippines was to transform Filipinos into the only predominantly Christian (Roman Catholic) population in Asia. Numerous non-literate groups continue to live in the mountainous interiors of Luzon, Panay, Negros, and Mindanao. Muslim Filipinos reside almost entirely in southern Mindanao and the Sulu archipelago.

In the late 19th Century Filipinos revolted against Spain and later made common cause with the United States in the Spanish-American war of 1898. From 1898 to 1946 the Philippines was America's sole possession in Southeast Asia. After the defeat of the occupying Japanese at the end of World War II, the Philippines became an independent nation in 1946. In 1972, as the result of a series of economic and political problems, Ferdinand Marcos, then serving his second elected term as president, declared martial law. In 1981 the facade of martial law was abolished by Marcos, although his one-man rule of the nation continues.

The Republic of the Philippines is politically divided into provinces that are subdivided into municipalities. The administrative center of a municipality, where the offices of various provincial and municipal officials are located, is called the *poblacion*. A typical *poblacion's* spatial organization is a plaza surrounded by the *municipio* (the building housing local officials), a public elementary school, the Catholic church and the priest's residence, and the marketplace (Hart 1955). The smallest political unit of the municipality is the *barangay*, until recently called *barrio* or village.

The major islands south of Luzon and north of central Mindanao is a geographical and cultural region known as the Bisayas. The three major Bisayan groups are known after their languages, Cebuan, Panayan, and Samarnon. Cebuan Filipinos live in Central Bisayas (Cebu, eastern Negros, Bohol, western Leyte, and coastal northern Mindanao). Samarnons occupy the Eastern Bisayas (eastern Leyte and Samar). The third major Bisayan group is Panayans, who live in the Western Bisayas (western Negros and Panay islands). Together these three Bisayan cultural-linguistic groups represent the majority of Christian Filipinos. (See Map 1.)

The Eastern Bisayas has been and remains today a region largely marginal to the nation's economic and cultural life. Reasons for this relative neglect is

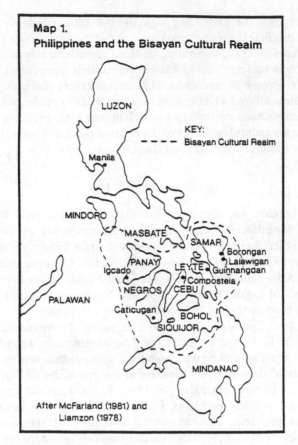

Map 1.
Philippines and the Bisayan Cultural Realm

KEY:
- - - - Bisayan Cultural Realm

LUZON

Manila

MINDORO

MASBATE   SAMAR
                              Borongan
         PANAY   Lalawigan
    Igcado   LEYTE   Guinhangdan
                         Compostela
         NEGROS CEBU
PALAWAN
    Caticugan   BOHOL
              SIQUIJOR

                    MINDANAO

After McFarland (1981) and
Llamzon (1978)

limited arable land, a largely subsistence agriculture, a small population, poor roads, and destructive typhoons. Leyte, the eighth largest island in the archipelago (Samarnons live only in the eastern part of the island), has the region's largest and most modern port, Tacloban, with a population of 80, 707 in 1975. Ferdinand Magellan and his expedition made their first landfall in the Philippines of Homonhon island off Leyte's southern coast.

Samar, the third largest island in the Philippine archipelago, has a rugged mountainous interior in which spurs from this highland partially separate small lowlands on the east coast. The major crops of the island are corn, rice, and coconuts. Lumber is an increasingly important product, although the exploitation of this natural resource is hindered by an inadequate network of roads. The island has no commercial airport.

Lalawigan is located on the east coast of Samar, about five miles south of the provincial capital, Borongan, with a population of 4,294 in 1975. Borongan is a typical Philippine provincial town with a plaza bordered by an old Spanish stone church, the *municipio* and public marketplace. Electricity is available only from sunset to early morning. Buses run daily to Tacloban and Manila. Passengers are ferried from northern Samar to the southern tip of Luzon to continue the trip to Manila (Hart 1974).

Lalawigan, a farming-fishing village, is located along the Borongan-Guiuan national road. The village, facing a section of the Pacific Ocean that is dotted with small rocky islands that fringe a rugged coastline, had 1,615 residents in 1975. By 1982 certain changes had been made in the village compared to 1955 when I first resided in the community. Lalawigan now has a high school and a resident priest. Fishermen no longer are limited to inshore fishing, since most of their boats have been motorized. Some residents are connected to the Borongan electrical system. Water is still obtained from wells scattered throughout the village. Daytime bus service and Honda pedicabs enable the residents to travel with some frequency to and from Borongan, where the nearest hospital is located.

Most residences in Lalawigan, typical of the rural Bisayas, are made of bamboo and plam thatch raised above the ground on sturdy poles. Lalawignons are Roman Catholics, and each house has a family altar with saint figures and picutres of the Holy Family. The household altar is the major center of household religious activities. Kinship in the Bisayas is traced bilaterally and the family is the most important social unit. Social life centers on occasions from the various life crises (baptisms, marriages, and funerals), the annual fiesta for the village's patron saint, and other Catholic church and public school ceremonies and programs.

Additional field data on this chapter's topic comes from other communities in the Central Bisayas. Compostela municipality is 30 kilometers north of Cebu City. The *poblacion's* commercial buildings line for several blocks one side of the national road running north to the tip of the island. In 1975 the *poblacion* had 3,459 residents. The municipality has no hospital and only one small drugstore. My research was done in the *poblacion* and two adjacent villages.

Negros, the fourth largest island of the archipelago, was named by the Spaniards after the Negritos who still live in its forested interior. The island is divided into two provinces; Negros Occidental is inhabited by Panayans, whereas Cebuans reside in Negros Oriental. Dumaguete (53,765 people in 1975) is the largest city of Negros Oriental. Siaton municipality is 50 kilometers south of Dumaguete. Siaton *poblacion* 3,366 persons in 1975) is the residence of the sole priest in the municipality. Here is also found a Catholic high school, a small community college, and the only hospital and drugstore in the town. Caticugan, a village of 909 persons in 1979 (personal census), is north of Siaton *poblacion* on the west bank of the Siaton river. The residents of this village are subsistence farmers raising corn and rice.

LANTI SYMPTOMS

There are numerous symptoms associated with *lanti*: a high fever that results in boils; loose, greenish excrement; cold extremities; *atas* (white-coated tongue sometimes including the inside of the mouth); *habas* (reddish bloches or skin eruptions where the skin folds on the arms, legs, thighs, and neck); *puno* (a skin disease of the scalp); rapid heart beats; stomach ache; incessant crying; dsire to be held by an adult; trembling; shouting during sleep (when awake the patient reports a sensation of falling); and a deepening of the fontanel (*bobon*). Those who treat *lanti* claim that of all these symptoms the three most recurrent ones are a high fever, boils, and *habas* (also see Makabenta 1979: 75).

LANTI: PATHOGENESIS AND ETIOLOGY

Pathogenesis describes the "agent or mechanism that produces or aggravates an illness", whereas etiology indicates the "circumstances that lead a particular patient to contract an illness" (Frake 1961: 125). In Lalawigan *lanti* is considered a natural illness caused by fright that, with a few exception, afflicts only infants or young children, and almost invariably the youngest child. If there are two children in the family, the youngest is most apt to be sickened by *lanti*, but it may strike the elder sibling. When this occurs the explanation given is that the elder sibling is "weaker than the youngest sibling". The usual restriction of *lanti* to the youngest child is not mentioned in our sources for two other similar illnesses to be discussed. Whether this feature of the illness is unique to Lalawigan or was missed by others studying the sickness is unknown. Although *lanti* usually is not fatal, if patients are not treated their physical conditions may deteriorate until they succumb from other complications.

The identical illness is mentioned, often briefly, in the literature on Samarnon Filipinos residing in eastern Leyte. Arens states that *ugmad* is a sickness caused by fright; the patient is *hinugmaran* or made ill by fear (1971: 116; also Makabenta 1979: 187). In a study of etiologies in Guinhangdan, a fishing village of 1,200 people in eastern Leyte, this illness is known as *kalas* (Nurge 1958: 1162). *Kalas* also means sudden emotion, surprise or astonishment (Makabenta 1979: 41). In Cebuan frightening experiences are called *lubatan* (Wolff 1972: 601). It should be noted that illness rarely occurs in the Bisayas as the putative result of other strong emotions such as anger, jealousy, or hysteria.

The pathogenetic cause of *lanti* is severe fright caused by natural events or experiences. Lalawignons rarely blame *lanti* on supernatural agents, although some speculated the spirits, or *sigbin* (a mythological animal resembling a small kangaroo whose bite is venomous), may cause *lanti*. But when actual incidents resulting in *lanti* were collected, no supernatural beings were blamed. However, Arens does state that "a fairy" (environmental spirit) may be the cause of *ugmad*.

Soul loss is not a cause of illness in Lalawigan, Caticugan, and Compostela. However, it is a cause of sickness in elsewhere in the Philippines. In Tarong, an Ilokan village in northern Luzon, all or part of a child's soul insecurely fixed to its body may be detached by sudden shock or fright. As a result the victim suffers tremors, tics, and dizziness; and delirium followed by a coma may occur (Nydegger and Nydegger 1966: 83). When this sickness is diagnosed, the patient is first treated with a home remedy. If the child does not recover, a local curer is consulted, who performs an elaborate diagnosis-curing rite (Nydegger and

Nydegger 1966: 86–87). Soul loss is a frequent cause of illness, especially among infants and younger children in Igcado, Antique province, Panay (Magos 1978).

The fright considered causative of *lanti* may take various forms. Parents of Lalawigan children who became sick reported such experiences as being startled by a pig (when defecating outside the house); seeing two men fighting; hearing barking dogs; seeing a large fire with black clouds of swirling smoke; playing with a dog or chicken that frightened them; riding on a bus; almost falling out of an outrigger boat; being severely scolded or punished; falling into a ditch; tumbling out of a bamboo walker or a hammock in the house; and hearing the sudden noise of a passing bulldozer.

Typical incidents that startled a parent or another household member which resulted in *lanti* in the youngest child (the transferred fright referred to earlier) were: seeing or killing a snake; mistakening an eel inside a closed basket for a snake; shooting a gun; fishing with dynamite; being attacked by an angered carabao (water buffalo); climbing a tall tree; burning a swidden; catching an unusually large fish; stumbling into a newly-dug house post hole; transferring the body of a neighbor to a coffin or having difficulty in lowering a coffin into the grave; visiting a large cave; puddling a rice field with two carabaos; being fearful of falling from a tall building; and slaughtering a large pig or carabao. Some of these events did not frighten the persons involved, yet *lanti* occurred because the experience was sufficient to alarm the youngest child.

The general consensus is that *lanti* results indirectly only when the kinsman involved is a permanent member of the child's household. Others believe that kinship and household residence are not necessary as long as the individual involved has en enduring and affectionate relationship with the child such as "always holding the baby". A few informants claimed that parents cannot cause *lanti* once the child leaves home.

Birth order is the crucial factor in Lalawigan determining the victims of this illness; only the youngest is at risk. Sex is not a factor, for boys and girls become ill from *lanti*. Immunity to *lanti* occurs once a child is no longer the youngest in the family. However, an adult who is an only child may suffer *lanti* for, as one informant explained, "There is no one else to whom it can be transmitted". For example, a husband had a startling experience that resulted in his wife's becoming ill, since the couple was childless and she was the youngest sibling in her family.

Lalawignons believe an affinity with mystical qualities embraces all kinsmen to a greater or lesser extent. The bond is strongest between parents and children (especially the youngest child). In both Lalawigan and Guinhangdan "The tie between parent and child is considered so firm that what happens to the former will influence the latter; what the father does when he is away from home may affect his offspring" (Nurge 1958: 1162). It is weaker between nieces and nephews and their uncles and aunts and weakest between more remote relatives such as cousins.

The experiences of the father are also a frequent cause of *lanti*. Unlike the mother "The father usually is working outside the house, often goes fishing, visits a swidden in the forest, and is more apt to see or do things that scare him". Mothers usually are more house-bound, caring for the children, cooking, ironing, sewing, and doing various household chores. Their opportunities for experiencing fright are fewer than their husbands. Thus, fright of the mother is rarely a cause of *lanti*. However, a pregnant woman in Lalawigan must not deliver if her youngest child is ill with *lanti*. The frightening aspects of delivery cause the sickness of the youngest sibling to be transferred to the new-born infant. When such transference of fright causes *lanti*, it is said "sickness sits on the infant".

Similar beliefs about the fright generated by delivery and birth exist in the central Philippines. In Dumaguete and environs a new-born infant is steamed (a therapy called *tu-ub*) by the midwife and then shaken ". . . to shake off the fears which it may have acquired during birth" (Polson and Pal 1956: 47). The same treatment is then given the new mother to free her of fears created during labor and delivery. Unless this emotional element is eliminated, either or both may become sick.

Most Lalawignons are uncertain why *lanti* is restricted with rare exceptions to the youngest child. Many parents believe that of their children the youngest has a weaker heart, is unusually nervous, and the most easily frightened. In those instances where *lanti* afflicted an older child, the reason given was that the victim was physically weaker than the youngest sibling.

Lalawignon parents, like other Christian Filipinos, often have a favorite child, and usually

... the favorite is the youngest member of the family. The youngest child often experiences a prolonging of his childhood status and is the object of special attention, not only from his parents but from older siblings as well (Guthrie and Jacobs 1966: 94).

The belief that the youngest child is uniquely susceptible, both physically and emotionally, to *lanti* or similar illnesses resulting from fright may explain in part the parents' greater attention and concern for the welfare of this offspring.

Lalawignons do not clearly understand the process by which fright is displaced to another. One informant explained that the transference was a process like magic; another thought it was similar to magnetism. Most believe this diffusion of fright occurs because the involved individuals normally are kinsmen who live permanently in the same household and have a close intimate relationship with the victim.

Frazer's well-known contagious magic principle ("things once in contact with each other remain forever in association, even after separation") best explains this invisible affinity that channels fright from one member of the household to the youngest child.

In other societies this magical affinity is regarded as existing among related persons, among agemates, and among members of social groups of many other kinds. Whatever good or harm befalls objects of individuals of one class also befalls other members of the class without any necessary direct contact, unless magic preventive measures are taken (Norbeck 1961: 56).

This mystical bond reappears in other forms in Bisayan culture. Many Bisayans believe a supernatural competition may develop between two closely related kinsmen, usually siblings or twins. During this competition one of the individuals is defeated by the other, namely become ill or suffers frequent misfortunes. This concept is known in Cebuan and Panayan as *magdaug* (*daug*, to overcome, Wolff 1972: 207–08; Kaufmann 1935: 185–86) and in Samarnon as *abong* (Makabenta 1979: 1). In Lalawigan *abong* is thought limited to siblings, some say only to twins of the opposite sex. In Caticugan a twin was purposely sent to live with his uncle in the *poblacion* to prevent *magdaug* between the two siblings.

Another manifestation of *magdaug* is the tabu that prevents a pregnant woman from having any physical contact with a dying person or a corpse. Such contact also generates competition between the fetus (life) and the patient or cadaver (death) that results in the illness if not the death of the fetus (Tan 1962: 97–98). In Igcado, a village in Antique province, Panay, a special ceremony is held to equalize this competition between a married couple (Magos 1978).

PREVENTIVE MEASURES

Adults may take preventive measures to protect a child from *lanti* or *ugmad*.

In Eastern Leyte, for example, a father who on the way to the field meets a frightful object will, upon arriving home, embrace and kiss his children, and say: "May you not be afraid of the thing I was afraid of today". If he forgets to do so and one of the children thereafter gets sick, the sickness is termed *ugmad* (Arens 1971: 117).

(This statement, implying that any child, not only the youngest, may be sickened with *ugmad*, is different from the situation in Lalawigan.)

Some Lalawignon parents, in anticipation of fright, may invite the child to accompany them to the forest or participate in an activity that might startle them. "Come, join me in my work" or "Come, child, let's go to the forest to kill a snake". One informant advised that when persons have been frightened, they should, upon returning home, step forcefully on the top rung of the house's entrance ladder, grasp the hand rail, and repeat a "magic prayer" (*urasiyun*). Other adults, if they had a startling experience (or one they think may frighten the child) will have precautionary *paglo-on* (a *lanti* treatment to be discussed) for the youngest child on arrival home. A pregnant mother had her youngest child treated for *lanti* as a protection. She believed her fear during delivery would transfer to the child, resulting in this illness.

Yet it is often impossible to prevent *lanti*, particularly since parents "must go about our daily jobs so all can eat". One also never knows for certain what type of experience will frighten the child. Thus the epidemiologic background is laid for numerous people to be at risk.

TRADITIONAL CURERS IN LALAWIGAN

When a child is ill the parents, a curer, or a specialist in *lanti*, may diagnose and treat the sickness. There is considerable hesitation on the part of parents to select initially one of the *lanti* treatments. Usually a home remedy is tried, especially if the symptoms appear minor. This reluctance is explained by the belief that any *lanti* treatment becomes a habit. If the child is sickened again by *lanti*, which often happens, it is mandatory for the same ritual to be repeated. When these patients mature and marry, their youngest child is required to be treated by the same ritual when sickened with *lanti*. For example, one grandmother scolded her daughter for having the first *lanti* cure for her grandson: "Now this treatment will be necessary for your children and their descendants". As discussed later, *lanti* ceremonies are only one category of rituals where need for continuance is a forced inheritance from one's ancestors.

The curer (who may be a shaman), midwife, and masseur are the three traditional medical specialists in the Bisayas (also see Lieban 1967: 81). Lalawignons, in addition to the curer (*tambalan*), traditional midwife (*partira*), and messeur (*hilut*), may also consult the *parasuna* (who specializes in treating poisonous snake and insect bites), the *parangihu* (who extracts teeth using his hands and *urasiyun*), and those who limit their practice to treating *lanti* (Hart 1978). Aside from the *tambalan*, who also treats *lanti*, there are three types of specialists dealing with *lanti*: the *paratubod, paralo-on* and *parabirik*. Of these Arens has identified only the *paralo-on* who "is often a *tambalan* . . ." (1971: 117).

Of the eighteen curers for *lanti* in Lalawigan in 1955, only one performed all three associated curing rites; two others perform two of the ceremonies. The remaining fifteen were specialists in only one *lanti* rite apiece. Nine of these curers specialized in *paglo-on*, the most popular initial therapy for *lanti*, and three apiece specialized in *paralo-on* and *parabirik*. One male *tambalan* was also a *paralo-on* specialist. Twelve of the fifteen village masseurs (who not only massage but treat sprains, reduce fractures, remove foreign substances from the throat, and treat other illnesses caused by these injuries) were also *lanti* specialists. Three *lanti* specialists were also midwives. The number of specialists treating *lanti* in this relatively small village indicates the frequency of this sickness among the young.

Like most Bisayan traditional medical specialists, those in Lalawigan rarely demand a set fee for their services. The patient offers a donation or *patucas* (usually in cash, sometimes in food or drink) that is accepted without question. The typical donations for a *lanti* treatment varies from 25 to 50 American cents. Informants claim that the curative rituals are ineffective unless the paractitioner is given a donation. When asked why they do not charge a regular fee, like physicians, most curers explain they cure mainly to help the people in their communities. As one *lanti* specialist commented: "God cures without payment so why should not I?"

Urasiyun are a ubiquitous element of Bisayan ethnomedicine. One curer explained their effectiveness by stating "The *oracion* [*urasiyun*] is from God, and nothing is as powerful as God" (Lieban 1967: 31). Scheans and Hutterer correctly state that *urasiyun* often cannot be translated as prayer (which is its meaning in Spanish from where the term has been borrowed) since it is not a petition aimed at influencing the supernatural, but rather a formula which compels it to act (1970: 29).

Wolff's definition of *urasiyun* describes better a formulary than a prayer: "A magic formula in Latin or pseudo-Latin which has curative or other magical powers (especially as a *sumpa* or charm) that are effective only when used by the owner" (1972: 1107). Valmoria similarly defines an *urasiyun* as a ". . . magico-religious formula or spell . . ." that ". . . when recited by an *oraysonista* is believed to produce the desired effect" (1981: 13). When the *urasiyun* are taken from the Catholic liturgy, they are identified in this article as prayers. Otherwise, *urasiyun* is translated as "formulary".

In the Bisayas formularies often include a mixture of garbled Latin, Greek, Spanish, English and local languages. Their accurate translation into English is further complicated by their numerous nonsense words or phrases. Formularies probably originated when a curer asked a sacristan to copy prayers (especially those for illness) from the *Missale Romanum* or *Rituale Romanum*. The sacristan, in copying the texts, made errors in spelling and grammar and his handwriting may have been difficult to read. These formularies were memorized by individuals who did not understand Latin or the other languages or could not accurately read the written versions so words or syllables were omitted or contracted. Additional errors were introduced when the formularies were transmitted orally or copied by other individuals (Arens 1958: 40).

It is not surprising that some treatments for *lanti* and a variety of other illnesses in the Bisayas utilize the principle of fumigation and heat. Heat therapy is popular with curers throughout the world. It was widely used in ancient Egypt, and from there it is believed to have diffused to Europe. Fire (or heat) not only purifies the body but it creates smoke or steam that casts out evil influences or harmful substances and attracts the forces of good (Williams 1979: 36).

Palina and *tu-ub* are widespread fumigation-heat therapies associated with Bisayan ethnomedicine. In Lalawigan *palina* is also called *lo-on* or *haplas* (Nurge 1955–56; Villegas 1971: 81–83; Hart 1975), whereas in Panayan the procedure is known as *butbut* (Kaufmann 1935: 82; Ponteras 1980: 231–36).

In *palina* various ingredients such as herbs, animal hair, medicinal coconut oil (*lana*), native incense, beeswax, snake moult, and scrapings of religious objects are added to live coals to produce smoke or fumes (Villegas 1971: 81–82; Tiston 1978: 65–67). The fumes are either fanned on the body or the patient is covered with a blanket or mat under which is put the smoking container. *Palina* is a common treatment is Lalawigan to extract foreign objects shot into the patient's body by offended spirits.

Tu-ub is a similar therapy in which the patient is steamed by a pot of boiling water containing both herbal and non-herbal ingredients (Pal and Polson 1973: 202–03; Montepio 1978: 111–12; Hart 1965: 88; Llopes Ruiz 1968: 89–90). The steam is concentrated on the patient by a blanket covering; sometimes the ill person straddles the steaming pot. Both *palina* and *tu-ub* are used for illnesses with natural and supernatural causes and thus for *lanti*.

PAGTUBOD RITUAL

There are three *lanti* rituals in Lalawigan: *pagtubod, paglo-on*, and *pagbirik*. If the sick child is an infant ("They cannot explain why they are ill") or if no frightening experience can be recalled as having occurred to the patient or other household member, the *paratubod* is consulted. *Pagtubod* means to burn, scorch, or incinerate, (Makabenta 1979: 181).

The *paratubod* begins by divining the cause of the illness. A piece of alum (*pedlanomre* or *tawas*) is rubbed on the patient's soles, palms, body joints, mouth, forehead and fontanel. As this is done the curer inaudibly recites a formulary, mentioning the name of the patient. The alum then is placed on live coals in a coconut shell or metal container, where it bubbles and melts, always staying white, and eventually assumes the shape of the object or event causing *lanti* (also see Arreo 1956: 101–102). If an animal that frightened the child or second person is known, one of its hairs (if possible) is added to the coals. One *lanti* specialist remembers how her daughter became ill after her husband's father (who lived permanently in their household) killed a large pig. "It was good that he kept the tail so we had a hair to use. But he had plenty of experience with *lanti*". Like all *lanti* rituals, the *pagtubod* ceremony is not secret, although guests rarely are invited. The patient may be treated at home or taken (usually by the mother) to the residence of the specialist.

The burnt alum is powdered, rubbed on the various parts of the patient's body while some is administered orally. The *paratubod* then recites the following formulary.

(Juamiam Tuam) (?)
Angelurum Malum (The evil of the angels)
Tehedomini Dios Mium (You, my Lord)
Aderabo ad Templom (I shall adore at the temple)
Et compace Angelurum (With the peace of the angels)
Paslom teledomini Dios (?Lord God)
Meus in Nomeme (Mine, In the name [of Father, Son, Holy Ghost?])

Paytubod may be done three times (three is a magical number for most Bisayan Filipinos) during one day or for three consecutive days if the initial treatment is unsuccessful or inconclusive. When treatment is repeated three times during one day it is because the patient and the curer live some distance apart. The therapy is telescoped to minimize transportation costs. In Guinhangdan, "it [referring to *paglo-on*] is believed that the treatment should be repeated three times and preferably at the same time of the day as during the first meeting" (Nurge 1958: 1166). Another *paratubod* thoughtfully commented that she recommends only one treatment. If the child then seems better, the rite is not repeated. "This way they will need only one *pagtubod* in the future if the child is again sickened by *lanti*."

PAGLO-ON RITUAL

A second, and the most common, curing rite for *lanti* in Lalawigan is *paglo-on* (to fumigate; Makabenta 1979: 103). The specialist who conducts it is called *paralo-on*. The patient is first placed on a mat on the floor. If the sickness has been caused by a startling experience of another known person, nail clippings (frequently from the third finger called *waray ngaran* or without name) of this individual are added to the coals. Other ingredients put on the burning coals are a frond from a plam leaf blessed in church on Palm Sunday or shavings from a candle blessed on Candelaria. Candelaria, or Candlemas Day, occurs on the day the Catholic church celebrates the feast of the Purification of the Blessed Virgin, forty days after Christ's death; an official rite, the Blessing of the Candles, is held before mass (Eggan 1955 2: 557). The resulting fumes are fanned over the patient, bathing all parts of the body (also see Arens 1971: 118).

In eastern Leyte the *paralo-on* adds other items to the live coals. Some ingredients are a hair of the patient, a thread from the clothing of either the patient or the parents, native incense mixed with the sap of the *pili* tree, a piece of a palm frond blessed on Palm Sunday, or "part of the object the person was afraid of" (Arens 1971: 117).

Some *paralo-on* then recite two Catholic prayers: I Believe in God (*Natoo Ako*) and Hail, Holy Queen (*Maghimaya ka Hadi*). Others omit these two prayers and recite the following formulary which is mandatory for the cure. For each of the ten statements, the name of the patient is mentioned.

Usa: de kana mahapausa. (One: may you [name of the patient] never be frightened again.)
Duha: de kana magruhaduha. (Two: may you never hesitate again.)
Tulo: hintultulan ko na et palalanti. (Three: I have discovered the one causing your *lanti*.)
Upat: nanngignipat et mga palalanti. (Four: they who caused *lanti* have become cautious.)
Lima: nahiligmak et mga palalanti. (Five: they who caused *lanti* have stumbled.)
Unum: de kana paghininumduman het mga palalanti. (Six: may the one who caused *lanti* forget you.)
Peto: nagkapipitukan pala et mga palalanit. (Seven: they who caused *lanti* were badly hit.)
Walo: nahalulu hin usa nga uhang et mga palalanti. (Eight: everything that caused your *lanti* has fallen into a pit.)
Siyam: nauyam pala et mga palalanti. (Nine: they who caused *lanti* are bored.)
Napulo: nagkapu-puan na et nga mga palalanti. (Ten: they who caused *lanti* have become armless and legless.)

The *paralo-on* then repeats three times: *Mapalus na et nga emo lanti nga cahuwasan ka na* (May whatever caused your *lanti* be removed and may you now get well). This curing rite is done for three consecutive afternoons.

The full meaning of these formularies often is obscure. Their mere utterance is believed curative. But they have additional functions. They reassure the accompanying parent that the source of the patient's illness has been identified, and until the exact etiology is known, an appropriate treatment cannot be selected. The formularies also reflect that frightening experiences often result from encounters with animals so they are captured ("fallen into a pit") or dismembered ("armless and legless"). Since humans may be causative agents, they are urged to be more "cautious" in the future.

Arens cites an eastern Leyte *paglo-on* formulary that is remarkably similar in form (ten statements) and content to the one used in Lalawigan. (For a complete version of Aren's formulary, see Hart 1975: 17). In fact, the first two statements in Aren's formulary are identical with those in the previously cited Lalawigan formulary. In these formularies the fear causing *lanti* (or *ugmad*) is personalized. The *paralo-on* demands that "*you* [italics added] disappear as the smoke disappears from the body of the sick person" or "*they* [italics added] who caused *lanti* have been badly hit".

Another variation of *paglo-on* in Lalawigan is that the *paralo-on* may make the sign of the cross on the various parts of the patient's body. When possible the patient is also requested to do this (also see Arreo 1956: 101). When making the sign of the cross, the *paralo-on* uses the third finger dampened with saliva. Saliva often is used for curative purposes in other treatments, for it absorbs the supernatural qualities of the prayers and formularies recited by the curer. Sometimes the sign of the cross is made with water in a coconut shell. If the patient may bathe the following day, this water used in the rite in Leyte is added to the bath.

If no bath is to be taken, the *paralo-on* throws the coconut shell outside, saying: "May all the things that scared you go with the throwing of this coconut shell" (Arens 1971: 119).

Arens adds that "In cases where the patient is not cured in the first ceremony, the fumigation is continued every day until the patient is well" (1971: 119).

PAGBIRIK RITUAL

The third and most elaborate curing rite for *lanti* in Lalawigan is *pagbirik* (to rotate, revolve; Makabenta 1979: 25); the curer is known as *parabirik*. *Pagbirik* is considered the most effective curing ceremony, perhaps because it is more complicated and time-consuming than the other two treatments. A bamboo basket (*sarasas*), used to carry coconuts or firewood, is suspended upside down by twine from a roof beam so that its opening is only a foot or so above the house floor. A lighted lamp or candle is put on the floor directly under the basket. The *parabirik* explain that the basket is suspended because it must be turned during the rite. Later it is lowered over the light to indicate that the ceremony is over.

The ceremony begins when the *parabirik* rotates the basket once clockwise while repeating the first statement of the formulary. It is turned clockwise again as the second statement is repeated. This is continued for each of the ten statements. The following formulary, used by most *parabirik* in the village, is similar to the one recited for *paglo-on*.

Usa: nanhipausa et palalanti, pauugmad nga deri na et bata paghinilanti-an. (One: whatever caused *lanti* has begun to wonder, and may the child [the patient's name] not get sick of *lanti* anymore.)

Duha: nagruhaduha na et palalanti, pauugmad nga deri na et bata paghinilanti-an. (Two: they become hesitate and may the child [the patient's name] not get sick of *lanti* anymore.)

Tulo: pinanhitultulan ko na et mga palalanti, pauugmad ngan deri na et bata paghinilanti-an. (Three: I know where they are now and may the child not get sick of *lanti* anymore.)

Upat: nanngignipat na et mga palalanti, pauugmad ngan deri na et bata paghinilanti-an. (Four: they have become cautious and may the child not get sick of *lanti* anymore.)

Lima: nanhiligmak na et mga palalanti, pauugmad ngan deri na et bata paghinilanti-an. (Five: they have stumbled and may the child not get sick of *lanti* anymore.)

Unum: deri na et maghenumdum et mga palalanti, pauugmad nga deri na et bata paghinilanti-an. (Six: may whatever is causing *lanti* forget you and may the child not get sick of *lanti* anymore.)

Peto: nagkapipitukan na et mga palalanti, pauugmad ngan deri na et bata paghinilanti-an. (Seven: they were badly hit and may the child not get sick of *lanti* anymore.)

Walo: nanhilulu na het mga beto et mga palalanti, pauugmad ngan deri na et bata paghinilanti-an. (Eight: they have fallen into different pits and may the child not get sick of *lanti* anymore.)

Siyam: nauyam na et mga palalanti, pauugmad ngan deri na et bata paghinilanti-an. (Nine: they finally got bored and may the child not get sick of *lanti* anymore.)

Napulo: pagkapupupu-an na et mga palalanti, pauugmad ngan deri na et bata paghinilanti-an. (Ten: may all those who caused *lanti* become armless and legless and may the child not get sick of *lanti* anymore.)

After repeating the tenth statement the curer rotates the basket counter-clockwise once, saying: "*Badbad, kabadbaran et bata hit iya lanti*" or "Turn in the opposite direction and may this *lanti* also turn away from the child". The *parabirik* then holds the basket stationary, repeating: "*Taknong! sugad pala et bata het etenaknong hin deri na casarakitan*" or "Stop! like the child has been stopped of being sick". Then the basket is quickly lowered over the lamp on the floor, united from the twine and put in a corner of the dwelling. The first part of the *pagbirik* ritual is finished.

The second part of the *pagbirik* ceremony requires the patient to be gently whipped once with each of sixteen leaves. Each leaf is used in a set order. As the patient is whipped with a leaf, the *parabirik* says a formulary that mentions both the names of the leaf and the patient while requesting that the person be cured. The names of these plants have additional meanings or are similar in sound to other words. Their therapeutic value is not herbal, but consist solely in the imitative magical quality of their names. For example, one plant is known as *payao*. *Hayao* refers to an "undefeated chicken [one that pecks all other chickens] that roams freely", implying that the child in the future may roam the village "undefeated" by *lanti*.

When all the 16 leaves have been used, the treatment is over. If the first treatment does not show results, the curing ritual is repeated. Some *parabirik* are hesitant to duplicate the ritual unless absolutely necessary. For if the child is sickened again with *lanti* the ceremony must be repeated the identical number of times.

There are several additional treatments for *lanti*, or as it is known in other localities, *ugmad* or *kalas*. While the *paglo-on* ritual is widespread in the Eastern Bisayas, the other two ceremonies described for Lalawigan are unreported in the literature. In Nurge's unpublished field notes for Guinhangdan (1955–56), a ceremony called *paghuwas* is used to treat *kalas*. The patient, sometimes when asleep, is intentionally frightened as the curer says: "Now, don't go anymore with your father". Another method, called *bagnaw*, includes a *paghuwas* that is followed by pouring water in which herbal materials have soaked over the patient. Nurge also states if the father is the cause of the patient's fright, a corner of his undershirt is put in water which the patient drinks as a cure.

If the cause of *lanti* is unknown, the patient usually is first treated by the *paratubod* to determine the nature of the frightening experience. If the cure is delayed, the patient may have also *paglo-on* and *pagbirik*. Several *lanti* specialists stated that some parents had their child treated by all three rituals in succession. When this is the case the treatments begin with *pagtubod* and end with *pagbirik*.

OTHER ILLNESSES RESULTING FROM FRIGHT

Bisayan illnesses traced to fright or fear are not limited to *lanti, ugmad* or *kalas*. This traumatic emotional experience is also given as the reason for some skin ailments and boils, fever, convulsions, measles, or digestive upsets (Llopes Ruiz 1968: 122–23; Aparece 1960: 40–41; Galleon 1971: 42–43, 79, 218; Merced-Rivera 1982; Gaabucayan 1969: 41). In Compostela a 11-year old boy was frightened when his aunt warned that unless his incessant crying stopped, a supernatural creature would carry him away to the forest. The next day boils appeared on his head that the curer blamed on his terror of a supernatural kidnapping. In this municipality a startling experience is also believed to cause a fatal relapse (*bughat sa tingag*) of a new mother (Wolff 1972: 1018).

Admiration by ancestral souls unintentionally may cause illness, especially in young children, when their "visit to welcome" the new family member frightens the child (Galleon 1971: 163). In Compostela this sickness is labelled *gihangad sa apuhan* or *balu*. *Hangad* means to look upward or to turn the head up, whereas *apuhan* refers to grandparents (Wolff 1972: 100). In other words, the child's attention is attracted to the hovering souls.

If the child is a male, the spectral visitors are the parents' grandfathers; if a female, the grandmothers come. Most children are terrified, for they "can see the souls" who give them "affectionate" but painful pinches. As a result, convulsions often follow, the skin becomes clammy, and eyes roll upward "until only the whites can be seen". The cure is an elaborate food offering during which the curer marks a cross with chicken blood on the patient's forehead to prevent future fright by the souls.

In Caticugan *ikala-uy* (*kala-uy*, to pit) is an illness with the same etiology as *gihangad sa apuhan*. Again children are sickened from fright when visited by friendly ancestral souls. An identical etiology in this village but limited to adults is known as *ikalgan* or *iyangud*. However, sometimes the illness resulting from visiting souls spares the adult but boomerangs to a child (Wolff 1972: 1135).

NIGHTMARE FRIGHT

Death is also traced to frightening nightmares (*urum*, Wolff 1972: 1109; *hupa*, Kaufmann 1935: 322; *ngarat*, Makabenta 1979: 130). This puzzling disorder is best known in the medical and anthropological literature by its Tagalog name, *bangungot* (nightmare). A popular account of *bangungot* states that 460 victims who died from this malady were autopsied between 1915–1938 in the Department of Pathology of the University of Santo Tomas, Manila. An additional 84 Filipino fatalities from *bangungot* occurred between 1937–48 in Honolulu (Ventura 1978 9: 2446–48). Women, old people and children do not suffer *bangungot* (Ventura 1978a: 2448).

Interestly, a series of similar mysterious deaths were recently reported by the U.S. Center for Disease Control. All of these fatalities were Asians who "died in their sleep apparently without any demonstrable cause. Before their death, they were all heard groaning, gasping, and breathing noisily" (Guerrero 1982). Except for one female, Hmong refugees who have died from nightmare fright in this country were males. Their average age was the early 30s. All victims were in good health before their deaths that occurred between 11 p.m. – 8 a.m. (Marshal 1981: 1008).

Various etiologies have been suggested (and rejected) for this sudden and often lethal affliction: acute hemorrhagic pancreatitis, cardiac failure, arrhythmia, or fermentation or putrefaction of a heavy meal causing autotoxication (Guerrero 1982; Ventura 1978a: 2448). Another suspected cause is that nightmares produce in the individual an unbearable stress causing the skeletal muscles to contract, forcing a greater volume of blood, at an increased rate of speed, through the heart (Ventura 1978a: 2448). It is speculated that Hmong deaths in the United States may have resulted from past inbreeding among the group (an assumption rejected by Munger and Hurlick 1981: 952), resulting in a congenital weakness of the autonomic system. This condition causes the heart to beat irregularly or possibly to fibrillate during times of intense emotional stress (Marshal 1981: 1008).

This illness among Bisayans has both natural and supernatural etiologies, although the former are more common. Some informants explain that nightmares occur when one sleeps without a pillow or with the head lower than the rest of the body. This position causes the blood to rush to the brain because the heart speeds up circulation. Overeating, another reason for nightmares, hinders the circulation of the blood, and as a result the blood stagnates in the abdomen. Nightmares also originate with a personal frightening experience, of either a natural or supernatural nature, in which the reaction may be delayed for days.

Informants also believe this illness can be traced to God who is punishing individuals for sins, insincere prayers, or failure to cross themselves before retiring at night. Several cases in Caticugan and Compostela were traced to hostile environmental spirits. In one of these instances, however, the patient's description of her illness episode indicated a possible imbalance of hot-cold elements (humoral pathology) in the body (Hart 1969). In Lalawigan *ngarat* may develop from an ordinary dream when one is ill or exhausted by the day's work.

The symptoms of nightmare fright include an inability on the part of the Bisayan patient to move or speak: "One feels nailed to the sleeping mat".[2] Violent spasms occur and breathing is labored. A Lalawignon said the best way to prevent *ngarat* when sleeping alone is to lie on one's back with the arms extended sideways and the feet overlapping — "like a crucifix". Other informants advised crossing one's self before going to sleep.

The sole remedy for this illness is to wake the person before death occurs. A curer in Compostela recommended massage after the person is awaken. Most curers, however, admit they had no experience in treating this sickness, for the patients either are awakened and recover or die before they can be called. For this reason it is dangerous to sleep alone in the house. A widowed healer in Compostela remarried because he did not want to "sleep alone, for if I suffer *urum* there would be no one to awaken me". He also said it is possible to diagnose the cause of death from nightmare fright, when the victim died alone, because "many bubbles appear in the mouth".

It was not difficult to obtain information on numerous cases of this affliction in the three communities I investigated. During World War II a Caticugan man was captured by the Japanese soldiers. He escaped after two days but several nights later died alone in his sleep. His death was blamed on nightmare fright resulting from this experience, for he had feared recapture and execution by the Japanese. Another Caticugan man joked about the spirits with his companion before retiring. "During my sleep I dreamt that an *ingkantu* [spirit] was choking me. I think maybe it was trying to steal my soul. I struggled and fought but I could hardly breathe. My companion heard me groaning so he woke me up." Other survivors report they were attacked during their nightmares by a spirit or witch (*aswang*). Several fatalities from nightmare fright were reported for villages adjacent to Caticugan.

One case of *urum* was investigated that involved a young female whose treatment appears unique. A woman in Caticugan was noticed with a large scar on each of her inner arms. She explained that by stating that one day, when 11-years old, she returned home after playing vigorously all afternoon. She was hungry and hot. After eating she slept nude without any covering or a mat to cool off. Later in the evening her mother heard the young girl shouting in her sleep. She then became stiff. Violent spasms followed that made it difficult for family members to restrain her. Finally she could not move or speak.

Fortunately a curer was visiting in a nearby house. He was called to the girl's residence and diagnosed the illness as the result of *urum*. He applied a red-hot metal ladle to her inner arms to awaken the patient. (Later the informant said the scars were caused because the curer left the ladle on her arms too long.) The girl, who felt no pain when the hot ladle was applied, awoke and recovered. The curer claimed she had also offended the environmental spirits who had caused her nightmare. A thanksgiving payment (food offering) for her recovery was later held.

Kabuhi is another widespread illness often traced to the patient's experiencing shock or fright (Lieban 1967: 81; Aparece 1960: 39–40; Demetrio 1970 2: 441–42). *Kabuhi* may be caused by the victim's seeing a snake, a ferocious animal, or learning of the death of a close kinsman, (Demetrio 1970 2: 441; Aparece 1960: 39–40; Nurge 1958: 1162). However, this illness may also be the result of food allergies, punitive environmental spirits, or follow child birth (Arens 1971: 121; Demetrio 1970 2: 442; Hart 1965: 57–58). One treatment for *kabuhi* is for the curer to shake the patient, saying: "Jesus, Mary, Joseph, fear disappear" (Demetrio 1970 2: 442).

A Filipino physician who has investigated the *kabuhi* syndrome identified it as a gastro-intestinal neurosis.

This syndrome [which is found "everywhere in the country under different names"] is characterized by a gnawing pain in the epigastric region which may or may not be associated with vaso-motor manifestations such as cold sweating, especially in the hands and feet, chest oppression and a cold sensation in the epigastrium. The incidence of this clinical complex is very high among women, especially in the older age groups either near or past menopause and in the aged (Canoy 1960: 503).

ANALYSIS

Lieban has commented that medical anthropology "encompasses the study of medical phenomena as they are influenced by social and cultural features, and social and cultural phenomena as they are illuminated by their medical aspects" (1977: 15). This generalization has been chosen for analysis based on the examination of illnesses originating with the patient's fear or fright, experienced directly or indirectly. Bisayan ethnomedicine reflects many facets of the world view of Filipinos and underlying principles that influence how they cope with life's numerous problems. Three major features of Bisayan culture, exemplified by this illness syndrome, are selected for comment: imitative magic aspects of Bisayan culture; the double standard for the sexual behavior of males; and cultural persistence.

Imitative magic is a ubiquitous thread running through all segments of Bisayan culture. This principle of magic best explains the therapeutic value of whipping the patient during the *pagbirik* ritual. Mental patients, more in the past than at present, once were severely whipped to expel the demonic forces possessing them. The *parabirik's* rotation of the basket (an action naming the ceremony) unties the sickness from the patient so receovery is possible. As indicated earlier, the 16 leaves used in this ritual are neither applied to the patient as a poultice nor brewed as a tonic, but rahter brought into contact with the patient by being used as whips. Their curative powers are based on the sympathetic association of their names, sometimes to similar sounding terms. For example, the names of three leaves used in *pagbirik* display such a linkage; *balukas* (*lakas*, to take off); *arigbangun* (*bangun*, to rise); and *talibangan* (*tabang*, to help or relieve). In other words, the use of these leaves assists the patient in shedding the fright causing *lanti*, to rise from the sick bed, or relieves the symptoms. (Hart 1975: 17 gives a complete listing of these 16 leaves and their suggestive names.)

A wider perspective of Bisayan culture quickly demonstrates the pervasiveness of this major principle of magic. In building a new house in Caticugan, rattan used to tie nipa shingles to the roof must not be cut with the teeth, or else the dwelling, on completion, will always be inhabited by biting insects. *Kalipay* leaves (also meaning happiness) are one item used in the post-hole ritual for a new house to ensure future harmonious relations among the occupants (Hart 1959: 40). Similar practices are associated with fishing. For example, sand or pebbles are thrown at the opening of a new bamboo fish trap so when submerged in the sea it will catch as many fish as "the grains of sand or pebbles" (Hart 1956: 70). *Malapgus*, a wild plant with beady heads, are part of the ritual held when rice is planted in the seed bed in Caticugan so the plants on maturity will produce similarly full tassels of rice (Hart 1954: 304–05). Many taboos associated with pregnant women are based on the principle of imitative magic such as avoiding ascending the house entrance ladder when someone is sitting on a rung to prevent a delayed or difficult delivery (Hart 1965: 42–47).

One cause of *lanti* (or *kalas*) reflects the widespread double standard governing the sexual life of males. In Guinhagndan *kalas* often is blamed on the father's illicit sexual activities. In this village ". . . the moment the father begins illicit intercourse . . . his child will have a tendency to be easily frightened, will jerk his head backwards, and, in serious cases, will have convulsions" (Nurge 1958: 1162). Although *lanti* is not usually associated with the father's infidelity, it is considered a cause when a child is stricken with his illness, expecially if the father is away on a trip. The possible unfaithfulness of the mother is ignored as originating *lanti* or *kalas*.

The double standard culturally permits males greater sexual freedom than females, both before and after marriage. As a Caticugan husband boasted: "A husband's love is free; a wife's love is bound." The Filipina often is regarded as

the temptress, the seductress, whom the man, by virtue of his maleness, is physically unable to resist. In fact, a man who fails to respond to a woman's advances is considered abnormal. His *pagkalalaki* (manhood) is suspect; he would be a *bayut* (effeminate or homosexual) (Yu and Liu 1980: 185).

A man is also supposed to be innately more sexually aggressive than a woman. Pal writes that in the rural areas of southern Leyte the masculinity of young men is regarded with serious question if they do not actively pursue young ladies, either as an individual or in roving male groups (1956: 392). The popularity and acceptance of the *querida* (mistress or kept woman) system is eloquent testimony to this double standard (Yu and Liu 1980: 179–202).

It is this cultural norm that explains in part the primacy of the father as a source of *kalas* or *lanti*, for he is more often in fact unfaithful than the mother. This particular etiology is also one example of the social control function of Bisayan ethnomedicine, which in this instance indirectly punishes infidelity and at the same time stresses the importance of a stable family (Nurge 1958: 1162).

Lanti offers a new explanation, hitherto unreported in the literature for Bisayan

Filipinos, for the persistence of some curing ceremonies. As indicated earlier, *lanti* rituals become a habit or are a mandatory inheritance of the patient when this illness recurs. Once started, the rituals must be continued (including the identical number of performances initially held) if this sickness returns to a former victim. When a former *lanti* patient matures and marries, if the youngest child is sickened by *lanti*, the ceremony that cured the parent must be held.

It may also be noted that the inheritance of rituals in Lalawigan and elsewhere in the Bisayas is not limited to those associated with *lanti*. An additional example in Lalawigan is the *katig-uban* (*tig-ub*, to add, *katig-uban*, a gathering) and *katu-igan* (*tu-ig*, year). Two overt and covert functions of these annual ceremonies are to celebrate the death anniversaries of one's ancestors and to reinforce existing bonds among their living descendants, many of whom do not interact regularly. This illustrates once again interrelatedness of etiologies with other segments of Bisayan culture, and requires an explanatory digression.

Beside fright, a frequent cause of illness in the Bisayas is angered or neglected ancestral souls. As one informant explained: "Souls (*kalug*) may punish the living since they can talk with God". Although displeased souls bring sickness and misfortune, properly honored souls reward their living kinsmen with abundant harvests, good health, and general prosperity. For most Bisayans the dead are not gone from their lives: they are merely living beyond. Souls retain their sense of responaibility and pride in their living descendants; they participate in their kinsmen's achievements and shame. If a relative brings honor or dishonor to the family, the souls equally share in the event.

The most common way to maintain a harmonious relation with one's dead, or to repair damaged relations, is to hold one of a variety of ceremonies associated both with the Catholic liturgy or folk Catholicism. These particular rituals may be a novena, rosary, a memorial mass in the church, or folk Catholic ceremonies that require either a simple or elaborate food offering. These rituals may be limited to family members, whereas others include neighbors and friends. A curer often officiates at these rituals; others are directed by a lay specialist in Catholic prayers.

Ritual inheritance in Lalawigan, therefore, includes both noncalendrical (or crisis) and calendrical (or regular) ceremonies. *Lanit* rituals are an example of former, while the *katig-uban* and *katu-igan* represent the latter. Ideally, persons whose participation in the family ceremonies is required by their relations to the souls must try to attend the rituals. Many Lalawignons, born in other communities in eastern Samar, return annually to their natal community to attend these ceremonies.

However, there are alternatives for Lalawignons, a practical people, who live in more distant villages or have jobs in other islands that make it difficult if not impossible to return home for these occasions. Some send money to help pay for the costs of the two rituals. Others hold a substitute rosary in their home on the appropriate date or "light a candle in church [in the place where they live] on this day and say a little prayer". Yet some Lalawignons who reside in Cebu city or Manila return to the village for their family's *katig-uban* or *katu-igan*, especially if they are sickly or "suffer sleepless nights thinking about their home". Informants cited instances of persons who became sick because of non-attendenace at these ceremonies.

Ritual inheritance is not restricted to the Eastern Bisayas. In Caticugan some families hold a celebration on November 1st or All Saints Day which is called *tangkalag* or *harang*. The ceremony, honoring one's ancestral souls, also protects family members from future illness and misfortune and cures those who are sick (also see Tan 1962: 78). However, another function of the ceremony (to which are invited friends, neighbors, and sometimes local political leaders) is to entertain assembled kith and kin in a community event that reinforces the sponsoring family's social position.

If one's parents held the *tangkalag*, it must be continued by their children (and their children), since the obligation is inherited. If the ceremony is not held, the responsible persons are sickened by offended ancestral souls. One informant resumed the *tangkalag* after a curer told her its abandonment was the reason three young sons had died.

An additional inherited ritual in Caticugan is the *kasal-kasal* (*kasal* means wedding; reduplication of the term implies not real) which is held to prevent or cure the illness of a spouse (often of a newly-wedded couple), their children (including those yet to be born), and close kinsmen. This ritual may include a sacrificed pig — cooked and reassembled in a way reported for pre-Hispanic rituals — that the curer offers to the couple's ancestral souls. During one *kasal-kasal* that I witnessed the couple announced that they did not want their children to continue the ritual. The souls were humbly requested to excuse them from this future obligation. The husband later explained he wanted to stop the ceremony because if his children forgot to hold it some of them would become ill. Additional reasons for stopping the traditional ritual include the time required to organize it and the cost of the food offering.

Ritual inheritance involves not only the souls but also the invisible environmental spirits who often cause illness when angered or even unintentionally offended. Such ceremonies are represented by two linked annual rituals held in Compostela called *sugat* and *pakigan*. The first ceremony (*sugat*) is a food offering to welcome the local spirits and those from other places invited by the curer to participate in the event. The second ceremony (*pakigan*) is also a food offering held to bid them farewell. The purpose of these ceremonies is to honor and entertain the spirits so they will not bring sickness and other misofrtunes to the sponsoring families. When the spirits depart they "take away all the bad things in the community". As typical of the other rituals, the obligation to continue the *sugat* and *pakigan* is inherited from one's parents. If the rituals are stopped, the irate spirits punish with illness the responsible persons. In 1980 eight of these ritual cycles were held in various villages in Compostela; one ritual was sponsored by twenty cooperating families, another by forty-eight families.

While these various ritual obligations are inherited, some Bisayans discard them. They may plead with the souls to be relieved of this ceremonial obligation. If one marries and moves to another community, the ritual may not be held, particularly if the other spouse has no similar obligation. Several informants said they took a chance, stopped the required ceremony and had not suffered any supernatural sanction. Yet supporters of these rituals believe that such persons may be only temporarily spared punishment by the souls and spirits. If they escape misfortune or sickness, their children (or even grandchildren) may be victims. Moreover, if a serious illness occurs, the curer may trace the affliction to the failure of the patient to uphold an inherited responsibility. The only cure for the patient is resumption of the abandoned ceremony. While this belief does not guarantee the perpetuation of these rituals from one generation to another, it is a powerful stimulus encouraging their persistence.

Individuals also inherit the role of curer. These persons must submit to this obligation that Ponteras describes as transmitted in the family line (1980: 201). If the call to heal is rejected, the person suffers a serious lingering illness; recovery occurs only when the person agrees to become a curer. One latent function of this belief, widespread in the Bisayas, is that it provides a socially acceptable explanation for becoming a healer. Nearly all curers, especially those in the rural areas, vociferously repudiate the accusation of some that they heal solely for money. They become curers, often against their will, in service of their communities because of forced role inheritance.

Various change-inhibiting factors or barriers to culture change have been identified, including fatalism, cultural ethnocentrism, motor patterns, incompatibility of traits, vested interests, caste, and class (Foster 1973; Barnett 1953). This aspect of Bisayan culture illustrates how cultural persistence may also be based on nonvoluntary ritual inheritance reinforced by supernatural sanctions. It explains, in part, the retention of rituals whose origin and many features can be historically traced to the Philippines' pre-Hispanic past.

This analysis of *lanti* and associated illnesses augments the literature describing sicknesses attributed to various strong and violent emotional experiences. *Lanti* is not an isolated etiology but part of a larger syndrome explaining symptoms associated with maladies varying in seriousness from minor ailments to fatalities. This chapter is an addition to the increasing number of studies that indicate that numerous etiologies are conceptualized, based on their cultural matrix. Not only do these investigations illuminate how medical concepts are influenced by culture and society, but they also furnish new insights for the interpretation of the social fabric of the group under scrutiny. Such research reinforces the recommendation of others of the necessity of giving greater attention to the emotive dimension of human behavior of which the *lanti* complex is but a single example (Ohnuki-Tierney 1981: 147).

NOTES

1. Research for this article was made possible by the Fulbright Program, a Social Science Research Council – Ford Foundation Southeast Asia award, Northern Illinois University Graduate School, and the Wenner-Gren Foundation for Anthropological Research. *Barangay*

(village) Lalawigan was first studied in 1955 and revisited in 1982. Caticugan, a village in southern Negros Oriental Province, Negros, was first investigated in 1950–51, revisited in 1955, 1964–65, 1972, 1979, and 1982. Several villages and *sitios* in Compostela, a municipality in eastern Cebu, were studied in 1979 and 1982. This article incorporates material first published in San Carlos University's *Philippine Quarterly of Culture and Society* (1975).
2. See pp. 114–148, this volume for descriptions of other examples of *Sleep Paralysis* from other cultures.

BIBLIOGRAPHY

Aparece, Francisco T.
　　1960　The Care of the Sick and the Burial of the Dead in the Rural Areas of the Bohol and Their Educational Implications. Cebu City, Philippines. M. A. thesis in education, San Carlos University.
Arens, Richard S. V. D.
　　1958　"Tambalan" and His Medical Practices in Leyte and Samar Islands, Phillippines. The Philippine Journal of Science: 86: 121–30.
　　1971　The "Lo-on" or Fumigation Ceremony on Leyte and Samar. Leyte-Samar Studies 5: 116–21.
Arreo, Antonino L.
　　1956　Llorente, Samar Since 1900: A Brief Survey of the Social, Political and Economic Life of the People. Manila. M. A. thesis in history, University of Manila.
Barnett, Homer G.
　　1953　Innovation; The Basis of Cultural Change. New York: McGraw-Hill.
Cannon, W. B.
　　1942　"Voodoo" Death. American Anthropologist 44: 169–81.
Canoy, Nestor R.
　　1960　Gastro-Intestinal Neurosis. Journal of the Philippine Medical Association 30: 503–12.
Demetrio, Francisco, S. J.
　　1970　Dictionary of Philippine Folk Beliefs and Customs. Cagayan de Oro, Philippines, Xavier University. Pasay City: Modern Press. 4 vols.
Eggan, Fred (ed.)
　　1955　The Philippines. New Haven, Conn. Human Relations Area Files. 4 vols.
Foster, George M.
　　1973　Traditional Societies and Technological Change. New York: Harper & Row, Publishers. 2nd Edition.
Frake, Charles O.
　　1961　The Diagnosis of Disease Among the Subanun of Mindanao. American Anthropologist 63: 113–32.
Gaabucayan, Samuel
　　1969　A Preliminary Study: Toward the Developmental Aspect of Folk Medicine in Barrio Agusan. M. A. thesis in folklore, Xavier University.
Galleon, Warlita K.
　　1971　Case Studies of Fifteen Medicine-Men ("Tambalans") of Maasin, S. Leyte. Cebu City, Philippines. M. A. thesis in anthropology, San Carlos University.
Gieser, Ruth and Joseph E. Grimes
　　1972　Natural Clusters in Kalinga Disease Terms. Asian Studies 10: 24–32.
Guerrero, M. X.
　　1982　"Bangungot" Puzzles U.S. Physicians. Times Journal [Manila]: June, 20.

Guthrie, George M. and Pepita Jimenez Jacobs
 1966 Child Rearing and Personality Development in the Philippines. University Park,
  Penn. The Pennsylvania State University Press.
Hart, Donn V.
 1954 Barrio Caticugan: A Visayan Filipino Community. Syracuse, New York. Dissertation
  in Anthropology, Syracuse University. University Microfilms, Ann Arbor, Mich.:
  Publication No. 10,075.
 1955 The Philippine Plaza Complex: A Focal Point in Culture Change. Yale University,
  New Haven, Conn. Southeast Asia Studies, Cultural Report Series No. 3.
 1956 Securing Aquatic Products in Siaton Municipality, Negros Oriental Province,
  Philippines. Manila: Bureau of Printing, Monograph No. 4. Institute of Science
  and Technology.
 1959 The Cebuan Filipino Dwelling in Caticugan: Its Construction and Cultural Aspects. New Haven, Conn.: Yale University, Southeast Asia Studies. Cultural Report
  Series.
 1965 From Pregnancy Through Birth in a Bisayan Filipino Village. *In* Donn V. Hart,
  Phya Anuman Rajadhon, and Richard J. Coughlin. Southeast Asian Birth Customs.
  Three Studies in Human Reproduction. New Haven, Conn.: Human Relations Area
  Files Press, pp. 1—113.
 1969 Bisayan Filipino and Malayan Humoral Pathologies. Folk Medicine and Ethnohistory
  in Southeast Asia. Ithaca, New York. Southeast Asia Program, Cornell University.
  Data Paper No. 76.
 1974 Culture in Curing in Filipino Peasant Society. Contributions to Asian Studies 5:
  15—25.
 1975 *Lanti*: Sickness by Fright: A Bisayan Filipino Peasant Syndrome. Philippine Quarterly
  of Culture and Society 3: 1—19.
 1978 Disease Etiologies of Samarnon Filipino Peasants. *In* Peter Morley and Roy Wallis
  (eds.), Culture and Curing: Anthropological Perspectives on Traditional Medical
  Beliefs and Practices. Pittsburgh, Penn.: University of Pittsgurgh Press, pp. 57—
  98.
Howells, William W.
 1950 The Heathens. Primitive Man and His Religions. New York: Doubleday and Co.
Janzen, John M.
 1978 The Quest for Therapy. Berkeley, Calif.: University of California Press.
Kaufmann, H. M. H. M.
 1935 Visayan-English Dictionary (Kapulungan Binisaya-Ininglils). Iloilo: La Editorial.
Lambeck, Michael
 1981 Human Spirits: A Cultural Account of Trance in Mayotte. Cambridge, London:
  Cambridge University Press.
Lieban, Richard W.
 1967 Cebuano Sorcery. Malign Magic in the Philippines. Berkeley, Calif.: University of
  California Press.
 1977 The Field of Medical Anthropology. *In* David Landy (ed.), Culture, Disease and
  Healing. Studies in Medical Anthropology. New York: Macmillan Publishing Co.,
  Inc., pp. 13—31.
Llamzon, Teodoro A.
 1978 Handbook of Philippine Language Groups. Quezon City: Ateneo de Manila Univer-
  sity Press.
Llopes Ruiz, Angeles
 1968 A Study of Cebuano Folk Medicine. Cebu City, Philippines. M. A. thesis in anthropology, San Carlos University.
McFarland, Curtis D.
 1981 A Linguistic Atlas of the Philippines. Manila: Linguistic Society of the Philippines.

Magos, Alicia F.
    1978   The "Ma-aram" in a Kinaray-a Society. Quezon City. M. A. thesis in anthro-
                pology, University of Philippines.
Makabenta, Eduardo Q.
    1979   Binisaya-English, English-Binisaya Dictionary. Quezon City: Emandonz.
Marshall, Eliot
    1981   The Hmong: Dying of Culture Shock? Science 212 (May 29): 1008.
Merced-Rivera, Barbara
    1982   Ethnomedicine in Tubigon, Negros Oriental, Philippines. Dumaguete, Philip-
                pines. Preliminary draft of M. A. thesis in anthropology, Silliman University.
Montepio, Susan N.
    1978   Folk Medical Practices in a Barrio: Their Implications for the Rural Health
                Program. Quezon City: M.A. thesis in anthropology, University of Philippines.
Munger, Ronald G. and Marshal G. Hurlich
    1981   Hmong Deaths. Science 213 (August 28): 952.
Murdock, George Peter
    1967   Ethnographic Atlas. Pittsburgh, Penn.: University of Pittsburgh Press.
    1980   Theories of Illness. A World Survey. Pittsburgh, Penn.: University of Pittsburgh
                Press.
Norbeck, Edward
    1961   Religion in Primitive Society. New York: Harper and Row.
Nurge, Ethel
    1955–56   Unpublished Field Notes for Guinhangdan.
    1958   Etiology of Illness in Guinhangdan. American Anthropologist 60: 1158–
                72.
Nydegger, William F. and Corinne Nydegger
    1966   Tarong: An Ilocos Barrio in the Philippines. New York: John Wiley and Sons.
                Six Cultures Series: Vol. 6.
Ohnuki-Tierney, Emiko
    1981   Illness and Healing Among the Sakhalin Ainu. A Symbolic Interpretation.
                Cambridge, London and New York: Cambridge University Press.
Pal, Agaton P.
    1956   A Philippine Barrio: A Study of Social Organization in Relation to Planned
                Cultural Change. The University of Manila Journal of East Asian Studies 5:
                333–489.
Polson, Robert A. and Agaton P. Pal
    1956   The Status of Rural Life in the Dumaguete City Trade Area, Philippines, 1952.
                Ithaca, New York: Southeast Asia Program, Cornell University. Data Paper
                No. 21.
Ponteras, Moises S.
    1980   Folk Healing in Iloilo. Quezon City. Dissertation in anthropology, University
                of Philippines.
Rubel, Arthur J.
    1964   The Epidemiology of a Folk Illness: susto in Hispanic America. Ethnology
                3: 268–83.
Saito, Shiro
    1972   Philippine Ethnography. A Critically Annotated and Selected Bibliography.
                Honolulu, Hawaii: The University of Hawaii Press.
Scheans, Daniel J. and Karl Hutterer
    1970   Some "Oracion" Tattoos from Samar. Leyte-Samar Studies: 4: 29–45.
Tan, Crispina A.
    1962   A Study of Popular Beliefs and Practices on Death and Burial in Rural Cebu.
                Cebu City, Philippines. M.A. thesis in education, San Carlos University.

Tiston, Rebecca C.
    1978 The "Tambalan" (Folk Medicine Practitioner) of Northern Leyte: Their Practices
          and Psychological Implications. Tacloban City, Philippines. M.A. thesis in education,
          Divine World University.
Valmoria, Henry R.
    1981 A Comparative Study of the Philippine Magical Prayers in the Collection of Xavier
          Folklife Museum and Archives, Xavier University, Cagayan de Oro, Philippines.
          M.A. thesis in comparative religion, Xavier University.
Ventura, Sylvia Mendez
    1978 The Baffling "Bangungot". The Philippine Heritage: The Making of a Nation. Lahing
          Pilipino Publishing, Inc.: Singapore 9: 2246–49.
Villegas, Maria G. R. S. M.
    1971 Superstitious Beliefs and Practices in the Coastal Towns of Eastern Leyte. Unitas
          55: 29–95.
Williams, Paul V. A.
    1979 Primitive Religion and Healing: A Study of Folk Medicine in North-East Brazil.
          Cambridge: D. W. Brewer, Rowman and Littlefield.
Wolff, John U.
    1972 A Dictionary of Cebuano Visayan. Ithaca, New York: Southeast Asia Program,
          Cornell University. Data Paper No. 87. 2 vols.
Yu, Elena and William T. Liu
    1980 Fertility and Kinship in the Philippines. Notre Dame, Ind.: University of Notre
          Dame Press.

STEPHEN FRANKEL

MOGO LAYA, A NEW GUINEA FRIGHT ILLNESS

The syndromes commonly referred to as culture-bound are in the main behavioral disorders and illnesses explicable in terms of the somaticization of psychological distress. Illnesses such as these are highly plastic, and so are particularly amenable to analysis in terms of cultural influences. All illness is culturally patterned, but in these culture-bound syndromes the patterning is so marked that the illness category may be said to be unique to the society in question. Fright illnesses are conventionally included amongst the culture-bound syndromes, though they differ from such florid syndromes as *latah* and *amok* in that the diagnosis in a fright illness commonly depends upon the interpretation of symptoms which are not in themselves pathognomonic of the diagnosis. Fright illnesses in children may be folk diagnoses for the common illnesses of childhood (cf. Kleinman 1980: 196). The illness described here is of this sort. Sufferers are typically infants. They are usually suffering from common childhood complaints, such as diarrhoea and respiratory infections. These are universal illness problems, but the precise nature of the threat that these symptoms may represent is particular to each society. This New Guinea fright illness is an expression of the social and cultural concerns of those responsible for the sick child, as well as a response to the phenomenology and natural history of particular disease processes.

EMOTIONS, ILLNESS AND THE SPIRIT

The Huli people of Papua New Guinea are subsistence farmers, growing their staple sweet potato in the broad valleys of the Tari area of the Southern Highlands Province. I will begin by outlining some of the concepts that are expressed in the Huli diagnosis *mogo laya* ('startled'). Hulis often speak of the emotions as if these are autonomous forces within the individual. Liability for the effects of emotional states may be assigned to the person held responsible for eliciting strong feeling in another. Emotions are said to arise from the *bu. Bu* has the everyday meaning of 'breath', but in its wider sense *bu* is the life force, the drive which activates all other functions. It is also the source of the emotions and desire. In anger and other strong feelings it is said to rise into the throat and head and fall back as the emotion subsides. The individual experiences emotional states as a rising and falling of the *bu* within the body. This intimate association between emotions and the basic drive is one factor in the relationship between illness and the emotions. Another is the effect of strong emotion, particularly fright, upon the spirit.

Hulis see life as a fragile state, and its fluctuations are parallelled by the ebb and flow of the spirit. During sleep it may wander, and the images of its journey

399

Ronald C. Simons and Charles C. Hughes (eds.), The Culture-Bound Syndromes, 399–404.
© 1985 *by D. Reidel Publishing Company.*

are seen in dreams. In illness the spirit may detach itself from the body, or conversely illness may follow if the spirit becomes detached. It may be said of a sickly person, 'His spirit has gone, just an empty skin is left'. Particularly in children the spirit is skittish. It is easily frightened out of the body, leaving the person weakened and at risk. This fear of the vulnerability of children is well grounded as infant mortality is high. The rite known as *angawai* was performed traditionally to recall the spirit into the body. It is thought to leave through the anterior fontanelle in babies, and the same area in adults. *Angawai* involves ministrations to this area, and the hair over this part of the crown may be held when someone is thought to be dying. This prevents the spirit leaving, thus allowing the person to recover.

Fright is particularly dangerous in children. The word for startled, *mogo laya*, carries the implication that the spirit has fled the body. Especially during the first few months of life mothers attempt to protect their babies from this danger by keeping them away from crowds and clamour. Illness and death can be ascribed to fright, and the individual responsible for startling the child held liable for compensation payments.

THE DIAGNOSIS OF *MOGO LAYA*

I will first illustrate the common features of illnesses ascribed to fright by describing one case:

Case One. A man gave his second wife some money (K6). His first wife objected to her co-wife being favoured in this way, and a quarrel developed. Both the husband and second wife struck her while she was holding her baby of nine months. The next day the baby developed diarrhoea, followed by fever and shortness of breath. He became severely ill (with pneumonia), and was admitted to the Health Centre. The mother said that the child had started with fright (*mogo laya*) when she had been struck, and so his spirit had fled his body. He recovered, and there were no repercussions.

I saw a total of ten cases of illness ascribed to this cause. They all occurred in children under the age of four years. Seven of these were under one year of age, the period when the attachment of the spirit to the body is particularly tenuous.

The characteristic feature of these illnesses is that the child was caused to start, and soon afterwards became ill. Such an experience is essential for this diagnosis to be selected. But the nature of the illness may also be important. All these illnesses were acute and severe. Six were cases of lower respiratory infections, three of diarrhoea (two with blood), and one child became unconscious:

Case Two. A boy of three became feverish, and then increasingly sleepy. His limbs shook briefly and he became quite unconscious. His mother thought that he had started (*mogo laya*) in church that morning, and attributed his illness to this. They held a prayer meeting at which they killed some chickens and sprinkled holy water around their house. The child improved a little, but they were still concerned. They took him to the Health Centre, where he was treated for cerebral malaria. He recovered.

This illness was ascribed to *mogo laya* though nothing dramatic had occurred to frighten the child. The key symptom here is the fit. In three of these ten cases the mothers knew of no particular events which had precipitated their children's illnesses. Besides the case I have just described, one mother thought that her son of ten months may have been dropped when she had left him to be looked after by other children, though the children denied this. Another thought that her daughter of seven months may have been frightened by a dream. But one of these three children shook and the other two had convulsions. There is thus an interaction between ideas concerning the concepts of causation of this illness and expectations of what constitutes its typical expression.

The Huli recognize a number of discrete illness categories which are supported by detailed theoretical views as to their causation, typical symptomatology, and likely natural history. Fright illness is one of these. In this illness the child is usually known to have been startled. But when the symptoms are 'typical', that is including fitting or shaking, the child is assumed to have been startled, by a dream for example. The relative stress that is placed upon the aetiology or the manifestations of these illnesses varies with the certainty of knowledge about its cause and the nature of the symptoms. This relationship is shown diagrammatically in Figure 1.

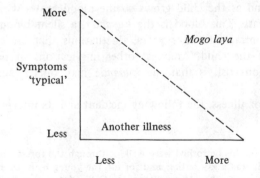

Fig. 1. Symptomatology and preceding experience in the diagnosis of *mogo laya*.

The believed fragility of children, the tenuous attachment of their souls, is one expression of the incorporation of the startle reaction into a Huli theory of pathogenesis. A second concerns the nature of the symptoms of this illness. The Moro reflex, with its jerky movements of rapid abduction and extension of the arms with opening of the hands, and the startle response which replaces it by the fourth month, have some similarities with convulsions and rigors. When children have these symptoms parents may suspect that the child has been startled. I would suggest that these neurophysiological responses provide some phenomenological basis for this diagnostic category.

It is interesting to note that convulsions may be a feature of fright illness in children elsewhere. The symptoms of the Chinese fright illness *haàk-ts'an* described by Topley (1970) include crying, a raised temperature and irritability, but it is also characterized by convulsive jerks. Hong Kong mothers also fear that fright will cause the child's soul to leave the body. Like Huli mothers they are particularly careful to protect their children from this threat for the first hundred days of life, and it may be worth noting that the Moro reflex is lost after this period.

However, the symptomatology in *mogo laya* is only one feature amongst the others I will go on to examine, and convulsions are not pathognomonic of this condition. All convulsions are not attributed to fright, and those diagnosed as suffering from *mogo laya* may not have convulsions. The key feature of the diagnosis is the belief that the soul has depart the body.

FRIGHT AND FEMALE POLLUTION

By adulthood the spirit is less easily dislodged. Where fright has serious ill effects that person is presumed to be especially vulnerbale for an additional reason. Any particular sensitivity to fright is held to indicate that such a person must harbour *kuyanda*. *Kuyanda* is a manifestation of the polluting power of female blood. If a child swallows any of its mother's blood at birth this blood is said to settle in the child's chest, and as the child grows so the blood grows within it as an amorphous parasitic mass. This blood is the *kuyanda*, a silent bloodsucker that leechlike swells and contracts in later years, fluctuations that are expressed in the rate of growth of the child. Amongst other implications of harbouring a *kuyanda* the most serious risk is that the *kyuanda* may burst, causing sudden death.

Though not a case of illness. the following incident and its interpretation illustrate this view.

Case Three. A young man and his betrothed were walking through the forest with some other people of their own age. It was a gay outing, and for fun the young man secretly cut ahead of the others to surprise them further down the track. He jumped out at the girl who was so terrified that she fainted. She soon recovered, and the incident was treated as a joke. But when he told his mother about it later she advised him not to marry the girl, as she probably had *kuyanda*. If he beat her or worried her the *kuyanda* might burst causing her to die. He would then have to compensate her clan. He took her advice, and broke off the engagement.

The aspect of the diagnosis I discussed above, the vulnerability of children expressed in terms of the loose attachment of their spirits, is congruent with Huli ideas. But it is this second feature, the incorporation of ideas about female pollution, that is quintessentially Huli. Most New Guinea societies are characterized by some concern with the polluting powers of female sexuality, but for the Huli this cultural trait is highly developed (see Frankel 1980). *Mogo laya* can be a serious illness, but alone it is not held to be fatal. Only with the additional hazard of harbouring a *kuyanda*, the parasitic mass that grows from ingesting the birth flow, is it possible, in Huli terms, to be startled to death.

FRIGHT, CONFLICT AND REDRESS: THE WIDER SOCIAL CONTEXT

Mogo laya differs from many of the folk illnesses that relate in some way to fright or startle, such as *susto* and *latah*, in that the cultural constructions are expressed almost exclusively in the responses of the observers and not those of the patient. As this is primarily an illness of young children this is to some extent inevitable. However, the way that the illness may extend into the affairs of parents and others raises a third characteristically Huli feature of this diagnosis: the interest in attributing personal responsibility for illness and in securing redress.

The presence of any illness raises doubts as to the threat that it may represent and questions as to the proper course of action. In most cases Hulis are willing to consider illnesses as random dicontinuities in normal functioning. They may theorize about the process underlying the illness, but they do not in general come to definite conclusions concerning the reasons why particular patients became sick when they did. One set of circumstances where people do put forward specific diagnoses is when the illness is seen to extend into the patient's or parent's social relations. The simplest example of this is where a victim demands compensation for trauma unequivocally caused by an assault. But an intercurrent illness that might otherwise have been disregarded may take on great significance where the parent or patient has an outstanding grievance. This occurs in illnesses attributed to *mogo laya*. The diagnosis can be understood in terms of Huli views of the soul, of children's fragility, of the dangers of female pollution. These are the mechanisms deemed to underlie the condition, its folk pathology. But the attribution of illness to these processes is often a vehicle for other concerns, and the diagnosis *mogo laya* in a child may also be understandable as an expression of conflict between the adults concerned.

Whoever is held to be responsible for startling the child may be liable for compensation. We must therefore consider the possibility that the ascription of these illnesses to fright may be influenced by such implications of the diagnosis. If we look at the relationship between the mother and the person whose actions frightened her child, we find that in four cases the husband was held responsible. These followed quarrels between the spouses, three of which ended with the husband striking his wife while she was holding the child that subsequently became sick, and one where the husband set fire to his wife's house. She escaped with her daughter, but the fright the child had suffered caused her to become ill. As with illnesses ascribed directly to assault, this preponderance of violence against wives by husbands in the causation of these children's illnesses may simply reflect the patterns of disturbance in Huli society. But the ascription of illness to such incidents should also be seen as a means of redress by wives in an unequal relationship with their husbands. Had any of these four children died, the mother's clan could be expected to demand compensation from the father. In fact, the only child in this series with the diagnosis who did die was one of those who had no clear history of a shock (the baby girl whose mother thought she may have been frightened during a dream). There was therefore no ascription of blame, and no legal repercussions. Discussions concerning compensation were initiated in some of the cases where someone was held to be culpable, but these were dropped when the sick child recovered. To show that the threat of compensation demands in such cases is real, I will describe an incident that occurred some ten years before.

Case Four. A group of adolescent boys shared a house. One of them was always afraid to go out at night. When there were chores to be done, such as fetching more firewood, he always refused to leave the house. They planned a trick for him. One of the boys stayed out one night and covered himself with phosphorescent fungus. The others told the nervous boy that there was some cooked pig for him, but they had left it in a shelter outside. The thought of pork caused him to overcome his fear of the dark, and he went out. While he was looking for the pork, the fluorescent boy came towards him, picked him up, and carried him towards the forest. The victim of the prank collapsed. He was later found to be dead. 'His *kuyanda* peeled open, and he died', though he had not been suspected of having *kuyanda* previous to this. All the boys in the house were held responsible for his death. Compensation of one hundred and twenty pigs was paid to the dead boy's clan.

Huli fright illness, like other folk diagnoses, condenses a range of concerns. This diagnosis is grounded in Huli understanding of bodily processes and of the agents that threaten normal functioning. It can be an expression of conflicts inherent in Huli social organization. It is also a response to particular sorts of diseases, primarily the common diseases of childhood, and it can be seen as a cultural elaboration upon a neurophysiological response, the startle reaction. This study underlines the need to take account of all these perspectives in the analysis of folk illnesses.

ACKNOWLEDGEMENTS

Fieldwork in 1977—9 was funded by the Social Science Research Council of Great Britain, and in 1982 by the Leverhulme Trust. I am most grateful to these bodies for their support. I shouls also like to thank Dr. Gilbert Lewis for his helpful suggestions on an earlier draft of this paper.

REFERENCES

Frankel, S. J.
    1980 I Am Dying of Man: The Pathology of Pollution. Culture, Medicine and Psychiatry
          4: 95—117.
Kleinman, A.
    1980 Patients and Healers in the Context of Culture. University of California Press.
Topley, M.
    1980 Chinese Traditional Ideas and the Treatment of Disease: Two Examples from Hong
          Kong. Man (N.S.) 5: 3: 421—437.

CHARLES C. HUGHES

FRIGHT-ILLNESS TAXON

Commentary

Fright is the fundamental experience that binds together the papers and cases reported in this taxon, but beyond saying that, the specifics vary. In some instances, fright may be followed by a variety of symptoms, both physical and psychological, in the person who initially experienced the stimulus. In other instances, however, the relationship between fright and symptoms is more indirect and the designated victim is not the person who initially suffered the startling experience, but rather someone closely related, such as a child. Moreover, the symptoms may be either acute or relatively chronic.

Obviously the question of whether DSM-III concepts can help standardize discussions of this putative syndrome will depend first upon defining what it is we are talking about — the person experiencing fright who subsequently displays symptoms of some type; or the particular cultural beliefs which in some instances are brought to bear in explaining observed symptoms of distress in someone else. While in the preceding papers the authors have taken a holistic approach to the phenomena, one that combines both behavior, symptoms, and belief into a composite pattern for analysis, here the attempt will be made to fractionate out the elements of that pattern and assess the utility or non-utility of a DSM-III approach. That attempt will not include examination of the psychopathologic characteristics or implications of the belief itself — its delusional attributes — for issues of mental health or psychpathology lie at the level of the functioning person, not that of standardized beliefs in a given group.

For the victim for whom the fright is reflexive, that is, who himself experiences subsequent symptoms, an obvious possible diagnostic concept is "Generalized Anxiety Disorder", in which the

... essential feature is generalized, persistent anxiety of at least one month's duration.... Although the specific manifestations of the anxiety vary from individual to individual, generally there are signs of motor tension, autonomic hyperactivity, apprehensive expectation, and vigilance and scanning (p. 232).

Another potentially relevant category is that of "Adjustment Disorder", having as an essential feature

... a maladaptive reaction to an identifiable psychosocial stressor, that occurs within three months after the onset of the stressor. The maladaptive nature of the reaction is indicated by either impairment in social or occupational functioning or symptoms that are in excess of a normal and expected reaction to the stressor ... (p. 299).

A specific type of adjustment disorder is 300.24 (Adjustment Disorder with Anxious Mood), "... used when the predominant manifestation involves such symptoms

405

Ronald C. Simons and Charles C. Hughes (eds.), The Culture-Bound Syndromes, 405–407.
© 1985 *by D. Reidel Publishing Company.*

as nervousness, worry, and jitteriness" (p. 301). Finally, again depending upon the particular data of a labelled case, it may be appropriate to use either the general or more specific diagnostic labels of the Somatoform Disorders.

One of the cases Rubel discusses may be used to illustrate the reflexive type of fright illness (see p. 336), the case of Antonio:

Axis I: 300.24 Adjustment Disorder with Anxious Mood (". . . appetite deterio-
            rated . . . became fretful and he felt his body involuntarily 'jump' ")
Axis II: Insufficient data
Axis III: Diagnosis of double pneumonia (recovering)
Axis IV: *Psychosocial stressors*: double-pneumonia; extremely poor; migratory
            farm laborer; speaks only Spanish even though sometimes works in
            non-Spanish-speaking areas; inadequate living conditions for family;
            saw ward-mate die in hospital; felt impotent in his attempts to get
            help; lay in presence of the corpse.
            Severity 5? — Severe (Operationalized definitional elements include
            "Serious illness in self or family . . .")
Axis V: *Highest level of adaptive functioning past year*: 3? — Good (defined
            as "No more than slight impairment in either social or occupational
            functioning".)

With regard to the indirect type of relationship between the fright stimulus and the person experiencing symptoms, as in the case of the children designated the victims in both *lanti* and *mogo laya*, unless those symptoms are clearly of a psychiatric nature (and those cited in cases discussed, such as diarrhea, can easily be ascribed to other causes given health conditions in Third World countries), the focus of a DSM-III assessment can still remain that of the adult whose fright experience is believed to have initiated the somatic symptoms in the child. Al-though psychodynamic data on the adults are lacking in these particular cases, their responses to seeing symptoms in the child and the actions they take suggest a derivative fright (perhaps guilt?) from what they interpret as an illness which something happening to them has brought about in a loved one. In effect, what may be happening is that, through their complicity in the series of events, the feedback loop of that initial fright experience has now been completed and creates a secondary fright or concern. If that is the case, perhaps the diagnostic label "Atypical Anxiety Disorder" (300.00) would be appropriate when that anxiety appears to exceed normal expectations.

This type of case also is a good illustration of the interactive nature of psy-chopathology, in which a stimulus can become caught up in the interpersonal process, often having implications that extend beyond the original victim and his perceptions. Such a "social psychiatric" perspective is what Mezzich (1979) had in mind when, an indicated earlier, he suggested the possible value of adding other axes to the DSM-III multiaxial analytic format, e.g., an axis concerned with "family relationships" or one dealing with "interaction with other individuals and groups".

REFERENCE

Mezzich, Juan E.
1970 Patterns and Issues in Multiaxial Psychiatric Diagnosis. Psychological Medicine 9: 125–137.

B. THE CANNIBAL COMPULSION TAXON

RONALD C. SIMONS

INTRODUCTION: *THE CANNIBAL COMPULSION TAXON*

In an important monograph published by the American Ethnological Society in 1960 and reprinted in 1971, Morton Teicher defined *windigo* psychosis as follows:

The outstanding symptom of the abberation known as *windigo* psychosis is the intense compulsive desire to eat human flesh. In many instances this desire is satisfied through actual cannibal acts. . . . One who develops this craving for human flesh or is considered to be in the process of doing so is called a Windigo.[1]

As Dr. Marano's bibliography amply attests there are many accounts of *windigos* and a fair number of analyses of the psychological, anthropological, and even biological causes and correlates of *windigo* behavior. *Windigo* is included in most lists of culture-bound syndromes and probably would have been considered an interestingly highly localized culture-bound psychiatric syndrome for many years to come if it were not for the publication in 1982 of Marano's highly influential paper, '*Windigo* Psychosis: The Anatomy of an Emio-Etic Confusion". Reviewing reports of *windigo* and focusing on behavior actually observed, Marano concluded that *windigo* psychosis as an actual behavioral event has never occurred! Instead, he believes the *accusation* that some unfortunate person was a Windigo and therefore fair game for ostracism, isolation, and in some cases execution was part of the Northern Algonkian culture, much as accusation of witchcraft, the evil eye, and communist or capitalist leanings have been used in other societies. Marano argues that *windigo* as "a culture-specific psychotic syndrome, the victims of which are obsessed by a compulsive desire to eat human flesh" is "a child of twentieth century anthropology". It is no understatement to say that Dr. Marano's paper revolutionalized thinking about *windigo*!

As is the usual practice in *Current Anthropology*, the paper was followed by commentaries, in this case 21 of them, and by Dr. Marano's replies to his critics. Most of the commentators were complimentary and accepted the validity of Marano's thesis. Here in addition to the original paper we have reprinted three of the more critical papers, those of H. B. M. Murphy, Hazel Weidman, and Robert Brightman, and Dr. Marano's responses to them.

The phenomenon called *windigo* would, if it existed, surely qualify as a culture-bound psychiatric syndrome, quibbling about "psychosis" versus "neurosis" aside. It would lie uniquely in a taxon by itself since a parallel syndrome has not been reported in other culture areas. But does it exist at all? I, for one, am convinced by the data Marano presents and by the logic of his argument. Thus, I believe that, like members of the *Fright Illness Taxon*, *windigo* should no longer be listed among the culture-bound psychiatric syndromes.

Ronald C. Simons and Charles C. Hughes (eds.), The Culture-Bound Syndromes, 409–410.
© 1985 *by D. Reidel Publishing Company.*

NOTES

1. Teicher, Morton
   1960   *Windigo* Psychosis. American Ethnological Society, University of Washington, Seattle.
2. In addition to Brightman, Murphy, and Weideman, commentators included:
   Bishop, Black, Bolman, Brown, Hay, Hurlich, Landes, McGee, Paredes, Preston, Rindington, Rohrl, J. Smith, R. Smith, Teicher, Waisberg and Meyer.

LOU MARANO

WINDIGO PSYCHOSIS: THE ANATOMY OF
AN EMIC-ETIC CONFUSION[1]

"*Windigo* psychosis"[2] has been the most celebrated culture trait of the Northern Algonkian peoples for almost half a century. As a classic example of "culture-bound psychopathology", its capacity to inspire theorization in anthropology and the related disciplines seems inexhaustible. This paper is a review of the voluminous *windigo* literature enlightened by five years' field experience[3] among the Northern Ojibwa and the Cree and extensive archival research. The conclusion reached is that, although aspects of the *windigo* belief complex may have been "components in some individuals' psychological dysfunction" (Preston 1980: 128), there probably never were any *windigo* psychotics in the sense that cannibalism or murder was committed to satisfy an obsessional craving for human flesh. It is argued, rather, that *windigo* psychosis as an etic/behavioral form of anthropophagy is an artifact of research conducted with an emic/mental bias.

Looking at the *windigo* phenomenon from the point of view of group sociodynamics rather than individual psychodynamics reveals that the crucial question is not what causes a person to become a cannibalistic maniac, but under what circumstances a Northern Algokian is *likely to be accused* of having become a cannibalistic maniac and thus run the risk of being executed as such. Upon close scrutiny the *windigo* curiosity discloses itself to be not a culturally isolated anthropophagic obsession, but instead a rather predictable – though culturally conditioned – variant of the triage homicide and witch hunting typical of societies under stress. In this process, as in all witch hunts, the victims of the aggression are socially redefined as the aggressors. Here the specific form of the redefinition was determined by the constant threat of starvation, a situation in which cannibalism has proved to be a tempting recourse for persons of all cultures throughout history. By attributing society's most salient fear to the scapegoat, the group was able to project its modal anxiety onto the individual, thus generating a rationale for homicide with which everyone could identify.

It is this recurrent transmogrification – once a reality of Northern Algonkian mental life – that anthropology has seized upon and reified. The importance of understanding the emics of our subject populations cannot be overstated, but to confuse these with their etic/behavioral history is an invitation to ethnological disaster (Harris 1979: 31–41). This paper argues that such a confusion has been made systematically in anthropological writings on the *windigo* phenomenon.

The present work focuses on published explications of the "psychosis"[4] and shows that there is insufficient evidence for the etic/behavioral existence of the mania in this literature. A full analysis of the ethnohistoric and ethnographic data will be presented elsewhere, but a brief summary is in order here.

Some 70 "cases of *windigo* psychosis" can be tabulated (70 are summarized

Ronald C. Simons and Charles C. Hughes (eds.), The Culture-Bound Syndromes, 411–448.
© 1982 *by The University of Chicago Press.*

in Teicher's [1960] anthology alone). None of these "cases" provide firsthand accounts of cannibalism, and some are so far removed from the events they purport to describe that they can most charitably be classified as rumor. In other words, the data are almost all emic inputs from informants who were not themselves involved in, or witnesses to, the events at issue; etic inputs are absent. Some — about 10% — of these cases, however, can be studied both emically and etically by reading court records, trial transcripts, and police investigation reports. In these documents the words of the principals are recorded, as well as the reports of outside investigators whose business it was to determine the behavioral facts as best they could. The value of these cases is far superior to that of the others for two reasons: the emic inputs come from those personally involved, and etic inputs are also present.

In only one of the documentary cases did cannibalism occur, and this was a case of murder-cannibalism under starvation conditions. This is hardly evidence of psychosis, nor is such behavior culture-specific. The man in this case was not confronted by his fellow Indians, but arrested by the Mounted Police and executed by the Dominion Government (Public Archives of Canada [hereafter PAC] 1879). The remaining executions of *windigo* "psychotics" were carried out by Indians and appear to be thinly disguised rationalizations for triage homicide (Annual Archaeological Report 1907 [1908]; PAC 1907–8, 1907–9). One of these was accompanied by a particularly strong element of scapegoating and witch hunting (Annual Archaeological Report 1903 [1904], PAC 1899, Edmonton Court Files 1899), and another appears to be the case of a man who, for reasons of his own, engineered his own death (Manitoba Court of Queen's Bench 1899).

It seems likely that the 10% sample these documented cases constitute is representative of the "*windigo*" universe. This statistical finding is reenforced by my ethnographic observations. In five years in the boreal forest I saw frequent instances of scapegoating and heard countless witchcraft accusations but never encountered one shred of evidence for cannibalistic yearnings. It was also patent that the Northern Algonkian *windigo* is a much more inclusive folk taxon than the *windigo* of anthropology. I contend that there is no good documentation for *windigo* psychosis and that the hearsay reports and folktales that have served as points of departure for contrary conclusions do not constitute a reliable body of evidence.

BACKGROUND TO THE LITERATURE REVIEW

Having arrived at this determination via the intellectual peregrination outlined above, I set out to research this review comprehensively. Much to my surprise, I discovered that Honigmann (1967: 401) had reached essentially the same conclusion. While he had been generally cautious and temperate in his treatment of the *windigo* in *Culture and Personality* (1954: 379–82), by 1967 he was able to write of Teicher's (1960) assemblage of windigo accounts (1967: 401, emphasis added):

Some of [Teicher's] cases describe individuals whom famine had driven to cannibalism, but who felt no emotional compulsion to eat human flesh and came away from their desperate act without suffering any notable personality disorder. They can hardly be considered victims of *Wiitiko* disorder, regardless of what their neighbors darkly suspected. *As for the other cases, I can't find one that satisfactorily attests to someone being seriously obsessed by the idea of committing cannibalism.* By "satisfactory" I mean a trustworthy observer's eyewitness report of a person who in his own words or by his own actions clearly admits to a compulsion to eat human flesh. All cases on record fall short of my standard. Often they recount what others told a writer, sometimes as an informant whose creditability itself remains in doubt. Sometimes, as I have already said, such hearsay evidence simply reports uncomplicated famine cannibalism. Other hearsay accounts describe people being killed, perhaps at their own behest, for their dangerous preoccupation with cannibalism, but the reporter didn't himself hear their admission. Hence I can't help but wonder if in those executions the Indians, rather like Euroamerican witch hunters, didn't simply suspect the victims, in conformity with their firm belief about compulsive cannibalism. Some instances are court cases involving men tried for murder, but the trial accounts don't clearly prove obsessive-compulsive behavior.

These singular perceptions have been almost completely overlooked in anthropology. (Barnouw [1979: 340–43], for example, ignores them utterly.) A partial explanation may be found in the fact that the passage quoted is embedded almost as an aside within an entirely conventional discussion of the *windigo* (Honigmann 1967: 399–403). Honigmann never specifically denied the existence of the "psychosis", and his consideration of etic/behavioral data is limited to Teicher's compendium of "cases". My investigation into the court cases referred to by Honigmann reveals unpublished material indicating a complete absence of psychotic cannibalism. Moreover, my reading of archival sources indicates that, from an etic perspective, all executed "windigo victims" met death at the hands of their fellow Indians for reasons unrelated to the threat of their committing cannibalism.

This review critically traces the development of the "*windigo* psychosis" from its inception to the present. It will be shown that by the time Honigmann published his insightful reflections in 1967, "windigo psychosis" had achieved such a reified status in anthropology that it was easy to ignore his signal contribution through the inertia of received wisdom. Nevertheless, those who have published on the subject since 1967 without reference to Honigmann's work must ultimately bear the responsibility for their omission.

CATEGORIES OF *WINDIGO*

When speaking of the *windigo*, we may distinguish at least three categories. The first is Windigo as superhuman monster(s), who may or may not have had human antecedents. (For a stylized portrayal, see Guinard 1930.) The second is a category of human beings the members of which may or may not be considered to have been possessed by the spirit of the cannibal monster. The practice of attributing cannibal possession to others is now a thing of the past, but those who were adjudged possessed were thought to have lost their essential human qualities, and this paved the way for their possible execution. The third category is a culture-specific psychotic syndrome the victims of which are obsessed by a compulsive desire to eat human flesh. The first two categories are Northern Algonkian; the third is a child of 20th-century anthropology. The main purpose of the present work is to review critically the evolution of this third category.

On the subject of Windigo as a woodland ogre I have little to add to what has already been written. It is associated with terrifying windstorms and uprooted trees (cf. Hallowell 1955: 257–59) and is metaphorically extended to the even more terrifying expression of uncontrolled human rage. Hallowell (1955: 145) and Preston (1975: 180) are among those who have shown that the Northern Algonkians prize emotional restraint and disciplined affect. Self-indulgent displays not only are upsetting to one's companions, but betray a possible inability to deal with the harsh Subarctic environment in a masterful way.

Among the Northern Ojibwa of the 1970s, "almost turning to *windigo*" meant something very close to "being driven to distraction", "being overcome by grief", "being out of one's mind from worry", and "being at one's wit's end". The *windigo* concept is closely associated with the fear of being lost in the bush and especially with the idea of being assumed into the sky to wander wraithlike between heaven and earth. Writing of the James Bay Cree, Preston (1980: 126–27) says that *windigo* scares "are often related to the mystery and great concern over lost persons". I believe Preston to be right on the mark here, and his observation applies equally well to the following *windigo* tales gathered from following *windigo* tales gathered from the contemporary Northern Ojibwa.[5]

The people in the village in which I lived related this story of a *windigo* event which began in a different village: Some years ago, a young man became angry because his mother did not return home when he expected her (cf. Parker 1960). When the woman did return home, her son was gone. The woman and others who were helping her search for him followed the young man's tracks down to the shore of the lake. At first his tracks were clearly visible in the sand; then they abruptly vanished. The people concluded that he had been assumed into the sky; he had become *windigo*. As time went by, people in other settlements could hear disembodied voices in the firmament. It was believed that one of the voices was that of the missing young man, but the sounds were etheral and the words hard to understand. Years went by, and one day when a man was working alone in the bush, the missing young man materialized in front of him. The young man told this person that others should not worry about him any more. He was happy in another world, where he was married to the daughter of K. B. (K. B. was a white trapper who was married to an Indian woman; years ago his young daughter had disappeared in the forest.)

Recently a middle-aged woman received word that her youngest son had been killed in a train accident down south. Friends and relatives sat with her as she mourned, but she managed to leave her cabin unseen. For a short time she was missing, and everyone was very concerned. Finally she was found in the woods, barefoot and disheveled. Her muscles were rigid, and she seemed disoriented. She had "almost turned to *windigo*" and had nearly floated up to the sky. Had the people found her in time? Her sister's husband, a man thought to have shamanistic powers, talked to her kindly, firmly, and at length. Through his ministrations and the support of her other relatives and friends, she made a full recovery.

The first part of the next story was reported by Rogers (1962: B39–40). Over 40 years ago a little girl was lost in the bush. She had been missing for three days when her father was paddling along the shores of a lake "as though in a daze' not really cognizant of his surroundings" (p. B39):

Suddenly he heard a voice cry out. . . . He stopped, looked in the direction of the voice, and there on the bank was his daughter, whom he hardly recognized. He just sat there and looked, thinking it was a spirit he saw and that he was crazy and imagining it all because of his grief. The little girl cried out again. This time her father went to her and took her into the canoe.

The father was very much afraid of losing her again, partly because it was believed that she had almost (or temporarily) become *windigo* (p. B40). The incident was still being discussed during the period of Rogers's fieldwork (1958–59), and it is still being discussed today. Whenever the woman – now a middle-aged matron – absents herself from the village and goes off into the woods under any circumstances other than the most routine, the story of her childhood disappearance and close brush with *windigo* is recalled.

Not long ago a young woman went into a severe depression after the birth of her first child. She became afraid of the west wind and was reluctant to leave her cabin, although she did occasionally do so. People on the village paths seemed threatening to her, and she experienced fright reactions as she passed them (cf. Saindon 1933). Her cabin was situated on the shores of a lake where the prevailing winter wind blew icy blasts out of a cobalt blue sky in which hung a low Subarctic sun. "One of these times after I go outdoors", she told her husband, "you will see my tracks in the snow and then my tracks will just disappear. The west wind will have carried me away." She feared she was becoming *windigo*. Village elders came to visit her. They showed sympathy and concern but no alarm. An elder from another village who was also an Anglican lay leader visited her and prayed with her. On examining the young woman he found that the muscles in her forearms were unnaturally rigid. He suggested that with the help of prayer and faith the situation would eventually correct itself. As the months passed, the woman's condition gradually improved.

WINDIGO PSYCHOSIS, 1933–67

Windigo was first identified as a "sickness" by J. E. Saindon, an Oblate missionary who worked among the Cree of western James Bay in the early part of this century. Saindon has the singular distinction of being the first and only individual to *observe* a *windigo* victim and report those observations in print (1928: 28; 1933: 11–12). The experience was quite unspectacular and corresponds very closely to the Northern Ojibwa accounts I have just given. Like the principals in the Northern Ojibwa stories, F., the victim of Saindon's account, showed no inclination whatever that she wanted to eat anyone. Her symptoms were that she did not wish to see anyone outside her immediate family because strangers looked like wild animals to her and she experienced urges to kill them in self-defense. Saindon assured F. that she would get well and she responded immediately to the suggestion (1933: 12).

It is intersting to note the similarities between Saindon's firsthand account and the *windigo* incident to which I was an eyewitness. Both cases involved married women who had become reclusive. Both women expressed fear of all but their closest relatives, and both were led to recovery by the assurances of religious leaders. It is also interesting that Saindon makes no mention at all of cannibalism in relation to *windigo*, but calls it a "psycho*neurosis*" which is "in certain cases an obsession and in others hysteria . . . characterized by an unbalanced imagination and an excessive impressionability" (1928: 27, emphasis added).[6]

Honigmann, a scant page away from his unique contribution, nevertheless overlooks the most valuable piece of information now recoverable from Saindon's account when he writes: "Unfortunately, when the priest entered her tent he didn't give her a chance to describe her symptoms; so there went a rare opportunity for an inquirer with a good knowledge of Cree to interview a victim of *Wiitiko* disorder" (1967: 400). But Honigmann here misses the main point. Of course it would have been desirable to have more background information on F., but the most diagnostic symptom of all in the case was the fact that the patient was cured (or at least went into indefinite remission) by a suggestion from an authority figure. This is not behavior characteristic of a psychosis. If psychoses were that easy to cure, our mental hospitals would be empty. We must also consider the possibility that F.'s symptoms were nothing more or less than the ones Saindon reported. F. appears to have been phobic and neurotic but not at all homicidal or cannibalistic.

From this narrow data base has come a torrent of interpretive elaboration. Saindon was urged to publish his observations by his friend and fellow priest, anthropologist John M. Cooper (Saindon 1933: 1). In the same issue of *Primitive Man* in which Saindon's modest reports appeared, Cooper (1933) published the brief communication in which the word "psychosis" was first applied to the *windigo* phenomenon. Although it was Cooper's contention that "the factual data here given are, except where otherwise stated, from the present writer's field notes taken among the eastern and western Cree and other Algonquian-speaking peoples" (p. 20), he did not present a single specific instance of *windigo* psychosis or any evidence of firsthand observation of such behavior. His initial description of the "psychosis" (1933: 21) set the tone for two generations of scholarship on the subject:

Cannibalism was resorted to by the Cree only in cases where actual starvation threatened. Driven to desperation by prolonged famine and often suffering from mental breakdown as a result thereof, the Cree would sometimes eat the bodies of those who had perished, or, more rarely, would even kill the living and partake of the flesh. This solution, however, of the conflict between hunger and the rigid tribal taboo often left, as its a aftermath, an "unnatural" craving for human flesh, or a psychosis that took the form of such a craving. More rarely such a psychosis developed in men or women who had not themselves previously passed through famine experience.

That "cannibalism was resorted to by the Cree only in cases where starvation threatened" seems to me to be a perfectly reasonable statement, but that crisis cannibalism should result in a psychotic craving for human flesh is a contention that demands specific verification. It has never resulted in an obsessive psychosis in any other part of the world. Survivors of the Donner party did not stalk the California gold fields searching for unsuspecting prospectors to eat (McGlashan 1947 [1880]: 236–61; Stewart 1960 [1936]: 280–93). It is probably true that breaking a taboo on one occasion lowers the threshold for breaking it on subsequent occasions. For this reason the Indians doubtless tried to avoid getting themselves into a food crisis with those who had already broken it.

Cooper's statements may be contrasted with those of Hudson's Bay Company officer and explorer Samuel Hearne, who lived for 20 years among the Cree. In reporting the extreme hunger he and his party experienced on his second expedition in search of the Coppermine River and Northwest Passage, he wrote (1971 [1795]: 34):

The relation of such uncommon hardships may perhaps gain little credit in Europe; while those who are conversant with the history of Hudson's Bay, and who are thoroughly acquainted with the distress which the natives of the country about it frequently endure, may consider them as no more than the common occurrences of an Indian life, in which they are frequently driven to the necessity of eating one another.

By the time Hearne wrote these words in 1770 the Hudson's Bay Company was already celebrating its first centenary. Whether or not eating one another was a frequent necessity for the Cree before the fur-trade epoch is a matter for further research, but in a footnote added later to the quoted passage, Hearne continued (pp. 34–35):

It is the general opinion of the Southern [i.e., Cree] Indians, that when any of their tribe have been driven to the necessity of eating human flesh, they become so fond of it, that no person is safe in their company. And though it is well known they are never guilty of making this horrid repast but when driven to it by necessity, yet those who have made it are not only shunned, but so universally detested by all who know them, that no Indians will tent with them, and they are frequently murdered slily [*sic*]. I have seen several of those poor wretches who, unfortunately for them, have come under the above description, and though they were persons much esteemed before hunger had driven them to this act, were afterward so universally despised and neglected, that a smile never graced their countenances: deep melancholy has been seated on their brows, while the eye most expressively spoke the dictates of the heart, and seemed to say, "Why do you despise me for my misfortunes? The period is probably not far distant, when you may be driven to the like necessity!"
    In the Spring of the year 1775, when I was building Cumberland House an Indian, whose name was Wapoos [Hare], came to the settlement, at a time when fifteen tents of Indians were on the plantations: they examined him very minutely, and found he had come a considerable way by himself, without a gun or ammunition. This made many of them conjecture he had met with, and killed, some person by the way; and this was the more easily credited,

from the care he took to conceal a bag of provisions, which he had brought with him, in a lofty pine-tree near the house.

Being a stranger, I invited him in, though I saw he had nothing for trade; and during that interview, some of the Indian women examined his bag; and gave it as their opinion that the meat it contained was human flesh; in consequence it was not without the interference of some principal Indians, whose liberality of sentiment was more extensive than in the others, the poor creature saved his life. Many of the men cleaned and loaded their guns; others had their bows and arrows ready; and even the women took possession of the hatchets, to kill this poor inoffensive wretch, for no crime but that of travelling about two hundred miles by himself, unassisted by fire-arms for support in his journey.

Psychologically oriented anthropologists will recognize in this account an example of the human tendency to condemn most vigorously in others that which is most feared in oneself and the propensity to project those fears onto vulnerable others. I suggest that the *windigo* belief complex evolved among the Northern Algonkians as a way to help minimize the chances of getting caught in a famine with those who had already broken the taboo against cannibalism, to minimize the liabilities imposed by the incapacitated, and to focus group anxieties and aggressions upon individuals adjudged socially expendable. It is not central to my argument whether this cultural configuration was aboriginal or a postcontact elaboration of pre-Columbian cosmology which developed in response to deteriorating infrastructural conditions. My judgement is that there is more evidence for the latter position, but in either case we need not accept the emic categories and concepts of our informants as our own. A lowered threshold to breaking a taboo against cannibalism in a crisis is a far cry from an obsessive cannibalistic compulsion.

Cooper's statement that "more rarely such a psychosis developed in men or women who had not themselves previously passed through famine experience", if taken seriously, directly contradicts his assertion of an exclusively nutritional impetus for Cree cannibalism. While Saindon's informants told him that the *windigo* sickness was "[a] strange malady that is rare today, but was formerly more frequent" (1933: 11), Cooper asserts that it is "[a] common psychosis among the eastern Cree and kindred tribes show[ing] two peculiar characteristics: the victim develops an 'unnatural' craving for human flesh: he turns into an ice-hearted Witiko" (1933: 24).

From these beginnings the misunderstandings snowballed. It could even be argued that the *windigo* phenomenon is more of an example of mass suggestibility among anthropologists than among Northern Algonkians. Hallowell (1934) quickly confirmed the existence of the disorder among the Berens River Saulteaux, a Northern Ojibwa group. Taking the information provided by his informants at face value, Hallowell identified the physical symptoms of the disease (a distaste for ordinary foods, nausea, vomiting). He reported that "if there were no improvement the afflicted one would often ask to be killed and this desire was usually gratified" (p. 8). He also distinguished between early and late stage of the disorder, even though he had no firsthand knowledge of either. If in the first stage the victim was depressed and nauseous, in these later cases (*of which I have no specific records*) the individual does not merely develop a fear of becoming cannibalistic but may exhibit a positive desire for human flesh, or even take steps to satisfy this desire. . . . But the cases of which I have knowledge were only in the initial anxiety stage and the persons affected were either killed or they recovered (p. 8, emphasis added).

Since Hallowell's informants could give him no specific instances of the cannibal-psychotic stage of the disorder, it would have been appropriate for him to have been more skeptical of its existence. Moreover, Hallowell did not attempt to ascertain the conditions under which anxious and anorexic Ojibwa were killed and those under which they were allowed to recover. The statement that they would "often ask to be killed" cannot be taken seriously in an etic/behavioral sense without a sample of cases.

Hallowell recognized that the Ojibwa, in making attributions of windigo cannibal possession, failed "to rationally consider alternative causes of the physical symptoms" and that the *windigo* victim became "the object of the projected fears" of others (p. 7). He also realized that "all reputed cases of this 'psychosis' may not be pathological" (pp. 8–9) and that if a series of cases were well-studied some of them might prove to be only mildly abnormal and not at all specific to Northern Algonkian culture (p. 9). But although he succeeded in discovering that Cooper's "*windigo* psychosis" was not a unitary type of mental disorder, his conclusion was that "the cannibalistic pattern functions as a cloak for a variety of mental processes" (1936: 1309). Better had he concluded that the pattern whereby a series of individuals is accused of cannibal possession functions as a cloak for a variety of social processes.

The next Algonkianist to take up the *windigo* theme was Landes, who based her conclusions on information gathered during visits to the Manitou Reserve, on the Rainy River in southwestern Ontario, in the summers of 1932 and 1933 and from an extensive correspondence with her principal informant, Mrs. Maggie Wilson (Landes 1937a, b, 1938a, b). Landes's descriptions of the *windigo* phenomenon are the most elaborate of the period, and it is probably for this reason that her writings seem to be the ones most often referred to by those who have attempted to comment on "*windigo* psychosis" by means of secondary sources alone (e.g., Parker 1960; Teicher 1960; Arieti and Meth 1959; Linton 1956; Lewis 1958 [quoted in Wing 1978: 72–73]; Bolman and Katz 1966). Her most estimable contribution to the *windigo* issue has, however, been wholly neglected, for she wrote that "from the psychiatric point of view . . . all Ojibwa neuroses and psychoses fall under the one category: *windigo*" (1938a: 30) and that "all [Ojibwa] insanities are generically termed *windigo*" (1937a: 46). The far-reaching implications of these statements seem never to have given pause to subsequent researchers. If what Landes was saying is that the Ojibwa tend to apply the term "*windigo*" to just about any form of mental disturbance, then she was correct, as I can confirm from my own observations. But if that is what she meant, it becomes at once obvious that the Ojibwa emic category is not isomorphic with the then newly emerging etic anthropological category (cf. Preston 1980). The difference between the emic and etic meanings of *"windigo"* is much greater than one of spirit possession versus psychosis. The difference is that the Indians apply the term to cases in which no cannibalism or murder is suspected or anticipated and the anthropologists do not. If anthropologists had taken this aspect of Landes's work seriously, we would have been forced to conclude that, emically speaking, *"windigo"* is a very inclusive term. In my own experience, in the vast majority of cases in which the Indians employ the term there is no psychosis by either Algonkian or European criteria, much less a psychosis involving murder and cannibalism. Unfortunately, anthropologists zeroed in on the bizarre, the grotesque, and the macabre in Landes's reports rather than on their inconsistencies and their second-hand nature. This bias toward the exotic in anthropology has been identified and criticized in other contexts by Naroll and Naroll (1963).

While Landes's identification of the broad nature of the Algonkian *windigo* concept is praiseworthy, her description of the phenomenon is problematic in other respects. In one paper she writes that the disorder is pretty much confined to males with shamanistic power who attribute failure in the hunt to the curses of rival shamans, women being relatively free from the condition (1938a: 31). In a book appearing in the same year (1938b: 213–26), however, she not only recounts tales of many female windigowak, but also states that babies and even dogs are considered susceptible to the affliction.

The *windigo* literature got to be the way it is because early 20th-century ethnologists in general and Algonkianists in particular failed to make explicit the distinction between data about which the observer is the ultimate judge of the adequacy of categories and concepts (etics) and data about which the informant is the ultimate judge of same (emics). More precisely, their work also suffered from the failure to distinguish thought from behavior (Harris 1979: 27–45). Further evidence for the necessity of making these distinctions can be found in the following passage (Landes 1938b: 217, emphasis added, parenthetical remarks Landes's):

An infant son of the great shaman Great Mallard Duck was viewed by his mother's co-wife and by his half-sisters and brothers as a windigo, and was therefore killed. *This happened during a period of starvation, when seven out of Duck's family of sixteen persons died of hunger.* "The baby that was nursing was just crazy. He was eating his fingers up (this is considered cannibalistic) and biting off the nipples of his (dead) mother's breasts. They knew he was to become a little *windigo*. His eyes were blazing and his teeth rattling (*windigo* symptoms indicating fever, privation, and neurotic fury), so the old woman killed the baby boy."

So strong was Landes's commitment to a psychological interpretation of *windigo* that she failed to see that there might be reasons other than the belief in cannibal monsters for killing an infant in a family in which seven out of sixteen people had already died of starvation. Can a starving baby be etically categorized as being in a "neurotic fury"? Is there any scientific basis for diagnosing infants as psychotic?

Referring to Landes's (1938a: 25) two-stage progression from melancholia to obsessive murder-cannibalism, Honigmann (1954: 380) wrote: "It does not appear that Landes ever directly observed the progressive deterioration about which she writes". It would have been better for anthropology as well as for the global reputation of the Cree and Ojibwa if Honigmann had shown less restraint in his commentary. As we have seen, by the time he pursued this line of thought to its logical conclusion 13 years later, no one was listening.

If it can be said that Saindon knew the *windigo* at the first level of abstraction and Cooper, Hallowell, and Landes knew it at the second, then successive writers have typically known it at ever more remote levels of abstraction. Cooper, Landes, and especially Hallowell were accomplished fieldworkers, even if none of them had ever observed a case of the ghoulish psychosis about which they wrote so confidently. Subsequent analysts have tended to be those who have either worked among highly acculturated reservation Indians or, more commonly, have never seen a bush Indian in their lives.

Parker's 'The *Wiitiko* Psychosis in the Context of Ojibwa Personality and Culture' (1960) is a prime example of *windigo* analysis at a third level of abstraction. Referring to the accounts of Hallowell, Landes, and Cooper, he writes (p. 603). "Unfortunately, none of these investigators had an opportunity to obtain detailed or reliable life history data about an actual wiitiko victim". (Neither did they obtain reliable case-history data, as we have already seen.) Having offered this caveat, Parker embarks at once on a long, convoluted, neo-Freudian fishing trip. Accepting Landes's (1938a: 31) statement that *windigo* psychosis is confined mainly to men, Parker ultimately concludes that *windigo* is an obsessive cannibalistic psychosis which is the result of frustrated dependency cravings of little Ojibwa boys for their stern and rejecting mothers. Following the ideas of Kardiner (1939, 1953), he suggests that with frustration comes the transformation of the nurturing object into the persecuting object. Thus the prototype for the cannibal giant is the mother figure. When "the victim feels that he has been possessed by the spirit of a cannibalistic *wiitiko* monster . . . he must serve the appetite of the *wiitiko* as his own" (p. 619). The dependency that Parker considers the salient feature of the Ojibwa modal personality presumably constitutes a predisposition to *windigo* insanity because "dependent and aggressive phantasies are often two sides of the same coin" (p. 612). At the same time as he characterizes the Ojibwa as having excessive dependency needs, Parker calls our attention to Ojibwa individualism, apathy, passivity, and paranoia, traits that have been debated elsewhere under the category of Northern Algonkian social "atomism" (James 1954, 1970; Friedl 1956; Hickerson 1960, 1967; Barnouw 1961; Smith 1979).

Teicher (1960) makes a heroic attempt to compile all the available source material on *windigo* "psychosis", apparently including, in addition to published sources, Hallowell's ethnographic field notes (p. 74). The questionable assumption throughout his work is that "belief stands in respect to behavior as does cause to effect" (p. 13). Of the 70 cases he catalogues, 26 involved no cannibalism. At first Teicher is cautious in his analysis: "It is probable in some of these instances that cannibalism would have occurred had death [from execution] not intervened. On the other hand these twenty-six cases constitute a fairly high proportion of the total number of cases reported as *windigo* psychosis" (p. 109). On the very next page, however, he ignores his own warning (p. 110):

A Northeastern Indian, convinced that he has become or is becoming *windigo*, inevitably turns to cannibalism as the appropriate behavior, an appropriateness determined by the cultural belief system. Regardless of the ailment he may actually have, once the common diagnosis of *windigo* has been applied, his future path of action is clearly demarcated by the culture; there is no alternative path.

With the exception of Saindon's timid parishioner, not one of Teicher's cases is drawn from a firsthand report. From the nature of his case material one must assume that had the man in Hearne's 1795 account been executed and had the Cree version of the tale been recorded later by one less sophisticated than Hearne, yet another instance of "*windigo* psychosis" would have been added to the literature. Almost all of Teicher's "cases" may be called into question on this account. Of his 70 "cases", 5 come from well-documented trial records (Annual Archaeological Reports 1903 [1904] and 1907 [1908]), but Teicher's belief in the "inevitability" of cannibalism once the *windigo* label has been applied severely limits his capacity for critical analysis.

Fogelson's (1965) 'Psychological Theories of *Windigo* "Psychosis" and a Preliminary Application of a Models Approach' is a more cautious and at the same time more ambitious attempt to explicate the *windigo* phenomenon at the third level of abstraction. Fogelson begins by saying that the *windigo* syndrome may have an organic etiology, but because there are insufficient data to generate, let alone test, specific physiological and genetic hypotheses, his report concentrates on psychological aspects of *windigo* (pp. 74—75). In referring to some early sources cited by Cooper (1934b), Fogelson makes a valuable contribution by pointing out that among the 18th-century Cree of Hudson Bay, Wiitiko appears to have been an Algonkian deity of evil principle. This malign god and his minions were a source of menace and danger to humans and had always to be propitiated. Manitou, on the other hand, was a benign deity but rather uninterested in human affairs (pp. 76—77). Fogelson's paper is important in that he was the first to suggest that the *windigo* complex had changed over time: "interesting to note is the absence in these early accounts of characteristics which were later associated with the Windigo being: as his gigantic stature, his *anthropophageous propensitics*, and his symbolic connection with the north, winter, and starvation" (1965: 77, emphasis added). (Hearne also makes no mention of the term in association with Cree beliefs surrounding cannibalism in the (1770s.) Moreover, Fogelson points out that

the fact that only seventy fairly well-authenticated cases of *windigo* disorder have found their may into the literature — from a population of over thirty thousand over a period of three centuries — suggests strongly that *windigo* disorder may be a relatively rare phenomenon, notable more for its spectacular features than for its chronicity (p. 88).

In making these discerning statements, Fogelson comes very close to scoring a major breakthrough in our understanding of the *windigo* phenomenon. In fact, most of Teicher's cases are very poorly authenticated, and the few that are well-documented Teicher systematically misinterprets. And, as we have seen above, in more than a third of Teicher's "cases" no cannibalism occurred even if we take the Indian accounts at face value. Unfortunately, Fogelson chooses not to pursue this line of thought and elects instead to create a psychological typology of questionable utility. Expanding on a model developed by A. F. C. Wallace, himself, and unnamed others at the Eastern Pennsylvania Psychiatric Institute in 1959, Fogelson arranges the tenuous *windigo* data base into five conceptual slots. "The analytic technique has been labeled the 'N-U-P-model' " (p. 89), in which N stands for "Normality", U for "Upset", and P for "Psychosis". Type 1 is the "Classic Three-Stage" *windigo* in which the victim degenerates from a normal Indian to a brooding melancholic to a cannibalistic killer (pp. 90–91). Type 2 is the "Two-Stage" variety, in which the sufferer is killed while "Upset" (pp. 91–92). Type 3 is the "Nonmelancholic Two-Stage", in which the crafty cannibal does in his unsuspecting relatives and has them turning over a slow fire before they even have time to know that they have an Upset person on their hands (p. 93). In Type 4 the victim begins a transformation into a *windigo* as the result of a shaman's curse but is cured through the ministrations of relatives (pp. 94–96), and in Type 5 a shaman begins to become a *windigo* from the conjuring of a rival shaman but fights off his enemy shamanistically and returns to Normality. Fogelson admits he had trouble in deciding whether to classify the shamanistic combat fantasy as an Upset or a Psychotic state but opted for the latter (p. 97). Little confidence can be placed in Fogelson's diagnosis in view of the fact that trained psychiatrists on different sides of the Atlantic cannot agree as to what constitutes a psychotic state even when they have the opportunity to examine patients for extended periods (Wing 1978: 98–139).[7]

Bolman and Katz's (1966) 'Hamburger Hoarding: A Case of Symbolic Cannibalism Resembling *Whitico* Psychosis' is the case history of a woman who, in addition to having other problems, hoarded food. She began by carrying around a cooked hot dog in her purse. Later she switched to raw hamburger. For two years she bought 2–5 lb. of hamburger a day; then she increased her purchases to about 60 lb. per day, by her own estimate. (The authors do not say if they ever confirmed her statement by observation.) This she carried with her in her car and had trouble parting with it even when it became rotten.[8] "Just as the Ojibwa hunter roamed the dark woods in search of prey, so the patient would spend night after night driving about the darkened streets of the city searching for open stores where she could buy hamburger" (p. 428). Needless to say, the woman did not kill or eat anyone, nor did she even eat the raw hamburger. She did hesitantly mention a fantasy impulse she had (once?) had: "while looking at a supermarket display of hamburger [s]he felt a sudden impulse to bury her face into this display full of meat and devour it" (p. 425). Evidently this was sufficient to convince the two psychiatrists who coauthored the paper that their patient was a "symbolic cannibal". (Following this line of reasoning, it might have been safer to conclude that the woman's fantasy about eating raw meat was an indication that she was a symbolic Eskimo. In fact, the authors twice identify those susceptible to *windigo* psychosis as "Cree Eskimos" [pp. 424, 427], a blunder they have apparently adopted from an earlier psychiatric paper [Arieti and Meth 1959: 558]). The patient was confined involuntarily to a mental hospital, where she switched from hoarding hamburger to hoarding bread. Eventually she gave up hoarding food and was released.

Also far removed from the primary source data are Rohrl's (1970, 1972) attempt at an organic explanation and the responses to it (Brown 1971; McGee 1972). On the basis of Teicher's "cases" and a letter from a Minnesota Chippewa informant, Rohrl (1970) suggests that the etiology of *windigo* psychosis may have a nutritional component. By this she does not mean hunger as such or protein-calorie malnutrition. It appears that she thinks of *windigo* as being in part a deficiency disease – like beriberi or pellagra – that can be cured by ingestion of fatty meats, particularly bear fat. She never specifices, however, the missing nutrient or nutrients that bear far might supply. In addition to the fat itself she suggests that "at least some proteins and B vitamins including thiamine" might be involved (p. 99). She goes on to state that "bear far *is believed* [my emphasis] to contain Vitamin C, or ascorbic acid, probably derived from berries and other foods in their diets". Vitamin C is a water-soluble vitamin, the inability of which to be stored in fat is the reason humans and other primates need a continuous supply. The B-complex vitamins, including thiamine, are also water-soluble. Rendered animal fat is a poor source of protein. While making her venturesome conjectures. Rohrl at no time questions the reality of the assumption of a culture-specific, etic/behavioral psychopathology.

In response to Rohrl's suggestions, McGee (1972: 244) has written: "That the . . . *windigo* melancholy may be caused by the absence of this enzyme or that vitamin is accepted. But why do these black-Irish fits manifest themselves as the *windigo* psychosis among the Northern Algonkians and not among their Dene, Siouan, Iroquoian and Eskimo neighbors when the latter undergo similar nutritional deprivation?"[9] Why indeed? What neither Rohrl, McGee, nor almost anyone else who has written on the *windigo* has suggested is that if the *windigo* "psychosis" does not exist among these contiguous populations, *perhaps it does not exist among the Northern Algonkians either.*

Brown (1971) rejects Rohrl's dietary hypothesis on the grounds that the attempt to cure *windigos* by feeding them fat was rare and that when it was undertaken it was done not nutritively but emetically, in order for the victim to be able to disgorge the intrusive heart of ice (cf. Bloomfield 1934: 155; McGee 1975: 114). Although Brown questions the idea of a nutritive cure for *windigo* obsession, her main quarrel with Rohrl turns out to be over the issue of Northern Algonkian rationality. Rohrl believes that the Indians subliminally grasped the importance of fat as a remedy, while Brown holds that they were attempting to administer a psychological cathartic when they bothered with the bear fat at all. Like Rohrl, Brown never questions the etic/behavioral reality of *windigo* psychosis.

Brown has made a valuable contribution to the *windigo* question in her discovery of a letter by the Methodist missionary Egerton Ryerson Young, dated Rossville, Norway House, July 29, 1871. Young wrote of an event that had occurred about 100 miles away from the post. A 15-year-old Cree boy was alleged to have gone crazy "and in his ravings kept asking for flesh to eat. At last he said, 'I will surely kill somebody and eat them if I can!' One day he attacked his father and tried hard to bite him. The father and an elder brother of the crazy one then deliberately strangled him and burnt the body to ashes" (Young 1871: 37, quoted in Brown 1971: 21). Brown cites Young to make the point that the "*windigo*" victim was strangled and cremated rather than fed hot bear grease, but more important than this are Young's comments that follow: "Poor boy, he was only a lunatic, and perhaps a few months in an asylum would have restored reason to its throne. I took my canoe and went and visited the family. [They had since come in to the settlement.] They are now in deep sorrow at what they have so rashly done."

The reader is entitled to a different interpretation of the quoted passages than the one I am about to make, but what it says to me is that a mentally ill boy was killed by his family. The story has a ring of implausibility to it. The phrase "tried hard to bite" implies that the boy was unsuccessful in his attempt to bite his father. How is it possible for a crazed 15-year-old male to fail at least to get in a nip while "attacking"? The Northern Algonkians are not immune to mental illness. No one disputes the fact that they fall victim to psychiatric disorders at least the rate of other populations. The question is, what are the options open to a small family hunting group in the vast boreal hinterland in dealing with a disruptive or burdensome individual? Young was one of many early observers who never doubted what seemed to them to be an obvious fact: the *windigo* belief complex was an ideological and superstructural rationalization for homicide, i.e., the execution of the alleged "*windigo*". It was not until the anthropological writings of the early 1930s that the balance shifted in favor of an explanation that held the executed parties responsible for having brought death upon themselves through their cannibalistic frenzy.

An example of the numerous references that can be cited in support of this argument is a latter written by John Kennedy McDonald (1907), a retired Chief Trader of the Hudson's Bay Company, to the editor of the *Manitoba Free Press* regarding the *windigo* execution of Wa-sak-apee-quay by the Fiddler brothers:

I lived among these people for 35 years and never locked my door unless when going on a distant trip. I have again to say that had there been an asylum or doctor near by that the band would have been only too glad to hand over the unfortunate woman, as once off their hands the men could leave to hunt and provide for their families, which they could not do when they had to watch her.

A demented or delirious person cannot be loaded into a birch-bark canoe and is a distinct liability on hunting trips.

Rohrl's (1972) rejoinder to Brown deepens the confusion: she cautions her to "consider the source" (p. 243). It is not clear if she means to impeach the reliability of missionary sources in general or that of Young in particular. Assuming the latter, it must be noted that Young wrote a series of popular books that contain obvious exaggerations and a fair amount of 19th-century sensationalism. But what is Rohrl's point? Is it that the boy was not killed, or that he was fed hot bear fat as a specific for *windigo* possession and Young failed to report the treatment? Her statement that "cultural phenomena, including *windigo* psychosis, are multi-factorial" (p. 243) is a truism that accepts the existence of the culture-bound psychopathology as a demonstreated fact. Five years earlier Honigmann had suggested strongly that this is an unwarranted assumption. Close scrutiny of the archives yields evidence of an etic/behavioral nature that documents the correctness of Honigmann's suggestion.

Almost as distant from the etic/behavioral data base as Bolman and Katz's work is Hay's 'The *Windigo* Psychosis: Psychodynamic, Cultural, and Social Factors in Aberrant Behavior' (1971). Hay argues that "the dynamics of the *windigo* disorder are essentially similar to the psychodynamics which apparently produce ritual cannibalism in some societies" (p. 1). With this he asks us to believe that funerary endocannibalism, the eating of parts of slain (or living) enemies, and *windigo* "psychosis" all have their origins in the same canniblaistic "impulse". Hay postulates the existence of such an impulse on the imputed desire to resolve the following problems cannibalistically: "(1) 'preserving' a relationship with some loved one who has been 'lost', (2) 'solving' ambivalent feelings toward some one, or (3) acquiring some property, such as vitality or courage" (p. 3). Is this impulse panhuman? On this subject Hay equivocates. From what he says, we must assume that had the Ojibwa and Cree behaved in a civilized manner and developed symbolic expressions of the cannibalistic impulse (e.g., the Christian Eucharist), they would have been spared the necessity of killing and eating each other (p. 4). (Hay's model would lead us to the conclusion that the symbolic manifestation of the Hamburger Hoarder's cannibalistic impulse was refined in therapy to a farinaceous form more appropriate to a member of an advanced civilization.)

The Northern Algonkians, according to Hay, must act on their cannibalistic impulse by means of an obsessive-compulsive psychosis because (1) they attach extraordinary importance to following one's dreams without consulting others and (2) they lack "alternative patterns for displacing cannibal desires from members of the band and expressing them symbolically" (p. 8). According to Hay, "the typical personality of the Northern Algonkians is such that most people should be expected to have deeply hidden cannibalistic impulses, the presence of which would tend to produce fear in the presence of a person struggling to control his own heightened cannibalistic tendencies" (p. 14).

Why should we expect the Northern Algonkians to be especially endowed with cannibalistic impulses? Hay does not enlighten us on this subject, although he begins his paper with the statement "To the Indians, the desire to eat human flesh was incomprehensible except as the result of sorcery or possession by the mythical *windigo* spirit" (p. 1). This is simply untrue. The Indians comprehend crisis cannibalism very well.[10] Hay believes that European chroniclers of the *windigo* phenomenon skewed their reports in such a way as to *overemphasize* the importance of starvation (p. 10):

The importance of the patterns of cannibalistic behavior available to the folklore of a society is indicated by the apparent distortions of events in the reports of the *windigo* cases by the Whites who recorded them. In our folklore, cannibalism is a last resort in famine and is used minimally to sustain life until other sources of food can be found. This pattern in Western folklore is so strong that the Whites who recorded these cases attributed second and later acts of cannibalism to starvation although no indication is given of any effort to obtain any food but human flesh and one recorded case even reports waste of some parts of one victim.

Hay believes that, while we practice cannibalism only as a last resort, Algonkians do it as the fulfillment of a basic "impulse", an impulse they have especially strongly either as an ethnic characterisitc or because they lack the wit to invent symbolic safety values that would enable them to vent their cannibalistic impulses harmlessly.

Hay (1971: 5) cites Teicher (1960: 91), who in turn refers to Ballantyne (1848: 50–55) for a story in which a starving mother kills her child and eats it. The data base for this tale is externely poor, and Hay's interpretation of the available data is questionable. If, however, we assume that the facts of the case were as he assumes them to be, we may question whether they justify his conclusion (p. 5): "It seems probable that this act was motivated at least as much by the desire to keep the relationship with the child as by hunger. If not, why should the woman not have begun with someone less dear?" Hay writes from the comfortable perspective of someone who has never faced a food crisis. The assumption tht children are the most "dear" under such circumstances is an ethnocentric prejudice not supported by anthropological evidence (see Turnbull 1972, 1978 for an extreme example; also West 1966 [1824] : 128). An ethnographic grounding indicates that if the child was eaten at all it was because it was most helpless and least able to resist or most expendable in terms of group survival, not because it was most dear. Hay's thesis that the Cree and Ojibwa kill and eat their loved ones in order to preserve a relationship or to eliminate frustrating interpersonal feelings demeans them and belittles the privations they have had to endure, their sufferings being in part the result of the fur trade and other European disruptions. Northern Algonkian parents love their children as much as parents anywhere love their children, a fact that only compounds the poignancy of the tragedies that did from time to time occur.

An interesting paper based on original interviews is Paredes's 'A Case Study of a "Normal" *Windigo*' (1972). In 1966 Paredes set about taping the life history of an elderly Minnesota woman of mixed Chippewa and Euro-American ancestry (p. 99):

Her father was a White lumberjack and camp cook; her mother was Chipewa and died before the informant can recollect. She spent her childhood in her maternal grandmother's house; also in the household were her "step-grandfather" and her mother's sister. Her father occasionally saw her but on the whole had little interaction with her.

The woman had lived a difficult life. She had not been well treated by her maternal relatives and in her earlier years had experienced a recurrent dream in which she was being chased by a giant. The giant failed to catch her, however, because she was protected by 12 men. In the dream she took refuge with an old woman who welcomed her warmly and fed her. Later she went out and gathered money and gave it to the kind old woman. She was also allowed to gather up all the clothing she wanted to wear. According to Paredes's informant, the giant who chased her in her dream had two names: Misabe and "weindiigo" (p. 102). Misabe quite literally means "giant" in Ojibwa. As a hero in folklore, Misabe is an enemy of Windigo and sometimes a slayer of windigowak. Paredes goes to some trouble in trying to explain why his informant combined the two legendary personages in her dream. He suggests that the composite giant might represent her step-grand-father (p. 105), her father (p. 106), her policeman uncle (p. 106), her dead mother (p. 106), her first husband (p. 107), one of several white people she had known as a child (a school superintendent's wife, a steamboat engineer, a male school employee [p. 107]), or some comination of the above.

Paredes classifies his informant as a "normal *windigo*" and believes that her case "show[s] that Teicher's [1960] assertion that *windigo* belief causes *windigo* behavior is simply untrue and does not hold at the individual level" (personal communication). At the same time, he points out that an application of Fogelson's (1965) N-U-P model to his data illustrates the fact that a person can be "Upset" by *windigo* fantasies, yet never progress to a "Psychotic" state, and in fact remain essentially "Normal" (personal communication). I agree with Paredes but suggest that this case has something far more direct to tell us. The works of Saindon, Landes, Honigmann, Ridington (1976: 109, 126, 128), and Preston (1980: 124–29) all indicate in different ways that "*windigo*" is a much more inclusive mental and phenomenological category for Northern Algonkians than the cannibal-psychotic obsession of anthropological renown. My own field experiences confirm and amplify the thoughts of these writers. Never in modern contexts did I hear the word "*windigo*" associated with cannibalism or aggression, but of course conditions and concepts change over time. Starvation is no longer a threat, and village life has for the most part replaced the seminomadic hunting-and-trapping cycle. Mentally impaired individuals no longer pose a danger to group survival. Treatment by nurses, physicians, and mental-health professionals is often available, and serious cases are flown out to hospitals (see Armstrong and Patterson 1975; Goldthorpe 1977; Young n.d.). The cannibal theme may be less important than it once was, but the work of Saindon and Landes provides evidence that the features of the *windigo* belief complex I observed in the 1970s survive virtually intact from an earlier period.

Paredes's characterization of his informant as a "normal *windigo*" is not the contradiction in terms it first appears to be; rather, it lends support to my thesis that *windigos* as individuals within a category of persons are more normal than we have thought. (Her being chased in her dreams by a *windigo* is no more abnormal than a Euro-American's series of nightmares involving werewolves or other cultural-ly defined bogeymen.) Certainly by the observed cases — Saindon's, Paredes's, and the three Northern Ojibwa women I have described above — they are much more normal than the bulk of anthropological writing on the subject would lead us to believe. And that, of course, is my main point.

Paredes's tongue-in-cheek attempt to link his informant's dreams to deeply repressed cannibalistic urges via Ojibwa folklore (pp. 110–11) is an exercise in irony irrelevant to the question of whether *windigo* psychosis is etically real. Yet his search for an explanation for the Windigo-Misabe dream composite leads him to some very sound and valuable conclusions. He shows that a close examination of Woodland Ojibwa folklore and the folklore of the related Plains Ojibwa and Plains Cree reveals that the name Windigo (or its cognates) is applied to a surprisingly wide range of mythological figures (1972: 107–8). Paredes believes the evidence suggests that, "considered in its broadest ethnological context, the *windigo* idea of mythology has complex associations with other characters, has benign even comical aspects, and, thus, cannot be summarily dismissed by simple characterization as a cannibalistic monster" (p. 108). Paredes, then, makes a geographical contribution to the literature similar to Fogelson's (1965: 76–77) temporal one. Together they show that the *windigo* complex is remarkably flexible in space and time. Their work suggests that the ideational configuration of *windigo* as a cannibal spirit-monster capable of taking possession of human bodies may be limited to rather specific sets of infrastructural contexts in the history of the Northern Algonkian peoples. (Space does not permit me to present these specific contexts here; see Bishop 1974, 1976, 1978; cf. Rogers n.d.).

Paredes goes on to caution against allowing culturological explanations to supersede situational explanations, especially when we must deal with fantasy material from other societies. He quotes Malinowski to the effect that in anthropology we often "neglect somewhat those elemental phases of human existence, just because they seem to be obvious and generally human, non-sensational and non-problematic" (Malinowski 1960 [1944]: 72). Thsi admonition is just as valid today as it was when it was first written.

"Secondly", writes Paredes (pp. 112–13),

the data presented here indicate that the whole complex of *windigo* belief may need reexamination. Is, for example, the *windigo* lore of southern Ojibwa significantly different from that of the sub-Arctic? What have been the effects of several centuries of acculturation on the *windigo* syndrome? How is it that the horrible cannibal monster is terminologically identified with the ludicrous clown-shamans of the plains Ojibwa and plains Cree [Skinner 1914: 500–505, 528–29; Mandelbaum 1940: 274–75]? What relationship does the *windigo* idea have to other folklore characters – is *windigo* a character, a *characterization*, or both? Precise answers to these and related questions should provide important insights into our understanding of "*windigo*".

Here Paredes is clearly on the right track.

The *windigo* and the infrastructure are closely linked by Bishop (1975), who suggests that while belief in an evil deity called Windigo may have been aboriginal (cf. Fogelson 1965), the emergence of the *windigo* complex as we have come to know it is the result of disruptions and depletions caused by the fur trade. He reports that, of the two 17th-century Montagnais incidents cited by Teicher (1960:

107) as conclusive evidence of the aboriginal existence of *windigo* psychosis, one involves a group (the Montagnais near Tadoussac and Three Rivers [Quebec]) whose "subsistence base ... had been drastically disrupted by trade and environmental depletion, processes that had been going on for at least 100 years" (pp. 239—40). In the other, reputed to have occurred near Lake St. John in the winter of 1660—61, "the Indian deputies of the Jesuits were supposedly seized with madness and a desire for human flesh for which they were put to death by others", but the Jesuits expressed doubt about the veracity of the report at the time and continued with their missionary activities undeterred (p. 242). Bishop points out that "the deputies had gone to summon Indians who resided near James Bay. This would threaten the trade monopoly of the Lake St. John Indians. They may have spread the rumor to prevent the Jesuits from continuing on their journey; or they may actually have murdered the deputies lest they reach the Indians to the north."

Bishop speaks of regional and episodic faunal depletions and holds that starvation became a much more serious danger for the Northern Algonkians in the 19th century than formerly. The 19th century was a period of peak *windigo* activity, although I must concede that it is possible that the phenomenon was simply better reported then than in earlier centuries. According to Bishop (p. 246), "despite the horror and repugnance expressed by Indians, the data demonstrate that cannibalism was potentially normal in an abnormal situation in the face of starvation". Thus changing infrastructural conditions interacting with a constantly evolving belief system "gave rise to the practice of killing actual or potential Human Windigos with no necessity to justify the act" (p. 247).

For all the merits of his paper, Bishop is yet another who fails to question the etic/behavioral reality of the obsessive-compulsive cannibal psychosis (p. 246): "It is ... necessary to distinguish between famine cannibalism and *Windigo* cannibalism: The former occurs under conditions of extreme famine; the latter may be exhibited in times of plenty as well as during food shortages." He finds convincing Speck's (1935: 43) argument that famine cannibalism could lead to *windigo* cannibalism at a later date. As has been said above, a close reading of original sources does not support a belief in the etic/behavioral existence of *windigo* cannibalism in any form.[11]

Waisberg's (1975) attempt to refute an earlier paper by Bishop (1973) on the grounds that starvation could occur under precontact conditions is unsuccessful because Bishop's position (like mine, which is not identical) hinges not on the existence of an aboriginal Algic Arcadia, but on the fact that conditions grew appreciably *more* difficult and unstable for these Indians as the fur-trade period progressed. I speak here not only of nutrition, but also of eipdemiology and demography.

Smith (1976) presents a more serious challenge to the historical interpretations Bishop and I favor. Smith, who has worked among the Rocky Cree of northern Maintoba and Saskatchewan, argues that "the ecological dynamics of the aboriginal Subarctic environment west of Hudson Bay offered the necessary preconditions for the entire Wittiko complex of cannibal giant and psychosis" (p. 28). My major point is that the Northern Algonkians have used the *windigo* cannibal theme to scapegoat or otherwise divest themselves of the sick, the weak, the marginal, and the disruptive under trying circumstances, Whether they have been doing this form time immemorial or only since contact is of secondary importance. Much more threatening to my thesis is Smith's contention that psychotic *windigo* cannibalism can be documented *"amidst abundant game"* (p. 22). His documentation comes from the Hudson's Bay Company "post journal of Fort Churchill" (Hudson's Bay Company 1741):

February ... Down yᵉ river two Indian [Cree] women, in a most miserable Condition of hunger, one of them is yᵉ mother of yᵉ other & they relate yᵉ following Tragical Story, yᵉ daughter had a husband & 3 Children, & was one of our goose Hunter Spring & fall Sometime last month this family was in such a Starved Condition that yᵉ man murthered his youngest Child & Eat it, And in 4 Days after he murthered his Closest Son who was about 12 Years of age, the women fearing he would murder them all they Left him wᵗʰ yᵉ dead Boy, taking wᵗʰ them their Second Child wᶜʰ was a girl about 7 or 8 years old, & male for yᵉ factory, they thn being about 150 miles Distance from hence, 3 Days after he pursued them and Coming up wᵗʰ them he Endeavoured to arrest yᵉ Girl from yᵉ mother but both yᵉ Women Endeavoruing to preserve yᵉ Child, he throatled it in it's mothers hands & after that Seized his wife to Murder her also, but yᵉ two women over Come him & his wife Knocked him on yᵉ head wᵗʰ a hatchet after they had Slue him they Buried him & his Daughter together under yᵉ Snow & came for yᵉ factory & in 16 Days time they got here, what is very Surprising at yᵉ time of this Disaster there was Plenty of Deer [caribou] about them & he had amunition & might have Kild Vension wᶜʰ his family Strongly Desired him to do, but he gave no manner of Care to their Sollicitations but his mind seemed to be fixed upon what is above related, yᵉ Subsistence yᵉ women got to bring them forward, was for Severall Days Deer Dung wᶜʰ they Picked up and Desolved in warm water & So Drank it till at Length providence flung in their way yᵉ Scraps of a Deer that yᵉ wolves had Killed & Left.

For purposes of argument I will assume that the chronicler was proficient in Cree and recorded the women's story essentially as they told it. The veracity of the women then becomes the central issue. If they were telling the truth, their story is very damaging to my position. After 240 years it is probably not possible to say with any degree of certainty what the truth of the matter was. Although they may have been telling the truth, I would like to suggest an alternative interpretation.

It is agreed by all that the events at issue began when "this family was in . . . a Starved Condition". The reasons for the starvation situation are open to question. The surviving women state that the situation developed because the man ignored their pleas to hunt the abundant caribou, being preoccupied with thoughts of mayhem and cannibalism. But Smith himself makes the case that the ecological dynamics of the Subarctic were such that famine was an ever present danger, even in precontact times (pp. 27–31). I think it is possible that starvation conditions developed in this situation because the man had a run of bad luck. A hunter can go into a "slump" for many reasons: an injury, an illness, scarcity of game, or simple misfortune. It is suspicious to me that the women were able to overpower and kill the man only *after* he had allegedly throttled the third child in the arms of its mother, especially since – according to them – he had been living on flesh while they had been making do on dissolved caribou dung. If the women were lying, the following scenario suggests itself: Starvation conditions developed because, for whatever reason, the man was unsuccessful in the hunt. The women – mother and daughter – were the initiators of the homicides and the cannibalism. They survived to tell the tale, and their version was accepted. Here again, as in so many cases, it is the story of the killers of the alleged *windigo* that is handed down. The stories of the executed parties are lost to posterity. We will probably never be certain of the facts in this case, but what is certain is that the conceptualization Smith employs to analyze the data needs to be refined. For Smith "the Wittiko 'psychosis' or disorder . . . involved an individual believing that he or she is or is becoming a Wittiko, *or the belief of others that he or she is exhibiting characteristic Wittiko and non-human behavior*. In extreme form, the individual actually becomes a cannibal, killing and eating his victims" (p. 20, emphasis added). By thus failing to distinguish emics from etics, Smith opens a veritable Pandora's box. Are the diagnostic features of *windigo* "psychosis" to be found in equal measure in the behavior of the "psychotics" and in the minds of the social authorities? Is there any scientific justification for classifying people as they appear in the nightmares and fantasies of their accusers (cf. Harris 1974: 214, 221, 235, 251)?

From his observations at Shamattawa, Manitoba, Turner (1978; Turner and Wertman 1977) correctly concludes that Cree social organization is "incorporative". For Turner the incorporation of individuals into Cree social groupings is symbolically analogous to the incorporation of individuals cannibalistically (Turner 1977). He contrasts Cree social organization with that of the Australian Aborigines,[12] and in doing so he constructs a typological dichotomy that describes, according to him, "two hunter and gatherer ways of life as they *probably* existed prior to modification by Europeans" (1978: 195). The Australians group themselves into totemic, exogamous clans on the exclusionary principle: a person cannot belong to more than one clan and remains in the birth clan throughout the life cycle. With the Cree, however, "outsiders could be incorporated into the band through residence and work association, and required no prior kinship, marriage, or symbolic ties to be acceptable as in Australia" (p. 202). Space does not permit a full treatment here to Turner's binary model, the components of which he has named "production group unity" (e.g., Cree) and "production group diversity" (e.g., Australian), but it merits our attention. It must suffice here to say that Turner's claim (p. 210) that such systems, once established, are relatively unresponsive to variations in population and resources requires careful *diachronic* verification by means of a sample drawn from a universe arger than two.

For Turner (1977: 65), cannibalism in Cree folklore "is taken as a metaphor for incorporation into (becoming part of) a social grouping; the various acts and relations described in the story can be seen as attempts at mediating opposed tendencies toward autonomy at the domestic, brotherhood and band levels". It is difficult to counter structuralist arguments with etic/behavioral and materialist refutations because structuralism concerns itself above all with mental sets. The study of mental sets seems at first to be a goal worthy of some effort — comparable and related to learning the languages of the people we study — until we realize that it is not necessarily the mental structures of the *natives* that are explicated by the structuralist. Lévi-Strauss (1969: 13, quoted in Harris 1979: 169) says, "it is in the last resort immaterial whether . . . the thought processes of the South American Indians take shape through the medium of my thoughts, or whether mine take place through the medium of theirs", and Turner himself has told me that ideas are "created" and need not be accounted for. Who, then, creates them? Turner concedes that in the last analysis he does not know.

For these reasons we are fortunate to have the critique of Preston (1980: 120), who has done extensive fieldwork among the James Bay Cree and has specialized in Northern Algonkian mental life:

[Turner's] use of the structural theory and the metaphorically extended notion of incorporation highlights, in my opinion, our tendency to overpower a very poorly known *Witiko* phenomenon with our own intellectual creation. The problem of translating the Algonkian idiom
of experience into terms that are understandable and worthwhile within our own tradition
of urbane intellectual inquiry is poorly served by psychodynamic and structuralist theories,
unless the effort includes the judicious use of Algonkian phenomena. Both Hay and Turner,
in my opinion, have created intellectual monstrosities in imposing elegant arguments upon
dubious data.

Again it must be stressed that the data to which Preston refers are the emic/mental Algonkian data. When etic/behavioral and historical data are added to this, the case against conventional interpretations of the windigo phenomenon is overwhelming.

It seems at first puzzling that Turner's analysis of the windigo — one of the most involuted over written — was produced by an anthropologist who has done fieldwork (albeit of brief duration) among the Northern Cree. The lesson to be learned here is that exposure to primary data source opportunities does not often lead to valid conclusions when inadequate research strategies are employed.

Turner's contribution reveals the most serious weakness of structuralism: its ahistorical and antievolutionary synchrony. He contends that Cree social organiza-tion is one of at least two hunter-gatherer production-group types that probably survive without modification in precontact form. Windigo myths, in turn, provide "clues to the kinds of social structures possessed by the Algonkians, both in the recent past and in the more distant past — perhaps even in the pre-Cartier past" (Turner 1977: 71). A growing literature addresses the issue of possible postcontact changes in the social structures of various Algonkian groups, but that is beyond the scope of this review. More to the point is whether Algonkian religion, especially the *windigo* belief complex as expressed in the Cree oral tradition, has undergone change. As we have seen, Fogelson's work gives a strong indication that it has changed and that the Windigo figure was probably not associated with anthropophagy until the end of the 18th century. For Algonkian groups to the south, Bishop (1975: 244) tells us: "Nowhere in the early Jesuit accounts relating to the Ojibwa and Ottawa is there a specific devil form recognizable as the Windigo, a rather remarkable fact considering the apparent preoccupation in the nineteenth century with the phenomenon". This is especially remarkable considering the Jesuits' natural interest in religious matters.

The stories on which Turner bases his analysis were collected ca. 1970 at Sandy Lake, Ontario (Ray and Stevens 1971). As will be shown in a forthcoming paper, the Sandy Lake "Cree" (actually Northern Ojibwa) underwent a nutritional and demographic crisis in the late 19th and early 20th centuries. A materialist analysis predicts that this situation will be reflected in their folklore (Marx and Engels 1977 [1846]: 47), and this proves to be the case. One of the stories, 'The Death of Pe-cequan', is the mythologized form of a *windigo* execution that took place in 1906 and its aftermath (Annual Archaeological Report 1907 [1908]; PAC 1907–8, 1907–9). A close examination of the archival data stronly indicates that the story as collected by Ray and Stevens (1971: 128–9) and cited by Turner (1977: 68) is one of the most recent — and perhaps one of the final — manifestations in the process identified by Fogelson (1965: 76–77).

A more ingenuous use of the structuralist paradigm is McGee's 'The Windigo Down-East, or The Taming of the Windigo' (1975). McGee does a structural analysis of an unusual Micmac myth collected in 1859 (Rand 1971 [1894]: 190–99). In this myth, "Chennoo" — the Micmac homologue of Windigo — is found in a distant northwestern forest by a family and treated with care and affection rather than with fear and revulsion. Through the family's nurturance Cheenoo gradually becomes more human and less monstrous. After killing an enemy Cheenoo with the aid of his new "son-in-law", Cheenoo accompanies the family southeast to Micmacland (McGee 1975: 17):

The farther south they go the weaker Cheenoo becomes. When they reach their village he is nearly dead. He has been transformed to look like an old but whole man. He has become human but he is not a Christian. A priest is sent for and he instructs Cheenoo. Cheenoo listens, is baptised, then dies in the Catholic faith.

McGee's central contention is that "the *windigo* myth functioned to define the concept of human personness for the north-eastern Algonkians" (p. 113). (A similar thought is expressed by Fogelson [1980: 148].) This is an entirely reasonable suggestion, but McGee does not follow up on it. He believes that "what is needed is an attempt to understand the *windigo* with respect to the mentally balanced, rather than to the psychotic" (p. 112). With this I heartily concur, but from an etic/behavioral perspective we cannot assign as high a priority to understanding how cultures transform monsters into humans as to understanding how cultures transform humans into social monsters. When, why, and under what circumstances are human beings socially redefined as nonpersons, thus legitimizing their persecution and possible execution? How is the Northern Algonkian process of divesting individuals of their humanity similar to or different from those of other groups? Can predictive or retrodictive generalizations be made cross-culturally? I will return to these questions.

Culturological treatments of the *windigo* complex are often supported by the claim that the Northern Athapaskans who share the boreal forest with the Northern Algonkians lack a cultural configuration comparable to the *windigo* (e.g., Parker 1960: 618–19). This claim is used to counter ecological and historical explorations into the *windigo* curiosity. Ridington, in 'Wechuge and *Windigo*: A Comparison of Cannibal Belief Among Boreal Forest Athapaskans and Algonkians' (1976), shows that the belief systems of these two macrogroups of Subarctic Indians are not as different as they may seem and that the *windigo* as we have come to know it may be an artifact of our own projections (a point also made by Preston [1980: 117–18]) as well as the result of the unique culture history of the Northern Algonkians since the 16th century.

The Athapaskan Beaver Indians (Dunne-za) of the Peace River district believe in a personage they call Wechuge. Wechuge, like Windigo, is an invincible, ice-gutted cannibal who eats his own lips as a preliminary to more substantial fare. In Dunne-za cosmology, Wechuge is associated with giant animals that hunted people in the mythic past, but now "it is these giant People-eaters who confer supernatural power to the child on his or her vision quest. Contact with this power gives a person the ability to find and transform animals into food" (Ridington 1976: 109). Wechuge exists as a legendary figure who tracks people down, kills them, and eats them (pp. 110–14), but ordinary people too can "become Wechuge" (pp. 114–23). Unlike becoming *windigo*, in which the victim is possessed by an entity alien to him or her (sometimes as the result of an enemy's curse), becoming Wechuge occurs when one loses control of one's own supernatural power through the violation of a taboo. (For example, people with "Frog power" cannot eat fly-blown meat; people with "Spider power" cannot hear any sound made by a stretched string.)

Becoming Wechuge, then, means becoming "too strong". People in the transformation phase are "cured" by the application of their own "medicine" and the "medicine" of others. If a person is not cured, the mythological precedent is for the victim to be killed and the body burned in order to melt the visceral ice and to prevent the body from returning to life. To Ridington's knowledge, things have never come to such a pass among the Dunne-za. As for actual "Wechuge cannibalism", Ridington heard of one case that was supposed to have happened late in the 19th century (p. 114). We do not know how much credence to give this or how to interpret it if it did occur.

Assuming for the time being that these correspondences between Northern Athapaskan and Northern Algonkian belief systems are not the result of diffusion, what can we make of them? Ridington has observed (pp. 107–8) that "the diagnosis of Windigo behavior as psychotic has not been seriously questioned in the literature even though all authors recognize that in none of the reported cases has there been first-hand information on individual case histories let alone analysis of subject's lives by observers with experience in psychiatric diagnosis". This is a good insight, and Ridington follows up on it. While taking note of other possibilities, he suggests that the belief systems of these two groups of boreal-forest Indians on the cannibal theme may have started out similarly and then diverged in historic times. "In general the Algonkians have experienced a longer period of disruptive influence from contact with Europeans than the Dunne-za" (p. 126). "It seems significant that the story of Tsekute, the only actual person said to have become a cannibal Wechuge, occurred at a time of maximum social upheaval and was linked to the elaboration of the Plateau Prophet Dance as described by Spier (1935) among the Dunne-za" (p. 125). Ridington deserves praise for making these points and also for indicating that witch fear (including the belief in cannibal monsters) is symptomatic of societies under stress.

To the best of my knowledge, the only Algonkianist to have benefitted directly from Honigmann's scholarship on *windigo* is Preston. In 'The *Witiko*: Algonkian Knowledge and Whiteman Knowledge' (1980), he makes the point that "the *Witiko* psychosis in the literature is not a very adequate approximation to the Algonkian emotional dynamics or to the great variability in Algonkian oral tradition on this topic" (p. 128). Preston believes it to be abundantly clear that, in both Algonkian and Western cultures, the experts fail to agree on the nature of the *windigo* phenomenon (pp. 127–28):

Apparently while some Algonkians are prepared to accept the possibility of the monstrous, some Algonkianists prefer to tacitly assert the necessity of fantasy and then to exaggerate with false concreteness some aspects of symbolic implication they have culled for this purpose from a variety of narratives. I concur with Honigmann and Ridington that, on the evidence, the case has not been made for *Witiko* belief and behaviour being diagnosed as a psychosis, although particular aspects of *Witiko* may be components of some individuals' psychological dysfunction. Nor can [*Witiko*] be realistically accepted as a category of persons, unless we can specify a category with boundaries allowing frequent realignment and with a content allowing great variance and transformative potential.

About the "psychosis" Preston writes (pp. 112, 114):

We have made the diagnosis without seeing the patient. . . . Some kind of compulsion and transformation is believed in by Northern Algonkians, but their words are too often taken as literal (rather than imagic or symbolic) representations of events, which we then use to construct our definition of a *Witiko* psychopathology. . . . It seems that we have taken an exotic notion out of its native context of the images of terror, and with much seriousness we have overinterpreted the meagre data.

Referring to Cooper (1933), Hallowell (1936), and Landes (1938a), Preston writes (p. 114): "One has the sense that these scholars (and later ones), in treating of the *Witiko*, suspended their normal standards of critical and judicious interpretation, being for some reason drawn to make imaginative suggestions without a positive factual basis". He asks if transplanted Europeans have been "simply finding the familiar in exotic settings", for "the Wild Man of the wilderness, often a hairy and solitary being who lurks just out of sight, is one of the oldest and most persistent folk beliefs in Western culture" (p. 117).

In an attempt to account for Euro-North American fascination with a very poorly documented *windigo*, Preston constructs a model that parodies psychiatric and structural explanations and calls it "*Witiko* and Psychic Unity" (p. 118). In it he suggests satirically that *windigo* psychosis "is an Algonkian reenactment of Freud's primal parricide" and that *windigo* cannibalism is "a recapitulation of the Oedipal *fête*". "The plot is absurd, if rationally plausible, and leaves us ... wondering why we write so much and make such a mess, on a topic about which we know so little". He concludes (pp. 127–28) with a quote from Evans-Pritchard (1962: 175) that reads in part: "If the specificity of a fact is lost, the generalization about it becomes so general as to be valueless". This is a basic principle of science and a piece of plain common sense that is ll too often overlooked in anthropology. I am in emphatic agreement with Preston that this truism has been for the most part ignored by analysts of the *windigo* phenomenon.

Preston's paper has many strengths, but it fails to explain why the Algonkian "ecology of *mind*" (p. 117) – poorly understood as it may be – should have evolved the belief in a cannibal spirit-monster capable of taking possession of ordinary humans, thereby necessitating the execution of those so "possessed". In his critique of Bishop's (1973) observation that reports of *windigo* cannibalism are positively correlated with starvation and ecological degradation on the Canadian Shield in the 1800s, Preston astutely points out that "we are not here faced with a simple task of filling empty stomachs, but rather with the elaboration of an implicitly symbolic system of belief" (pp. 116–17). He is quite correct in contending that starvation and other infrastructural crises cannot account for the existence of *windigo* cannibalism as distinguished from "lifeboat" cannibalism, but this is not the problem that confronts us. He himself considers the evidence for psychotic *windigo* cannibalism insufficient (p. 128). His view is confirmed by my investigations into archival sources, which indicate that *windigo* cannibalism probably never occurred in an etic/behavioral sense. The task remaining before us is to answer the question why *windigo accusations and executions* are positively correlated with starvation, ecological degradation, and other crises in the material sphere. How, in other words, can we account for the elaboration of Preston's implicitly symbolic system of belief?

This is a task to which the research strategy of cultural materialism – which grants, as a matter of theoretical principle, research priority to the study of infrastructural variables as determinative (Harris 1979: 46–76) – lends itself very well. Honigmann's comparison of *windigo* executions to Euro-American witch hunting was a shrewd one. Harris has been foremost among those who have shown that fluctuations in the frequency and severity of witchcraft accusations are not capricious, but the results of practical and mundane causes (1974: 207–66; 1980: 404–5; cf. Mair 1969). Preston's inability to deal with the evolution of the *windigo* belief complex illustrates the limitations of phenomenology and other ideographic strategies.

Ridington (1976: 126) has given us important clues toward an understanding of why the religion of the Northern Algonkians might have diverged in important ways from the symbolic belief systems of their Subarctic neighbors. My own ethnohistorical inquiries are congruent with Bishop's (1974, 1976) and will show how the specific culture history of the Northern Algonkian peoples since the 1500s is compatible with the evolution of the *windigo* belief system.[13]

While every culture history — like every life history — is unique, recurrent patterns can be identified, and it is the business of social science to make generalizations based on those patterns. A generalization we can make with some confidence is that witch fear (as differentiated from shamanism) is characteristic of traumatized societies. Kluckhohn (1944) showed that Navaho witch fear and executions were the consequences of a devastating military defeat followed by mass incarceration at Fort Sumner, "the full calamity of which it is difficult to convery to white readers" (pp. 64, 68):

During the post-Fort Sumner period, the chiefs in power took care of advocates of renewed resistance to whites by spreading the word that these people were witches. Many were killed. There seems evidence that a correlation exists between the amount of fear and talk about witches and the general state of tension prevailing among the Navaho. Thus, during the last difficult years of controversy over the stock reduction program [beginning in 1933 and continuing through the New Deal years] there has been appreciably more witchcraft excitement than for some time past.

Kluckhohn concludes his monograph by reprinting a 1942 New Mexico newspaper account of a particularly gruesome triple murder and suicide that was the result of Navaho witch fear (p. 142).

In 'Witch-Fear in Post-Contact Kaska Society' (1947). Honigmann documents the wave of torture, maimings, and killings that swept over the Kaska from about 1897 until suppressed by the Royal Canadian Mounted Police and the British Columbia Provincial Police in the mid-1920s. Most of the victims were children, many whom were persecuted by their closest relatives. Honigmann attributes the outbreak to the development of a situation in which "the Kaska found their survival imperiled" (p. 236). This resulted from "the influx of strangers [who] had upset the balance of game", the introduction of new illnesses, and an increased dependence on trapping, the trading post, and non-native foods.

Carpenter (1961 [1953]: 509) has demonstrated how the introduction of deadly diseases, the decimation of game herds, an economy based more and more on an uncertain fox-fur trade, and competition with hostile Inuit groups for women and an ever decreasing food supply caused the Aivilik Inuit to become preoccupied by witch fear. By 1950 the aboriginal pattern of magic for controlling game, disease, weather, etc., had been almost completely replaced by the constant fear of malevolent witchcraft: "every man's hand was suspected of being against every nonrelative" (p. 508).

Lindenbaum (1979) has shown how the mounting importance of sorcery in the ideology of the South Fore of New Guinea "simultaneously registered and aggravated the social inequalities and demographic imbalances" occurring in their area in the 1950s and 1960s (p. viii). "Between 1957 and 1968, over 1,100 kuru deaths occurred in a South Fore population of 8,000. . . . Since kuru is primarily a disease of adult women — the childbearers, hog tenders, and gardeners — its effects on Fore society have been particularly deranging. When the incidence of kuru reached a peak, in the 1960's, the South Fore believed their society was coming to an end" (p. 6). "To this day, Fore universally believe that kuru is caused by malicious sorcerers in their midst" (p. 28). The ethnographic record indicates that the ideology of sorcery among the Fore became elaborated in a brief period between 1951 and the 1960s (p. 74). This situation is complicated by novel social relations that resulted from three decades of exposure to Australian authorities. "A new way of life gave rise to greater manipulation of the environment, and to differences in rank requiring the coercion of others in order to maintain an elevated position" (p. 7). The ubiquitous sorcerers, then, are considered by the superordinate to be those who "might willfully use their private technology to up-end the social order" (p. 143). Fore big-men "seek to discredit political rivals both in their own community and in a more general sense" by accusing them of sorcery and calling them "rubbish men" (p. 126). "In a masterly illusion projected by an egalitarian ethic, the dispossessed are characterized as a threat, a casuistic line of argument we share with the Fore. People in marginal positions are portrayed as a danger to the establishment. If kuru becomes the prototype for studies of slow virus infections, Fore beliefs about mystical danger may contribute to our understanding of the emergence of social inequality" (p. 146).

CONCLUSIONS

Although the particular manifestatios of the Northern Algonkian stress response are specific to them alone, *windigo* witch fear has much in common with that of the Navaho, the Kaska, the Aivilik, and the Fore. By the time *windigo* accusations reached their peak, the Northern Algonkians had been involved in the fur trade for more than two centuries. Trapping began as a supplementary activity that provided luxury European goods, but by this time most of these Indians were bound to the trading posts by a system of debt peonage. Regional and episodic depletions of such important animals as the moose and the beaver resulted in widespread suffering (Bishop 1974, 1976, 1978). For the group I know best — the Northern Ojibwa — these depletions, combined with an increased dependence on the trading posts, caused a shift in the basic mode of production away from big-game hunting toward the capture of fish, small game, and whatever fur-bearers were available (cf. Rogers 1966; Rogers and Black 1976). This new mode of production put a premium on the labor of children, who could become net producers at an early age (cf. Mamdani 1973; White 1973, 1975; Nag, White, and Peet 1978). Consequently there was a substantial rise in population among rhe Northern Ojibwa throughout the 19th century in the face of a deteriorating resource base (Bishop

1976: 48; 1978: 225—26). This apparent paradox put even more strain on Northern Ojibwa society as the new mode of production and reproduction was intensified past the point of dimishing returns (cf. Boserup 1965; Harris 1977; 1980: 188—92). European diseases took a terrible toll and imposed severe hardships on a seminomadic people that could not provide protracted nursing care to its sick. I contend that the *windigo* belief complex was the Northern Algonkian manifestation of the collective witch fear that is predictable in traumatized societies, not an obsessive cannibalistic psychosis of individuals.

Although unrepresentative of the professional literature, a recent article in the popular journal *Science Digest* serves as a grim example of how legitimate anthropological inquiry can be warped for public consumption. In this paper Lindholm and Lindholm (1981: 52) tell of a fictional Indian named Red Bear:

[he] sits up wild-eyed, his body drenched in sweat, every muscle tensed. . . . He has dreamed of the *windigo* — the monster with the heart of ice — and the dream sealed his doom. Coldness gripped his own heart. The ice monster had entered his body and possessed him. He himself had become a *windigo*, and he could do nothing to avert his fate.

Suddenly the form of Red Bear's sleeping wife begins to change. He no longer sees a woman, but a deer. His eyes flame. Silently he draws his knife from under the blanket and moves stealthily toward the motionless figure. Saliva drops from the corners of his mouth, and a terrible hunger twists his intestines. A powerful desire to eat raw flesh consumes him.

Anthropologists who have worked on the *windigo* phenomenon are understandably eager to disassociate their work from this kind of vilification. In fairness to Lindholm and Lindholm, however, it must be said that they have merely followed conventional interpretations to their logical, if imaginative, conclusion.

In a review article on psychiatric anthropology, Kennedy concludes his summary of the *windigo* question with these thoughts (1973: 1158—59):

What is so exasperating about the *windigo* literature, as about all the discussions of the "exotic disorders", is the vast amount of interesting speculation on the basis of such slender evidence. Since Fogelson [1965], Linton [1956: 61—67], Parker [1960], Roehrl [*sic*; 1970, 1972], Teicher [1960], Wallace [1961: 175], and Yap [1951, 1969] have never reported observing an actual case of *windigo*, and have made their diagnoses, classifications, and analyses from fragmentary accounts, most of the discussion amounts only to speculative hypotheses that may now be untestable.

I hold Kennedy to be right on the first count but wrong on the second. Relatively hard data are recoverable from archival sources. These data in combination with a thorough ethnographic grounding yield a plausible and likely uniformitarian solution to the *windigo* puzzle. It is a solution that confirms the suspicions expressed by Honigmann in 1967.

NOTES

1. I am grateful to Charles Wagley for his comments on an earlier version of this paper. It was he who pointed out the significance of Kluckhohn's *Navaho Witchcraft* (1944) to

my study. J. Anthony Paredes's response to an earlier draft was most gracious, and I thank him for bringing Smith's 'Notes on the Wittiko' (1976) to my attention. In a meticulous critique of a different paper, Jean Briggs made me aware of Carpenter's 'Witch-Fear among the Aivilik Eskimos' (1953). CA referee Raymond Fogelson generously sent a valuable critique that gave me the benefit of his long-standing expertise in the fields of psychological anthropology and *windigo* studies. His comments and those of an anonymous referee have been extremely useful and are much appreciated.

My special thanks go to Marvin Harris, whose analysis of the European witch craze (1974) helped me while still in the field to make the mental connections from which this paper grew. His comments and criticisms have greatly improved the manuscript. It is difficult to express the value of the intellectual stimulation I have received from association with him or of his personal generosity and support. I alone, however, am responsible for possible inadequacies or excesses.

2. *Windigo* [wIndIgo] is the most common Ojibwa pronunciation and *wiitiko* [witIko] is most common among the Cree, but the voiced or voiceless quality of stops is not phonemic in either language. For purposes of this paper the allomorph /*windigo*/ is used except within direct quotes. The word begins with an upper-case letter when it refers to the Algonkian mythological personage and with a lower-case letter elsewhere, quotes excepted.

3. This includes time spent as an anthropological fieldworker, agent for a bush plane company, teacher, husband, father, son-in-law, and fully functioning member of the kinship system.

4. For reasons of space I make almost no mention of the scores of passive references to "*windigo* psychosis" by writers who claim no special competence on the subject and whose comments are obviously based on the work of others.

5. Only in the last case did I witness the *windigo* episode, but all three women are well known to me.

6. Translation from the French by Kimberly Head.

7. Wing confines his discussion to the diagnosis of schizophrenia.

8. It should be noted in passing that in the part of the United States in which these events presumably took place (Wisconsin) a car trunk serves as a good deep freezer for many months of they year and is used as such by many completely normal and rational people.

9. In a later paper McGee writes that "the reason fat was used as a cure for the *windigo* psychosis is because it is the most human of foods [in a structural sense], and not because it contains vitamin B_{12}. The motivation was to re-humanize the psychotic – not to 'cure' him. Anyone who rejected fat had surely ceased to be human and should be destroyed; as long as fat was taken, there was hope for transformation" (1975: 124).

10. I do not deny that Northern Algonkians are likely to attribute the development of a food crisis to the sorcery of an enemy, but they are also quite capable of recognizing the urgency of metabolic necessity.

11. The fact that the Jesuits' Indian deputies were accused of having been overcome by cannibal-madness by the Lake St. John Indians could be taken as evidence for the belief in *windigo* insanity among the mid-17th-century Algonkians even if the accusation was false and the deputies were murdered for purely mundane reasons. This militates against my argument that the belief is a relatively recent one. I believe, however, that since boreal-forest subsistence is precarious – particularly after the fur-trade period, which began very early in Quebec – the taboo against cannibalism was elaborated at an early juncture and antedates the belief in *windigo* possession. Therefore it would not be surprising to find those seeking to justify murder doing so by accusing their victims of having been on the verge of violating the strongest taboo.

12. The prototype for the Australian form appears to be the Aranda (Turner 1978: 196).

13. The culture histories of the various Northern Algonkian groups that share the *windigo* belief system are far from uniform, but their similarities seem to outweigh their differences.

REFERENCES

Annual Archaeological Report 1903
  1904 The Killing of Moostoos the Wehtigoo. (Summary of legal proceedings held at Fort Saskatchewan and Edmonton, July—August, 1899.) Appendix to the Report of the Minister of Education, Ontario, Toronto: King's Printer, pp. 126—138.

Annual Archaeological Report 1907
  1908 The Killing of Wa-sak-apee-quay by Pe-se-quan, and others. (Transcript of trial held at Norway House, October 7, 1907.) Appendix to the Report of the Minister of Education, Ontario, Toronto: King's Printer, pp. 91—121.

Arieti, Silvano, and Johannes M. Meth
  1959 Rare, Unclassifiable, Collective, and Exotic Psychiatric Syndromes. *In* Silvano Arieti (ed.), The American Handbook of Psychiatry. New York: Basic Books, pp. 546—563.

Armstrong, Harvey and Paul Patterson
  1975 Seizures in Canadian Indian Children: Individual, Family, and Community Approaches. Canadian Psychiatric Association Journal 20: 247—255.

Ballantyne, Robert M.
  1848 Hudson's Bay. Edinburgh: William Blackwood.

Barnouw, Victor
  1961 Chippewa Social Atomism. American Anthropologist 63: 1006—1013.
  1979 Culture and Personality. Third Edition. Homewood: Ill.: Dorsey Press.

Bishop, Charles A.
  1973 Ojibwa Cannibalism. Paper prepared for the IXth International Congress of Anthropological and Ethnological Sciences, Chicago, Ill., August—September.
  1974 The Northern Ojibwa and the Fur Trade: A Historical and Ecological Study. Toronto: Holt, Rinehart and Winston of Canada.
  1975 Northern Algonkian Cannibalism and *Windigo* Psychosis. *In* Thomas R. Williams (ed.), Psychological Anthropology. The Hague: Mouton, pp. 237—248.
  1976 The Emergence of the Northern Ojibwa: Social and Economic Consequences. American Ethnologist 3: 39—54.
  1978 Cultural and Biological Adaptations to Deprivation: The Northern Ojibwa Case. *In* Charles D. Laughlin, Jr. and Ivan A. Brady (eds.), Extinction and Survival in Human Populations. New York: Columbia University Press, pp. 208—230.

Bloomfield, Leonard
  1934 Cannibal-possession. *In* Plains Cree Texts, Publications of the American Ethnological Society 16, pp. 152—155.

Bolman, William M. and Alan S. Katz
  1966 Hamburger Hoarding: A Case of Symbolic Cannibalism Resembling *Whitico* Psychosis. Journal of Nervous and Mental Disease 142: 424—428.

Boserup, Ester
  1975 The Conditions of Agricultural Growth: The Economics of Agrarian Change under Population Pressure. Chicago: Aldine.

Brown, Jennifer
  1971 The Cure and Feeding of *Windigo*: A Critique. American Anthropologist 73: 20—22.

Campbell, William
  n.d. The Diary of "Big Bill" Campbell. MS, Thomas Fisher Rare Book Library, University of Toronto. Also in Confederation College Library, Thunder Bay, Ont.

Carpenter, Edmund S.
  1961 Witch-fear among the Aivilik Eskimos. *In* Yehudi A. Cohen (ed.), Social Structure (1953) and Personality: A Casebook. New York: Holt, Rinehart and Winston, pp. 508—516. (Reprinted from American Journal of Psychiatry 110: 194—199.)

Cooper, John M.
   1933   The Cree *Witiko* Psychosis. Primitive Man (now Anthropological Quarterly) 6: 20–24.
   1934a Mental Disease Situations in Certain Cultures: A New Field for Research. Journal of Abnormal and Social Psychology 29: 10–17.
   1934b The Northern Algonquian Supreme Being. Washington, D.C.: Catholic University of America.
Dawson, Kenneth C. A.
   n. d.   Pre-history of the Interior Forest of Northern Ontario. *In* A. T. Steegmann, Jr. (ed.), Boreal Forest Adaptations: The Algonkians of Northern Ontario. New York: Plenum.
Edmonton Court Files
   1899   The Queen vs Pay-i-uu and Nap-i-so-sis. Cr. 157 (Old Series).
Evans-Prichard, E. E.
   1962   Social Anthropology and Other Essays. New York: Free Press.
Fogelson, Raymond D.
   1965   Psychological Theories of *Windigo* "Psychosis" and a Preliminary Application of a Models Approach. *In* Melford E. Spiro (ed.), Context and Meaning in Cultural Anthropology: Essays in Honor of A. Irving Hallowell. New York: Free Press, pp. 74–99.
   1980   *Windigo* Goes South: Stoneclad among the Cherokees. *In* Marjorie M. Halpin and Michael M. Ames (eds.), Manlike Monsters on Trial: Early Records and Modern Evidence. Vancouver: University of British Columbia Press, pp. 132–151.
Friedl, Ernestine
   1956   Persistence in Chippewa Culture and Personality. American Anthropologist 58: 814–825.
Goldthorpe, W. Gary
   1977   Submission to the Royal Commission on the Environment by Canada Health and Welfare Medical Services Branch, Sioux Lookout Zone Hospital, Royal Commission on the Environment, 55 Bloor St. W., Room 801, Toronto, Ont. M4W 1A5.
Guinard, Joseph E.
   1930   *Witiko* among the Tête-de-Boule. Primitive Man (now Anthropological Quarterly) 3: 69–71.
Hallowell, A. Irving
   1934   Culture and Mental Disorder. Journal of Abnormal and Social Psychology 29: 1–9.
   1936   Psychic Stresses and Culture Patterns. American Journal of Psychiatry 92: 1291–1310.
   1955   Culture and Experience. Philadelphia: University of Pennsylvania Press.
   1963   American Indians, White and Black: The Phenomenon of Transculturalization. Current Anthropology 4: 519–531.
   1976   Contributions to Anthropology: Selected Papers of A. Irving Hallowell. Chicago: University of Chicago Press.
Harris, Marvin
   1974   Cows, Pigs, Wars, and Witches: The Riddles of Culture. New York: Random House.
   1977   Cannibals and Kings: The Origins of Cultures. New York: Random House.
   1979   Cultural Materialism: The Struggle for a Science of Culture. New York: Random House.
   1980   Culture, People, Nature: An Introduction to General Anthropology. Third edition. New York: Harper and Row.
Hay, Thomas H.
   1971   The *Windigo* Psychosis: Psychodynamic, Cultural, and Social Factors in Aberrant Behavior. American Anthropologist 73: 1–19.

Hearne, Samuel
  1971   A Journey from Prince of Wales's Fort in Hudson's Bay to the Northern Ocean.
  (1795) Rutland, Vt., and Tokyo: Charles E. Tuttle.
Hickerson, Harold
  1960   The Feast of the Dead among the Seventeenth-century Algonkians of the Upper
          Great Lakes. American Anthropologist 62: 81–107.
  1967   Some Implications of the Theory of the Particularity, or "Atomism", of Northern
          Algonkians. Current Anthropology 8: 313–343.
Honigmann, John J.
  1947   Witch-fear in Post-contact Kaska Society. American Anthropologist 49: 222–243.
  1954   Culture and Personality. New York: Harper.
  1967   Personality in Culture. New York: Harper and Row.
Hudson's Bay Company Archives
  1741   Entry in Post Journal of Fort Churchill (HBCA B 42/a/22).
  1830   Lac la Pluie District Report (HBCA, B105/e/9/f11).
James, Bernard
  1954   Some Critical Observations Concerning Analyses of Chippewa "Atomism" and
          Chippewa Personality. American Anthropologist 56: 283–286.
James, Bernard
  1970   Continuity and Emergence in Indian Poverty Culture. Current Anthropology 11:
          435–452.
James, Edwin (ed.)
  1956   A Narrative of the Captivity and Adventures of John Tanner during Thirty Years
  (1830) Residence among the Indians in the Interior of North America. Minneapolis: Ross
          and Haines.
Kardiner, Abram
  1939   The Individual and His Society. New York: Columbia University Press.
  1953   The Relation of Culture to Mental Disorder. In Paul H. Hoch and Joseph Zubin
          (eds.), Current Problems in Psychiatric Diagnosis. New York: Grune and Stratton,
          pp. 157–179.
Kennedy, John G.
  1973   Cultural Psychiatry. In John J. Honigmann (ed.), Handbook of Social and Cultural
          Anthropology. Chicago: Rand McNally, pp. 1119–1198.
Kluckhohn, Clyde
  1944   Navaho Witchcraft. Papers of the Peabody Museum of American Archaeology
          and Ethnology, Harvard University, 22(2).
Knight, Rolf
  1974   Grey Owl's Return: Cultural Ecology and Canada's Indigenous Peoples. Reviews
          in Anthropology, August, pp. 349–359.
Landes, Ruth
  1937a   The Personality of the Ojibwa. Character and Personality 6: 51–60.
  1937b   The Ojibwa of Canada. In Margaret Mead (ed.), Cooperation and Competition
          among Primitive Peoples. New York: McGraw-Hill, pp. 87–126.
  1938a   The Abnormal among the Ojibwa Indians. Journal of Abnormal and Social Psy-
          chology 33: 14–33.
  1938b   The Ojibwa Woman. New York: Columbia University Press.
Lévi-Strauss, Claude
  1969   The Raw and the Cooked. New York: Harper and Row.
Lewis, Sir Aubrey
  1958   Social Psychiatry. In Lectures on the Scientific Basis of Medicine, London: Athlone
          Press, pp. 116–142.
Lindenbaum, Shirley
  1979   Kuru Sorcery: Disease and Danger in the New Guinea Highlands. Palo Alto: Mayfield.

Lindholm, Charles and Cherry Lindholm
    1981   World's Strangest Mental Illnesses. Science Digest 89(6): 52–57.
Linton, Ralph
    1956   Culture and Mental Disorders. Springfield: Thomas.
McDonald, John Kennedy
    1907   The Norway House Murders – A Plea for Mercy. Letter to the Editor of the Mani-
            toba Free Press dated Nov. 21. Clipping found in the John Maclean Papers, Box 50,
            File 22, United Church of Canada Archives, Victoria University in the University
            of Toronto, M5S 2C4 Canada.
McGee, Harrold Franklin, Jr.
    1972   *Windigo* Psychosis. American Anthropologist 74: 244–246.
    1975   The *Windigo* Down-East, or The Taming of the *Windigo*. Proceedings of the Second
            Congress, Canadian Ethnology Society, Vol. 1. Jim Freedom and Jerome H. Barkow
            (eds.), National Museum of Man, Mercury Series, Canadian Ethnology Service Paper
            28, pp. 110–132.
McGlashan, C. F.
    1947   Second edition. History of the Donner Party: A Tragedy of the Sierra. Stanford:
  (1880) Stanford University Press.
Mair, Lucy
    1969   Witchcraft. London: World University Library.
Malinowski, Bronislaw
    1960   A Scientific Theory of Culture and Other Essays. New York: Galaxy Book.
  (1944)
Mamdani, Mahmood
    1973   The Myth of Population Control: Family, Caste, and Class in an Indian Village.
            New York: Monthly Review Press.
Mandelbaum, David G.
    1940   The Plains Cree. Anthropological Papers of the American Museum of Natural
            History 37: 155–316.
Manitoba Court of Queen's Bench
    1899   The Queen vs Toosh-e-naum and Ah-ne-o-kizhick. MS, No. 14, Fall Assize.
Marano, Louis A.
    n.d.   Boreal Forest Hazards and Adaptations: The Present. *In* A. T. Steegmann, Jr. (ed.),
            Boreal Forest Adaptations: The Algonkians of Northern Ontario. New York:
            Plenum.
Marx, Karl and Frederick Engels
    1977   The German Ideology. Pt. 1. New York: Interational Publishers.
  (1846)
Masson, Louis F. R.
    1960   Les bourgeois de la compagnie du Nord-Ouest: Récits de voyages, lettres, et
  (1889– rapports inédits relatifs au Nord-Ouest canadien. New York: Antiquarian Press.
  90)
Nag, Moni, Benjamin N. F. White and R. Creighton Peet
    1978   An Anthropological Approach to the Study of Economic Value of Children in
            Java and Nepal. Current Anthropology 19: 293–306.
Naroll, Raoul and Frada Naroll
    1963   On Bias of Exotic Data. Man 25: 24–26.
Nelson, George
    1823   Letter journal, Lac la Rouge, English River district. MS, Metropolitan Toronto
            Public Library, Toronto.
Paredes, J. Anthony
    1972   A Case Study of a "Normal" *Windigo*. Anthropologica 14: 97–116.

Parker, Seymour
    1960   The *Wiitiko* Psychosis in the Context of Ojibwa Personality and Culture. American
            Anthropologist 62: 603–623.
Preston, Richard J.
    1975   Cree Narrative: Expressing the Personal Meanings of Events. National Museum
            of Man, Mercury Series, Canadian Ethnology Service Paper 30.
    1980   The *Witiko*: Algonkian Knowledge and Whiteman Knowledge. *In* Marjorie M.
            Halpin and Michael M. Ames (eds.), Manlike Monsters on Trial: Early Records
            and Modern Evidence. Vancouver: University of British Columbia Press, pp. 111–
            131.
Public Archives of Canada
    1879   The Queen vs Ka-ki-si-kutchun, "The Swift Runner". MS, Department of Justice
            File CRG 13, C-1, Vol. 1417.
    1899   RCMP Investigation and Arrest File, Moostoos Case. MS, File RG 18, Vol. 1442,
            No. 166.
    1907–   Department of Justice Capital Case File on Joseph Fiddler. MS, File RG 13, C-1,
    1908   Vol. 1452.
    1907–   RCMP Investigation into the Homicide by Jack and Joseph Fiddler. MS, File
    1909   RG 18, Vol. 3229, HQ-781-G-1.
Rand, Silas T.
    1971   Legends of the Micmacs. New York: Johnson Reprint (Longmans, Green).
    (1894)
Ray, Arthur J.
    1974   Indians in the Fur Trade. Toronto and Buffalo: University of Toronto Press.
Ray, Carl and James Stevens
    1971   Sacred Legends of the Sandy Lake Cree. Toronto: McClelland and Stewart.
Ridington, Robin
    1976   *Wechuge* and *Windigo*: A Comparison of Cannibal Belief among Boreal Forest
            Athapaskans and Algonkians. Anthropologica 18: 107–129.
Rogers, Edward S.
    1962   The Round Lake Ojibwa. Art and Archaeology Division, Royal Ontario Museum,
            Occasional Paper 5.
    1966   Subsistence Areas of the Cree-Ojibwa of the Eastern Subarctic: A Preliminary
            Study. *In* Contributions to Anthropology 1963–64, pt. 2, pp. 59–90. National
            Museum of Canada Bulletin 204.
    n.d.   Cultural Adaptations: The Northern Ojibwa of the Boreal Forest 1670–1980. *In*
            A. T. Steegmann, Jr. (ed.), Boreal Forest Adaptations: The Algonkians of Northern
            Ontario. New York: Plenum.
Rogers, Edward S. and Mary B. Black
    1976   Subsistence Strategy in the Fish and Hare Period, Northern Ontario: The Weaga-
            mow Ojibwa, 1890–1920. Journal of Anthropological Research 32: 1–43.
Rohrl, Vivian J.
    1970   A Nutritional Factor in *Windigo* Psychosis. American Anthropologist 72: 97–
            101.
    1972   Comment on 'The Cure and Feeding of *Windigos*: A Critique'. American An-
            thropologist 74: 242–244.
Saindon, J. Emile
    1928   En missionnant: essai sur les missions des Pères Oblats de Marie Immaculée à la
            Baie James. Ottawa: Imprimerie du Droit.
    1933   Mental Disorders among the James Bay Cree. Primitive Man (now Anthropological
            Quarterly) 6: 1–12.

Skinner, Alanson Buck
    1914   Political Organization, Cults, and Ceremonies of the Plains-Ojibwa and Plains-Cree
            Indians. Anthropological Papers of the American Museum of Natural History
            11: 475–542.
Smith, James G. E.
    1976   Notes on the *Wittiko*. *In* William Cowan (ed.), Papers of the Seventh Algonquian
            Conference, 1975. Ottawa: Carleton University, pp. 18–28.
    1979   Leadership among the Indians of the Northern Woodlands. *In* Robert Hinshaw
            (ed.), Currents in Anthropology: Essays in Honor of Sol Tax. The Hague: Mouton,
            pp. 305–324.
Speck, Frank G.
    1935   Naskapi. Norman: University of Oklahoma Press.
Spier, Leslie
    1935   The Prophet Dance of the Northwest and Its Derivatives: The Source of the Ghost
            Dance. American Anthropologist General Series in Anthropology 1.
Stewart, George R.
    1960   Ordeal by Hunger: The Story of the Donner Party. New edition. Cambridge:
    (1936) Riverside Press.
Teicher, Morton I.
    1960   *Windigo* Psychosis: A Study of a Relationship between Belief and Behavior among
            the Indians of Northeastern Canada. Seattle: University of Washington Press.
Tucker, Sarah
    1958   The Rainbow in the North: A Short Account of the First Establishment of Christi-
            anity in Rupert's Land by the Church Missionary Society. London: James Nisbet.
Turnbull Colin
    1972   The Mountain People. New York: Simon and Schuster.
    1978   Rethinking the Ik: A Functional Non-social System. *In* Charles D. Laughlin, Jr.
            and Ivan A. Brady (eds.), Extinction and Survival in Human Populations. New
            York: Columbia University Press, pp. 49–75.
Turner, David H.
    1977   *Windigo* Mythology and the Analysis of Cree Social Structure. Anthropologica
            19: 63–73.
Turner, David H.
    1978   Hunting and Gathering: Cree and Australian. *In* David H. Turner and Gavin A. Smith
            (eds.), Challenging Anthropology. Toronto: McGraw-Hill Ryerson, pp. 195–213.
Turner, David H. and Paul Wertman
    1977   Shamattawa: The Structure of Social Relations in a Northern Algonkian Band.
            Ottawa: National Museum of Man, Mercury Series.
Waisberg, Leo G.
    1975   Boreal Forest Sussistence and the *Windigo*: Fluctuation of Animal Populations.
            Anthropologica 17: 169–185.
Wallace, Anthony F. C.
    1961   Culture and Personality. New York: Random House.
West, John
    1966   The Substance of a Journal during a Residence at the Red River Colony. New
    (1824) York: Johnson Reprint (London: L. B. Seeley).
White, Benjamin
    1973   Demand for Labor and Population Growth in Colonial Java. Human Ecology 1:
            217–236.
    1975   The Economic Importance of Children in a Javanese Village. *In* Moni Nag (ed.),
            Population and Social Organization. The Hague: Mouton, pp. 127–146.

Wing, J. K.
    1978   Reasoning about Madness. Oxford: Oxford University Press.
Yap, Pow Meng
    1951   Mental Diseases Peculiar to Certain Cultures: A Survey of Comparative Psychiatry.
            Journal of Mental Science (now British Journal of Psychiatry) 97: 313–327.
    1969   The Culture-Bound Reactive Syndromes. *In* William Caudill and Tsung-yi Lin (eds),
            Mental Health Research in Asia and the Pacific. Honolulu: East-West Center Press,
            pp. 33–53.
Young, Egerton Ryerson
    1871   Letter dated Rossville, Norway House, July 29, 1871. Personal Scrapbook.
Young, T. Kue-hing
    n.d.   Indian Health Care in Northwestern Ontario: Health Status, Medical Care, and
            Social Policy. Unpublished Master's Thesis, Department of Community Health,
            University of Toronto, Toronto, Ont.

COMMENTARIES AND REPLIES

Commentaries

A. H. B. M. MURPHY

The main questions to which this paper addresses itself are (a) What were the behaviors to which the term *"windigo* psychosis" now applies? (b) Were these behaviors exhibited or merely attributed? (c) Did they merit the label "psychosis"? and (d) Does *"windigo* psychosis" deserve to be treated as a distinct entity? I leave the first two of these questions to persons with field experience with northern Amerindians, which I lack, and address myself to the second two, on which I have more competence.

In medical anthropology and transcultural psychiatry, as in so many research areas in which disciplines overlap, one of the persisting problems is the way in which terms deriving from the one discipline are understood by researchers in the other. Even within a single discipline terms can be used idiosyncratically, but the risk of honest misunderstanding is greater when two or more apply to the same problem. Marano states that because Saindon's patient responded promptly to the assurance that she would get well, this was "not behavior characteristic of a psychosis", since "if psychoses were that easy to cure, our mental hospitals would be empty". This is a misunderstanding of the term psychosis in its present-day and certainly in its transcultural use. Although some psychoses are chronic, many of them, particularly in developing societies, can exhibit quite rapid improvement, and even chronic schizophrenics can show marked but temporary remission (and we do not know how long the remission in Saindon's patient lasted) when given strong reassurance and encouragement. Moreover, there is not nearly as clear a distinction between psychosis and neurosis as the nonpsychiatrist assumes and as some psychiatric authorities would have us believe. Psychosis implies the greater degree of interference with adaptive functioning and is the less easy to understand, but the idea of there being a sharp distinction is false. Insofar as the expression of a desire to eat human flesh, except under conditions of extreme starvation, is likely to incur adverse social sanction, it must be considered as maladaptive, and a diagnosis of psychosis would certainly need to be considered when this was reported, as in cases cited by Teicher on pp. 46, 49, and 54 of his monograph. That many of the alleged cases of *windigo* psychosis could be given another psychiatric label — involutional depression, for instance — does not preclude our applying that special term to those which exhibit certain characteristics.

To merit such a distinctive label, the cases to which it is applied need to exhibit one or more of a set of distinctive characteristics which may be behavioral, such as eating human flesh, but can also be ideational such as feeling a strong temptation

449

Ronald C. Simons and Charles C. Hughes (eds.), The Culture-Bound Syndromes, 449–462.
© 1983 *by The University of Chicago Press.*

to eat such flesh. If a mother states she has an urge to kill her newborn infant, which is not so uncommon, one does not wait until she kills it before calling her psychotic even though one would also not diagnose psychosis on that statement alone. For a psychiatrist, what appears distinctive about most of the case Teicher and Marano cite (other than those of anthropophagy under starvation conditions) is that eating human flesh is thought about, whereas such ideas are almost never expressed by the insane, regardless of how disturbed, in other societies. That the reason may be situational is beside the point.

Marano's paper is welcome in that it reminds us of the fragility of the evidence on which the etic label of *windigo* psychosis has been based, and his challenging of the label is legitimate. I am less happy about his introductory reference to "witch hunts" as an alternative explanation, and I feel that he needs to read more about witches and witch hunts in general. However, that is an aspect I leave to my anthropologist colleagues to comment on.

B. HAZEL H. WEIDMAN

Marano is to be congratulated for his critical review of the *windigo* literature. His contribution is an important and corrective one which raises a whole new set of theoretical issues.

After following his argument through to its conclusion, it is easy to see how different Marano's etic posture is from that of some of the earlier writers on the subject. It is also easy to see how assumptions from a different etic tradition, which emphasizes relationships between culture, personality, and psychopathology, could lead to the ready acceptance of the reality of a "*windigo* psychosis". There is a large body of anthropological and psychiatric literature which, given the cultural beliefs about "*windigo*", would support the likelihood of the existence of some type of *windigo*-related psychiatric syndrome. Whether such a syndrome would have the characteristics of an orthodox medical "psychosis" is another matter, and it is precisely these symptomatological details which are missing from the emic data.

Marano has not only shifted from a culture-and-personality tradition of inquiry (which includes psychiatric anthropology and cultural psychiatry) to that of cultural materialism; he has also shifted the focus of attention from "*windigo*"/victim to "murderer"/survivor. He has not, however, avoided emic-etic confusion in his own work.

The emic-etic confusion is most apparent in Marano's treatment of a tale about a 15-year-old "lunatic" boy who was strangled and cremated by his family. Marano accepts the probability that this person was mentally ill but rejects the possibility that his illness might have been, etically, a "psychosis". Furthermore, he fails to consider the possibility that the boy's behavior may have been consonant with *windigo* imagery and beliefs and, therefore, in emic terms, the functional equivalent of an etic "psychosis". In addition, he fails to question whether, from an emic perspective, the family's behavior might have been appropriate for dealing with dysfunction explained by *windigo* imagery and beliefs. Instead, Marano holds to an etic interpretation that there was no "psychosis"; there was only "mental illness". He also implies that early observers were correct in never doubting what seemed to be an "obvious" fact, that "the *windigo* belief complex was an ideological and superstructural rationalization for homicide", which Marano further assumes to be required for group survival because of cultural, ecological, and economic circumstances of the period involved.

Marano builds a good case for understanding the latent functions of "*windigo*"/homicides for goup survival; however, he appears to project his etic analysis of latent functions into the conscious awareness and motivational system of the Northern Algonkians themselves. This is a rationalistic approach, indeed, which disregards the affective and psychodynamic parameters of incidents such as those reported in this article. Marano underscores very well one type of etic projection onto emic data in his tracing of the origins of the "*windigo* psychosis". He is unaware of the same process in his own work, and we are now confronted with another type of etic projection onto emic data: the transformation of "self-defensive behavior because of mental illness in another" into "deliberate homicide based upon economic need and matters of group survival".

One point Marano seems to overlook is that under severe ecological, acculturative, intragroup, and interpersonal stress, similar culturally patterned ego-defensive psychological processes would be expected to be utilized by anyone involved in a crisis situation leading to a "*windigo*" incident. If only two parties are involved in a situation of starvation, for example, and both are adults, each will be inclined to perceive the other as becoming "*windigo*", and each will be building to a final "protective" action which may lead to the murder of the other. One is destroyed; the other survives to tell the tale of being attacked by someone whose behavior was becoming more and more "*windigo*"-like. From a psychologically oriented etic perspective that does not disregard emic views, one might argue plausibly as follows: (a) Through processes of repression, denial, and projection, the "murderer" was the more psychologically impaired of the two, perceiving "*windigo*"-like behavior in the other but in fact *being* more "*windigo*"-like than the other, or (b) the "murderer" simply used the culturally patterned ego-defense mechanisms more efficiently than the "victim". Efficient use in this instance would imply the process of disowning one's own unacceptable impulses, identifying them in the other individual, acting to destroy that identified source of distress, and, possibly, becoming better integrated psychologically as a consequence of that action. These types of issues are unaddressed by Marano because of his materialistic orientation and focus upon "murderer"/survivor in contrast to "*windigo*"/victim. Nevertheless, he has argued for the acknowledgment of similarities between "*windigo*" phenomena and "witchcraft" phenomena, and such issues, inevitably, arise if this is achieved.

It appears that we might now expect a flurry of activity in response to the challenge of Marano's work. It is inadequate as it stands, but an acceptable theoretical formulation will need to integrate aspects of his approach along with more psychologically centered ones.

C. ROBERT A. BRIGHTMAN

Marano's survey of the *windigo* literature will have the positive effect of prompting reflection on the credibility of both recorded cases and existing interpretations. However, in the light of material contained in the better-documented cases, his arguments seem unduly categorical, and the summary explanation of *windigo* as an "ideological rationalization" for homicide overlooks evident variation in socio-ecological context and resolution.

Marano suggests that *windigo* psychotics never existed, raising thereby the question of what behaviors we should take as diagnostic of a psychosis. If we take as symptomatic of this disorder the expressed desire to eat human flesh, together with behavior directed towards this objective, Marano is in the position of having to dismiss the many cases in which these elements figure. Granted that non*windigos* were sometimes executed, it is difficult to suppose that the threats and attacks noted in so many accounts were *all* hallucinations or fabrications of the survivors. For example, in Young's case (Brown 1971), Marano finds it implausible that the afflicted youth failed to bite his father and so rejects the testimony. Unsuccessful attempts at biting are mentioned elsewhere (Teicher 1960: 93); anorexia might explain the victims' weakness, and in neither case does this criterion seriously discredit the evidence.

Since Algonquians did not become *windigo* cannibals, all cases of cannibalism are explained by famine, and it becomes necessary to disallow Smith's (1976: 22) case in which murder and cannibalism took place amidst abundant game. Marano redefines the case as famine cannibalism, reversing in the process the identities of aggressor and victim. It would, of course, be possible to reinterpret all of the cases so as to conform to Marano's premise. However, the cumulative evidence suggests a distinctively Algonquian mental disorder: Algonquians defined *themselves* as incipient windigos when food was available (Teicher 1960: 45—46, 49, 81, 93), and this suggests the occurrence of murder and cannibalism without famine as in the Smith and second Anderson cases. The causal relationship, both emic and etic in Harris's idiom, between famine and *windigo* cannibalism is well known. However, as in the Wiskahoo case, *windigo* psychosis could develop without precedent famine cannibalism; the latter is a culturally important but not necessary precondition.

Turning from *windigo* to their executioners, Marano understands the complex to have "evolved" as a precipitate of its latent functions: belief rationalizes homicide, but the homicides are unmotivated by fear of cannibal monsters. This entails at least one contradiction, since the elimination of practiced cannibals, who might become "repeaters" in case of famine, is specified as one function of the complex. It is, however, clear that execution did not follow automatically *either* from famine *or* from *windigo* cannibalism. Wiskahoo was subject to transitory psychotic episodes for three years; his relatives would tie him up at such times, and he was executed only when his moods became chronic. The Oak Bay *windigo* observed by Henry was an admitted famine cannibal, but he was executed only after his remarks about the plumpness of the children suggested that the condition was chronic. In some cases (Thompson 1916: 104; Isham 1949: 100–101), famine cannibals were neither killed nor apparently ostracized. It appears probable that neither famine cannibals nor potential *windigo* cannibals were precipitously executed without evidence that they posed a continuing threat to the band and that self-identification as *windigo* was often the critical element.

Among other functions, Marano notes the elimination of mentally or physically dysfunctional persons and the projection onto these of anxieties related to social and ecological change. These are important and neglected components of the complex, but it is unclear whether the Algonquians are understood as unconscious of their ecological scapegoating or as self-conscious prevaricators, activating folklore to rationalize acts of murder. The argument, despite superficial resemblance, shows none of the primitivism of Arens's (1979) essay on cannibalism and anthropology. On the contrary, in defining the complex as a rationalization for killing the dangerous or dysfunctional, Marano's portrait is hardly more flattering than the most colorful existing accounts of the psychosis. Rather underemphasized are the "emic" emphasis on *curing* rather than summarily executing potential *windigo* and also the very real fears provoked by such individuals. It takes a skeptical reading of the depositions in the Moostoos case to suppose that the participants were not gravely frightened throughout the whole tragic process of attempted cure and execution.

Thompson's (1916: 261) report, "I have known a few instances of this deplorable turn of mind, and not one instance could plead hunger, much less famine as an excuse of it", confirms the native "emics": Algonquians became mentally ill and reacted to the mentally ill within the context of distinctively Algonquian premises. These premises were reactive with, but not derivative of, famine cannibalism and ecological expedience.

Replies

A. TO H. B. M. MURPHY

Murphy declines to address the issue of the behavioral *windigo*, proceeding directly to the questions of whether this possibly nonexistent syndrome merits the designation "psychosis" and whether "*windigo* psychosis" deserves to be treated as a distinct entity. I fail to see how this line of inquiry can logically be justified without granting at least hypothetical existence to certain exhibited (not merely attributed) behaviors. But what are these behaviors? Are they "the expression of a desire to eat human flesh"? or "eating human flesh"? or the ideational "feeling a strong temptation to eat such flesh"? What Murphy finds most distinctive about the *windigo* literature is that "eating human flesh is thought about". I have gone to some effort to demonstrate that the evidence for *windigo* cannibalistic behavior is inadequate. If, as I maintain, evidence for cannibalism on the part of alleged "*windigo* victims" is insufficient, how much confidence may we place in reports of their cannibalistic thoughts? I can well believe Murphy's statement that cannibalistic ideas "are almost never expressed by the insane, regardless of how disturbed, in other societies". This reinforces my skepticism about their alleged expression by Northern Algonkians.

If Murphy's comments on the definition of "psychosis" are correct, they serve to strengthen my belief that this poorly operationalized term should never again be applied to a category of people — especially in a culture-bound context — without rigorous behavioral and empirical justification. Certainly we should *never* apply the label "psychotic" to a group of executed persons on the basis of information provided by their executioners.

B. TO HAZEL H. WEIDMAN

I see Weidman's comments as generally supportive, but she attributes to me a position I do not and could not hold. She believes that there is an emic-etic confusion in my own work and illustrates this belief by reference to E. R. Young's 15-year-old "lunatic" boy. She claims that I reject "the possibility that his illness might have been, etically, a 'psychosis' ", that I hold "to an etic interpretation that there was no 'psychosis'; there was only 'mental illness' ". This is entirely incorrect. However "psychosis" may be defined etically (and this appears to be an ongoing process), I believe it to be quite possible that the boy was psychotic. My use of the term "mental illness" was not to deny the possibility of psychosis, but because I lack the evidence (and the training) necessary to make such a diagnosis, especially since the person in question died over a hundred years ago.

Weidman states that I project my "etic analysis of latent functions into the conscious awareness and motivational system of the Northen Algonkians themselves". A more precise phrasing is that I engage in some etic analysis of both conscious and unconscious Northern Algonkian motivational dynamics. I make these etic/mental formulations reluctantly and minimally, because I have no other alternative. It is not true, however, that I have done so by "disregard[ing] the affective and psychodynamic parameters" of the *windigo* incidents as they can be reconstructed from the data still available to us. I have tried to heed Harris's (1979: 40) warning that "anthropologists should use the etic approach to mental life sparingly", and when I have been forced to do so it has been with a full appreciation of the affective and psycho-dynamic parameters of an emic/mental universe in which I participated for five years. (Most of my analysis is, of course, etic/behavioral.) And it seems, too, that Weidman criticizes me for dabbling in the etics of Northern Algonkian mental life and then chides me for leaving more issues of this type "unaddressed". Her own etic/mental formulations are provocative and welcome.

C. TO ROBERT A. BRIGHTMAN

Brightman's comments are predicated on what I believe to be misplaced confidence in what he terms "the better-documented cases". He holds that "the cumulative evidence suggests a distinctively Algonquian mental disorder". What is the nature of the evidence he marshalls in support of this belief?

Brightman refers to the Smith (1976) and second Anderson (Teicher 1960: 49) cases as evidence for "the occurrence of murder and cannibalism without famine". Unless I misread Smith's (Current Authropology 23: 404) most recent thoughts on the case, he is no longer convinced that the archival account he discovered (Hudson's Bay Company 1741) warrants this interpretation. The factual reliability of the Anderson letters is open to question. Anderson was not a witness to the events about which he corresponded and clearly relied on information supplied by others. Anderson writes, "they were not destitute of food as he [the alleged cannibal] had just returned from fishing and brought a good supply". In a similar pronouncement on the Swift Runner case, Teicher (pp. 85–86), following J. P. Turner (1950: 499–501), reproduces a completely fanciful version of the events. Among the errors is the statement (Teicher 1960: 86): "What made his act even more barbarous was the fact that while he was indulging in his ghastly orgy he had plenty of dried meat hanging around the camp".

Turner's popularization notwithstanding, the Swift Runner case was well investigated and well documented by the Northwest Mounted Police. A 58-page Department of Justice file exists in the Public Archives of Canada (1879). While there is some question about whether Swift Runner could have reached help, there is no question about the fact that the family was starving and that the eldest boy had died of hunger before the killing began. The case is cited to illustrate the fact that reports of noncrisis (or "windigo") cannibalism must be reviewed very critically and that there is no evidentiary basis for Brightman's statement that "the causal relationship . . . between famine and windigo cannibalism is well known".

Brightman admits that "the Oak Bay windigo observed by Henry was a . . . famine cannibal" but two centuries after the fact displays more certainty as to the existence of a derivative cannibalistic obsession than Henry showed at the time. Overlooked are Henry's reflective qualifications (Bain 1901: 200): "It is probable that we saw things in some measure through the medium of our prejudices. . . ." Referring to the young man's observations on the "fatness" of the children in the camp in which he sought refuge, Henry wrote (pp. 200–201):

It was perhaps not unnatural that after long acquaintance with no human form but such as was gaunt and pale from want of food, a man's eyes should be almost riveted upon anything where misery had not made such inroads, and still more upon the bloom and plumpness of childhood; and the exclamation might be the most innocent, and might proceed from an involuntary and unconquerable sentiment of admiration.

I agree with Brightman that cannibals were not always "precipitously executed without evidence that they posed a continuing threat to the band". More research is needed to determine the circumstances under which cannibals were likely to be executed and those under which they were likely to remain unmolested (though perhaps suffering some degree of ostracism). There is, however, more than one way to pose "a continuing threat to the band", and I think Brightman overstates the importance of "self-identification as *windigo*" as the critical element determining execution.

If the data are correct in the Wiskahoo case, Wiskahoo (who ate no one) apparently suffered from a psychological dysfunction conditioned by Northern Algonkian culture, including the *windigo* belief complex. I note the possibility of such cases at the outset of my paper (Current Anthropology 23: 385). Thompson (1916: 125) states that "Wiskahoo was naturally a cheerful, good natured, careless man, but hard times had changed him. He was a good Beaver worker and trapper, but an indifferent Moose Hunter, now and then killed one by chance, he had been twice so reduced by hunger, as to be twice on the point of eating one of his children to save the others, when he was fortunately found and relieved by the other Natives". After these experiences he deaded being alone and when under the influence of alcohol grew sad and thoughtful, saying "Nee weet to go" (I [am] *windigo*). My reading of the evidence suggests that Wiskahoo suffered from an entirely justified fear, that his inadequacy as a hunter could again result in starvation for his family, with all of its terrible implications. His depression, then, had a rational foundation and was grounded in inter-subjectively verifiable reality. I therefore question Brightman's diagnosis that "Wiskahoo was subject to transitory psychotic episodes for three years".

In reference to the Moostoos case, Brightman suggests that I "suppose that the participants were not gravely frightened throughout the whole tragic process" and gives it as my position that the homicides of alleged *windigo* victims were "unmotivated by fear of cannibal monsters". This is a serious misreading of my work. what would be the sense of positing a functional-materialist explanation for the evolution of a belief if no one could reasonably be expected to be affected by, or act upon, that belief?

Brightman states that my analysis leaves it unclear "whether the Algonkians are understood as unconscious of their ... scapegoating or as self-conscious prevaricators, activating folklore to rationalize acts of murder". In my reply to Weidman (Current Anthropology 23: 409) I try to show the perils inherent in this kind of etic/mental speculation. How many of us are sufficiently aware of our own motivations, or those of our relatives, friends, and associates? We can write with correspondingly less confidence about the consciousness and motivations of people from another culture who long ago lived through crises alien to our experience.

I *am* reasonably certain that the psychic dynamics of *windigo* slayers were not uniform. Ethnohistorical case materials suggest wide variation, with two apparent patterns emerging from the data. The Moostoos (Louison) and Mapanin (Francis Auger) cases both occurred in northern Alberta within 200 miles and three years of each other (Annual Archaeological Report 1903 [1904]; Edmonton Court Files 1899; PAC 1899, 1896). There seems to be little doubt that the individuals involved in these cases experienced stark terror, and executions of the accused "windigos" were grisly. In five northwestern Ontario cases, however,

ranging from ca. 1880 to 1906, there is no indication of fear of the "windigos"'
who appear to have been put to death as quickly and painlessly as possible (AAR
1906 [1907]; PAC 1907–8, 1907–9; Manitoba Court of Queen's Bench 1899).
In the best-documented of these cases, the Wasakapeequay (Mrs. Thomas Fiddler)
execution, concern over cannibal possession seems to have been secondary if not
tertiary in the motivations of the executioners. There is no dispute about the
fact that Mrs. Fiddler showed not the slightest inclination to kill or eat anyone.
Evidence gathered in 1907 shows only that the woman was very sick; she was
delirious, weak, incoherent, and not expected to recover (AAR 1907 [1908]:
103). Witness Angus Rae testified at the trial in October 1907 that Mrs. Fiddler
was strangled to "put her out of her misery" (p. 104). It is hard to say exactly
what the people camped at Sandy Lake believed about possession by cannibal
monsters in September of 1906, but by their own best accounts they were not
afraid of Mrs. Fiddler, and euthanasia was the primary motive for her execution.
From the testimony of Angus Rae (p. 109):

Q. Did you ever hear the chief give any reason for having people put to death who were sick?
A. When they are sick and so long in misery they put them out of their misery.
Q. Did you hear the chief say that? A. Yes.
Q. What chief? A. Jack.
Q. Give the exact words.
A. Jack said when anyone was sick like that and is so miserable they might as well put them
to an end.

Angus Rae's testimony suggests that the issue of cannibal possession may have
first been raised *after* Mrs. Fiddler's execution (pp. 106–7, emphasis added).

Q. Do you know why the woman was put to death?
A. My wife told me that the people were saying that the woman was going to turn into a
cannibal. The people in the wigwam were saying this.
Q. Was it before or after the death that your wife told you this?
A. *Two days after the death.*

By the time Hallowell did his fieldwork, about thirty years later, the process
had moved inexorably along. No contemporaneous report indicated that Mrs.
Fiddler had uttered a single intelligible word during her illness, but Hallowell
"was told by his informants that Wasakapeequay could not eat and that she
vomited everything. He was also told that she begged to be killed since she was
firmly convinced that she was turning into a cannibal" (Tiecher 1960: 74, based
on Hallowell's unpublished field notes).

In my paper (Current Anthropology 23: 391) I found it implausible that the
allegedly crazed and raving 15-year-old boy reported by Young (Brown 1971:
21) tried and failed to bite his father. Brightman believes my skepticism to be
unjustified and cites the Moostoos case (Tiecher 1960: 93) in support of his position. It is true that Moostoos's executioners said he had tried unsuccessfully to
bite (AAR 1903 [1904]: 127, 129, 136) and that this was one of the reasons

they had to sink an axe into his head. They also said, however, that Moostoos "floated up right off the ground, and . . . it was hard to reach up to seize him" (p. 130).[1]

Brightman believes that I underemphasize attempts to "cure" rather than execute potential *windigos* and again cites the Moostoos case as an example. The Annual Archaeological Report 1903 (1904) makes reference to attempts to cure Moostoos shamanistically (pp. 131, 133–135, 137–38). The thrust of these passages is that although several of the men were thought to possess some measure of personal "medicine", Entominahoo the "headman" was the group's acknowledged shaman. As principal secular and religious leader, Entominahoo certainly must have played a major role in identifying Moostoos as one possessed by a cannibal demon and in leading the group toward the consensus culminating in Moostoos's execution. He also was the major actor in shamanistic attempts to "cure" Moostoos.

A full analysis of this case will be presented elsewhere, but it seems appropriate to examine the role of Entominahoo here. It appears unlikely to me that Moostoos would have been killed had not Entominahoo either pronounced or confirmed the condition of cannibal possession. Entominahoo's wife testified (AAR 1903 [1904]; 134): "It is only my own husband that knows anything about Wehtigoos". According to Entominahoo's testimony (p. 133, emphasis added), Moostoos said: " 'If you don't hold me down, I'll kill you all'. He [Moostoos] said that twice. *It was only I that heard him say that before they got hold of him.* He and I were alone in the morning. I then tried to cure him with the medicine. It was late at night that we commenced to hold him down. Nothing was wrong with him in the daytime lying asleep."

But in the margin of page 12 of the Edmonton Court Files (1899), the justice of the peace notes that Entominahoo is "deaf". It is curious that Moostoos's initial threats of murder (and cannibalism?) were first heard only by a man with a noticeable hearing impairment. Harris has written (1975: 527) that "shamans are usually personalities who are predisposed toward hallucinatory experiences". This was certainly true, at least episodically, of the Northern Algonkian shaman I knew best. Entominahoo also stated. "Then in the evening we saw he was thinking something wrong about us" (ECF 1899: 7; AAR 1903 [1904]; 128). How could Entominahoo "see" what Moostoos was thinking? The camp had been hit by a deadly epidemic, and Moostoos was only one of its victims (ASR 1903 [1904]: 131–33). His struggles, ravings, and teeth-grindings are consistent with delirium caused by high fever. It is possible that the specific manifestations of his delirium were culturally conditioned by the *windigo* belief complex. I find it intriguing, however, that Moostoos, who was an Athapascan Beaver Indian, was killed by a group of Algonkian Crees on the grounds that he had become possessed by a spirit-monster that existed in their cosmology, not his.[2]

The issue of collective suggestibility with regard to the *windigo* phenomenon was first raised in print in 1860 by Khol (pp. 357–58) and is cited extensively by Fogelson (1965: 79–81). Kohl (p. 357) found it to be "very natural that in a country which really produces isolated instances of such rumors [famine cannibalism], and with a nation so devoted to fancies and dreams, superstitions should be mixed up in the matter, and that at last, through this superstition, wonderful stories of windigos should be produced, as among us, in the middle ages, the belief in witches produced witches". Kohl (p. 358) also believed that "this fear and the general opinion have so worked upon some minds, that they believe themselves to be really windigos, and must act in that way". This last is a position I question with respect to cannibalistic behavior, but Kohl's perspicacious observation that the windigo phenomenon is characterized by "a certain epidemic tendency, and a spontaneous self-production and propagation" puts him far ahead of his time.

I agree with Brightman that despite superficial resemblance my analysis is dissimilar to Arens's (1979) monograph on cannibalism and anthropology, but I question the purport of Brightman's statement that my "portrait is hardly more flattering than the most colorful existing accounts of the psychosis". I do not seek to "flatter", but to understand. My thesis is that the Northern Algonkian peoples are not culturally or psychologically aberrant, but respond to stress in much the same way as do ethnographically similar populations.

Meyer's supportive comments are appreciated, but some clarifications are necessary.[3] Meyer states that since "etic information on actual *wihtiko* 'events' is sparse, it is apparent that anthropologists should concentrate on emics — what Northern Algonkians believe — in this regard". In response I must reaffirm the importance of etics in general and in *windigo* studies in particular. Incomplete as they are, ethnohistorical case materials are crucial to our understanding of the *windigo* phenomenon. The pronouncements of fieldworkers and data analysts must be distinguished in a systematic way from those of informants.

A current example of this necessity is an article that appeared after my paper went to press. In '*Witiko* Accounts from the James Bay Cree'. Flannery, Chambers, and Jehle (1981) present narratives collected between 1932 and 1938 by John M. Cooper and Regina Flannery and provide commentary on these narratives. This paper is limited by the same emic-etic confusion that flawed so many of its precursors. Second- and thirdhand informant accounts of compulsive cannibalism are received uncritically, and the existence of "*windigo* psychosis" is accepted as a given.

Nevertheless, Flannery, Chambers, and Jehle provide us with welcome source material and valuable insights. Among the latter is the realization that "the hazards of bush life in the winter require flexibility on the part of the subsistence unit and the consequences of errors in judgment can be severe" (p. 59). "Nearly every older informant [in the 1930s] recalled that a relative had starved to death" (p. 70). According to the theory put forth in my paper (Current Anthropology 23: 285, 388, 391, 397), individuals who reduce the flexibility of the group are likely candidates for windigo accusations and executions.

The authors divide the narratives into three categories: "tales of primeval times when animals spoke and behaved like men, ... stories of 'long ago' in which the exact locale or persons involved are unclear", and "true stories' of [informant's] own experience or those of relatives" (p. 57). Only three of the twelve "historical witiko incidents" (pp. 70–77), however, purport to be accounts of informants' own experiences. Of these one was 'a hoax" in which a "family from the Albany area ... conspired to drive the Moose Factory Indians from their hunting and trapping lands by creating a false Witiko alarm" (p. 75). Another was "a clear case of starvation cannibalism" in which "there is no evidence of [the woman's] having later developed a craving for human flesh" (p. 74). The third case was related by a woman who as a child lived for a time in the same domestic unit as her mother's uncle, a man said to be "crazy for human flesh" (p. 72). In a 70-year retrospection, however, Flannery's informant could not say how dangerous the man actually was. He was physically abusive to his four-year-old daughter when the child had a tantrum, but such behavior is not peculiar to Northern Algonkian Indians, as any police officer, social worker, or psychotherapist can attest. There is no indication that the informant ever heard the man express a desire to consume human flesh, and, of course, there is no indication that she witnessed any move to satisfy this attributed desire. The man probably did suffer from a psychological disturbance, but his wife is reported to have said: "I am never afraid of him. It is only when he is sick [that] I don't like it" (p. 72).

In spite of the recognition that "[starvation] cannibalism did not lead inevitably to mental disturbance or aberrant behavior" (p. 70) and the acknowledgment of "folkloristic elements" (p. 71) in the accounts, such as *windigo* victims with ice in their chests and those who could not be killed by gunfire (cf. pp. 72, 75), the authors consider their twelve "historical witiko incidents" to be essentially true stories that "recount actual events which occurred in the latter half of the nineteenth century" (p. 70). The stories, in turn, presumably illuminate "aspects of the human witiko psychosis" (p. 71), which is implicitly accepted as an established fact. Obviously I do not believe that the interesting data presented in this paper justify any such conclusion.

NOTES

1. The scope of Moostoos's levitation seems to have increased over time. Moostoos was killed in March 1899, and the testimony quoted above was given in July or August. In a deposition made on April 24, however, the same witness stated that Moostoos "seemed at the time to be standing on air about 2 feet off the ground" [ECF 1899].
2. On the other hand, June Helm (personal communication) believes that there has been significant and long-standing cultural diffusion between some Northern Athapaskan groups and the Western Woods Cree.
3. Meyer's comments have not been reproduced here. They can be found in Current Anthropology 24 (1): 121, 1983 (CCH).

REFERENCES

Annual Archaeological Report
1903– The Killing of Moostoos the Wehtigoo. (Summary of legal proceedings held at
1904 Fort Saskatchewan and Edmonton, July–August, 1899.) Appendix to the Report of the Minister of Education, Ontario, Toronto: King's Printer, pp. 126–138.

Annual Archaeological Report
1907–   The Killing of Wa-sak-apee-quay by Pe-se-quan, and others. (Transcript of trial
1908   held at Norway House, October 7, 1907.) Appendix to the Report of the Minister
        of Education, Ontario. Toronto: King's Printer, pp. 91–121.
Arens, W.
1979   The Man-eating Myth. New York: Oxford University Press.
Bain, J. (ed.)
1901   Travels and Adventures in Canada and the Indian Territories between the Years
        1760 and 1776, by Alexander Henry. Toronto: George N. Morang.
Brown, J.
1971   The Cure and Feeding of Windigos: A Critique. American Anthropologist 73:
        20–22.
Day, G. M.
1967   Historical Notes on New England Languages. In Contributions to Anthropology:
        Linguistics I (Algonquian), National Museum of Canada, Bulletin 214, Anthropolo-
        gical Series 78, pp. 107–112.
Edmonton Court Files
1899   The Queen vs Pay-i-nu and Nap-i-so-sis. MS, Cr. 157 (Old Series).
Flannery, R., M. E. Chambers, and P. A. Jehle
1981   Witiko Accounts from the James Bay Cree. Arctic Anthropology 18: 57–77.
Fogelson, R. D.
1965   Psychological Theories of Windigo 'Psychosis' and a Preliminary Application of
        a Models Approach. In M. E. Spiro (ed.), Context and Meaning in Cultural An-
        thropology: Essays in Honor of A. Irving Hallowell. New York: Free Press, pp.
        74–99.
Gerard, W. R.
1904   The Tapehanek Dialect of Virginia. American Anthropologist 6: 313–330.
Hallowell, A. I.
1942   The Role of Conjuring in Saulteaux Society. Publications of the Philadelphia
        Anthropological Society 2. Philadelphia: University of Pennsylvania Press.
Harris, M.
1975   Culture, People, and Nature: An Introduction to General Anthropology. Second
        Edition. New York: Thomas Y. Crowell.
Isham, J.
1949   Observations on Hudson's Bay. Toronto: Champlain Society.
Kohl, J. G.
1860   Kitchi-Gami: Wanderings round Lake Superior. London: Chapman and Hall.
Landes, R.
1938   The Abnormal among the Ojibwa Indians. Journal of Abnormal and Social Psy-
        chology (now Journal of Abnormal Psychology) 33: 14–33.
Manitoba Court of Queen's Bench
1899   The Queen vs Toosh-e-naun and Ah-ne-o-kizick. MS, No. 14, Fall Assize.
Preston, R.
1975   Cree Narrative: Expressing the Personal Meaning of Events. National Museum of
        Man, Mercury Series, Canadian Ethnology Service Paper 30.
Public Archives of Canada
1879   The Queen vs Ka-ki-si-kutchin, "The Swift Runner". MS, Department of Justice
        File C RG 13, C-1, Vol. 1417.
1896   Northwest Mounted Police Preliminary Investigation File into the Killing of Mapanin
        (Francis Auger) at Trout Lake (Alberta) on January 22, 1896. MS, RG 18, Vol.
        152, File 242.
1899   Northwest Mounted Police Investigation and Arrest File, Moostoos Case. MS, File
        RG 18, Vol. 1442, No. 166.

1907– Department of Justice Capital Case File on Joseph Fiddler. MS, File RG 13, C-1,
1908 Vol. 1452.
1907– RCMP Investigation into the Homicide by Jack and Joseph Fiddler. RCMP Inquiry
1909 into the Escape and Suicide of Jack Fiddler. MS, File RG 18, Vol. 3229, HQ-
781-G-1.

Smith, J. G. E.
1976 Notes on the *Wittiko*. *In* W. Cowan (ed.), Papers of the 7th Algonquian Conference,
1975. Ottawa: Carleton University, pp. 18–38.

Teicher, M.
1960 *Windigo* Psychosis. *In* V. Ray (ed.), Proceedings of the 1960 Annual Spring Meeting
of the American Ethnological Society. Seattle: American Ethnological Society,
pp. 1–129.

Thompson, D.
1916 David Thompson's Narrative, 1784–1812. J. B. Tyrrell (ed.). Toronto: Champlain
Society.

Tooker, W. W.
1904 Some Powhattan Names. American Anthropologist 6: 670–694.

Turner, J. P.
1950 The North-West Mounted Police. Ottawa: King's Printer.

THE CANNIBAL COMPULSION TAXON

Commentary

The generalized picture of *windigo* is that of a person who becomes obsessed with the compulsion to kill other people and eat human flesh, often under the belief of being possessed by a mythical monster. Such anthropophagy may or may not occur, but out of fear that it might, the victim is sometimes killed by members of the group.

But the questions persist: *what is it* and at what level should it be analyzed? What phenomena lie behind the label and the generalized picture? As Marano's discussion clearly brings out, there is considerable ambiguity and heterogenity in the primary data on which various etiological and explanatory formulations have been based. There are anecdotal reports, hearsay accounts of incidents, formal legal actions, an occasional report from a reputed sufferer, and much cultural material relating to the belief syndrome. One striking feature is that most of the basic cases do not include actual homicide or cannibalism, but rather, the *belief* that it did or might occur.

Given Marano's theoretical interests, such an omission of possible psychopathology is understandable; but this is not to say that no psychopathology may exist in these accounts. The next question, then, if that possibility is accepted, is whether a powerful set of cultural *beliefs* per se (i.e., that some persons are likely to kill and cannibalize) might be an appropriate focus of analysis for the attribution of psychopathology. As has been indicated before, such an exercise has long been discredited on the basis of its simplistic mixing of levels of analysis as well as its failure to take a functional approach to understanding personality dynamics.

Furthermore, in order for the discussion to be as congruent as possible with the usual psychiatric appraisal, the data employed should be those at the level of primary behavioral information pertaining to an individual person. For this reason, whatever other theoretical approaches may or may not help explain the total range of elements entering into this putative "syndrome", it seems to me worthwhile to examine the kinds of behavior that is considered prototypical for the syndrome even though, as Marano and others indicate, the incidence of such cases may have been grossly exaggerated.

As with the earlier section on the *Startle Matching Taxon*, the articles included in this volume do not contain behavioral accounts with sufficient detail for an informed appraisal to be made. In his discussion, Marano makes frequent reference to the best single source of primary data, the 70 "cases" compiled by Teicher (1960); and a case from that collection recorded by Father Saindon which contains more psychiatrically-relevant data than most will be used here for an examination in the DSM-III format (Teicher 1960: 89–90):

463

Ronald C. Simons and Charles C. Hughes (eds.), The Culture-Bound Syndromes, 463–465.
© 1985 *by D. Reidel Publishing Company.*

On one of my missionary tours the people told me that F. was sick. She would not go out; she did not wish to see anyone. However, she looked after her household duties. I made inquiries. Finally, they told me that she was attacked with the *"Windigo* sickness". "What is that?" I asked. "A strange malady that is rare today, but was formerly more frequent." The Indians stood in great fear of patients attacked by this malady, such fear that in the last stages of the malady they thought it necessary to kill the patient. It was thus at Moose Factory many years ago, where there was an execution of this kind by hanging.

F. had the *windigo* malady. She did not want to see anyone except her husband and her children, because strangers became metamorphosed in her mind into wild animals – wolves, bears, lynxes. These animals are dangerous to life. To protect herself she was driven by the desire to kill them. But this was repugnant to her, because these animals are human beings.

She fought against the obsessing idea that found lodgement in her consciousness. She wished to kill and she didn't wish. The idea became stronger and more compelling. As a solution of her conflict, she fled from reality and took the stand of not wishing to see anyone or to speak with anyone. Walled up in her tent, she was resigned to her condition. She was taciturn. She almost always held her eyes cast down. She struggled against this situation. She couldn't sleep.

Along with the above data Teicher includes another incident which he infers may also pertain to the same person; but since there may be doubt, and since one might question the suddenness of the remission on the basis of an authoritarian command reported in the additional material, only the above will be used here.

A DSM-III assessment of the case might be as follows:

Axis I: 300.30   Obsessive Compulsive Disorder ("The essential features are recurrent obsessions or compulsions. *Obsessions* are recurrent, persistent ideas, thoughts, images, or impulses that are ego-dystonic, that is, they are not experienced as voluntarily produced, but rather as thoughts that invade consciousness and are experienced as senseless or repugnant. Attempts are made to ignore or suppress them. . . . The most common obsessions are repetitive thoughts of violence (e.g., killing one's child). . . . Depressions and anxiety are common [associated features]. . . . The course is usually chronic, with waxing and waning of symptoms. . . . Impairment is generally moderate to severe" (p. 234); and "The obsessions or compulsions are a significant source of distress of the individual or interfere with social or role functioning" (p. 235).

Axis II: Insufficient data

Axis III: Insufficient data

Axis IV: *Psychosocial stressors*: fear from peers believing she was a Windigo and might kill her?
            Severity: 5 – Severe (Operational definition – "serious illness in self or family; major financial loss; marital separation. . .". In this patient she "fought against the obsessing idea . . . wished to kill and didn't wish . . . the idea became stronger and more compelling . . . she fled from reality . . .")

Axis V: *Highest level of adaptive functioning past year*: 6 – Very Poor ("Marked by impairment in both social relations and occupational functioning";

this person did not wish '. . . to see anyone or to speak with anyone . . .
walled up in her tent . . . almost always held her eyes cast down . . .")

REFERENCE

Teicher, Morton I.
  1960 *Windigo* Psychosis: A Study of a Relationship Between Belief and Behavior Among
       the Indians of Northeastern Canada. American Ethnological Society. Seattle: Uni-
       versity of Washington.

APPENDIX

CHARLES C. HUGHES

GLOSSARY OF 'CULTURE-BOUND' OR FOLK PSYCHIATRIC SYNDROMES

INTRODUCTION

As suggested by Hughes in his Introduction to this volume, the term "culure-bound syndromes" has an elusive meaning; in fact, the several conceptual elements that might imply a focused and exclusive reference for the phrase vanish upon examination, leaving a phrase that still has currency but little discriminable content. What remains appears to be more a feeling tone about certain patterns of behavior so unusual and bizarre from a Western point of view that, regardless of definitional ambiguities, they have continued to be accorded by some writers a reified status as a different "class" *sui generis* of psychiatric or putatively psychiatric phenomena.

Even if such a unique class were defensible, the topic is beset with sheer notational confusion. A reader may wonder, for example, whether terms resembling each other in spelling (e.g., *bah tschi, bah-tsi*) are reporting different disorders or simply reflecting differences in the authors' phonetic and orthographic transcription styles for the same disorder. Or perhaps the various renderings are accurately transcribed but represent *dialectical* differences in names used for a given syndrome by various groups having the same basic cultural orientation (e.g., *windigo, witiko, wihtigo, whitigo, wiitiko*)? In addition, of course, there may be entirely different terms for what is claimed to be essentially the same condition in diverse cultural groups (e.g., *koro* and *shook yang*).

Dr. Simons noted in the foreword to this book that, as colleagues at Michigan State University over ten years ago, we began to think about such a volume. Out of those early discussions came recognition of several important conceptual and format problems that had to be resolved. One was the question of the most useful type of framework for grouping and sorting the phenomena that receive the label of "culture-bound syndrome"; others were the issue of appropriate terminology for such syndromes, as well as the boundaries of this purported special class of disorders.

More recently he suggested that a "glossary" of the folk terms used for the syndromes would be a useful addition to the substantive chapters in the book. We agreed that at this stage of knowledge it would be most useful to sort the syndromes listed in the glossary on the basis of gross descriptive features. I agreed to take on the task and for some time wrestled with formulating terms of reference and a succinct method of indexing the material. What eventually emerged as this appendix may be seen as a preliminary way of sorting other "culture-bound syndromes" consistent with the concept of "taxon" which Dr. Simons has used as a first-order sorting device applied to the syndromes specifically dealt with in the book.

Ronald C. Simons and Charles C. Hughes (eds.), The Culture-Bound Syndromes, 469–505.

This glossary is, in the first instance, an attempt (obviously only a beginning) to systematize and bring some cross-referenced order to the names used for the various conventional "culture-bound syndromes". Actually, although called a "glossary", it is intended to function at the same time as a brief synonymy, gazeteer, and index to the various names.

But systematizing the names for these syndromes is only part — and the most easily handled part — of ordering the content and integrating the concept of "culture-bound syndromes" into other conceptual schemes. An even more significant issue is whether what have heretofore been called the "culture-bound" syndromes are not, in fact, simply a sub-set of a broader domain, that of *folk psychiatric disorders*. There is one difference, however: namely, that, though generically the same, these particular disorders have become *better publicized* than other disorders in that group; but, as demonstrated in the material following in this glossary, when examined synoptically and with *symptomatic behavioral detail*, the phenomena of what have traditionally been delimited as the "culture-bound" syndromes resolve imperceptibly into the general array of folk-conceptualized disorders of psychiatric interest.

I began assembling data for this glossary using only those "conventional" culture-bound disorders for which there was a distinctive non-English name (e.g., *amok*). But it soon became apparent that to remain with so circumscribed a format would be to lose the chance to undergird discussions of 'what are culture-bound syndromes?' with substantive, comparable data. For this reason I began, for example, to include instances of reputedly witchcraft-caused types of disorders, such as among the Shona reported by Gelfand (1964), the reason for inclusion being the *character of the behavioral symptoms* displayed in the syndrome, not the reputed cause. In fact, throughout the glossary any reference to cause (whether "folk" or scientific) is irrelevant for this cataloguing; the essential point is clusterings of observable data conceptualized as a disorder by the group itself.

In the same light, I have also included syndromes which authors themselves may not have explicitly called "culture-bound" and some for which there may be no specific *native* term but which seem comparable to the essential spirit of the idea (e.g., significant cultural influence in the genesis and expression of a patterned disorder). An example is *brain fag* as seen among Nigerian students (Prince 1960); others are the *crazy sickness* among the Navaho (Kaplan and Johnson 1964: 216–220) and *ghost sickness* among the Kiowa Apache (Freeman et al. 1976). Of course, an indigenous word may well exist to describe such behavior, and a author with interests lying in the psychodynamic and not the linguistic aspects of the phenomena may simply have chosen not to include it for English reader. But, again, as with notions of cause, it is not existence or non-existence of the *word* that is important, but rather it is the patterned, observable *data*.

In some instances a non-Western name has become widely adopted into English (and other) usage to designate an obviously similar condition appearing in a different cultural context (as with *amok*). And the reverse holds as well — an English or other term used in referring to disorders in other societies; *Arctic hysteria* is an example, or *kayak angst* (in this case, of course, neither word being of English derivation). When such a term is used the reader is referred to the cognate indigenous term (if one exists) for fuller details of synonyms, location, symptomatology, and bibliography. If the disorder occurs in an English-speaking folk tradition and is named, the English term is used, e.g., *falling out* among American blacks (Weidman 1979).

Several articles have recently appeared in the literature that demonstrate the plasticity of a taxonomic idea such as "culture-bound", as well as the appeal of the phrase. It has been suggested, for instance, that obesity is a "culture-bound disorder" in American society (Ritenbaugh 1982); that the post-partum *blues* constitute another such syndrome in the same group (Stern and Kruckman 1983); that protein-energy malnutrition represents the influence of "culture-binding" on the process of biomedical scientific conceptualizing itself (Cassidy 1982); and that the disease hypertension is a good illustration of the intersection of two different domains of disease labelling, the folk or popular and the scientific/biomedical (Blumhagen 1980). Although I have not included any of these in the glossary, given the interactive nature of disease as well as disease nosology with a given cultural context, the omission may well be arguable. Citation of these examples occurring in a modern society does, however, underscore the point that while every society has its folk or "popular" concepts of disorder, superimposed over those ideas in some groups is another (and contending) system, the conceptual scheme of modern medicine and psychiatry, and such a juxtaposition is what much of the presumed controversy concerning that status of the "culture-bound syndromes" is about.

The sheer abundance and variety of cross-cultural data pertaining to mental disorders or apparent mental disorders obviously disallows a complete inventory in this glossary, and some exclusions are necessary for limiting what otherwise could become unmanageable. For example, a term is excluded if it is simply a generic term for "crazy" without any further specification, e.g., *were* among the Yoruba (Leighton et al. 1963) or *caduco* on Guam (Penningroth and Penningroth 1977). In some instances, however, where it has been an author's preference to list specific disorders following the generic term for mental illness, that practice has been followed here, e.g., *gila mengamok* ("crazy") ("random running and violence toward other people")

The phenomena of possession and trance pose major challenges in regard to this glossary. For one thing, the behaviors and experiences are so ubiquitous that there could be no end to the listing of relevant published materials. There is already a substantial literature dealing with such matters as formal, ritualized healing cults and periods of "out of awareness" phenomena prescribed by various social and ceremonial occasions (e.g., Bourguignon 1976; Langness 1976; Prince 1968; Crapanzano and Garrison 1977, and many more). Sometimes, of course, behavior of persons in such situations is of psychiatric relevance (i.e., demonstrates pathology at the behavioral level), but often it is simply the playing of a publically-viewed and socially-prescribed role.

What is included in this glossary from such a vast array of descriptive data are those behavioral episodes labelled disorder by the folk tradition itself when the explanation for the behavior is that the person is "possessed", i.e., as described by the author, the behavior fits the other general criteria for culturally-structured pathology in that it has psychopathologic features and is not simply a *pro-forma*, ritually-prescribed public performance. Further, there may be a distinctive folk term, and the author may or may not label it as "culture-bound" (e.g., *phii pob*). But even in this respect data are not available in sufficient detail to be confident of including the behaviors defined as "possession" and denoted by distinctive terms in the eleven major languages of India (Rao 1978: 7).

Unless there are specific *symptomatic data* given, other disorders often discussed as "culture-bound" but commonly referred to by English terms are excluded because of their abstractness, e.g., "malignant anxiety", "voodoo death", or "thanatomania". Nor is bewitchment as a *cultural category* included, although when it is entered as a folk rationalization for psychiatrically-relevant symptoms in a person it is recorded so long as there is a distinctive folk term for it (e.g., *el dano*, Ponce 1965). Of course, the behavioral and psychological effects on the victim are certainly of psychiatric import (e.g., Gaviria and Wintrob 1976; Weimer and Mintz 1966–67).

Perhaps it is in trying to match the conventional definition of a "culture-bound" syndrome" with bewitchment, voodoo death, and other cultural patterns that the most telling argument against thinking of the "culture-boud syndromes" as a distinctive class of disorders becomes most apparent. For such cultural patterns (like other aspects of the socio-cultural environment) exist in a dialectic relationship with the personality level of behavior, sometimes serving a role causative of pathology, sometimes ameliorative. But in all instances the forms of such interaction can be varied.

The implicit model for the "culture-bound" disorders is based on an ontologic and specific concept of disease applied to the rather dramatic instances of deviance. But a more comprehensive perusal of literature relevant to the issue, especially literature offering material as close as possible to the level of "micro-detailed" phenomena and primary observation suggested by Simons in his Introduction to this volume, makes the point that out of the behavioral continua that comprise the daily round of human existence (*all* influenced by a cultural setting), some patterns of disorder become stereotyped and so extreme — so obviously displaying "sick" symptoms — that they are socially recognized and even named. Others, while recognized, may not receive the distinction of bearing a singular name and remain uncodified linguistically.

Regardless of the issue of a distinctive name, however, if the behavior is sufficiently striking and deviant from normal expectations, it seems a truism that people in *any* group will have *some* language by which they refer to the behavior we might, for example, call "possession", even if it be circumlocutional language comparable to our "acute situational reaction" (see also J. Murphy 1976). What seems suggested is that, based on individual behavioral data, regardless of the pre-packaging of data implied by use of a specific name, efforts in this area should proceed as soon and as systematically as possible from the culturally "emic" to the psychiatrically "etic" level of conceptualization and analysis of relevant cultural patterns. The existence or non-existence of a *distinctive* name should become irrelevant.

The basic format for information about each entry in this glossary is organized as follows:

(A)　Alternative spelling(s) of the same term, and syndromes with other names purportedly exhibiting essentially the same pathology or behavior as does the key entry term. Where it seems obvious that terms spelled slightly differently are basically the same word, I have placed all spellings in the key position, e.g., *ufufunyane, ufufunyana, ufufuyane*. Citation of the source for the alternative spelling or putatively similar disorder is also included if known.

(B)　Either the geographic locale of the group in which the term is found, or the *cultural* context of the term if simple geographic localization would not be sufficiently specific (as in the culturally heterogenous, multi-group situation in southeast Asia).

(C)　Symptoms commonly reported in cases and/or discussions of the syndrome.

(D)　Suggested bibliographic sources. If there is more than one reference available (and the paucity of multiple sources on a number of the syndromes is quite apparent, at least in my review of the literature), then several entries are included. The list is short, highly selective, and likely to annoy some readers because of what I have failed to include. The suggestions are intended simply to help a neophytic reader get into the literature available on the particular syndrome. If there is more than one source, criteria for including others include authoritativeness of the source, presumed availability, and recency of publication (or, on the contrary, status as a classical, "bench-mark", or "first report" entry, such as Beard's article on *jumping Frenchmen*). Finally, the reference given may be either to a source in which the term is discussed *inter alia* (e.g., Czaplicka 1914; Landy 1983; Kleinman and Lin 1981; or a bibliographic source such as Favazza and Oman 1977), or else to an article which focuses on the particular syndrome (e.g., Yap 1952).

When a given key entry (e.g., *lulu*) is considered by an author to be a synonym for another term (e.g., *negi-negi*) and is used by the same group, the reader is referred to the latter entry for full details of other synonyms and symptoms. If, however, the entry term refers to a cognate condition in a different society, the reader is referred to the basic term for full information about symptom patterns, but the geographic localization and references specific to the entry term are given under its own heading (e.g., for *saladera* the reader is referred to the basic information on *susto*, while under *saladera* itself are noted the group or region where *saladera* is used instead of *susto*, along with references dealing specifically with *saladera*).

Readers are encouraged to challenge this initial formulation by raising questions of completeness, accuracy, mis-assignment of a term to a described condition, spelling, and the like, as well as to suggest additions. Those wishing to enter into such dialogue are invited to contact either editor of this volume:

RONALD C. SIMONS, M.D., M.A.
Department of Psychiatry,
Michigan State Univeristy,
East Lansing, MI 48824–1316,
U.S.A.

CHARLES C. HUGHES, Ph.D
Department of Family and
Community Medicine,
University of Utah Medical Center
Salt Lake City, UT 84132
U.S.A.

GLOSSARY

abisinwin
- A. –
- B. Nigeria (Yoruba)
- C. postpartum psychosis; exictement, irrationality; woman may have to be chained down and child taken away
- D. A. Leighton et al. (1963: 106); Prince (1964: 87)

afota
- A. –
- B. Nigeria (Yoruba)
- C. hysterical blindness
- D. Prince (1964: 88)

ahade idzi be (see *amok*)
- B. New Guinea highlands (Kovena, Kuma, Benabena, Manga, Siane, Huli peoples; see Salisbury 1968)
- D. Newman (1964)

agua (*el*)
- A. –
- B. Peru
- C. numerous complaints attributed to "cold" water – colds, bronchial congestions, digestive and cardiac symptoms
- D. Ponce 1965: 42)

aire (*el*)
- A. –
- B. Peru
- C. wide variety of physical and psychological symptoms attributed to "vapors" – eczema, dermatitis, urticaria, epilepsy, convulsions, and hysteria; also pains in various part of the body, paralysis of the extremities and face, conjunctivitis, pleurisy, pneumonia, and gastrointestinal disturbances
- D. Ponce (1965: 42)

aire-orunsun
- A. –
- B. Nigeria (Yoruba)
- C. restlessness, sleeplessness
- D. A. Leighton et al. (1963: 110)

aiyiperi
- A. *warapa, giri* (Prince 1964: 88)
- B. Nigeria (Yoruba)
- C. hysterical convulsive disorders, posturings and tics, psychomotor seizures, probably tetanus
- D. Prince (1964: 88)

aluro
- A. *egba, ategun* (Prince 1964: 88)

B. Nigeria (Yoruba)
C. organic or hysterical paralyses
D. Prince (1964: 88)

amok, amuck

A. *ahaDe idizi Be* (Newman 1964); *cafard* (Yap 1951: 319); *cathard* (Kiev
    1972: 86); *soudanite, pseudonite* (Yap, 1951: 319; Kiev 1972: 86); *mal
    de pelea* (Rothenberg 1964; Yap 1974: 98); *colera* (Yap 1974: 98); *iich'aa*
    (Yap 1974: 77, 99); *gila mengamok* (Chen 1970: 207); *ngamok* (Schmidt
    1964: 148); *gila besi* (Schmidt 1964: 149)
B. Malaysia, Indonesia
C. dissociative episode(s); outburst(s) of violent and aggressive or homicidal
    behavior directed at people and objects; persecutory ideas; automatism;
    amnesia; exhaustion and return of consciousness following the episode (for
    amok runners who are not killed during the episode)
D. chapters by Carr, Westermeyer, Burton-Bradley, Arboleda-Florez in this
    volume; van Loon (1926/27); van Wulfften Palthe (1936: 529–531); Yap
    (1974); H. Murphy (1973); Kiev (1972); Teoh (1972)

amurakh (see *latah*)

A. *irkunii* (Yukaghir; Czaplicka 1914: 315); *olan* (Tungus; Czaplicka 1914:
    315); *menkeiti* (Koryak; Czaplicka 1914: 315)
B. Yakuts (paleo-Siberian group)
D. Czaplicka (1914: 307–325)

anfechtung

A. –
B. Hutterites, Manitoba
C. withdrawal from social contact; feeling of having sinned; rumination on
    religious unworthiness; great concern with the devil; temptation to commit
    sucide; somatic symptoms
D. Kaplan and Plaut (1956)

anthropophobia (see *taijin kyofusho*)

apoda

A. *danidani, edani* (Prince 1964: 87)
B. Nigeria (Yoruba)
C. mental deficiency; "village idiot"
D. A. Leighton et al. (1963: 107)

Arctic hysteria (see *pibloktoq*)

asinwin

A. –
B. Nigeria (Yoruba)
C. acute psychotic episode, sudden onset; likelihood of suicide or homicide
D. Prince (1964: 86)

ategun (see *aluro*)

bah-tsi, bah tschi (see *latah*)

B. Thailand

    D. Suwanlert (1976); Yap (1974: 97)

banga

    A. *bangu; misala* (Kiev 1972: 75; Yap 1951: 319)

    B. Congo, Malawi (formerly Nyasaland)

    C. speech disturbances; convulsions; undifferentiated excitement, weeping, and laughter; running away

    D. Kiev (1972: 75), Yap (1951: 319), Yap (1969: 40)

bebainan

    A. –

    B. Bali

    C. patient suddenly begins to cry, tries to run away, fights off anyone who attempts to restrain him; abruptly falls to ground exhausted; amnesiac after the attack

    D. Dean and Thong (1972)

benzi mazurazura

    A. *benzi remu kuhwa* (Gelfand 1964: 166)

    B. Shona and related peoples, southern Africa

    C. believed caused by witchcraft; victim strikes others without realizing what he has done until after the episode; in *benzi rema kuhwa* victim continually tells lies

    D. Gelfand (1964: 166)

black out (see *falling out*)

bilis

    A. –

    B. Hispanic populations

    C. following a fit of anger and rage, person experiences symptoms of acute nervous tension, chronic fatigue, and malaise

    D. Clark (1959: 175); Kay (1977: 164)

boxi

    A. –

    B. Nepal

    C. physical symptoms such as headache, stomach pain, giddiness, vomiting, tingling sensations in extremities; feeling of being strangled, knocked down, severely beaten or pressed on back of neck; exhibitionistic in behavior

    D. Sharma (1966)

brain fag (see also *gila ilmu*)

    A. –

    B. Nigerian and east African students

    C. pain, heat or burning sensations, pressure or tightness around head; blurring of vision; inability to assimilate what is read, poor retentivity, inability to concentrate when studying; anxiety and depression; fatigue and sleepiness despite adequate rest

    D. Morakinyo (1980); Prince (1960)

boufée delirante aigüe

    A. –

    B.   Haiti
    C.   sudden onset aggressive behavior, marked confusion, psychomotor excite-
         ment; sometimes visual and auditory hallucinations
    D.   Kiev (1972: 88–89)

brujeria (see *mal puesto*)
buduh kedewandewan
    A.   –
    B.   Bali
    C.   person is afflicted with "blessed madness" – prays and mediates in sacred
         places, purportedly encountering divinities; wears ceremonial clothing on
         ordinary occasions; withdraws from friends and relatives and wanders in
         the bush
    D.   Connor (1982: 257)

cafard, cathard (see *amok*)
    B.   Polynesia
    D.   Yap (1951: 319); Kiev (1972: 86)

caida de (la) mollera (mollera caida)
    A.   –
    B.   Mexican-America groups
    C.   symptoms of crying, fever, vomiting, and diarrhea in infants believed caused
         by fall in which an infant's incompletely closed fontanelle is depressed
    D.   Kay (1977: 135); Rubel (1960); Clark (1959)

celos
    A.   *jealousy*
    B.   Chile
    C.   envy, anger, aggressivity; sadness and crying; disobedience; nervousness;
         quarrelsomeness or rage; loss of appetite
    D.   Grebe and Segura (1975)

chisara chisara
    A.   –
    B.   Shona and related people, southern Africa
    C.   psychotic symptoms believed caused by witchcraft; victim lives alone
         in woods
    D.   Gelfand (1964: 165)

chucaque (el)
    A.   –
    B.   Peru
    C.   nausea, vomiting, diarrhea, diffuse pains in abdomen
    D.   Ponce (1965: 42)

colera (see also *amok*, per Yap 1974: 98)
    A.   *colerina* (Ponce 1965)
    B.   Guatemala
    C.   nausea, vomiting, diarrhea, fever; severe temper tantrum with screaming
         generally suppressed; unconsciousness and dissociative behavior

D. Paul (1967)

colerina (la) (see *colera*)

B. Peru

D. Ponce (1965: 42)

crazy violence

A. *crazy drunken violence*

B. Navajo Indians

C. violent or assaultive behavior with complete awareness and consciousness; deliberate recklessness and willingness to take consequences; sometimes associated with drunkeness

D. Kaplan and Johnson (1964)

danidani, edani (see *apoda*)

dhat (see also *shen-k'uei*)

A. *jiryan* (Carstairs 1956); *sukra prameha* (Obeyesekere 1976: 207)

B. India

C. severe anxiety and hypochondriasis associated with discharge of semen; whitish discoloration of the urine; feelings of weakness and exhaustion

D. Malhotra and Wig (1975); Wig (1983: 89); Carstairs (1956); Obeyesekere (1976)

dindinrin

A. —

B. Nigeria (Yoruba)

C. withdrawn, suspicious, uncommunicative, chronic schizophrenic behavior

D. Prince (1964: 87)

djukat

A. —

B. Sarawak (Iban people)

C. toxic-infective delirium and puerperal psychosis

D. Schmidt (1964: 150)

ebenzi

A. —

B. Shona and related people, southern Africa

C. during an attack, person suddenly starts talking nonsense and performing senseless acts; after spell, victim is lucid and able to carry out normal expectations; believed caused by witchcraft

D. Gelfand (1964: 166)

egba (see *aluro*)

empacho

A. —

B. Hispanic groups

C. gastro-intestinal blockage believed due to food clinging to intestinal wall; believed caused by person having been required to eat against his will

D. Rubel (1960: 798–800); Rubel (1966: 165–167); Clark (1959: 179–180); Kay (1977: 135)

Eskimo sleep paralysis (see *uqamairineq*)
espanto (see *susto*)
espirituamento de susto
  A. —
  B. Chile
  C. disturbed sleep, nightmares, somnambulism
  D. Grebe and Segura (1975)
evil eye (see *mal ojo*)

falling-out, black out
  A. *indisposition* (Wiedman 1979: 96)
  B. Southern Blacks (U.S.A.) and Bahamians (for "Black Out")
  C. dissociative behavior; sudden collapse, sometimes without warning, some-
      times preceded by feelings of dizziness or "swimming" in the head; eyes
      are usually open but victim claims inability to "see"; usually hears and
      understands what is occurring around him but is powerless to move
  D. Weidman (1979); Lefley (1979a, 1979b); Rubin and Jones (1979)
frigophobia (see *pa-leng*)

gahsum-ari (see *hwa-byung*)
  B. Korea
  D. Lee, B. S. (1983)
gbohungbohun
  A. —
  B. Nigeria (Yoruba)
  C. hysterical aphonia
  D. Prince (1964: 88)
ghost sickness
  A. —
  B. Kiowa Apache Indians (southern plains, U.S.A.)
  C. during period of mourning victim is hypersensitive to sounds and touch
      of presumed ghost of dead relative, becomes terror-stricken; fears that
      if he turns head back to look over his shoulder the ghost will cause partial
      bodily palsy; cannibalistic fantasies, epileptiform spells, severe eating and
      psychophysiological disturbances
  D. Freeman, Foulks, and Freeman (1976)
ghost sickness
  A. —
  B. Navajo Indians
  C. varied symptoms attributed to witchcraft, including weakness, bad dreams,
      feelings of danger, confusion, feelings of futility, loss of appetite, feelings
      of suffocation, fainting, dizziness, fear and anxiety, sometimes hallucina-
      tions and loss of consciousness
  D. Kaplan and Johnson (1964)

gila babi (*gila* means "madness")
  A. –
  B. Rural Malaysia (Malays)
  C. epileptic convulsions
  D. Chen (1970: 207)

gila besi (see *amok*)
  A. *ngamok* (Schmidt 1964: 149)
  B. Sarawak (Iban people)
  D. Schmidt (1964: 149)

gila bejako
  A. –
  B. Sarawak (Iban people)
  C. autistic talk as predominant feature
  D. Schmidt (1964: 149)

gila buatan orang
  A. (symptoms similar to *gila kena hantu*; attribution of cause differs)
  B. Rural Malaysia (Malays)
  C. fits of violence, superhuman ability to cause physical destruction, auditory hallucinations believed caused by witchcraft
  D. Chen (1970: 207)

gila ilmu, gila mangaji, gila isin
  A. (the above names are interchangeable); see also *brain fag* and *gila untak*
  B. Rural Malaysia (Malays)
  C. person displays symptoms attributed to excessive mental concentration and serious study; unable to stop reciting verses of the Koran or mystical incantations; often refuses to eat, drink, sleep, or rest
  D. Chen (1970: 207)

gila isin
  A. *gila urat* (Schmidt 1964: 148, 149)
  B. Sarawak (Iban people)
  C. quick-tempered and sometimes violent behavior
  D. Schmidt (1964: 149)

gila kejubong
  A. –
  B. Sarawak (Iban people)
  C. person laughs to himself, tears off his clothes, dances by himself
  D. Schmidt (1964: 149)

gila kena hantu
  A. (symptoms similar to *gila buatan orang*; attribution of cause differs)
  B. Rural Malaysia (Malays)
  C. fits of violence, superhuman ability to cause physical destruction, auditory hallucinations believed caused by evil spirits
  D. Chen (1970: 207)

gila ketawa
  A. –

B. Sarawak (Iban people)
C. victim talks and laughs to himself, wanders about aimlessly, cannot sleep
D. Schmidt (1964: 1949)

gila mengamok

A. *amuck, amok*
B. Rural Malaysia (Malays)
C. sudden, unprovoked outburst of frenzied rage; indiscriminant killing or maiming of all persons and animals before person is overpowered or killed; the extreme form of gila kena hantu and gila buatan orang
D. Chen (1970: 207)

gila merian

A. –
B. Rural Malaysia (Malays)
C. postpartum depression, auditory hallucinations, insomnia, confusion
D. Chen (1970: 207)

gila nganu

A. –
B. Sarawak (Iban people)
C. scolding and hitting other people
D. Schmidt (1964: 149)

gila ngaransi

A. –
B. Sarawak (Iban people)
C. person who throws his belongings away and destroys his property
D. Schmidt (1964: 149)

gila nyadi

A. –
B. Sarawak (Iban people)
C. state of continuous violence
D. Schmidt (1964: 149)

gila talak

A. –
B. Rural Malaysia (Malays)
C. "insanity due to divorce"
D. Chen (1970: 207)

gila untak (see also *brain fag*)

B. Sarawak (Iban people)
D. Schmidt (1964: 149)

gila urat

A. see also *gila isin* (Schmidt 1964: 148, 149)
B. Sarawak (Iban people)
C. social withdrawal; weakness and child-like babble; blood-shot eyes "from too much concentration"
D. Schmidt (1964: 148, 149)

giri
  A. *aiyiperi, warapa* (Prince 1964: 88)
  B. Nigeria (Yoruba)
  C. convulsions without foaming or falling to ground; nonsensical talk; irrational behavior
  D. A. Leighton et al. (1963: 106–107); Prince (1964: 88)

grisi siknis (see *pibloktoq*)
  B. Miskito Indians (Honduras, Nicaragua)
  D. chapter by Dennis, this volume

guria
  A. *vailala madness* (Hoskin et al. 1967)
  B. New Guinea
  C. dissociation; shaking
  D. Hoskin et al. (1967); Yap (1974: 99)

hex
  A. *voodoo death*
  B. world-wide in incidence; case reported here from Baltimore, Maryland
  C. patient admitted with shortness of breath and episodes of chest pain and syncope of one month's duration; patient had been "hexed" since birth and was doomed to die before her 23rd birthday; manifestly terrified. Patient died day before her 23rd birthday.
  D. Clinicopathologic Conference (1967)

haak-tsan (see *susto*)
  B. Canton
  D. Yap (1974: 98); Topley (1970)

hiwa: itck
  A. –
  B. Mohave Indians
  C. loss of appetite, sleeplessness, depressed behavior
  D. Devereux (1961); Kiev (1972)

hsieh-ping
  A. *windigo* (Yap 1969: 41, 48)
  B. Taiwan
  C. prodromal depression, anxiety, feeling of being possessed, disorientation, tremor, glossolalia, visual and auditory hallucinations
  D. Rin and Lin (1962); Yap (1969; 41, 48); Kiev (1972: 87); Lin, Kleinman, and Lin (1981: 256)

hwa-byung
  A. *anger syndrome; wool-hwa-byung* (Chang 1983); gahsum-ari (? see Lee, B. S. 1983)
  B. Korea
  C. insomnia, excessive tiredness, acute panic, morbid fear of impending death, dysphoric affect; indigestion, anorexia, dyspnea, palpitation, generalized

pains and aches, feeling of a mass in the epigastrium; attributed to suppression of anger

D. Lin (1983a, 1983b); Lee, S. H. (1977); Lee, B. S. (1983); Chang, S. C. (1983)

iich'aa (also see *amok*, per Yap 1974: 77, 99)

A. *moth craziness* (Kaplan and Johnson 1964: 210)

B. Navajo Indians

C. epileptiform behavior; loss of self-control; fits of violence and rage

D. Kaplan and Johnson (1964); Neutra et al. (1977); Yap (1974: 77, 99)

ikota, ihota, ilota (see *latah*)

B. paleo-Siberian groups

D. Yap (1951: 318; 1952: 516)

imu (see *latah*)

B. Ainu (Hokkaido Island, Japan)

D. chapter by Ohnuko-Tierney in this volume; Winiarz and Wielawski (1936)

inarun

A. –

B. Nigeria (Yoruba)

C. weakness and burning or itching of the body, skin rashes, dimness of vision, impotence, deadness of feet and paralysis of the legs; occasionally psychotic symptoms

D. Prince (1964: 88)

indisposition (see *falling-out*)

B. Haiti

D. Philippe and Romain (1979)

ipa were

A. –

B. Nigeria (Yoruba)

C. psychosis associated with epilepsy

D. Prince (1964: 88)

irijua (*la*)

A. –

B. Peru

C. children's disease; symptoms appearing after the birth of a sibling or following weaning; sadness, melancholy, irritability, hyper-sensitivity, anorexia, tearfulness, loss of weight.

D. Ponce (1965: 42)

irkunii (see *amurakh*)

B. Yukaghir (paleo-Siberian group)

D. Czaplicka (1914: 315)

itiju

A. –

B. Nigeria (Yoruba)

C. extreme bashfulness; fear of being among people
D. A. Leighton et al. (1963: 110)

iwara

A. –
B. Nigeria (Yoruba)
C. excessive eagerness, tenseness; wants things done in a hurry
D. A. Leighton (1963: 110–111)

jayau

A. *mamau laban jayau*
B. Sarawak (Iban people)
C. lack of sleep, loss of appetite, tendency to suicide; attributed to love charms, frustration in love, desire for revenge
D. Schmidt (1964: 150)

jinjinia bemar (see *koro*)

B. Assam
D. Dutta (1983)

jiryan (see *dhat*)

jugau

A. –
B. Sarawak (Iban people)
C. dim-witted and foolish behavior
D. Schmidt (1964: 150)

jumping, jumping Frenchman (see *latah*)

B. northeastern United States; eastern Canada
D. Beard (1880); de la Tourette (1884); Yap (1951: 319; 1952: 519–521); Stevens (1965)

kaika (la)

A. –
B. Peru
C. general discomfort, loss of weight, anorexia, depression
D. Ponce (1965: 43)

kayak angst (see *nangiarpok*)

kiesu (see *saka*)

A. *Kenya*
D. Harris (1957)

koro

A. *shook yong, show yang* (van Wulfften Palthe 1936: 533); *shuk yang* (Pfeiffer 1982: 210); *su yang* (Yap 1951: 317); *suo yang; suk yeon* (Yap 1964); *suk yeong* (Yap 1974: 98); *rok-joo* (Keshavan 1983); *jinjinia bemar* (Dutta 1983; Nandi et al. 1983; Rosenthal and Rosenthal 1982)
B. South China, Chinese and Malaysian populations in southeast Asia; Assam (Hindus)

C. intense and sudden anxiety that the penis (or, for females, the vulva and breasts) will recede into the body; the penis is held by the victim or someone else, or devices are attached to prevent its receding

D. chapters by J. G. Edwards, J. M. Edwards, Ifabumuyi and Rwegellera, and Leng in this volume; van Wulfften Palthe (1936: 532–538); Ngui (1969); Yap (1964, 1965); Jilek and Jilek-Aall (1977); Dutta (1983); Nandi et al. (1983); Rosenthal and Rosenthal (1982); Tan (1981: 375–376); Lin, Kleinman, and Lin (1981: 255–256)

kupenga kwechitsiko

A. *menta ra mumba* (Gelfand 1964: 165)

B. Shona and related people, southern Africa

C. anxiety, dissociative symptoms; display of mental imbalance in front of others which improves when victim is alone; attributed to witchcraft

D. Gelfand (1964: 165)

lanti (see *susto*)

B. Philippines (Bisayan)

D. chapter by Hart (this volume)

lastimadura (*la*) (see *ticradura*)

B. Peru

D. Ponce (1965: 43)

latah, lattah

A. *Latha* (Ionescu-Tongyonk 1977: 154); *imu* (Yap 1951: 318); *ikota* (Yap 1952: 516); *ilota; ihota; mali-mali* (Yap 1951: 318); *myriachit, miryachit* (Yap 1974: 97); *yaun, young-dah-te* (Yap 1974: 97); *bah-tsi, bah tschi* (Yap 1974: 97); *amurakh* (Czaplicka 1914: 320); *jumping Frenchman* (Yap 1951: 319); *pibloktoq* (Yap 1974: 97); misala (Yap 1951: 319)

B. Malaysia and Indonesia

C. hypersensitivity to sudden fright or startle; hyper-suggestibility; echopraxis; echolalia; dissociative or trance-like behavior

D. chapters by Simons, Kenney, and Ohnuki-Tierney in this volume; de la Tourette (1884); Czaplicka (1914: 307–325); van Loon (1926/27); van Wulfften Palthe (1936: 531–532); Aberle (1952); Yap (1952); H. Murphy (1973, 1976)

latido

A. –

B. Latin-American, Mexican-American populations

C. great weakness; abdominal pulsations; emaciation brought on by person being unable (emotionally) to eat

D. Clark (1959: 178); Kay (1977: 135)

lulu (see *negi-negi*)

mal de pelea (see *amok*)

B. Puerto Rico

D. Rothenberg (1964)

mal (de) ojo
- A. *evil eye*
- B. Mediterranean; Latin American hispanic populations
- C. fitful sleep, crying without apparent cause, diarrhea, vomiting, fever in a child or infant explained as caused by fixed stare from an adult; sometimes adult as victim (especially females)
- D. Kiev (1972: 75–79); Clark (1959: 172); Rubel (1966: 157–161)

mal puesto
- A. *witchcraft illness* (Yap 1974: 59); *brujeria* (Clark 1959: 174)
- B. Latin America; hispanic populations
- C. multiple psychological and somatic symptoms explained as caused by witchcraft
- D. Rubel (1966: 167–171)

malgri
- A. –
- B. Wellesley Islands of the Gulf of Carpontarian, northern Australia
- C. anxiety, headache, fatigue, gastro-intestinal disorder, constipation
- D. Cawte (1974, 1976)

mali-mali (see *latah*)
- B. Philippines
- D. Yap (1951: 318)

mamhepo
- A. –
- B. Shona and related peoples, southern Africa
- C. believed to be caused by witchcraft; victim mimics a particular animal chosen by a witch, such as a snake; said to afflict victims who are selfish
- D. Gelfand (1964: 166)

manau
- A. –
- B. Sarawak (Iban people)
- C. senile dementia
- D. Schmidt (1964: 149)

maruru teruaien
- A. –
- B. Sarawak (Murut people)
- C. non-violent dementia; autistic talk, especially in teen-agers
- D. Schmidt (1967/68: 30)

melancholia (see *pension*)

menerik (see *pibloktoq*)
- B. Paleo-Siberian groups
- D. Czaplicka (1914: 307–325)

menkeiti (see *amurakh*)
- B. Koryak
- D. Czaplicka (1914: 315)

menta ra mumba (see *kupenga kwechitsiko*)
misala (see *latah*)
    B.   Malawi (formerly Nyasaland)
    D.   Yap (1951: 319)
mogo laya (see *susto*)
    B.   New Guinea (Huli)
    D.   chapter by Frankel (this volume)
myriachit, miryachit (see *latah*)
    B.   paleo-Siberian groups
    D.   de la Tourette (1884); Czaplicka (1914); Yap (1952: 521–523)
moth craziness (see *iich'aa*)

nangiarnek (see *nangiarpok*)
nangiarpok
    A.   *nangiarnek, kayak angst*
    B.   Greenlandic Eskimos
    C.   severe anxiety; dissociative reaction and psychophysiological symptoms while in a kayak on the open sea
    D.   Gussow (1963, 1970)
negi-negi
    A.   *lulu* (Yap 1969: 46)
    B.   New Guinea, Papua
    C.   dissociation; aggressive behavior, sometimes homicidal
    D.   Yap (1969: 41, 42, 46); Langness (1965)
nervios
    A.   –
    B.   Costa Rica
    C.   headaches, body pain; respiratory complaints, worries, depressions, disorientation; itching, lack of appetite, cough, fever, sore throat, runny eyes, fatigue, vomiting, congestion
    D.   Low (1981)
ngamok (see *amok*)
    A.   *gila besi*
    B.   Sarawak (Iban people)
    D.   Schmidt (1964: 148–149)

olan (see *amurakh*)
    B.   Tungus
    D.   Czaplicka (1914: 315)
old hag (see *uqamairineq*)
    B.   Newfoundland
    D.   chapter by Ness, this volume; Hufford (1982)
ori ode
    A.   –

B. Nigeria (Yoruba)
C. somatic complaints of burning, crawling, thumping in the head which often spreads throughout the body; dimness of vision and "dazzling" of the eyes; insomnia, dizziness, trembling
D. Prince (1964: 87)

otak miring
A. –
B. Rural Malaysia
C. eccentric behavior in aged persons; senile dementia
D. Chen (1970: 208)

pa-feng
A. –
B. Taiwan
C. excessive fear of the wind (associated with pa-leng)
D. Rin (1966)

pa-leng
A. *frigophobia* (Klev 1972: 71)
B. Taiwan
C. morbid fear of the cold; fear of loss of vitality; need to wear excessive clothing
D. Kiev (1972: 71); Rin (1966); Chang, Rin, and Chen (1975)

pasmo
A. –
B. Mexican-American groups
C. infection stimulated by rapid chilling of the body
D. Kay (1977: 135–136)

pataletas
A. –
B. Chile
C. temper tantrums, crying and screaming; falling to the ground; foaming, jumping or kicking; sometimes pain in stomach
D. Grebe and Segura (1975)

pension
A. *melancholia*
B. Chile
C. depressed symptoms – sadness, lack of appetite, loss of weight
D. Grebe and Segura (1975)

phii pob
A. –
B. rural Thailand
C. belief one is possessed by a spirit; numbness of limbs, followed by falling with or without convulsions; usually unconsciousness; sometimes clenched

fists and bodily rigidity; shouting out, screaming, weeping; speech confused; timidity and shyness

D. Suwanlert (1976)

pibloktoq

A. *arctic hysteria, piblokto, problokto* (Whitney 1910: 67, 83); *amurakh, menerik* (Czaplicka 1914: 307–325); *grisi siknis* (chapter by Dennis, this volume)

B. Eskimo (Arctic); paleo-Siberian groups

C. prodromal brooding; depressive silences; loss or disturbance of consciousness during seizure; tearing off of clothing; fleeing or wandering; rolling in snow; performing mimetic acts such as echolalia and echopraxia; glossolalia

D. chapters by Gussow, Foulks, and Dennis in this volume; Aberle (1952); Parker (1962); Foulks (1972); Czaplicka (1917: 307–325); Novakovsky (1924); Brill (1913)

pissu

A. –

B. Ceylon

C. burning sensations in stomach and underneath the navel; difficulty in standing and sitting; coldness in body; auditory and visual hallucinations; dissociative symptoms attributed to possession by spirit

D. Obeyesekere (1970)

problokto (see *pibloktoq*)

pujo

A. –

B. Mexican-American groups

C. term applied variously to abdominal griping, umbilical hernia, diarrhea

D. Kay (1977; 135)

qissaatuq

A. –

B. Central Eskimos (Hudson's Bay region)

C. compulsive passivity, withdrawal, depression, sometimes brief flurry of self-destructive activity; feelings of unworthiness and guilt

D. Vallee (1966)

quajimaillituq

A. –

B. Central Eskimos (Hudson's Bay region)

C. periods of hyperactivity with short episodes of quiescent normality; paranoid ideation and behavior; glossolalia and use of neologisms; compulsivity and anti-social acts and words

D. Vallee (1966)

qatari culture-bound neurosis

A. –

   B. Qatari women, Persian Gulf
   C. faintness, nausea, anorexia, palpitations, breathlessness, chest pain, fatigue, generalized aches and pains
   D. El-Islam (1974)

rabt
   A. —
   B. Egypt
   C. fear of loss of male sexual potency as a result of witchcraft activity
   D. El Sendiony (1977)

rok-joo (see *koro*)
   B. Thailand
   D. Harrington (1982)

ruden mebuyai ("Ruden" means "madness")
   A. —
   B. Sarawak (Murut people)
   C. change in behavior resulting in indecision, aimlessness, apathy, evasiveness in young people; ("mebuyai" means "stupid")
   D. Schmidt (1967–68: 29)

ruden meruai
   A. —
   B. Sarawak (Murut people)
   C. epileptic behavior; sometimes victim falls into fire and even dies from burns
   D. Schmidt (1967/68: 29)

ruden pa'lamai
   A. —
   B. Sarawak (Murut people)
   C. believed caused by sorcery to induce another person's love; victim cries and shouts, preoccupied with image of lover; appearance of misery; condition similar to ruden mebuyai
   D. Schmidt (1967/68: 29–30)

ruden rupan
   A. —
   B. Sarawak (Murut people)
   C. victim has visual and auditory hallucinations of crowds of people who want to catch him and kill him; indiscriminant running in attempt to get away; calling out names of alleged attackers; sometimes death from exhaustion and refusal of food and water, or from suicide; during remission victim is quiet and withdrawn; symptoms attributed to contact with or closeness to haunted well
   D. Schmidt (1967–68: 27)

ruden talai
   A. —
   B. Sarawak (Murut people)

    C.   tiredness and pain in limbs and trunk; sleeplessness; headaches and visual hallucinations of people who want to kill him; aggressive and violent behavior toward people (amok); attributed to contact with a particular tree
    D.   Schmidt (1967– 68: 28)

ruden sinoso
    A.   –
    B.   Sarawak (Murut people)
    C.   victim alternately feels cold and sits by fire, then feels hot and wants to cool himself; sits motionless without moving for long periods; refuses food and drink; attributed to witchcraft
    D.   Schmidt (1967/68: 29)

saka
    A.   *ufufuyane* (Yap 1974: 99); *kiesu* (Harris 1957: 1946)
    B.   Kenya (Taita people)
    C.   prodromal restlessness and anxiety; trembling and convulsive movements with closed eyes and expressionless face; sometimes monotonous, repetitive movements and neologisms; trance-like appearance and manner; sometimes bodily rigidity and loss of consciousness
    D.   Harris (1957)

saladera (see *susto*)
    B.   Amazonian Peru
    D.   chapter by Dobkin de Rios (this volume)

sangue dormido
    A.   –
    B.   Cape Verdean Islanders (Portuguese) and emigrants from that group
    C.   psychophysiologic disorders such as pain, numbness, tremor, paralysis, convulsion, stroke, blindness, heart attack, infection, miscarriage, and mental illness following traumatic injury
    D.   Like and Ellison (1981)

shen-k'uei (see also *dhat*)
    A.   –
    B.   Chinese populations
    C.   marked anxiety or panic; somatic complaints for which no organic pathology can be demonstrated, e.g., dizziness, backache, fatigability, general weakness, insomnia, frequent dreams, appearance of white hair and physical thinness; sometimes complaints of sexual dysfunction such as premature ejaculation and impotence; symptoms popularly associated with excessive semen loss from frequent intercourse, masturbation, nocturnal emission or passing of "white turbid urine" believed to contain semen
    D.   Wen and Wang (1981)

shinkeishitsu (see also *taijin kyofusho*)
    A.   –
    B.   Japan

C. fear of meeting people; feelings of inadequacy; anxiety; obsessive-compulsive symptoms; hypochondriasis

D. Kiev (1972: 71–72); Caudill and Schooler (1969: 116); Tanaka-Matsumi (1979)

shin-byung, sin-byung

A. *sin-byong* (Kim 1972)

B. Korea

C. initial phases characterized by somatic complaints (general weakness, dizziness, fear, anorexia, insomnia, gastrointestinal disorders) and anxiety; subsequent phases by dissociation and possession (by ancestral spirits), dreams, hallucinations

D. Kim (1972, 1974); Kim and Rhi (1976)

shook yong, shuk yang, su yang, suo yang, suk-yeon, suk yeong (see also *koro*)

B. South China, Chinese and Malay populations in southeast Asia

D. chapters by J. G. Edwards, J. M. Edwards, Ifabumuyi and Rwegellera, and Gwee in this volume; Yap (1964, 1965); Lin, Kleinman, and Lin (1981: 254–255)

soudanite, pseudonite (see *amok*)

B. Saharan peoples

D. Yap (1951: 319); Kiev (1972: 86)

suchi-bai

A. –

B. Bengal (Hindu) (especially widows)

C. obsessive-compulsive behavior regarding cleanliness and observance of ritual purity rules, e.g., washing too often; not eating anywhere outside; changing of street clothes; washing of money (including currency notes); bathing for four hours twice a day; hanging street clothes outside on a tree and entering house naked; hopping while walking (to avoid touching anything dirty in the streets); remaining immersed in the holy river for most of the day; sprinkling of cow-dung water on all visitors; washing furniture

D. Chakraborty and Baneriji (1975)

sukra prameha (see *dhat*)

B. Sri Lanka (Ceylon)

D. Obeyesekere (1976)

susto

A. *espanto, saladera* (Dobkin de Rios, this volume); *lanti* (Hart, this volume); *mogo laya* (Frankel, this volume); *haak-tsan* (Yap 1974: 98); *womtia* (Shutler 1977: 179); *narahati* (Good and Good 1982)

B. Central American and Andean groups; peoples of Mexican-American cultural descent in U.S.

C. anxiety, irritability, anorexia, insomnia, phobias, trembling, sweating, tachycardia, diarrhea, depression, vomiting in person attributed to fright to self or someone else

D. chapters by Rubel, O'Nell, and Collado; Dobkin de Rios; Hart; and Dennis
    in this volume. Also Kiev (1972: 69–70); Rubel (1964); Yap (1969, 1974);
    Bolton (1981); Uzzell (1974); Logan (1979); Foster (1953); Good and
    Good (1982); Ardon et al. (1983)

tabacazo
  A. –
  B. Chile
  C. agitation or mental confusion; despair; loss of consciousness; aggressivity
  D. Grebe and Segura (1975)

taijin kyofusho
  A. *anthropophobia* (Takahashi 1975); *shinkeishitsu* (Kiev 1972: 71)
  B. Japan
  C. interpersonal anxiety; fear that specific parts of body (e.g., eyes) or body
      odor give offense to other people
  D. Tanaka-Matsumi (1979); Takahashi (1975)

tawatl ye sni ("totally discouraged")
  A. –
  B. Dakota Sioux
  C. sense of deprivation and loss; wandering of thoughts and belief that one
      is with dead relatives; orientation to the past; thoughts of death; excessive
      drinking, thoughts of suicide, sometimes leading to suicide; preoccupation
      with ideas of ghosts or spirits
  D. Shore and Manso (1981: 7–8); Johnson and Johnson (1965: 141–143)

ticradura (la)
  A. *la lastimadura* (Ponce 1965: 43)
  B. Peru
  C. children's affliction believed caused by severe physical trauma, with sym-
      ptoms of sadness, feeling vaguely unwell, or loss of weight
  D. Ponce (1965: 43)

tripa ida
  A. –
  B. Mexican-American groups
  C. severe fright or trauma resulting in locking of the intestines
  D. Kay (1977: 135)

tuyo
  A. –
  B. Sarawak (Iban people)
  C. autistic talk, withdrawal, odd behavior in the young
  D. Schmidt (1964: 150)

ufufunyane, ufufunyana, ufufuyane (also see *saka*)
  A. *ukuphosela* (Loudon 1965); *saka* (Yap 1974: 99); *kiesu* (Harris 1957)
  B. Zulu, South Africa (especially females)

C. stereotyped nightmares with sexual content and symbolism; pains in lower abdomen, sometimes with accompanying paralysis; transient blindness; seizures with incoherent talk and neologisms; attacks of hysterical shouting and sobbing; epileptiform convulsions and temporary loss of consciousness over a period of days or weeks

D. Yap (1974: 99); DeVos (1974: 555); Loudon (1959: 360–363); Loudon (1965: 142)

ukuphosela (see *ufufunyane*)

B. Xhosa people, South Africa (Loudon 1965: 142)

D. Loudon (1965)

uqamairineq

A. *uqumanigianiq, Eskimo sleep paralysis* (chapter by Bloom and Gelardin, this volume); *old hag* (Ness, this volume)

B. Eskimo (Inuit and Yuit) peoples of Alaska

C. hypnagogic anxious and dissociative episode; sometimes visual hallucinations

D. chapters by Bloom and Gelardin, and by Ness, this volume

uqumanigianiq (see *uqamairineq*)

utox

A. –

B. Taiwanese aborigines (Atayal)

C. sudden fright followed by visual and auditory hallucinations, clouding of consciousness

D. Yap (1974: 96–97); Rin and Lin (1962: 141)

vailala madness (see *guria*)

vomiting sickness

A. –

B. Jamaican rural blacks, especially children

C. hypoglycemia; extended vomiting, often followed by collapse, convulsions, coma, and sometimes death.

D. Thomas and Krieger (1976)

wacinko

A. –

B. Oglala Sioux

C. anger, pouting, withdrawal, depression, psychomotor retardation, mutism, immobility, sometimes suicide

D. Lewis (1975)

wagamama

A. –

B. Japan

C. childish, negative, apathetic, irresponsible behavior punctuated with emotional outbursts

D. Caudill and Schooler (1969: 116–117)

warapa
   A. *aiyiperi, giri* (Prince 1964: 88)
   B. Nigeria (Yoruba)
   C. symptoms localized in stomach, body, feet, and brains; epileptic condition; amnesiac after event
   D. A. Leighton et al. (1963: 106); Prince (1964: 88)
waswas
   A. –
   B. Indonesia and other Islamic areas
   C. obsessive preoccupation with ablutions for prayer and with excessive repetitions of words and gestures
   D. Pfeiffer (1982)
were agba
   A. –
   B. Nigeria (Yoruba)
   C. senile dementia
   D. Prince (1964: 87)
were alaso
   A. –
   B. Nigeria (Yoruba)
   C. occasional psychotic episodes in a person displaying normal behavior usually, e.g., putting on best clothing when there is no obvious occasion for it, staring into space, sudden displays of generosity
   D. A. Leighton et al. (1963: 106); Prince (1964: 87)
wild man behavior (see *ahaDe idzi Be*)
windigo
   A. *wiitiko* (Parker 1960); *whitiko* (Manschreck and Petri 1978); *witiko, witigo* (Yap 1969: 47); *wihtigo* (Yap 1951: 320); *wechuge* (Ridington 1976)
   B. Cree, Ojibwa, Saulteaux and related groups of central and northeastern Canada
   C. prodromal depression; nausea, distaste for usual foods; feelings of being bewitched and possessed by a cannibalistic monster; homicidal (sometimes suicidal) impulses; reported cannibalistic ideation
   D. paper by Marano and commentaries by Murphy, Weidman, and Brightman in this volume; Parker (1960); Teicher (1960); Ridington (1976); Kiev (1972: 84–85); Yap (1951: 320)
womtia (see *susto*)
   B. Yaqui Indians
   D. Shutler (1977: 179)
wool-hwa-byung (see *hwa-byung*)
   B. Korea
   D. Chang (1983)

yaun, young-da-te (see *latah*)
B. Burma
D. (Yap 1951: 318; 1974: 97)

zar
A. –
B. Ethiopia, Egypt, Sudan, Iran
C. dissociative behavior; victim believes he is possessed by a spirit; shouting, dancing, hitting head against wall; sometimes sings and weeps; apathy and withdrawal, sometimes refusing to eat or carry out daily activities; occasional homicidal impulses
D. Modarressi (1968); Pavicevic (1966)

zuwadanda
A. –
B. Shona and related peoples, southern Africa
C. psychotic behavior attributed to witchcraft; victim continually steals from others and imagines that something is continually moving over his body
D. Gelfand (1964: 166)

REFERENCES

Aberle, David F.
 1952 *Arctic Hysteria* and *Latah* in Mongolia. The New York Academy of Sciences 14 (7): 291–297.
Ardon, Rolando Collado, Arthur J. Rubel, Carl W. O'Nell, and Raymond H. Murray
 1983 A Folk Illness (*Susto*) as an Indicator of Real Illness. Lancet, December 10, 1983: 1362.
Beard, G. M.
 1880 Experiments with the *Jumpers* or *Jumping Frenchmen* of Maine. Journal of Nervous and Mental Diseases 7: 487–490.
Blumhagen, Dan
 1980 Hyper-Tension: A Folk Illness with a Medical Name. Culture, Medicine, and Psychiatry 4: 197–227.
Bolton, Ralph
 1981 *Susto*, Hostility, and Hypoglycemia. Ethnology: 20 (4): 261–276.
Bourguignon, Erika
 1976 Possession and Trance in Cross-Cultural Studies of Mental Health. *In* William P. Lebra (ed.), Culture-Bound Syndromes, Ethnopsychiatry, and Alternative Therapies. Honolulu: The University Press of Hawaii, pp. 47–55.
Brill, A. A.
 1913 *Piblokto* or *Hysteria* Among Peary's Eskimos. Journal of Nervous and Mental Disease 40 (18): 514–520.
Carstairs, G. M.
 1956 Hinjra and Jiryan. British Journal of Medical Psychology: 29: 128–138.
Cassidy, Claire Monod
 1982 Protein-Energy Malnutrition as a Culture-Bound Syndrome. Culture, Medicine, and Psychiatry 6: 325–345.

Caudill, William and Carmi Schooler
    1969 Symptom Patterns and Background Characteristics of Japanese Psychiatric Patients.
          In William Caudill and Tsung-yi Lin (eds.), Mental Health Research in Asia and
          the Pacific. Honolulu: East-West Center Press, pp. 114–147.
Cawte, John
    1974 *Malgri*: A Culture-Bound Syndrome. *In* John Cawte (ed.), Medicine Is the Law:
          Studies in Psychiatric Anthropology of Australian Tribal Societies. Honolulu: The
          University Press of Hawaii, pp. 106–119.
    1976 *Malgri*: A Culture-Bound Syndrome. *In* William P. Lebra (ed.), Culture-Bound Syn-
          dromes, Ethnopsychiatry, and Alternate Therapies. Volume IV of Mental Health
          Research in Asia and the Pacific. Honolulu: The University Press of Hawaii, pp.
          22–31.
Chakraborty, Ajita and G. Banerji
    1975 Ritual, A Culture Specific Neurosis, and Obessional States in Bengali Culture. Indian
          Journal of Psychiatry 17: 211–216.
Chang, Suk C.
    1983 Letter. American Journal of Psychiatry 140 (1): 1268
Chang, Y. H., H. Rin, C. C. Chen
    1975 *Frigophobia*: A Report of Five Cases. Bulletin of the Chinese Society of Neurology
          and Psychiatry 1 (2): 9–13.
Chen, Paul C. Y.
    1970 Classification and Concepts of Causation of Mental Illness in a Rural Malay Com-
          munity. International Journal of Social Psychiatry 16: 205–215.
Clark, Margaret
    1959 Health in the Mexican-American Culture: A Community Study. Berkeley and Los
          Angeles: University of California Press.
Clinicopathologic Conference: Case Presentation
    1967 (BCH #469861) Bulletin of the Johns Hopkins Hospital (Johns Hopkins Medical
          Journal), 120: Jan.–June: 186–199.
Connor, Linda
    1982 The Unbound Self: Balinese Therapy in Theory and Practice. *In* A. Marsella and
          G. White (eds.), Cultural Conceptions of Mental Health and Therapy. Dordrecht,
          Holland: D. Reidel Publishing Co.
Czaplicka, M. A.
    1914 Aboriginal Siberia: A Study in Social Anthropology. *Arctic hysteria*, Oxford:
          Clarendon Press, pp. 307–325.
de la Tourette, G. Gilles
    1884 *Jumping, Latah*, and *Myriachit*. Archives de Neurologie 8: 68–74.
Dean, Stanley and Denny Thong
    1972 Folk Psychiatry in Bali – "Island of the Gods": Some Modern Implications. Trans-
          cultural Psychiatric Research Review IX: 30–32.
Devereux, George
    1961 Mohave Ethnopsychiatry and Suicide: The Psychiatric Knowledge and the Psychic
          Disturbance of an Indian Tribe. Bureau of American Ethnology, No. 175. Washington:
          The Smithsonian Institution.
DeVos, George A.
    1974 Cross-Cultural Studies of Mental Disorder: An Anthropological Perspective. *In* Silvano
          Arieti (ed.), American Handbook of Psychiatry, Vol. II (2nd ed.). New York: Basic
          Books, pp. 551–567.
Dutta, Deepali
    1983 *Koro* Epidemic in Assam. (Letter) British Journal of Psychiatry 143: 309–310.
El-Islam, M. Fakhr
    1974 Culture-bound Neurosis in Qatari Women. Transcultural Psychiatric Research News-
          letter XI: 167–168.

El Sendiony, Mohammed Farouk Mahmoud
   1977 The Problem of Cultural Specificity of Mental Illness: A Survey of Comparative Psychiatry. The International Journal of Social Psychiatry 23 (3): 223–230.
Favazza, Armando R. and Mary Oman
   1977 Anthropological and Cross-Cultural Themes in Mental Health: An Annotated Bibliography, 1925–1974. Columbia and London: University of Missouri Press.
Foster, George M.
   1953 Relationships Between Spanish and Spanish-American Folk Medicine. Journal of American Folklore 66: 201–217.
Foulks, Edward F.
   1972 The *Arctic Hysterias* of the North Alaskan Eskimos. Anthropological Studies, No. 10. Washington: American Anthropological Association.
Freeman, Daniel M. A., Edward F. Foulks, and Patricia A. Freeman
   1976 Ghost Sickness and Superego Development in the Kiowa Apache Male. The Psychoanalytic Study of Society 7: 123–171.
Gaviria, Moises and Ronald M. Wintrob
   1976 Supernatural Influence in Psychopathology: Puerto Rican Folk Beliefs about Mental Illness. Canadian Psychiatric Association Journal 21: 361–369.
Gelfand, Michael
   1964 Psychiatric Disorders as Recognized by the Shona. *In* Ari Kiev (ed.), Magic, Faith, and Healing. New York: Free Press, pp. 156–173.
Good, Byron, and Mary Jo D. Good
   1982 Toward a Meaning-Centered Analysis of Popular Illness Categories: Fright Illness and Heart Distress in Iran. *In* Anthony J. Marsella and Geoffrey M. White (eds.), Cultural Conceptions of Mental Health and Therapy. Dordrecht: D. Reidel Publishing Co., pp. 150–158.
Grebe, Maria Ester and Jose Segura
   1975 Psiquiatria Folklorica de Chile: Estudio Anthropologica de Seis Enfermedades Vigentes [Folk Psychiatry in Chile: An Anthropological Study of Six Current Illnesses], in Acta Psychiatrica Psicologica de America 20: 367–382, 1974. Abstracted and translated in Transcultural Psychiatric Research Review XII: 178–180, 1975.
Gussow, Zachary
   1963 A Preliminary Report of *Kayak-Angst* Among the Eskimo of West Greenland: A Study in Sensory Deprivation. The International Journal of Social Psychiatry 9 (1): 18–26.
   1970 Some Responses of West Greenland Eskimo to a Naturalistic Situation of Perceptual Deprivation: With an Appendix of 60 Case Histories Collected by Dr. Alfred Bertelsen in 1902–1903. Inter-Nord: Revue Internationale d'Études Arctiques et Nordiques 11: 227–262.
Harrington, J. A.
   1982 Epidemic Psychosis. (Letter) British Journal of Psychiatry 141: 99–100.
Harris, Grace
   1957 Possession "Hysteria" in a Kenya Tribe. American Anthropologist 59 (6): 1046–1066.
Hoskin, J. O., L. G. Kiloh, and J. E. Cawte
   1967 Epilepsy and *Guria*: The Shaking Syndromes of New Guinea. Social Science and Medicine 3: 38–48.
Hufford, David C.
   1982 The Terror That Comes in the Night. Philadelphia: University of Pennsylvania Press.
Ionescu-Tongyonk, John
   1977 Transcultural Psychiatry in Thailand: A Review of the Last Two Decades. Transcultural Psychiatric Research Review XIV: 145–162.
Jilek, W. and L. Jilek-Aall
   1977 A *Koro* Epidemic in Thailand. Transcultural Psychiatric Research Review XIV: 57–59.

Johnson, Dale L. and Carmen A. Johnson
    1965 Totally Discouraged: A Depressive Syndrome of the Dakota Sioux. Transcultural
         Psychiatric Research Review and Newsletter II (October): 141—143.
Kaplan, Bert and Thomas F. A. Plaut
    1956 Personality in a Communal Society: An Analysis of the Mental Health of the Hut-
         terites. Lawrence, Kansas: University of Kansas Publications, Social Science Studies,
         1956.
Kaplan, Bert and Dale Johnson
    1964 The Social Meaning of Navaho Psychopathology and Psychotherapy. *In* Ari Kiev
         (ed.), Magic, Faith, and Healing. New York: Free Press, pp. 203—229.
Kay, Margarita Artschwager
    1977 Health and Illness in a Mexican American Barrio. *In* Edward H. Spicer (ed.), Ethnic
         Medicine in the Southwest. Tucson: The University of Arizona Press, pp. 99—166.
Kiev, Ari
    1961 Spirit Possession in Haiti. American Journal of Psychiatry 118: 133—138.
    1972 Transcultural Psychiatry. New York: The Free Press.
Keshavan, M. S.
    1983 Epidemic Psychoses, or Epidemic *Koro*? (Letter) British Journal of Psychiatry
         148: 100—101.
Kim, Kwang-Iel
    1972 "Sin-byung"; a Culture-Bound Depersonalization Syndrome. Neuropsychiatry
         (Seoul) 11: 233—234.
    1974 Cultural and Mental Illness in Korea. Korea Journal 14 (2): 4—8, 23.
Kim, Kwang-Iel and Bou Young Rhi
    1976 A Review of Korean Cultural Psychiatry. Transcultural Psychiatric Research Review
         XIII: 101—114.
Kleinman, A.
    1980 Patients and Healers in the Context of Cultural. Berkeley: University of California
         Press, pp. 146—178.
Kleinman, Arthur and Tsung-Yi Lin (eds.)
    1981 Normal and Abnormal Behavior in Chinese Culture. Dordrecht: D. Reidel Publsihing
         Co.
Landy, David
    1983 Medical Anthropology: A Critical Appraisal. *In* Julio L. Ruffini (ed.), Advances
         in Medical Social Science. New York: Gordon Breach Science Publishers, pp. 185—
         314.
Langness, Lewis
    1965 Hysterical Psychosis in the New Guinea Highlands. Psychiatry 28: 258—277.
    1976 Hysterical Psychoses and Possessions. *In* William P. Lebra (ed.), Culture-Bound
         Syndromes, Ethno-psychiatry, and Alternate Therapies. Honolulu: The University
         Press of Hawaii, pp. 56—67.
Lee, Bom Sang
    1983 Is *Hwa-Byung* Really *Gahsum-Ari*, and Is It Culture-Bound? (Letter) American
         Journal of Psychiatry 140 (9): 1267—1268.
Lee, S. H.
    1977 A Study on the *Hwa-Byung* (anger syndrome). Journal of Korea General Hospital
         1: 63—64 (English abstract).
Lefley, Harriet P.
    1979a Prevalence of Potential Falling-Out Cases Among the Black, Latin and Non-Latin
          White Populations of the City of Miami. Social Science and Medicine 13B: 113—
          114.
    1979b Female Cases of Falling-Out: A Psychological Evaluation of a Small Sample. Social
          Science and Medicine 13B: 115—116.

Leighton, Alexander H., T. Adeoye Lambo, Charles C. Hughes, Dorothea C. Leighton, Jane M. Murphy, and David B. Macklin
    1963 Psychiatric Disorder Among the Yoruba. Ithaca: Cornell University Press.
Lewis, Thomas H.
    1974 A Syndrome of Depression and Mutism in the Oglala Sioux. American Journal of Psychiatry 132: 753–755.
Like, Robert and James Ellison
    1981 Sleeping Blood, Tremor and Paralysis: A Trans-cultural Approach to an Unusual Conversion Reaction. Culture, Medicine and Psychiatry 5: 49–63.
Lin, Keh-Ming
    1981 Culture-Bound Syndromes Among Overseas Chinese. In Arthur Kleinman and Tsung-Yi Lin (eds.), Normal and Abnormal Behavior in Chinese Culture. Dordrecht: D. Reidel Publishing Co., pp. 371–386.
    1983a Hwa-Byung: A Korean Culture-Bound Syndrome? American Jounral of Psychiatry 140 (1): 105–107.
    1983b Letter. American Journal of Psychiatry 140 (1): 1268–1269.
Lin, Keh-Ming, Arthur Kleinman, and Tsung-yi Lin
    1981 Overview of Mental Disorders in Chinese Cultures: Review of Epidemiological and Clinical Studies. In Arthur Kleinman and Tsung-yi Lin (eds.), Normal and Abnormal Behavior in Chinese Culture. Dordrecht: D. Reidel Publishing Co., pp. 237–272.
Logan, Michael H.
    1979 Variations Regarding Susto Causality Among the Cakchiquel of Guatemala. Culture, Medicine and Psychiatry 3: 153–166.
Loudon, J. B.
    1959 Psychogenic Disorder and Social Conflict Among the Zulu. In Marvin Opler, (ed.), Culture and Mental Health. New York: The Macmillan Comapny, pp. 351–369.
    1965 Social Aspects of Ideas About Treatment. In A. V. S. de Reuck and Ruth Porter (eds.), Transcultural Psychiatry. Boston: Little, Brown and Company, pp. 137–161.
Low, Setha
    1981 The Meaning of Nervios: A Sociocultural Analysis of Symptom Presentation in San Jose, Costa Rica. Culture, Medicine and Psychiatry 5: 25–47.
Malhotra, H. K. and N. N. Wig
    1975 Dhat Syndrome: A Culture-Bound Sex Neurosis of the Orient. Archives of Sexual Behavior 4: 519–528.
Manschreck, Theo C. and Michele Petri
    1978 The Atypical Psychoses. Culture, Medicine and Psychiatry 2: 233–268.
Modarressi, Taghi
    1968 The Zar Culture in South Iran. In Raymond Prince (ed.), Trance and Possession States. Montreal: R. M. Bucke Memoiral Society, pp. 149–155.
Morakinyo, O.
    1980 A Psychophysiological Theory of a Psychiatric Illness (the Brain Fag Syndrome) Associated with Study among Africans. Journal of Nervous and Mental Disease 168 (2): 84–89.
Murphy, H. B. M.
    1973 History and the Evolution of Syndromes: The Striking Case of Latah and Amok. In M. Hammer, K. Salzinger, and S. Sutton (eds.), Psychopathology: Contributions From The Biological, Behavioral, and Social Sciences. New York: John Wiley & Sons, pp. 33–53.
    1976 Notes for the Theory on Latah. In William P. Lebra (ed.), Culture-Bound Syndromes, Ethnopsychiatry, and Alternate Therapies. Volume IV of Mental Health Research in Asia and the Pacific. Honolulu: The University Press of Hawaii, pp. 3–21.
Murphy, Jane M.
    1976 Psychiatric Labeling in Cross-Cultural Perspective. Science 191: 1019–1028.

Nandi, D. N., G. Banerjee, H. Saha, and G. C. Boral
    1983 Epidemic *Koro* in West Bengal, India. International Journal of Social Psychiatry
          29 (4): 265–268.
Neutra, Raymond, Jerrold E. Levy, and Dennis Parker
    1977 Cultural Expectations Versus Reality in Navajo Seizure Patterns and Sick Roles.
          Culture, Medicine and Psychiatry 1: 255–275.
Newman, Philip L.
    1964 "Wild Man" Behavior in a New Guinea Highland Community. American Anthropo-
          logist 66: 1–19.
Ngui, P. W.
    1969 The *Koro* Epidemic in Singapore. Australian and New Zealand Journal of Psychiatry
          3: 263–265.
Novakovsky, Stanislaus
    1924 *Arctic* or *Siberian Hysteria* as a Reflex of the Geographic Environment. Ecology
          V (2): 113–127.
Obeyesekere, Gananath
    1970 The Idiom of Demonic Possession: A Case Study. Social Science and Medicine 4:
          97–111.
    1976 The Impact of Ayurvedic Ideas on the Culture and the Individual in Ceylon. *In*
          Charles Leslie (ed.), Asian Medical Systems: A Comparative Study. Berkeley and
          Los Angeles: University of California Press, pp. 201–226.
Parker, Seymour
    1960 The *Wiitiko* Psychosis in the Context of Ojibwa Personality and Culture. American
          Anthropologist 62: 603–623.
    1962 Eskimo Psychopathology in the Context of Eskimo Personality and Culture. Ameri-
          can Anthropologist 64: 76–96.
Paul, Benjamin D.
    1967 Mental Disorder and Self-Regulating Processes in Culture: A Guatemalan Illustration.
          In Robert Hunt (ed.), Personalities and Cultures. New York: The Natural History
          Press, pp. 151–165.
Pavicevic, Marinko B.
    1966 Psychoses in Ethiopia. Transcultural Psychiatric Research 3: 152–154.
Penningroth, Philip E. and Barbara A. Penningroth
    1977 Cross Cultural Mental Health Practice on Guam. Social Psychiatry 12: 43–
          48.
Pfeiffer, Wolfgang M.
    1982 Culture-Bound Syndromes. *In* Ihsan Al-Issa (ed.), Culture and Psychopathology.
          Baltimore: University Park Press, pp. 201–218.
Philippe, Jeanne and Jean Baptiste Romain
    1979 *Indisposition* in Haiti. Social Science and Medicine 13B: 129–133.
Ponce, Oscar Valdivia
    1965 Historia de la Psiquiatria Peruana. (Paper in Spanish abstracted in English.) Trans-
          cultural Psychiatric Research 2: 41–43.
Prince, Raymond
    1960 The *Brain Fag* Syndrome in Nigerian Students. Journal of Mental Science 106:
          559–570.
    1964 Indigenous Yoruba Psychiatry. *In* Ari Kiev (ed.), Magic, Faith, and Healing. New
          York: The Free Press of Glencoe, pp. 84–120.
    1968 Trance and Possession States, ed. Proceedings, Second Annual Bucke Memorial
          Society, 1966. Montreal: R. M. Bucke Memorial Society.
Rao, A. Venkoba
    1978 Some Aspects of Psychiatry in India. Transcultural Psychiatric Research Review
          XV: 7–27.

Ridington, Robin
1976   *Wechuge* and *Windigo*: A Comparison of Cannibal Belief Among Boreal Forest Athapaskans and Algonkians. Anthropologica 8 (2): 107–128.
Rin, Hsien and Tsung-Yi Lin
1962   Mental Illness Among Formosan Aborigines as Compared with the Chinese in Taiwan. Journal of Mental Science 108: 135–146.
Rin, Hsien
1966   Two Forms of Vital Deficiency Syndromes Among Chinese Male Mental Patients. Transcultural Psychiatric Research 3: 19–21.
Ritenbaugh, Cheryl
1982   Obesity as a Culture-Bound Syndrome. Culture, Medicine and Psychiatry 6: 347–361.
Rosenthal, Stuart and Perihan A. Rosenthal
1982   *Koro* in an Adolescent: Hypochrondriasis as a Stress Response. Adolescent Psychiatry X: 523–530.
Rothenberg, A.
1964   Puerto Rico and Aggression. American Journal of Psychiatry 120: 962–970.
Rubel, Arthur J.
1960   Concepts of Disease in Mexican-American Culture. American Anthropologist 62 (5): 795–814.
1964   The Epidemiology of a Folk Illness, *Susto*, in Hispanic America. Ethnology 3: 268–83.
1966   Across the Tracks: Mexican-Americans in a Texas City. Austin: University of Texas Press.
Rubin, Jeffrey C. and Judy Jones
1979   Falling-Out: A Clinical Study. Social Science and Medicine 13B: 117–127.
Salisbury, Richard F.
1968   Possession in the New Guinea Highlands. International Journal of Social Psychiatry 14 (2): 85–94.
Schmidt, K. E.
1964   Folk Psychiatry in Sarawak: A Tentative System of Psychiatry of the Iban. *In* Ari Kiev (ed.), Magic, Faith and Healing. New York: Free Press of Glencoe, pp. 139–155.
1967/68 Some Concepts of Mental Illness of the Murut of Sarawak. International Journal of Social Psychiatry 14 (1): 24–31.
Sharma, B. P.
1966   Report. Transcultural Psychiatric Research 3: 132–133.
Shirokogoroff, S. M.
1935   Psychomental Complex of the Tungus. London: Kegan Paul, Trench, Trubner and Co., pp. 246–256.
Shore, James H. and Spero M. Manson
1981   Cross-Cultural Studies of Depression Among American Indians and Alaska Natives. White Cloud Journal 2 (2): 5–12.
Shutler, Mary Elizabeth
1977   Disease and Curing in a Yaqui Community. *In* Edward H. Spicer (ed.), Ethnic Medicine in the Southwest. Tucson: The University of Arizona Press, pp. 169–237.
Snow, Loudell F.
1974   Folk Medical Beliefs and Their Implications for Care of Patients: A Review Based on Studies Among Black Americans. Annals of Internal Medicine 81: 82–96.
Stern, Gwen and Laurence Kruckman
1983   Multi-Disiplinary Perspectives on Post-Partum Depression: An Anthropological Critique. Social Science and Medicine 17 (15): 1027–1041.

Stevens, H.
1965   *Jumping Frenchman* of Maine. Archives of Neurology 12: 311–314.
Suwanlert, Sangun
1976   *Phii Pob*: Spirit Possession in Rural Thailand. *In* William P. Lebra (ed.), Culture-Bound Syndromes, Ethnopsychiatry, and Alternate Therapies. Honolulu: The University Press of Hawaii, pp. 68–87.
Takahashi, Tooru
1975   A Social Club Spontaneously Formed by Ex-Patients Who Had Suffered From *Anthropophobia* (Taijin Kyofu (Sho)). International Journal of Social Psychiatry 21 (2): 137–140.
Tanaka-Matsumi, Junko
1979   *Taijin Kyofusho*: Diagnostic and Cultural Issues in Japanese Psychiatry. Culture, Medicine and Psychiatry 3: 231–245.
Tan, Eng-Seong
1981   Culture-Bound Syndromes Among Overseas Chinese. *In* Arthur Kleinman and Tsung-Yi Lin (eds.), Normal and Abnormal Behavior in Chinese Culture. Dordrecht: D. Reidel Publishing Co., pp. 371–386.
Teicher, Morton I.
1960   *Windigo* Psychosis: A Study of a Relationship Between Belief and Behavior Among the Indians of Northeastern Canada. Proceedings of the 1960 Annual Spring Meeting of the American Ethnological Society. Seattle: University of Washington Press.
Teoh, Jin-Inn
1972   The Changing Psychopathology of *Amok*. Psychiatry 35: 345–351.
Thomas, Anthony and Laurie Krieger
1976   Jamaican Vomiting Sickness: A Theoretical Investigation. Social Science and Medicine 10 (3/4): 177–183.
Topley, Marjorie
1970   Chinese Traditional Ideas and the Treatment of Disease: Two Examples from Hong Kong. Man 5: 421–437.
Uzzell, Douglas
1974   *Susto* Revisited: Illness as a Strategic Role. American Ethnologist 1: 369–378.
Vallee, Frank G.
1966   Eskimo Theories of Mental Illness in the Hudson Bay Region. Anthropologica 8: 53–83.
van Loon, F. H. G.
1926/27 *Amok* and *Lattah*. Journal of Abnormal and Social Psychology. 21: 434–444.
van Wulfften Palthe, P. M.
1936   Clinical Textbook of Tropical Medicine. Batavia: G. Kolff and Company.
Weimer, Sanford R. and Norbett L. Mintz
1976/77 Health Practice at the Technologic/Folk Interface: Witchcraft as a Culture-Specific Diagnosis. International Journal of Psychiatry in Medicine 7 (4): 351–362.
Wen, Jung-Kwang and Ching-Lun Wang
1981   Shen-K'uei Syndrome: A Culture-Specific Sexual Neurosis in Taiwan. *In* Arthur Kleinman and Tsung-Yi Lin (eds.), Normal and Abnormal Behavior in Chinese Cultures. Dordrecht: D. Reidel Publishing Co., pp. 357–369.
Whitney, Harry
1911   *Hunting with the Eskimos*. New York: The Century Co.
Wiedman, Hazel H.
1979   Falling-Out: A Diagnostic and Treatment Problem Viewed from a Transcultural Perspective. Social Science and Medicine 13B: 95–112.

Wig, Narendra N.
    1983 DSM-III: A Perspective from the Third World. *In* Robert L. Spitzer, Janet B. W. Williams, and Andrew E. Skodol (eds.), International Perspectives on DSM-III: Diagnostic and Statistical Manual of Mental Disorders, Third Edition. Washington, D.C.: American Psychiatric Press, Inc., pp. 79–89.

Winiarz, W., and J. Wielawski
    1936 *Imu* – A Psychoneurosis Occurring Among Ainus. Psychological Review 23: 181–186.

Yap, P. M.
    1951 Mental Diseases Peculiar to Certain Cultures: A Survey of Comparative Psychiatry. Journal of Mental Science 97: 313–327.

    1952 The *Latah* Reaction: Its Pathodynamics and Nosological Position. The Journal of Mental Science XCVIII (413): 515–564.

    1964 *Suk-Yeon* or *Koro* – A Culture-bound Depersonalization Syndrome. The Bulletin of the Hong Kong Chinese Medical Association, 16 (1): 31–47.

    1965 *Koro* – A Cultural-Bound Depersonalization Syndrome. British Journal of Psychiatry 111·43–50.

    1969 The Culture-bound Reactive Syndromes. *In* William Caudill and Tsung-yi Lin (eds.), Mental Health Research in Asia and the Pacific. Honolulu: East-West Center Press, pp. 33–53.

    1974 Comparative Psychiatry: A Theoretical Framework. *In* M. P. Lau and A. B. Stokes (eds.). Toronto: University of Toronto Press.

LIST OF CONTRIBUTORS

Dr. Julio Arboleda-Florez, Department of Psychiatry, University of Calgary, Calgary General Hospital, 841 Centre Avenue, East Calgary, Alberta, CANADA, T2E 0A1.

Dr. Joseph D. Bloom, Department of Psychiatry, University of Oregon, Health Sciences Center, Portland, OR 97201.

Dr. Robert Brightman, Department of Anthropology, University of Wisconsin, Madison, WI 53706.

Dr. Burton G. Burton-Bradley, P. O. Box 111, Port Moresby, PAPUA NEW GUINEA.

Dr. John E. Carr, Department of Psychiatry and Behavioral Sciences, University of Washington, Seattle, WA 98195.

Dr. Rolando Collado, Francisco Benitez 12, Colonia Progreso Tizapan, Mexico 20, MEXICO.

Dr. Phillip A. Dennis, Department of Anthropology, Texas Tech University, Box 4549, Lubbock, TX 79409.

Dr. Marlene Dobkin deRios, Department of Anthropology, California State University, Fullerton, CA 92634.

Dr. J. Guy Edwards, Department of Psychiatry, Royal South Hants Hospital, Southampton & South West Hampshire, Health Authority, Graham Road, Southamptom, S09 4PE, ENGLAND.

Mr. James W. Edwards (Doctoral Candidate in Anthropology, Columbia University), 18 Prospect Place, Brooklyn, NY 11217.

Dr. Edward F. Foulks, Department of Psychiatry G1, 1149 Gates Pavilion, University of Pennsylvania, Philadelphia, PA 19104.

Dr. Stephen Frankel, Department of Social Anthropology, Free School Lane, Cambridge, CB2 RF, ENGLAND.

Mr. Richard D. Gelardin, Anchorage Community College, 2533 Providence Avenue, Anchorage, AK 99504.

Dr. Zachary Gussow, Department of Psychiatry and Behavioral Sciences, Louisiana State University Medical Center, School of Medicine in New Orleans, 1542 Tulane Avenue, New Orleans, LA 70112.

Dr. Gwee Ah Leng, Pacific Clinic, 536–537 Tanglin Shopping Center, Singapore, 1024, SINGAPORE.

Dr. Donn V. Hart†, Department of Anthropology, Northern Illinois University, DeKalb, IL 60115.

Dr. Charles C. Hughes, Department of Family and Community Medicine, University of Utah Medical Center, 50 North Medical Drive, Salt Lake City, UT 84132.

† deceased

Ronald C. Simons and Charles C. Hughes (eds.), The Culture-Bound Syndromes, 507–508.
© *1985 by D. Reidel Publishing Company.*

Dr. O. I. Ifabumuyi, Ahmadu Bello University, Teaching Hospital, Department of Psychiatry, Kaduna, NIGERIA.

Dr. Michael G. Kenny, Department of Sociology and Anthropology, Simon Fraser University, Burnaby, B.C., CANADA V5A IS6.

Dr. Lou Marano, Department of Anthropology, Drake University, Des Moines, IA 50311.

Dr. H. B. M. Murphy, Emeritus Professor, McGill University, Douglas Hospital Research Centre, 6875 Boul. LaSalle, Verdun, Quebec, CANADA H4H 1R3.

Dr. Robert Ness, Department of Psychiatry, University of Connecticut Health Center, Farmington, CT 06032.

Dr. Emiko Ohnuki-Tierney, Department of Anthropology, 5240 Social Science Building, University of Wisconsin, Madison, WI 53705.

Dr. Carl W. O'Nell, Department of Anthropology, University of Notre Dame, Notre Dame, IN 46556.

Dr. G. G. C. Rwegellera, Institute of Health, Ahmadu Bello University, Teaching Hospital, P.M.B. 2016, Kaduna, NIGERIA.

Dr. Arthur Rubel, Department of Family Medicine, University of California at Irvine, Irvine, CA 92717.

Dr. Ronald C. Simons, Department of Psychiatry, A-236B East Fee Hall, Michigan State University, East Lansing, MI 48824–1316.

Dr. Hazel H. Weidman, Professor of Social Anthropology and Director, Office of Transcultural Education and Research, Department of Psychiatry (D-29), P. O. Box 016960, School of Medicine, University of Miami, Miami, FL 33101.

Dr. Joseph Westermeyer, Department of Psychiatry, University Hospital, Box 393, Mayo Memorial Building, 420 Delaware Street, S.E. Minneapolis, MN 55455.

INTRODUCTION TO THE INDEX

The sheer number of references to certain ideas and to certain works (e.g. "deviance" and Yap's 1951 paper) make conventional subject and author indices more of a hindrance than a help. Since the papers in this book discuss a limited number of highly interrelated issues (level of analysis, biological factors, psychopathology, the part played by social and cultural factors in customary but unusual behaviors, etc.), many passages could conceivably be indexed almost anywhere! The very coherence of the debate which gives this book any interest it may have makes it impossible to index comprehensively. However we believe that the selective index we have provided will facilitate access to the book's main concepts and to the ways in which they are currently being debated.

In the pages which follow we have indexed a substantial selection of the concepts used by the contributors or implied in their papers. We suggest that readers use this index to access the main concepts of this book and use the preceding Glossary (pp. 469–505) as the index to the individually named syndromes. When we thought it useful, other terms were also indexed, e.g. names of the syndromes which, like *amok*, were discussed in papers not included in the section on their home taxon.

Though the meaning of most of the index categories will be clear, the following notes may be useful as a guide to what is listed under index categories whose contents may not be self-evident:

"Aggression" indexes references to aggressive behavior and thoughts in general, including socialization processes which modify or curtail aggression. It does not, however, include homicide, which is indexed under "Behavior, violent or homicidal".

"Analysis, level of" indexes discussions of the level of abstraction of the concepts and terms used, both those which speak of the need for a multilevel and hence interdisciplinary approach to the study of culture-bound syndromes and those which advocate a unilevel conceptual framework.

"Anxiety" is well nigh ubiquitous in the culture-bound syndromes. The index includes only selected references which seem especially useful. (Similarly, other analytic and diagnostic terms from psychiatry, such as "hallucinations" and "dissociative reactions", are included only selectively; such terms are used sparingly as index categories.)

"Behavior" as a general category consists primarily of authors' discussions of the importance of observing behavior and of using observed behavior as the primary source of inference. It also includes discussions of observed events *vs* hearsay reports, as in *windigo*. Sample descriptions of specific behaviors in certain syndromes are also indexed here.

Under the rubric "Cultural factors" are indexed not only specific cultural or ethnographic descriptions of groups being studied (not all chapters provide such descriptions), but also examples of various cultural factors used in the analyses of the syndromes – values, norms, beliefs, conceptualizations of the world, etc. This index category is obviously one of the critical points of entry into the central theoretical subject matter of the book.

Although the entire book is about culture-bound syndromes, "Culture-bound syndromes" as an index category brings together specific authors' references to and discussions of the term and its application.

"Demographic characteristics" indexes data on age and sex, and on social, educational, and similar characteristics of the populations in which a given condition is found.

"Diagnosis, psychiatric" refers to discussions and examples of the use of psychiatric diagnosis in explaining a syndrome.

"Disorder and Disease, concepts of" provides a niche for these two critical analytic constructs, here combined in a single index category. This category complements the category "Health and Illness", which includes indigenous conceptualizations of health and illness.

"Emic" and "etic" are much-used terms in current behavioral and social sciences. The first term describes conceptualizations or data as seen by a participant in the local culture, and the second describes an outsider's perception and analysis.

"Epidemiology" indexes data offered by authors on the incidence, prevalence and distribution of a syndrome, usually in relation to possible or putative etiologic factors.

"Etiology" includes not only the etic-minded outsider's analysis or assertions of cause, but also the emic explanations of the "folk" themselves.

"Folk illness" gathers together references to indigenous formulations of illness, its cause, treatment, etc.

"Folk taxonomy" indexes discussions of indigenous nosology.

"Psychodynamics" indexes psychodynamic (usually psychoanalytic) formulations, hypotheses, and speculations relating to the manner in which the variables discussed function in the natural history of a syndrome. Refutations of psychodynamic hypotheses and assertions are also indexed here.

"Psychopathology" includes not only indisputable instances of mental illness but also cases of explicit controversy about whether psychopathology or simply aberrant "normality" is being illustrated.

"Role" is a critical category in many discussions of the culture-bound syndromes, especially if looked at from a social-psychiatric perspective. This index category includes those instances in which authors discuss the differential role rights and responsibilities of women and men.

"Social factors" could be a ubiquitous category; in this index an attempt was made to limit it to selected references to social structural and social organizational factors, social status, socioeconomic and sociopolitical factors, whether presented as context for the discussion of a syndrome or as factors in its etiology.

Entries under "Stress" include both explicit discussions by authors and inferences from the data they present.

"Symptoms" as an index category includes the wide variety of symptoms discussed in the various chapters – a conglomerate category that underscores the variability in symptoms found in the syndromes. The set of symptoms typical of any specific syndrome or folk illness is listed in Section C of its glossary entry.

INDEX